Equine Fluid Therapy

This textbook is dedicated to the following. To Serop, Vana, Lara, Ania, and Karni – you are like the stars in the sky – reach for them! To my parents for their never-ending support and belief in me. To all of the veterinary students and residents who have inspired me. To my equine patients that have taught me so much. To Quizzy. And to Langdon, your perseverance is reflected within these pages – thank you. K.G.M.

This textbook is dedicated to my family and friends. C.L.F.

Equine Fluid Therapy

EDITED BY

C. Langdon Fielding DVM, DACVECC

Loomis Basin Equine Medical Center
Penryn, CA, USA

K. Gary Magdesian DVM, DACVIM, DACVECC, DACVCP

Henry Endowed Chair in Critical Care and Emergency Medicine
School of Veterinary Medicine, University of California, Davis, CA, USA

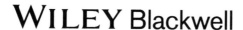

This edition first published 2015 © 2015 by John Wiley & Sons, Inc.

Editorial Offices

1606 Golden Aspen Drive, Suites 103 and 104, Ames, Iowa 50014-8300, USA

The Atrium, Southern Gate, Chichester, West Sussex, PO19 8SQ, UK

9600 Garsington Road, Oxford, OX4 2DQ, UK

For details of our global editorial offices, for customer services and for information about how to apply for permission to reuse the copyright material in this book please see our website at www.wiley.com/wiley-blackwell.

Library of Congress Cataloging-in-Publication Data

Equine fluid therapy / [edited by] C. Langdon Fielding, K. Gary Magdesian.
    p. ; cm.
  Includes bibliographical references and index.
  ISBN 978-0-470-96138-4 (cloth)
  1. Horses–Physiology. 2. Veterinary fluid therapy. I. Fielding, C. Langdon, editor.
II. Magdesian, K. Gary, editor.
  [DNLM: 1. Fluid Therapy–veterinary. 2. Horse Diseases–therapy. 3. Acid-Base Imbalance–veterinary. 4. Water-Electrolyte Imbalance–veterinary. SF 951]
  SF768.2.H67E675 2015
  636.1'08963992–dc23
                                        2014033181

A catalogue record for this book is available from the British Library.

Wiley also publishes its books in a variety of electronic formats. Some content that appears in print may not be available in electronic books.

Set in 8.5/12pt Meridien by SPi Publisher Services, Pondicherry, India

1 2015

Contents

List of contributors

Escolástico Aguilera-Tejero DVM, PhD, DECEIM
Dept. Medicina y Cirugía Animal
Universidad de Córdoba
Spain

Kevin Corley BVM&S, PhD, DECEIM, DACVIM,
DACVECC, MRCVS
Veterinary Advances Ltd
The Curragh, Co. Kildare, Ireland

Julie E. Dechant DVM, MS, DACVS, DACVECC
Associate Professor
Clinical Equine Surgical Emergency and Critical Care
School of Veterinary Medicine
University of California, USA

Thomas J. Divers DVM, DACVIM, DACVECC
Cornell University
Ithaca, NY, USA

Darien J. Feary BVSc, MS, Diplomate ACVIM,
Diplomate ACVECC, GradCertEd (HighEd)
Senior Lecturer in Equine Medicine
School of Animal and Veterinary Science
Equine Health and Performance Centre
The University of Adelaide, South Australia

C. Langdon Fielding DVM, DACVECC
Loomis Basin Equine Medical Center
Penryn, CA, USA

Laurie Gallatin DVM, DACVIM
Coppertop Clydesdales and Gallatin Veterinary Services LLC
Marysville, OH, USA

Diana M. Hassel DVM, PhD, DACVS, DACVECC
Associate Professor – Equine Emergency
Surgery & Critical Care
Department of Clinical Sciences
Colorado State University, USA

Jamie Higgins DVM, DACVS, DACVECC
Idaho Equine Hospital
Nampa, ID, USA

Sophy A. Jesty DVM, DACVIM (Cardiology and Large
Animal Internal Medicine)
Assistant Professor in Cardiology
University of Tennessee, USA

Marco A.F. Lopes MV, MS, PhD
Department of Veterinary Medicine and Surgery
College of Veterinary Medicine
University of Missouri, USA

K. Gary Magdesian DVM, DACVIM, DACVECC, DACVCP
Professor and Henry Endowed Chair in Critical Care and
Emergency Medicine
School of Veterinary Medicine, University of California,
Davis, CA, USA

Harold C. McKenzie III, DVM, MS, DACVIM
Associate Professor of Large Animal Medicine
Department of Veterinary Clinical Sciences
Virginia-Maryland Regional College of
Veterinary Medicine
Virginia Polytechnic and State University, USA

Margaret Mudge DVM, DACVS, DACVECC
The Ohio State University
Department of Veterinary Clinical Sciences
Columbus, OH, USA

Yvette S. Nout-Lomas DVM, PhD, DACVIM, DACVECC
Assistant Professor – Equine Internal Medicine
Department of Clinical Sciences
College of Veterinary Medicine and
Biomedical Sciences
Colorado State University, USA

Jon Palmer VMD, DACVIM
Director of Perinatology/Neonatology Programs
Chief, Neonatal Intensive Care Service
Graham French Neonatal Section
Connelly Intensive Care Unit
New Bolton Center
University of Pennsylvania, USA

Lucas Pantaleon DVM, MS, DACVIM, MBA
Board Certified Large Animal Internal Medicine Specialist
Industry Consultant
Director Technical Services, Ogena Solutions
Versailles, KY, USA

Allison Jean Stewart BVSc (hons),
MS, DACVIM-LAIM, DACVECC
Professor of Equine Medicine
Auburn University
Auburn, AL, USA

Brett Tennent-Brown BVSc, MS,
DACVIM, DACVECC
Senior Lecture in Equine Medicine
Faculty of Veterinary Science
University of Melbourne, Australia

Ramiro E. Toribio DVM, MS, PhD, DACVIM
Associate Professor
The Ohio State University
College of Veterinary Medicine
Columbus, OH, USA

Preface

Fluid therapy is a cornerstone of emergency medicine and critical care. It is the basis for the treatment of many forms of shock and metabolic derangements. The complex interplay of acid–base, electrolyte, and hemodynamic physiology, at the root of fluid therapy, is what sparked our passion for fluid therapy and initiated the idea of a textbook on this subject matter.

The motivation for developing *Equine Fluid Therapy* came from the realization that much of the basic and clinical research findings on this topic in horses is dispersed in numerous resources. Many of the seminal papers on equine fluid physiology can be difficult to access. Therefore, we strived to compile this information into one practical resource. *Equine Fluid Therapy* is the end result of this journey, addressing the topics of electrolyte, acid–base, and fluid balance in horses.

Our goals for *Equine Fluid Therapy* are (i) to provide a practical approach to fluid therapy for a variety of medical conditions in horses, and (ii) to provide a reference for specialists in anesthesia, surgery, internal medicine,

and emergency/critical care medicine who manage the electrolyte, acid–base, and fluid balance derangements in critically ill horses. *Equine Fluid Therapy* is organized into three sections: basic physiology, fluid therapy for common equine medical problems, and specialty topics in fluid therapy. It is our hope that the book is useful to practitioners, veterinary students, house officers, and specialists alike.

One of the greatest benefits of compiling this book has been the opportunity to work with and learn from many of our colleagues in this area of equine medicine. *Equine Fluid Therapy* brings together the research and clinical expertise of a large number of leaders in this field. We greatly appreciate their contributions to this text, and are honored by their participation.

Finally, and importantly, we hope that this textbook benefits the horses and foals that we treat, through improved fluid management.

C. Langdon Fielding
K. Gary Magdesian

SECTION 1
Physiology of fluids, electrolytes, and acid–base

CHAPTER 1

Body water physiology

C. Langdon Fielding

Loomis Basin Equine Medical Center, Penryn, CA, USA

Introduction

The topic of fluid therapy usually focuses on the ideal fluid type and rate that should be administered to equine patients for specific clinical conditions. While the remainder of this textbook addresses these important questions, a brief introduction to the distribution of administered fluids is needed as a basis from which to interpret subsequent chapters. Specifically, concepts including the physiologic fluid spaces, effective osmolality, and oncotic pressure are important foundations to understand prior to important foundations to understand prior to formulating a fluid therapy plan.

Physiologic fluid spaces

The physiologic fluid spaces are typically divided into total body water (TBW), extracellular fluid volume (ECFV), and intracellular fluid volume (ICFV) as shown in Figure 1.1. It is important to remember that these fluid spaces are both physiologic (not anatomic) and dynamic. They represent a volume estimate at a point in time and therefore are constantly changing based on a number of physiological principles. Much of the attention in clinical medicine is focused on the ECFV; blood sampling for laboratory testing comes from this fluid space.

Total body water (TBW)

Total body water represents the total volume of water within the animal. Values in adult horses have ranged from 0.55 to 0.77 L/kg depending on the measurement technique used (Dugdale et al., 2011; Fielding et al., 2004; Latman et al., 2011). A consensus from most of the research would suggest that a typical horse has a volume of TBW between 60 and 70% of its weight. A value of 2/3 is often used by many textbooks and is easy to remember. The majority of studies determining TBW have used deuterium oxide dilution, but this is not practical in a clinical setting. Acute changes in body weight are likely the best determination of changes in TBW in sick horses and foals. Monitoring of weight change should be done frequently (1–2 times per day if possible), in order to recognize acute loss or gain of body water.

Extracellular fluid volume (ECFV)

Extracellular fluid volume represents the volume of TBW that is not contained within the cells. This includes the plasma volume (PV), interstitial volume (IV), and transcellular compartments (gastrointestinal tract, joint fluid, etc.). The ECFV has also been measured using a number of different dilution techniques and reported values in adult horses have ranged from 0.21 to 0.29 L/kg (Dugdale et al., 2011; Fielding et al., 2004; Forro et al., 2000). A good approximation of the ECFV is about 1/3 of TBW.

In addition to evaluating fluid balance, monitoring the size of the ECFV is clinically useful in determining the dosage of some medications. In disease states, the ECFV is the space from which fluid losses often occur (e.g. sodium-rich fluid loss in diarrhea); it is also the space where fluids are administered and often remain (i.e. intravenous isotonic crystalloids). Three techniques that have been used clinically to monitor changes in the ECFV are bioelectrical impedance analysis (BIA), sodium dilution, and volume kinetics (Fielding et al., 2008; Forro et al., 2000; Zdolsek et al., 2012).

Equine Fluid Therapy, First Edition. Edited by C. Langdon Fielding and K. Gary Magdesian.
© 2015 John Wiley & Sons, Inc. Published 2015 by John Wiley & Sons, Inc.

Total body water

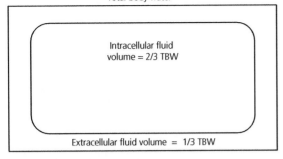

Figure 1.1 Relationship between total body water (TBW), extracellular fluid volume (ECFV), and intracellular fluid volume (ICFV) in a normal horse. Diagram represents a simplified "single cell" model.

Table 1.1 Physiologic fluid spaces in horses and foals.

Fluid space	Adult horse (L/kg)	Neonatal foal (L/kg)
Total body water	0.55–0.77	0.74
Extracellular fluid volume	0.21–0.29	0.36–0.40
Intracellular fluid volume	0.36–0.46	0.38
Plasma volume	0.052–0.063	0.09

Plasma volume is easier to estimate as compared to the other fluid spaces and has been reported as 0.052 to 0.063 L/kg in healthy adult horses (Marcilese et al., 1964). Clinical monitoring of the PV is essential as excessive expansion or contraction can lead to clinical derangements such as edema and shock, respectively. Changes in packed cell volume (PCV) over time may give an indication of PV alterations, but the role of splenic contraction makes the use of this measurement somewhat complicated in horses. Total plasma protein concentration may be a more useful tool for monitoring PV; however, abnormal protein losses can make interpretation problematic.

Intracellular fluid volume (ICFV)

Intracellular fluid volume is the volume of fluid contained within the cells. It is usually estimated as the difference between TBW and the ECFV. Bioimpedance technology has been used to make estimates of this fluid space in horses, but dilution techniques cannot be easily applied to the ICFV. Reported values for ICFV are between 0.356 and 0.458 L/kg in horses (Dugdale et al., 2011; Fielding et al., 2004; Forro et al., 2000). Monitoring of the ICFV is typically not performed in clinical practice, but BIA may offer the best assessment available at this time.

Physiologic fluid spaces in foals

Physiologic fluid spaces in newborn foals have been described (Table 1.1). In general, there is an increased size of the ECFV and TBW as compared to adults (Fielding et al., 2011; Spensley et al., 1987). Values of TBW in newborn foals appear to be larger (0.74 L/kg) as compared to adults, which is consistent with other

species (Fielding et al., 2011). Estimations of ECFV in foals are also significantly larger than in adults and have been reported to be between 0.36 and 0.40 L/kg in newborn foals; this decreases to 0.290 L/kg in foals at 24 weeks of age (Fielding et al., 2011; Spensley et al., 1987). The PV was estimated to be 0.090 L/kg (Fielding et al., 2011; Spensley et al., 1987), which represents an increase as compared to adults. Interestingly, the ICFV of foals is approximately 0.38 L/kg, which is similar to that in adult horses (Fielding et al., 2011). The ratio of ICFV to ECFV is approximately 1:1 in newborn foals as compared to adults with a ratio of approximately 2:1 (Figure 1.2).

These differences in physiologic fluid spaces in foals alter the volume of distribution for common medications that have a high degree of water solubility (i.e. aminoglycoside antibiotics). This is one reason why the dosing of some medications differs in neonates as compared to adult horses. Fluid therapy plans must also take into consideration the different fluid physiology of the neonate.

Concepts in fluid balance

Perhaps the two most important physiologic concepts in water balance and fluid therapy are:

1 *Effective osmolality* (*tonicity*) – this guides the intracellular to extracellular fluid balance.
2 *Starling's law of net filtration* – this guides the intravascular to interstitial fluid balance.

Osmolality

Osmolality refers to the number of osmoles per kilogram of solvent (or water). The osmotic effect exerted by solutes is based on the total number of particles regardless

Adult horse
Total body water

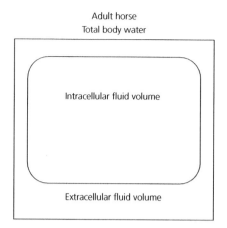

Intracellular fluid volume

Extracellular fluid volume

Neonatal foal
Total body water

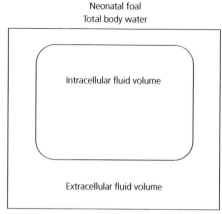

Intracellular fluid volume

Extracellular fluid volume

Figure 1.2 The relative sizes of the intracellular fluid volume, extracellular fluid volume and total body water in adults and foals.

of the size or weight of those particles. Osmolality is measured in serum by the method of freezing-point depression. Serum osmolality in adult horses was reported to range from 271 ± 8 to $281 \pm 9\,mOsm/kg\ H_2O$ (Carlson et al., 1979; Carlson & Rumbaugh, 1983; Pritchard et al., 2006). Serum osmolality in foals has been reported as 245 ± 19 to $267\,mOsm/kg\ H_2O$ (Brewer et al., 1991; Buchanan et al., 2005).

Osmolality in serum can also be estimated with a calculation that is based on the use of the primary osmotically active substances in serum. One of the available equations for calculation is:

ECF osmolality (mOsm/kg)

$$= 2 \times ([Na^+] + [K^+]) + [glucose]/18 + [BUN]/2.8 \quad (1.1)$$

The values for sodium and potassium are doubled to estimate the contributions of the anions (given that positive and negative charges are always balanced). Glucose and body urea nitrogen (BUN) are divided by their molecular weights in order to convert milligrams per deciliter to millimoles per liter. While not extensively reported, normal values for calculated osmolality in horses would likely range from 295 to $300\,mOsm/kg$ H_2O based on reported ranges for these ion concentrations in horses.

The osmolal gap is the difference between measured and calculated osmolality. Reference ranges for the osmolal gap in horses have not been reported; based on available information, it is anticipated that the calculated osmolality may be greater than the measured osmolality. This same observation has been reported in cats and has been attributed to laboratory error (Wellman et al.,

2012). A wide osmolal gap represents the presence of unidentified osmoles. The clinical usefulness of this test in horses may be more limited than in small animal medicine, as ethylene glycol toxicity is not commonly reported in horses. Other unidentified osmoles could be suspected using this calculation, however.

Effective osmolality (tonicity)

Effective osmoles are those that do not freely move across a membrane, and therefore exert tonicity. When considering horses (or other animals), the cellular membrane dividing the ECF from the ICF determines whether an osmole is effective. For example, sodium, potassium, and glucose that are distributed into the extracellular fluid space (e.g. by intravenous infusion) cannot freely move across the cell membrane into the cell (they all have specific mechanisms of transport). These are examples of effective osmoles. By contrast, urea (BUN) can freely move across the cell membrane and is therefore considered an ineffective osmole.

Tonicity refers to the effective osmolality of a solution. If the tonicity of an administered solution is the same as that of plasma, it is referred to as an isotonic solution. Conversely, a solution with an increased tonicity (i.e. 7.2% saline) as compared to plasma is referred to as hypertonic, and a solution with a decreased tonicity (i.e. 0.45% saline) is referred to as hypotonic.

Understanding the tonicity (effective osmolality) of different intravenous fluids as compared to plasma is critical to understanding fluid therapy. Many fluids (e.g. 0.9% saline) are referred to as "isotonic" even though they are slightly hypertonic (osmolality = 308 mOsm/kg H_2O) as compared to normal equine plasma (approximately 280 mOsm/kg H_2O). This mild hypertonicity of some supposedly "isotonic" intravenous fluids can lead to movement of water out of the cells and resulting cellular dehydration, as shown in Figure 1.3 (Fielding et al., 2008). This cellular "dehydrating" effect will be more significant when horses do not have access to free water.

Fluids that are hypotonic compared to normal plasma can result in movement of water into cells (Figure 1.4). This may be an important part of treatment in animals that have lost water from both the ECFV and ICFV. However, in cases of chronic hypernatremia, this movement of water into cells (when water is administered to the patient) can be life-threatening (see Chapter 2). These important concepts are further outlined in the discussion of transcellular fluid shifts below.

Effective osmolality is the main determinant of fluid balance between the ECFV and ICFV. All fluids that are lost must come from one or both of these spaces. In order to effectively provide fluid therapy, the clinician must recognize or estimate the source of fluid deficits (ECFV vs ICFV) and attempt to replace them from the respective location. Similarly, all fluids that are administered (intravenously, orally, etc.) will distribute to one or both of these spaces. Effective fluid therapy results when fluids are targeted to replace the missing fluid volume

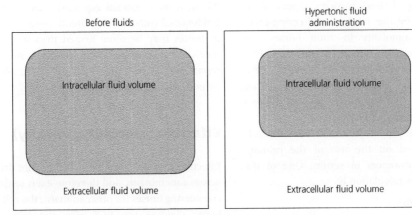

Figure 1.3 The effect of administering hypertonic fluids to the extracellular fluid volume (ECFV). There is an expansion of the ECFV and a shrinking of the intracellular fluid volume (ICFV).

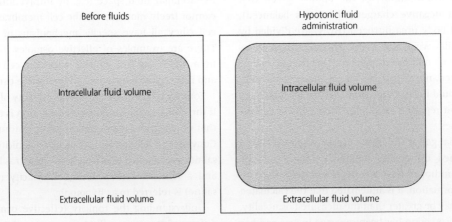

Figure 1.4 The effect of administering hypotonic fluids to the extracellular fluid volume (ECFV). There is an expansion of the ECFV and an expansion of the intracellular fluid volume (ICFV).

(e.g. a sodium-rich fluid is used to treat a hypovolemic horse with severe diarrhea that has ECFV deficits). However, ineffective fluid therapy results when fluids are misdirected to the inappropriate fluid space (e.g. a sodium-poor fluid such as 5% dextrose is used to treat the same hypovolemic horse with diarrhea).

In conclusion, the effective osmolality (tonicity) of a given fluid is extremely important for selecting the composition of a fluid to be administered to the patient. In general:

1 Administration of hypertonic fluids tends to expand the ECFV by an amount greater than the administered volume by drawing fluid from the ICFV.
2 Administration of hypotonic fluids tends to expand the ECFV by an amount less than the administered volume, as some fluid volume is lost to the ICFV.

Colloid osmotic pressure

Colloid osmotic pressure (COP) is the osmotic pressure generated by proteins within a fluid (typically plasma). It is also referred to as "oncotic pressure". The COP is one of the determinants (hydrostatic pressure also plays a role) of fluid balance between the vascular and interstitial spaces. Administered fluids that have COPs below plasma values will tend to move out of the vascular space and into the interstitial space. Conversely, fluids with COPs that are similar to or greater than plasma values will tend to "hold" fluid within the vascular space.

When fluids rich in protein are lost from a patient (i.e. severe blood loss), these fluids may be more effectively replaced with a fluid that has a normal to supranormal COP (i.e. whole blood). However, loss of fluids that are low in protein (e.g. prolonged, large-volume nasogastric reflux) can typically be replaced with fluids having a low oncotic pressure (i.e. an isotonic crystalloid).

Starling's law

The complex relationship described by Starling's law helps to govern the movement of fluid out of the vascular space into the interstitium. Figure 1.5 shows a simple model of Starling forces moving fluid out of the vascular space into the interstitial space.

$$\text{Net filtration} = K_f[(P_{cap} - P_{int}) - (\pi_{plasma} - \pi_{int})] \qquad (1.2)$$

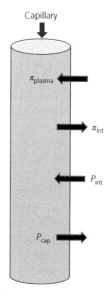

Figure 1.5 Starling factors affecting the fluid movement out of the vascular space into the interstitial space. P_{cap} refers to the hydrostatic pressure within the vascular space. P_{int} refers to the hydrostatic pressure within the interstitial space. π_{plasma} represents plasma oncotic pressure. π_{int} refers to the oncotic pressure within the interstitial space.

The term K_f represents the permeability of the capillary wall. In states of inflammatory disease, it is presumed that permeability significantly increases and results in movement of fluid and protein out of the vascular space (Levick & Michel, 2010). This fluid would then accumulate within the interstitial space resulting in edema that is observed clinically. Recent research has questioned the role of other factors, such as decreases in interstitial hydrostatic pressure, in addition to changes in K_f in the formation of edema (Reed & Rubin, 2010). Treatments designed to decrease K_f (i.e. some colloid solutions) aim to reduce the amount of fluid moving from the vascular space to the interstitial space.

The term P_{cap} refers to the hydrostatic pressure within the vascular space. Under normal circumstances, this pressure is generated by the heart. In experimental conditions, it can be increased by ligation of veins, with local increases in hydrostatic pressure. In heart failure or fluid overload, the P_{cap} increases thereby raising the pressure pushing fluid out of the capillary into the interstitial space. The role of P_{cap}, when designing a fluid therapy plan, should not be underestimated. Patients suspected of having an increased P_{cap} (sometimes in specific organs or local tissue regions) may need more moderate volume replacement (if any at all). Likewise, administering fluids with an increased oncotic pressure to volume overloaded patients can be particularly risky.

The term P_{int} refers to the hydrostatic pressure within the interstitial space. This can be considered the pressure that is "pushing back" against the inevitable flow of fluid out of the vascular space into the interstitium. The role of P_{int} was ignored for many years, but recent research has focused on its importance in the role of edema formation. Changes that occur in the structure (matrix) of the interstitium can cause a decrease in P_{int} (sometimes highly negative values) thereby "pulling" more fluid out of the vascular space and into the interstitium. A normal, healthy interstitium will hold a limited amount of fluid and as the volume increases, the hydrostatic pressure increases and resists further fluid movement out of the capillary. However, a diseased interstitium (i.e. as a result of inflammatory disease) may allow marked fluid expansion without creating significant pressure to resist further fluid entry. Under inflammatory conditions sometimes a negative pressure within the interstitial space can be generated, which may contribute to edema formation (Reed et al., 2010).

The term π_{plasma} represents plasma oncotic pressure and is described above. The normal plasma oncotic pressure has been reported as 22 to 25 mmHg (Boscan et al., 2007; Jones et al., 1997) in healthy horses. Horses that are sick and/or undergoing anesthesia may have plasma oncotic pressures as low as 12 mmHg (Boscan et al., 2007). Equations have been developed to estimate plasma oncotic pressure based on the value of total plasma protein, but these can have unacceptable accuracy (Magdesian et al., 2004; Runk et al., 2000). Plasma oncotic pressure was estimated to be approximately 19 mmHg in healthy neonatal foals (Runk et al., 2000). The oncotic pressures of the fluids commonly used in equine practice are discussed in Chapter 24. Rapid administration of a fluid with a low oncotic pressure (as compared to plasma) is likely to further drop the plasma oncotic pressure.

The term π_{int} refers to the oncotic pressure generated by the proteins and mucopolysaccharides within the interstitium. It is important to remember that the majority of protein is located within the interstitium (not the vascular space). Albumin, the primary determinant of plasma oncotic pressure, has an interstitial concentration lower than the plasma concentration. However, given the much larger size of the interstitial space, the absolute amount of protein within the interstitium is much greater than that within the vascular space.

Protein can move from the vascular space into the interstitium and then return through the lymphatic system. For this reason, administration of protein (in the form of plasma transfusion) into the vascular space will result in a distribution of some of the administered protein throughout much of the ECFV (i.e. into the interstitial space). This means that plasma administration is essentially ineffective at reducing fluid accumulation within the interstitial space (edema) and is unlikely to significantly change plasma oncotic pressure unless large amounts are administered. Interstitial colloid osmotic pressure is difficult to measure, but some estimates are in the range 12–15 mmHg in other species under experimental conditions (Wiig et al., 2003).

Changes in any of the terms of the Starling equation will likely affect other parameters as well. For example, when capillary hydrostatic pressure is increased experimentally, there is a subsequent drop in the interstitial oncotic pressure (Fadnes, 1976). This results from increased fluid moving into the interstitium, thereby lowering its oncotic pressure.

In a more expanded version of the Starling formula, the capillary reflection coefficient (σ) is included:

$$\text{Net filtration} = K_f[(P_{cap} - P_{int}) - \sigma\,(\pi_{plasma} - \pi_{int})] \qquad (1.3)$$

The reflection coefficient acts as a correction factor for the effective oncotic pressure given that some capillaries are more permeable to proteins than others. For example, capillaries in the glomerulus may be quite impermeable and have values close to 1. Conversely, capillaries in the pulmonary system are relatively more permeable to protein and have a reflection coefficient close to 0.5. The other variables are described above.

Fluid movement out of the vascular space

In a simplistic model, fluid should be considered to move continuously out of the vascular space (according to the Starling factors described above), then into the interstitial space, and finally into the lymphatic system. The fluid is returned to the vascular space by way of lymphatic flow (e.g. thoracic duct draining into left subclavian vein). A certain amount of protein is taken with this fluid and also moves continuously through the system.

Fluid accumulation within the interstitial space (interstitial edema) results when there is dysfunction of this continuous system (of fluid movement from the vascular space to the interstitium and to the lymphatics). Causes of edema in equine practice include the following:

1 Decreased plasma colloid osmotic pressure (hypoproteinemia).
2 Increased capillary hydrostatic pressure.
3 Increased capillary permeability.
4 Lymphatic obstruction.

However, it is likely that any type of systemic inflammation will result in changes to the interstitial hydrostatic pressure (as well as causing changes in capillary permeability) and that this also may contribute to edema formation. A single abnormality (e.g. hypoproteinemia) may have to be very severe in order to cause edema. However, when multiple derangements are present (e.g. hypoproteinemia, increased intravascular pressure due to excessive fluid administration or cardiac dysfunction, and decreased interstitial pressure due to inflammation), edema formation will be more likely to manifest, and will do so sooner than with an individual abnormality (Figure 1.6).

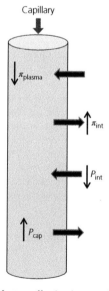

Capillary

Figure 1.6 Starling factors affecting increased fluid movement out of the vascular space into the interstitial space and resulting in interstitial edema. P_{cap} refers to the hydrostatic pressure within the vascular space. P_{int} refers to the hydrostatic pressure within the interstitial space. π_{plasma} represents plasma oncotic pressure. π_{int} refers to the oncotic pressure in the interstitial space.

Starling's law and fluid therapy

The practical implications of Starling's law underlie many of the basic concepts for fluid therapy. In choosing a fluid therapy plan, the clinician can influence the capillary hydrostatic pressure and the plasma oncotic pressure most directly. The two main concepts are:

1 Fluids with a high oncotic pressure relative to plasma are likely to raise both plasma oncotic pressure and capillary hydrostatic pressure.
2 Fluids with low oncotic pressure relative to plasma are likely to lower plasma oncotic pressure and raise capillary hydrostatic pressure.

Over time, administered fluids may also have an effect on the interstitial oncotic pressure, but likely play a minor role in changing the interstitial hydrostatic pressure. While the role of capillary permeability remains unclear, most intravenous fluid choices do not strongly influence this variable. Some synthetic colloids (depending on the size of the molecules) may have the potential to "plug" capillary walls that are more permeable. More information on this topic can be found in Chapter 24.

Optimal fluid therapy considers all of the components of Starling's law. For example, a newborn foal with bacteremia may be undergoing a severe systemic inflammatory response (SIRS), and would be expected to have reduced interstitial hydrostatic pressure and possibly increased capillary permeability and reduced oncotic pressure. This patient is a prime candidate for edema formation. Conversely, a severely dehydrated endurance horse is likely to have a high plasma protein concentration and a normal interstitial hydrostatic pressure. This horse is likely to tolerate aggressive fluid therapy well.

Summary of tonicity and colloid osmotic pressure

Based on the information above, potential fluids can be described as either hyper- or hypotonic and either hyper- or hypo-oncotic as compared to the patient's plasma. A fluid that is both hypertonic and hyperoncotic has the potential to shift fluid from the ICFV into the ECFV and expand the intravascular volume. This would potentially make a good resuscitation fluid as it expands the vascular space quickly; however, it would make a very poor maintenance fluid as it is likely to dehydrate the cells. A hypotonic and hypo-oncotic fluid such as 0.45% saline would be very poor at expanding the vascular volume, but might make a better long-term fluid (especially with some additives) for maintenance of hydration of cells, interstitium, and vascular space.

References

Boscan P, Watson Z, Steffey EP. (2007) Plasma colloid osmotic pressure and total protein trends in horses during anesthesia. *Vet Anaesth Analg* **34**:275–83.

Brewer BD, Clement SF, Lotz WS, et al. (1991) Renal clearance, urinary excretion of endogenous substances, and urinary diagnostic indices in healthy neonatal foals. *J Vet Intern Med* **5**:28–33.

Buchanan BR, Sommardahl CS, Rohrbach BW, et al. (2005) Effect of a 24-hour infusion of an isotonic electrolyte replacement fluid on the renal clearance of electrolytes in healthy neonatal foals. *J Am Vet Med Assoc* **227**:1123–9.

Carlson GP, Rumbaugh GE. (1983) Response to saline solution of normally fed horses and horses dehydrated by fasting. *Am J Vet Res* **44**:964–8.

Carlson GP, Rumbaugh GE, Harrold D. (1979) Physiologic alterations in the horse produced by food and water deprivation during periods of high environmental temperatures. *Am J Vet Res* **40**:982–5.

Dugdale AH, Curtis GC, Milne E, et al. (2011) Assessment of body fat in the pony: part II. Validation of the deuterium oxide dilution technique for the measurement of body fat. *Equine Vet J* **43**:562–70.

Fadnes HO. (1976) Effect of increased venous pressure on the hydrostatic and colloid osmotic pressure in subcutaneous interstitial fluid in rats: edema-preventing mechanisms. *Scand J Clin Lab Invest* **36**:371–7.

Fielding CL, Magdesian KG, Elliott DA, et al. (2004) Use of multifrequency bioelectrical impedance analysis for estimation of total body water and extracellular and intracellular fluid volumes in horses. *Am J Vet Res* **65**:320–6.

Fielding CL, Magdesian KG, Carlson GP, et al. (2008) Application of the sodium dilution principle to calculate extracellular fluid volume changes in horses during dehydration and rehydration. *Am J Vet Res* **69**:1506–11.

Fielding CL, Magdesian KG, Edman JE. (2011) Determination of body water compartments in neonatal foals by use of indicator dilution techniques and multifrequency bioelectrical impedance analysis. *Am J Vet Res* **72**:1390–6.

Forro M, Cieslar S, Ecker GL, et al. (2000) Total body water and ECFV measured using bioelectrical impedance analysis and indicator dilution in horses. *J Appl Physiol* **89**:663–671.

Jones PA, Tomasic M, Gentry PA. (1997) Oncotic, hemodilutional, and hemostatic effects of isotonic saline and hydroxyethyl starch solutions in clinically normal ponies. *Am J Vet Res* **58**:541–8.

Latman NS, Keith N, Nicholson A, et al. (2011) Bioelectrical impedance analysis determination of water content and distribution in the horse. *Res Vet Sci* **90**:516–20.

Levick JR, Michel CC. (2010) Microvascular fluid exchange and the revised Starling principle. *Cardiovasc Res* **87**:198–210.

Magdesian KG, Fielding CL, Madigan JE. (2004) Measurement of plasma colloid osmotic pressure in neonatal foals under intensive care: comparison of direct and indirect methods and the association of COP with selected clinical and clinicopathologic variables. *J Vet Emerg Crit Care* **14**:108–14.

Marcilese NA, Valsecchi RM, Figueras HD, et al. (1964) Normal blood volumes in the horse. *Am J Physiol* **207**:223–7.

Pritchard JC, Barr AR, Whay HR. (2006) Validity of a behavioural measure of heat stress and a skin tent test for dehydration in working horses and donkeys. *Equine Vet J* **38**:433–8.

Reed RK, Rubin K. (2010) Transcapillary exchange: role and importance of the interstitial fluid pressure and the extracellular matrix. *Cardiovasc Res* **87**:211–17.

Runk DT, Madigan JE, Rahal CJ, et al. (2000) Measurement of plasma colloid osmotic pressure in normal thoroughbred neonatal foals. *J Vet Intern Med* **14**:475–8.

Spensley MS, Carlson GP, Harrold D. (1987) Plasma, red blood cell, total blood, and extracellular fluid volumes in healthy horse foals during growth. *Am J Vet Res* **48**:1703–7.

Wellman ML, DiBartola SP, Kohn CW. (2012) Applied physiology of body fluid in dogs and cats. In: DiBartola SP (ed.) *Fluid, Electrolyte, and Acid–Base Disorders in Small Animal Practice*. St Louis, MO: Saunders, pp. 2–25.

Wiig H, Rubin K, Reed RK. (2003) New and active role of the interstitium in control of interstitial fluid pressure: potential therapeutic consequences. *Acta Anaesthesiol Scand* **47**:111–21.

Zdolsek J, Li Y, Hahn RG. Detection of dehydration by using volume kinetics. *Anesth Analg* 2012;**115**:814–22.

CHAPTER 2

Sodium and water homeostasis and derangements

C. Langdon Fielding

Loomis Basin Equine Medical Center, Penryn, CA, USA

Introduction

The intake of sodium and water has been extensively studied in horses as the topic has implications for routine husbandry, exercise, and the treatment of sick animals. Sodium and water are ingested and absorbed through the gastrointestinal system. The ingested salt and water are then excreted through the kidneys or undergo insensible losses (e.g. evaporation through sweat). Nearly all disorders of salt and water metabolism are due to abnormalities in intake or excretion. Often a combination of both will create a significant abnormality in sodium and water balance. The sodium concentration of common biological fluids in horses is shown in Table 2.1.

Sodium and water intake

Daily sodium intake for horses has been reported as ranging from 0.7 mmol/kg/day to 2.3 mmol/kg/day, but can be highly variable due to the environment, feed sources, etc. (Groenendyk et al., 1988; Tasker, 1967a). Approximately 75% of the sodium intake appeared to be absorbed in the gastrointestinal tract with the remainder lost in fecal output (Groenendyk et al., 1988). Sodium can be absorbed rapidly following oral administration with appearance in the plasma in as little as 10 minutes (Lindinger & Ecker, 2013). Sodium is absorbed through active transport in the proximal colon, cecum, and small colon (Clarket et al., 1992; Giddings et al., 1974). Sodium concentrations measured

throughout the intestinal tract of the horse indicated higher concentrations in the proximal portions of the intestine, with lower concentrations moving distally (Alexander, 1962). Sodium absorption is increased under the effects of aldosterone (Clarke et al., 1992). Medications, such as furosemide (frusemide), have been shown to increase fecal sodium content and therefore may affect absorption of the ion (Alexander, 1977).

Daily water intake has been described for normal horses at approximately 54–64 mL/kg/day (Groenendyk et al., 1988; Tasker, 1967a). In one study, however, it ranged from 54 to 83 mL/kg/day indicating a wide variation in normal horses (Groenendyk et al., 1988). Approximately 74% of water intake was absorbed through the gastrointestinal system with the remainder lost in fecal output (Groenendyk et al., 1988). However, water losses increase dramatically when diarrhea is present (Tasker, 1967b). Water intake is influenced by the thirst response, which is stimulated by both changes in osmolality as well as hypovolemia. This has been described in horses as it has been for other species (Houpt et al., 1989; Jones et al., 1989).

Sodium and water balance

In the kidneys, sodium and water are freely filtered by the glomerulus and then reabsorbed as they move through the rest of the nephron (Figure 2.1). Horses appear to conserve more sodium than humans, but this will significantly depend on the intake in a given animal (Rawlings & Bisgard, 1975).

Equine Fluid Therapy, First Edition. Edited by C. Langdon Fielding and K. Gary Magdesian.
© 2015 John Wiley & Sons, Inc. Published 2015 by John Wiley & Sons, Inc.

In the proximal tubule, approximately 67% of the filtered sodium and water is reabsorbed. Water and many organic solutes are coupled to the reabsorption of sodium in this segment. The loop of Henle reabsorbs approximately 25% of sodium and 15% of water. The water is absorbed through the descending limb while sodium (along with potassium and chloride) is absorbed in the ascending limb. The distal tubules and collecting ducts reabsorb approximately 8% of filtered sodium and 10–15% of filtered water. Sodium and water absorption throughout the kidney is shown in Figure 2.1.

Urine from normal horses has a sodium concentration ranging from 40 to 214 mmol/L depending on the study (Fielding et al., 2008; Robert et al., 2010; Roussel et al.,

Table 2.1 Sodium concentration of common biological fluids in horses.

Fluid	Sodium concentration	References
Serum	137–139 mmol/L	Watson et al. (2002); Fielding et al. (2008)
Urine	40–110 mmol/L	Roussel et al. (1993); Robert et al. (2010); Fielding et al. (2008); Watson et al. (2002)
Cerebrospinal fluid	145±2.0 mmol/L	Mayhew et al. (1977)
Sweat	110–249 mmol/L	Kingston et al. (1997); Rose et al. (1980); Spooner et al. (2010)
Peritoneal fluid	134±2 mmol/L	Latson et al. (2005)
Normal feces	127±33 mmol/kg DM	Ecke et al. (1998)
Saliva	54–56 mEq/L	Alexander (1966)
Mare's milk	12 mEq/L	Ullrey et al. (1966)

1993; Watson et al., 2002). The concentration of sodium in the urine depends both on the amount of sodium being reabsorbed by the kidney and the amount of water being excreted. The fractional excretion may be a more useful evaluation of sodium loss in the urine, with normal values being less than 1% (Robert et al., 2010; Roussel et al., 1993; Toribio et al., 2007). However, it has been proposed that values exceeding 0.5% may be indicative of renal disease in horses (Grossman et al., 1982). Fractional excretion values can be strongly influenced by diet and the concurrent administration of intravenous fluids (Roussel et al., 1993). Normal values for fractional excretion of sodium in foals on a consistent milk diet are similar to adult horses (Brewer et al., 1991). Increased fractional excretion values may be associated with abnormal renal tubular function and an inability to reabsorb adequate amounts of sodium.

The fractional excretion of sodium by the kidneys is given by the equation:

$$\text{Fractional excretion of Na}^+ = ([Cr_{plasma}]/[Cr_{urine}]) \\ \times ([Na^+_{urine}]/[Na^+_{plasma}]) \\ \times 100$$

$$(2.1)$$

where Cr_{plasma} is the concentration of creatinine in the plasma, Cr_{urine} is the concentration of creatinine in the urine, Na^+_{urine} is the concentration of sodium in the urine, and Na^+_{plasma} is the concentration of sodium in the plasma.

Factors affecting sodium balance

The reabsorption of sodium in the kidney is influenced by a number of mediators including aldosterone, angiotensin II, uroguanylin, catecholamines, and natriuretic peptides (Table 2.2).

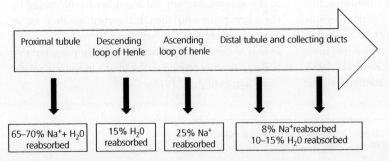

Figure 2.1 Sodium reabsorption in the kidney.

Table 2.2 Major factors affecting sodium reabsorption in the kidneys.

Factor	Effects on sodium reabsorption in the kidney
Angiotensin II	Increases reabsorption in proximal tubule
	Stimulates release of aldosterone
	Increases renal efferent arteriolar constriction
Aldosterone	Increases sodium reabsorption in distal tubule
Natriuretic peptides	Increase GFR
	Inhibit sodium reabsorption
Catecholamines	Increase reabsorption of sodium at multiple sites
	Activate RAAS system
	Increase renal vascular resistance
Uroguanylin	Inhibit sodium absorption

GFR, glomerular filtration rate; RAAS, renin-angiotensin-aldosterone system.

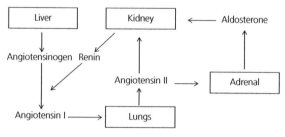

Figure 2.2 Simplified diagram of the renin-angiotensin-aldosterone system (RAAS).

Angiotensin II

Angiotensin II (AT II) is one of the important effectors in the renin-angiotensin-aldosterone system (RAAS) (Figure 2.2. Renin is released from the juxtaglomerular cells of the kidney in response to decreased perfusion pressure and decreased chloride delivery to the macula densa in the distal convoluted tubule. Stimulation of the sympathetic nervous system through β_1-adrenoceptors and numerous paracrine and endocrine factors also influence the release of renin.

Renin acts to convert angiotensinogen to angiotensin I. Angiotensinogen is produced primarily in the liver; its production is increased by a number of factors including acute inflammation and angiotensin II. Angiotensin I is converted to angiotensin II (AT II) by angiotensin-converting enzyme (ACE). The enzyme is located in numerous vascular beds but the main site of synthesis is in the pulmonary system. Numerous medications have been developed to block the effects of ACE, and these are discussed more thoroughly in the chapter addressing fluid therapy in heart failure (Chapter 17).

Angiotensin II (AT II) has a number of effects that produce changes in sodium and water balance. First, AT II primarily affects sodium balance by its effects on the Na^+/H^+ exchanger in the proximal tubule, where it increases the reabsorption of sodium (Wang & Chan, 1990). Second, AT II also directly stimulates the release of aldosterone and its effects on sodium reabsorption are discussed below in the next section. Third, AT II increases efferent renal arteriolar constriction (to a greater extent than afferent) thereby increasing the filtration fraction, which can indirectly lead to more sodium reabsorption in the proximal tubule (Denton et al., 1992). AT II has a number of other effects but these three are the primary ones affecting sodium and water balance.

Aldosterone

As mentioned previously, AT II is one of the major stimulants for the production of aldosterone by the adrenal cortex. Hyperkalemia is the other primary stimulant for increased aldosterone secretion. The effects of AT II and plasma potassium are synergistic. Additionally, AT II is needed for changes in the plasma potassium concentration to have their full effects on aldosterone production.

Aldosterone's major effect on sodium and water balance is to cause an increase in sodium reabsorption in the distal tubule. This indirectly leads to an increase in the extracellular fluid volume. As discussed in the chapter on potassium disorders (Chapter 3), aldosterone also augments potassium secretion in this same region of the kidney.

Natriuretic peptides

The natriuretic peptides – atrial natriuretic peptide (ANP) and brain natriuretic peptide (BNP) – increase glomerular filtration rate (GFR) by causing renal afferent arteriolar dilation and efferent arteriolar constriction (Loutzenhiser et al., 1988). They also inhibit sodium reabsorption in the collecting tubule and potentially in other segments of the kidney as well. As their name implies the natriuretic peptides act to increase

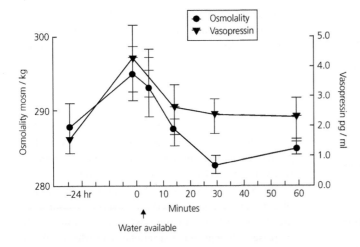

Figure 2.3 Changes in concentration of vasopressin and osmolality in plasma taken from six ponies prior to a period of water deprivation (water replete), after 24 hours of water deprivation (0) and 5, 15, 30, and 60 minutes after water was made available. Values are mean ± SEM. From Houpt KA, Thorton SN, Allen WR. Vasopressin in dehydrated and rehydrated ponies. Physiol Behav 1989;45:659–661. Reproduced with permission.

sodium loss through the kidneys. The release of atrial natriuretic peptide is primarily stimulated through distention of the atria, typically in response to volume overload.

Catecholamines

The release of epinephrine (adrenaline) and norepinephrine (noradrenaline) due to stimulation by the sympathetic nervous system causes changes in renal hemodynamics and increased reabsorption of sodium. First, catecholamines cause direct stimulation of sodium reabsorption in the proximal tubule and loop of Henle (Bello-Ruess, 1980). Second, catecholamines cause activation of the RAAS system, which increases sodium absorption as described earlier (Johnson et al., 1995). Finally, catecholamines cause an increase in renal vascular resistance (both afferent and efferent) that helps to limit the loss of sodium (Tucker et al., 1987).

Uroguanylin

Uroguanylin and guanylin are produced in the intestines in response to an ingested salt load. They travel through the bloodstream to the kidneys where they act to inhibit the absorption of sodium and water. They have not yet been identified in horses, but are present in a number of other species.

Factors affecting regulation of water balance

Arginine vasopressin

The single most important effector of water balance is arginine vasopressin (AVP). It is synthesized in the

hypothalamus in the supraoptic and paraventricular nuclei. It is released in response to increases in osmolality or to decreases in blood volume/blood pressure.

Cells within the hypothalamus alter their volume in response to changes in the extracellular fluid (ECF) osmolality. Increases in osmolality (and resultant cell shrinkage) will cause the subsequent release of vasopressin into the circulation, and this has been described in horses as well as other species (Figure 2.3) (Houpt et al., 1989; Irvine et al., 1989). Levels of AVP were correlated with serum osmolality in horses with dehydration (Sneddon et al., 1993). Similar to humans, there is likely a threshold effect for AVP release in horses. In other species, a 1 to 2% change in plasma osmolality can result in a 2–4-fold increase in AVP concentrations (Dunn et al., 1973).

The non-osmotic release of vasopressin (i.e. without an increase in osmolality) is primarily due to hypovolemia (hypotension). This non-osmotic release of vasopressin is mediated by baroreceptors though there continues to be investigation into other potential factors that may be involved in its release. As opposed to the very sensitive response of vasopressin to small changes in osmolality, much larger changes in volume status are needed to cause the release of vasopressin.

There are clinical situations in which the osmotic stimulus for vasopressin release is in opposition to the non-osmotic stimulus. For example, a patient may have severe hypovolemia but a decreased osmolality due to hyponatremia. In this situation, the non-osmotic stimulus (the drive to preserve normal circulating volume and blood pressure) will take precedence over the osmotic stimulus. To summarize, vasopressin release is more sensitive to small changes in osmolality but large changes in volume status will override changes in osmolality.

Vasopressin exerts its primary control over water balance through its effects in the collecting ducts of the kidney. Vasopressin binds to V2 receptors in this region which leads to the phosphorylation of the water channel protein aquaporin 2. This allows water movement out of the collecting ducts through the luminal membrane. Additional aquaporin channels (other than type 2) facilitate the movement of water out of the cell through the basolateral membrane.

Serum sodium concentration

The serum sodium concentration in normal horses has been reported to range from 137 to 139 mmol/L (Fielding et al., 2008; Lindner, 1991; Watson et al., 2002), although different laboratories vary in their provided normal ranges. Numerous point of care analyzers are available for use in equine practice and therefore the serum sodium concentration can be evaluated in both a hospital and a field setting. Both plasma and serum samples can be used for analysis and results do not appear to differ significantly (Lindner, 1991).

Understanding the meaning of the serum sodium concentration is one of the most difficult concepts in electrolyte and fluid therapy. The complexity originates from the different sodium and potassium concentrations in the varying physiologic fluid spaces (particularly intracellular vs extracellular). Even the intravascular and interstitial spaces (both part of the extracellular fluid volume) do not have the same exact sodium concentration due to the Gibbs–Donnan effect, although they are very close (Kurtz & Nguyen, 2005). Serum sodium really reflects the relationship between total body sodium, total body potassium, and total body water (Figure 2.4). One of the simplest ways of describing this relationship is by the formula (Edelman et al., 1958):

$$\text{Serum } [Na] = (\text{total body Na} + \text{total body K}) / \text{total body water} \quad (2.2)$$

Potassium is included in this formula because it is the primary cation of the intracellular compartment. More

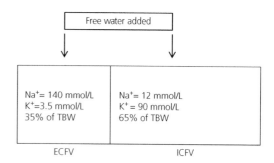

Figure 2.4 When free water is administered to the animal, it will distribute to the extracellular and intracellular fluid spaces in an unequal manner. Serum sodium concentration is not a simple relationship between sodium and water because the dispersion of sodium and water between the different fluid spaces is not equal. ECFV, extracellular fluid volume; ICFV, intracellular fluid volume; TBW, total body water.

complex models have been proposed, but it is not clear that they add significantly to the original formula (Nguyen & Kurtz, 2004). It is probably easiest to consider that changes in total body potassium or sodium without corresponding changes in total body water will result in abnormalities in the serum sodium concentration. When total body water (free water) is increased, it will distribute between the intracellular and extracellular fluid spaces. Its effects will be proportional to the combined amount of sodium and potassium, but not to the sodium concentration alone. The same is true when total body sodium or potassium is increased/decreased.

For simplicity, the serum sodium concentration is often evaluated without consideration of potassium. This may be an easier way to consider the relationship between sodium and water. However, when predicting changes in the sodium concentration in response to the addition of water and electrolytes, the more complete formula should be used.

Introduction to hyponatremia and hypernatremia

Nearly all derangements in the serum sodium concentration are the result of changes in intake or output of water and/or sodium. In most cases, a combination of abnormalities (e.g. concurrent water deprivation and renal disease) is needed in order to generate a significantly abnormal serum sodium concentration. Diagnosis of the primary problem leading to the serum sodium abnormality is important to safely and effectively treat the problem. In general, acute changes in serum sodium concentrations can be treated rapidly, whereas chronic changes must be treated more slowly.

Hyponatremia

Pseudohyponatremia is when the measured serum sodium concentration is below the true concentration. Commonly identified causes of pseudohyponatremia include hyperproteinemia and hyperlipemia. The reasons for this have been well described but, briefly, relate to the presence of increased lipid or protein causing alteration of the water concentration in the sample (Fortgens & Pillay, 2011). This could also potentially hide a patient with true hypernatremia by creating a "pseudonormonatremia".

There are two general concepts that contribute to hyponatremia:
1 Excess free water intake (by either ingestion or administration).
2 Inability to excrete free water.

Horses can ingest large amounts of free water for a variety of reasons including dehydration/hypovolemia, inappropriate thirst, and boredom. Simply ingesting large amounts of free water is not typically able to create a clinically significant hyponatremia unless the ingested volumes are extreme. The kidneys are able to excrete excess free water and maintain a normal serum sodium concentration under normal circumstances. However, rapid ingestion of large volumes of water after a period of water deprivation can cause a clinically significant decrease in serum sodium concentration, leading to clinical signs associated with cerebral edema.

The kidney may be unable to excrete an appropriate amount of free water due to renal failure or an inappropriate production/response to vasopressin. A combination of excessive free water ingestion and the inability of the kidneys to excrete this water, as occurs during hypovolemia, is often required for significant hyponatremia to develop. A classic example would be the loss of a high sodium-containing fluid (e.g. diarrhea) in a dehydrated animal. The patient would consume water to combat dehydration. Likewise, vasopressin will be released in response to hypovolemia in order to help prevent water

---

Box 2.1 Conditions that may lead to hyponatremia.

Diarrhea
Salivary losses
Renal failure
Ruptured bladder
Excess free water administration/consumption
Severe sweat losses
Adrenal insufficiency
Rhabdomyolysis
Syndrome of inappropriate ADH secretion

---

diuresis and maintain circulating volume. As free water is retained, the serum sodium concentration will continue to fall.

Hyponatremia is classically divided into cases that are hypovolemic, euvolemic, and hypervolemic based on clinical assessment and history. While some cases fit this grouping very well, many times the volume status of the patient is not immediately apparent. This chapter focuses on the underlying causes of hyponatremia and describes a general approach to treatment. Whenever possible, however, the volume status of hyponatremic patients should be estimated as it can aid in treatment decisions.

Hyponatremia is not a common abnormality in horses and only 2.7% of horses presenting to a referral hospital had plasma sodium concentrations below the normal range (C.L. Fielding, unpublished data). Clinically significant hyponatremia is even less common but may be suspected when one of the clinical conditions listed in Box 2.1 is present. As with many electrolyte abnormalities, multiple factors (diarrhea, kidney disease, etc.) may be responsible for the observed derangement.

Diarrhea

Experimentally induced diarrhea in horses resulted in significant fecal losses of sodium and water (Ecke et al., 1998; Tasker, 1967b). Fecal sodium losses can be severe and therefore hyponatremia results when water losses are replaced by drinking (free water). Unless animals are able to replace the sodium deficit, hyponatremia results. Hyponatremia has also been observed in clinical cases of colitis in horses, though the abnormality is often mild with values ranging from 125 to 130 mmol/L (Burgess et al., 2010; Magdesian et al., 2002; Stewart et al., 1995). Less commonly, the hyponatremia resulting from diarrhea can be more severe and result in clinically observed neurologic changes (Lakritz et al., 1992).

Salivary losses

Experimentally created esophageal fistulas resulted in clinical hyponatremia, though values were not low enough to cause neurologic deficits (Stick et al., 1981). Hyponatremia is not commonly described in cases of esophageal obstruction. The sodium concentration in the saliva of horses is approximately 55 mEq/L (Alexander, 1966). Given the low sodium concentration in saliva relative to plasma, large volumes of saliva would need to be lost and replaced by free water in order to generate a clinically significant hyponatremia.

Renal failure

Hyponatremia is a feature of acute renal failure in horses, though it does not appear to be present in all cases (Divers et al., 1987; Geor, 2007). The hyponatremia appears to be relatively mild with values not less than 124 mmol/L (Divers et al., 1987). Hyponatremia was also commonly described (65% of horses) with chronic renal failure; however, specific values were not reported (Schott et al., 1997). Horses that have access to salt and an intact thirst mechanism may be able to compensate for lack of appropriate renal function.

Uroabdomen (ruptured bladder)

Rupture of the urinary bladder or urachus with subsequent uroabdomen occurs most commonly in foals, but has also been described in adult horses (Beck et al., 1996; Behr et al., 1981; Dunkel et al., 2005; Genetzky & Hagemoser, 1985; Quinn & Carmalt, 2012;). A large volume of urine with a low sodium concentration accumulating in the abdomen will result in a significant decrease in serum sodium concentration. This urine accumulation effectively creates a dilutional hyponatremia where free water is not excreted from the body but retained within the abdominal cavity (Behr et al., 1981). This is particularly true in neonatal foals who consume mare's milk, which has a sodium concentration of 12 mEq/L (Ullrey et al., 1966).

Hyponatremia is a consistent feature of uroabdomen. However, administration of intravenous balanced electrolyte solutions may mitigate this; serum sodium concentration may be within the normal range in hospitalized foals that develop uroabdomen while concurrently being administered isotonic fluids for other reasons (Dunkel et al., 2005).

Free water administration/consumption

Administration of free water without access to sodium (free salt, feed) will result in hyponatremia (Lopes et al., 2004). This may be observed in horses that are feed deprived with continued access to fresh water (Freestone et al., 1991). It can also be observed when water is administered orally or intravenously without significant concentrations of sodium (Lopes et al., 2004). The administration of low-sodium intravenous fluids (i.e. 5% dextrose in water) may be dangerous in patients that are anorexic and not receiving sodium from other enteral sources.

Horses with certain neurologic diseases may also consume large quantities of free water inappropriately. The excessive drinking may be caused by a variety of factors, especially cerebral diseases, but all can result in hyponatremia. It may be difficult to maintain a normal sodium concentration in these patients despite treatment as the correction of the hyponatremia may not resolve the excessive water intake if the neurologic disease is still present. Water restriction is often required in such cases.

Sweat losses

Horse sweat has a sodium concentration ranging from 110 to 249 mmol/L (Kingston et al., 1997; Rose et al., 1980; Spooner et al., 2010). The majority of studies indicate that the sodium concentration is mildly decreased as compared to plasma, but factors such as type of feed and environment influence the values (Spooner et al., 2010). Sweat losses alone would be unlikely to create a hyponatremia. However, large volumes of sweat combined with on-going free water replacement could generate a hyponatremia when sodium intake is low. Competitive endurance exercise is associated with a mild decrease in serum sodium concentration; however, clinically significant hyponatremia is not evident in most horses (Fielding et al., 2009).

Adrenal insufficiency

A lack of mineralocorticoid production has been described in horses (Couëtil & Hoffman 1998; Dowling et al., 1993). Hyponatremia was only reported in one of these cases and concurrent gastrointestinal disease was present making interpretation of the cause of the serum sodium concentration difficult. Lack of mineralocorticoid production is typically associated with an increased urinary sodium concentration and concurrent hyperkalemia. As the extracellular fluid volume (ECFV) decreases, an increased vasopressin concentration helps to maintain the hyponatremia.

Rhabdomyolysis

Hyponatremia has been associated with cases of rhabdomyolysis in horses and other species (Katsarou & Singh, 2010; Perkins et al., 1998). Hyponatremia may result from secondary renal disease (pigment-induced renal failure), fluid shifting, or it may even be an inciting cause for the rhabdomyolysis (Katsarou & Singh, 2010; Perkins et al., 1998). Increased sodium concentration was observed in the urine of horses with rhabdomyolysis in one study (el-Ashker, 2011). In clinical cases, both hyponatremia and rhabdomyolysis need to be treated, with prevention of renal injury with fluid therapy in those with significant myoglobinuria.

SIADH (syndrome of inappropriate antidiuretic hormone)

While equine clinicians have suspected this syndrome to exist in foals and adult horses, there are no confirmed cases reported in the literature. As the name of the syndrome implies, concentrations of antidiuretic hormone (ADH; vasopressin) are increased despite the absence of either of the two major stimuli for its release (increased osmolality and hypovolemia). Criteria for the diagnosis of SIADH (Berl & Schrier, 2010) include:

1 ECFV osmolality is decreased.
2 Inappropriate urinary concentration.
3 Euvolemia.
4 Elevated urinary sodium concentration.
5 Absence of renal insufficiency or other endocrine disorder.
6 Absence of diuretic administration.

There are four proposed types of SIADH in humans; in general the syndrome is related to a defect in the osmoregulation of ADH (vasopressin). It is unknown whether different types of SIADH exist in horses.

Clinical effects of hyponatremia

As the serum sodium concentration decreases, water moves from the extracellular into the intracellular space in order to maintain osmolal equality between the two spaces. Movement of water into nerve cells of the brain can result in neurological signs. In humans, the clinical signs can develop at sodium concentrations less than 125 mmol/L if there is an acute change in the serum sodium concentration (Arieff et al., 1976). In chronic hyponatremia, humans may not develop clinical signs until the serum sodium concentration drops below 110 mmol/L (Biswas & Davies, 2007). Research in horses has not identified sodium cut-offs for producing clinical signs, but it is likely that similar values may be appropriate. In case reports of neonatal foals with hyponatremia, foals with serum sodium concentrations below 110 mmol/L exhibited significant neurologic deficits (Lakritz et al., 1992; Wong et al., 2007).

Many of the clinical signs in patients with mild hyponatremia may be related to the primary disease and not to the effects of a low serum sodium concentration. Mild hyponatremia is usually not associated with clinical signs. Headaches and restlessness may be observed in humans with mild derangements in sodium concentration, but these may be difficult to identify in horses. More severe hyponatremia can lead to dysphagia, focal or generalized seizures, coma, and even death as brain swelling progresses. Complete and serial neurologic examinations should be performed in foals or horses with hyponatremia to determine if mild neurologic deficits are present.

Treatment of hyponatremia

The rate of correction of hyponatremia is critical. Particularly in chronic cases, rapid correction of the serum sodium concentration can lead to dangerous movement of fluid out of brain cells. This decrease in brain cell volume can result in demyelination (central pontine myelinolysis)and permanent neurologic damage (Karp & Laureno, 1993).

Unfortunately, the cause and chronicity of hyponatremia are not always apparent when treatment must be initiated. After a thorough history and neurologic evaluation is obtained, it should be determined whether the patient is clinical. Ideally, some estimate of the duration of hyponatremia should be made. If it is impossible to determine the duration, it should be assumed to be chronic.

For acute cases with clinical signs attributable to hyponatremia, the administration of hypertonic saline may be warranted for careful correction of sodium concentration. In humans, a 3% hypertonic saline solution has often been used; however, 7.2% hypertonic saline is more commonly available in equine practice. The concentration of the fluid is not as important as the overall rate of total sodium administration (i.e. a slower rate for a more concentrated fluid). General guidelines for treatment are based on the observation in humans that demyelinating syndrome was avoided in severely hyponatremic patients by limiting correction rates to no more than 12 mEq/L in 24 h and 18 mEq/L in 48 h (Sterns et al., 1986, 1994; Sterns, 1987).

The Adrogué–Madias formula has been used to estimate the anticipated change in sodium concentration with the administration of hypertonic saline (Adrogué & Madias, 2000). However, it has been shown to underestimate the final serum sodium concentration, in some cases putting patients at risk for demyelination (Mohmand et al., 2007). The overcorrection may be due to a water diuresis that can be induced by hypertonic saline and was more common in patients that started with a lower serum sodium concentration (Mohmand et al., 2007). It is likely that equine clinicians should use particular caution when treating horses with an extremely low serum sodium concentration (<115 mmol/L) with hypertonic saline in order to avoid overcorrection.

The Adrogué–Madias formula for predicting the change in serum sodium concentration following infusion with hypertonic saline (Adrogué & Madias, 2000) is given here:

$$\text{Change in serum sodium concentration with 1 L infusate} = \frac{(\text{infusate sodium concentration} - \text{Patient serum sodium concentration})}{(\text{Total body water} + 1)}$$

$$(2.3)$$

A recent study evaluated the combination of 3% hypertonic saline and desmopressin for the correction of acute hyponatremia, but further research is needed in a controlled setting (Sood et al., 2012). The authors found this combination to be less likely to overcorrect the serum sodium concentration as it helped to prevent the water diuresis associated with hypertonic saline.

Significant hyponatremia is not common in horses and therefore most equine clinicians have very limited experience in treating the disorder. Given the severe consequences of an overly rapid correction of hyponatremia, it is prudent to target a very conservative approach to treatment:

1 In horses with hyponatremia and dehydration/volume deficits, administer an isotonic crystalloid (Normosol™-R, lactated Ringer's solution (LRS)) at approximately 2–4 mL/kg/h. LRS may have a slight advantage in that its sodium concentration is 130 mEq/L, whereas Normosol-R and Plasma-Lyte® A have a sodium of 140 mEq/L. LRS would allow for a slower rate of correction in horses with markedly low serum sodium concentrations. Re-check serum sodium concentration frequently (every 2 hours) targeting a change of approximately 0.5 mEq/h. If serum sodium concentration rises too rapidly, sterile water can be added to the infused fluid to decrease the rate of change.

2 In patients with hyponatremia and volume overload, furosemide can be administered as a continuous rate infusion (0.12 mg/kg/h) in combination with an isotonic crystalloid solution (Normosol-R, LRS) at approximately 2 mL/kg/h. Re-check serum sodium concentration frequently (every 2 hours) targeting a change of approximately 0.5 mEq/h. If serum sodium concentration rises too rapidly, sterile water can be added to the infused fluid to decrease the rate of change.

Hypernatremia

Hypernatremia is an uncommonly reported problem: only 0.2% of horses in a general hospital population had a serum sodium concentration above the normal range (C.L. Fielding, unpublished data, 2013). The incidence of hypernatremia is likely to be higher in critical cases and was reported as 2.5% in human patients in a surgical intensive care unit (Sakr et al., 2013). Derangements in serum sodium concentration have been reported to be associated with outcome in human patients (Sakr et al., 2013).

Pseudohypernatremia (measured serum sodium concentration that is above the true concentration) can be present; a commonly identified cause of pseudohypernatremia is hypoproteinemia. In humans, up to 25% of ICU patients had pseudohypernatremia that was primarily associated with low serum protein concentrations (Dimeski et al., 2012). This could also potentially hide a patient with hyponatremia by creating "pseudonormonatremia".

There are five general concepts that contribute in varying degrees to hypernatremia (Sam & Feizi, 2012):

1 The patient has lost the sense of thirst or does not have access to water.
2 Impaired ability to concentrate urine.
3 A high serum urea concentration may compete with sodium for elimination in the urine.
4 Large fecal or urine output of free water without significant sodium or potassium excretion.
5 Foals that are fed milk replacer that is inappropriately mixed, with an inadequate amount of water.

A lack of thirst or the inability to access free water is probably the most important factor in developing clinical hypernatremia. Otherwise, under normal circumstances an animal would simply drink water in order to resolve hypernatremia. One of the few described clinical cases of hypernatremia in an adult horse involved neoplasia affecting the thirst center (Heath et al.,1995). Despite a serum sodium concentration of 167 mEq/L, the horse did not show any desire to drink (Heath et al., 1995).

An impaired ability to concentrate urine is also important in the development of hypernatremia, but usually is coupled to lack of access to free choice water. In many cases, animals can compensate for an impaired ability to concentrate urine by increasing water intake. If renal function is adequate, the kidney can provide significant compensation for free water deficits. While conditions such as diabetes insipidus (DI) are reported in horses, they are not common (Schott et al., 1993). In reported cases of DI, horses did not have hypernatremia on presentation but only developed the abnormality once water was withheld (Schott et al., 1993). Renal failure may be a more common reason for the inability to concentrate urine. However, even with an inability to concentrate urine, an animal could compensate and prevent hypernatremia if allowed to consume enough free water.

The presence of a high serum urea concentration could limit the ability of the kidney to excrete adequate sodium. In very simple terms, if the kidneys are not able to concentrate urine adequately, urea may "take the place" of sodium as an excreted solute. This would therefore prevent a reduction in the serum sodium concentration through urinary excretion.

Large fecal or urinary losses of free water can exacerbate hypernatremia. If the lost fluid is hypotonic and does not contain a moderate to high concentration of

---

> **Box 2.2 Conditions that may lead to hypernatremia.**
>
> Water deprivation
> Iatrogenic administration of high-sodium fluids
> Lack of thirst mechanism
> Diuretic administration

---

sodium or potassium, it will result in worsening of the serum sodium concentration.

Clinical cases of hypernatremia often involve more than one of these contributing factors.

Causes of hypernatremia in horses

Box 2.2 lists the common causes of hypernatremia in horses.

Water deprivation

As discussed above, deprivation of free water alone would have to be fairly prolonged to result in hypernatremia because of the renal ability to concentrate urine. However, horses presented with dehydration following water deprivation should always have evaluation of the serum sodium concentration. Horses with severe dehydration and hypernatremia may rapidly consume large amounts of water if suddenly given access after a period of deprivation; this could result in dangerously rapid decreases in serum sodium, with subsequent cerebral edema.

An unusual form of water deprivation involves foals (often orphans) that are maintained on a milk replacer that is being mixed incorrectly. These foals may continue to drink the hypertonic milk replacer as it is the only source of feed available. They are effectively deprived of free water and can develop severe hypernatremia.

Iatrogenic

The use of hypertonic saline (particularly high volumes) for resuscitation and treatment of traumatic brain injury in horses has the potential to create hypernatremia. It is unlikely that hypertonic saline administration would result in clinically significant hypernatremia unless additional free water was not provided and there was impairment of the kidneys, leading to a reduced ability to concentrate urine. In a clinical study of dehydrated horses, hypertonic saline induced mild hypernatremia, but the effects on serum sodium diminished as additional isotonic fluids were administered (Fielding & Magdesian, 2011).

Any fluid administered intravenously or orally with high concentrations of sodium has the potential to induce transient hypernatremia (Gossett et al., 1990; Lopes et al., 2004; Rivas et al., 1997). Besides hypertonic saline, hypertonic sodium bicarbonate is the other commonly used intravenous fluid with the potential to induce hypernatremia. As with hypertonic saline, functional kidneys and access to free water should quickly restore the serum sodium concentration to normal after administration.

Lack of thirst mechanism

Any condition (often neurologic) that eliminates thirst has the potential to create hypernatremia. Under these circumstances, a horse would no longer sense the need to drink in order to combat plasma hyperosmolarity. There is one reported case where neoplasia near the thirst center of a horse was associated with hypernatremia (Heath et al., 1995). Neurogenic loss of thirst should be considered a differential in cases of hypernatremia that have had adequate access to water and no history of fluid administration.

Diuretics

Loop diuretics and osmotic diuretics have been associated with hypernatremia in humans (Liamis et al., 2013; Seo & Oh, 2010). The effect is reported in only approximately 10–20% of cases (Seo & Oh, 2010). These same medications are used in horses but clinically significant hypernatremia has not been a consistent finding, perhaps because patients in which these drugs are used are often monitored closely in terms of electrolyte and fluid balance (Fielding et al., 2008). Prior drug administration should be part of the relevant medical history in cases of hypernatremia.

Clinical consequences of hypernatremia

As hypernatremia develops, there is a tendency for water to move osmotically out of cells and into the circulation. This effectively dehydrates cells and prevention requires physiologic compensation. Generation of idiogenic osmoles within the cell helps to preserve cellular volume and prevent dehydration (Figure 2.5). A number of idiogenic osmoles have been identified and these fall into three main categories: polyols, trimethylamines, and amino acids and their derivatives (Somero, 1986; Yancey et al., 1982). The development of the idiogenic osmoles is delayed as compared to the increase in serum sodium concentration (Lien et al., 1990). Likewise, as the patient consumes free water and the serum sodium concentration falls, there is a delay in the disappearance of the idiogenic osmoles (Lien et al., 1990). This creates a risk for cellular swelling (as free water is added back to the system) and the neurologic sequelae that can develop.

Myoinositol is an osmole that remains intracellularly for prolonged periods and plays a significant role in protection from hypernatremia; however, it is also responsible in part for the subsequent damage once the serum sodium concentration begins to fall (Hijab et al., 2011; Lien et al., 1990). To summarize, idiogenic osmoles that are created

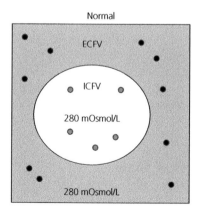 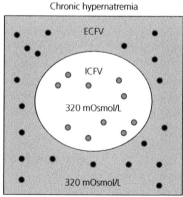 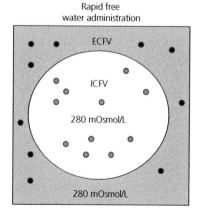

Figure 2.5 Changes in extracellular fluid volume (ECFV) and intracellular fluid volume (ICFV) osmolality and volumes associated with chronic hypernatremia and rapid free water administration.

or accumulated during the development of hypernatremia can be detrimental once water is added and the serum sodium concentration falls. For this reason, slow correction of hypernatremia is critical in allowing time for the idiogenic osmoles to disappear.

Mild hypernatremia (<160 mmol/L) may not be associated with clinical signs. Therefore, any present clinical signs may be related to the primary underlying disease and not to the hypernatremia. As the serum sodium concentration exceeds 160 mmol/L in humans, clinical signs are more likely to be evident (Peruzzo et al., 2010). In dogs, seizures developed in patients with serum sodium concentrations greater than 180 mmol/L (Barr et al., 2004). Few cases of hypernatremia are described in horses in the literature, and it is difficult to predict the level at which clinical signs develop. Similar to hyponatremia, the rapidity with which the serum sodium concentration changes is likely important.

Nearly all reported cases of hypernatremia in horses are in experimental animals (Gossett et al., 1990; Lopes et al., 2004; Rivas et al., 1997). Clinical signs from hypernatremia were not observed, but the changes in serum sodium were acute and mild. A clinical case due to neoplasia near the thirst center of a horse was reported and it had associated neurological signs (Heath et al., 1995). Clinical signs in this horse included prolapse of the third eyelid, myoclonus of head and neck muscles, and tail swishing (Heath et al., 1995). However, the clinical signs may not have been entirely attributable to hypernatremia.

Treatment of hypernatremia

Similar to hyponatremia, the treatment for hypernatremia is influenced by the pace at which the abnormality developed. Cases in which the hypernatremia developed rapidly (e.g. administration of hypertonic fluids) can often be corrected just as rapidly. When the duration of hypernatremia is unknown, the following guidelines can be used (Lee, 2010):

1 Half of the water deficit can be replaced in 12 to 24 hours as the neurologic status is carefully monitored.
2 The remaining deficit can be corrected over the subsequent 48 hours.
3 The maximum rate of decrease in plasma sodium concentration should not exceed 0.5 mEq/L/h.

It is important to account for ongoing losses of water during treatment as this will lead to a slower rate of serum sodium normalization. Serum and urine electrolytes should be monitored every 2 hours if possible. As neurologic signs improve, the rate of correction can be slowed as necessary.

During the treatment of hypernatremia, exogenous sodium sources should be considered carefully. Even fluids that have a low sodium concentration will contribute to total body sodium if the kidneys are not able to excrete sodium normally.

Diuretics may have a place in the treatment of hypernatremia if total body sodium is increased and sodium needs to be excreted. Furosemide is the most commonly used diuretic in horses and it is associated with the urinary excretion of sodium. Free water will still need to be administered along with diuretics. Most cases of hypernatremia in horses likely will respond to treatment with free water and therefore diuretics should be reserved as second-line treatments.

Practical recommendations for the treatment of hypernatremia in horses include:

1 In the dehydrated/hypovolemic patient with hypernatremia, initial volume deficits should be replaced with an isotonic or slightly hypertonic crystalloid (Normosol-R or 0.9% NaCl) at a rate of 2–4 mL/kg/h. In horses with markedly increased sodium concentrations, fluids may need to be made slightly hypertonic to prevent lowering of the sodium too quickly; for example, the fluid can be made to contain a sodium concentration 20 mEq/L below the patient's serum sodium concentration until the rate of decrease can be evaluated. The sodium content of the fluid is gradually lowered based on the rate of decrease. Serum sodium concentrations should be re-checked every 2 hours. Once volume deficits are replaced (over approximately 12 hours), a fluid containing more free water (0.45% saline) can be administered at a slower rate (1–2 mL/kg/h) with continued monitoring of serum sodium concentration.
2 In a patient with fluid overload and hypernatremia, furosemide (0.12 mg/kg/h) can be administered as a continuous infusion in combination with an intravenous fluid containing additional free water (i.e. 0.45% NaCl). Serum sodium concentrations should be re-checked every 2 hours.

Unique features of foals

Research evaluating sodium and water balance in newborn foals is available but the majority of data come from studies in humans and sheep. Premature foals

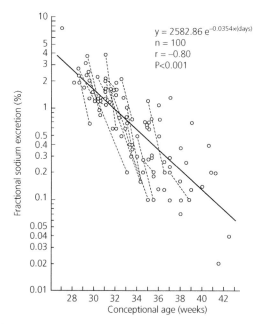

Figure 2.6 Fractional sodium excretion, expressed as percentage of filtered load, against conceptional age. The solid line is the calculated regression line; broken lines connect studies performed on the same infants on different days. From Al-Dahhan J, Haycock GB, Chantler C, et al. Sodium homeostasis in term and preterm neonates. I. Renal aspects. Arch Dis Child 1983;58:335–42. Reproduced with permission.

have a reduced ability to compensate for sodium loss when challenged with furosemide as compared to full-term foals (Broughton, 1984). It was speculated that this represents immaturity of the neonatal kidney in these premature foals. It has been shown that in humans fractional excretion of sodium is higher in pre-term neonates as compared to regular term neonates (Figure 2.6) (Al-Dahhan et al., 1983). If also true in pre-term foals, it would warrant modification of sodium and fluid supplementation in this group.

There is little research evaluating the ability of the newborn foal's kidney to handle a sodium challenge. Long-term infusion of an isotonic sodium-containing fluid resulted in mild hypernatremia in healthy foals, but did not appear to increase retention of body fluid (Buchanan et al., 2005). Research in humans indicates a lack of ability to appropriately excrete increased sodium loads in newborn and particularly premature infants (Hartnoll et al., 2000). Clinical experience suggests that critically ill neonatal foals are prone to retain both sodium and water, but more research is needed to

document and elucidate the mechanism behind this water retention.

The list of causes of hyponatremia in foals is similar to for adults (Box 2.1); however, certain conditions are more common in or unique to foals. The syndrome of inappropriate ADH secretion is speculated to occur in sick foals, though research documenting this has not been published. Other causes of hyponatremia that are more common in foals include uroperitoneum as occurs with ruptured bladder or urachus (Behr et al., 1981; Dunkel et al., 2005), particularly in foals not already receiving intravenous fluids. Errors in mixing milk replacers resulting in an overly dilute mixture or foals that have access only to water will also develop hyponatremia. As with adult horses, both renal failure and gastrointestinal disease can lead to a decrease in serum sodium concentration.

Hypernatremia is seen most commonly in foals that have not been allowed to nurse or drink water. Sodium concentrations can be markedly increased in foals, particularly those that are living in a hot climate.

References

Adrogué H, Madias NE. (2000) Hyponatremia. *N Engl J Med* **342**:1581–9.

Al-Dahhan J, Haycock GB, Chantler C, et al. (1983) Sodium homeostasis in term and preterm neonates. I. Renal aspects. *Arch Dis Child* **58**:335–42.

Alexander F. (1962) The concentration of certain electrolytes in the digestive tract of the horse and pig. *Res Vet Sci* **3**:78–84.

Alexander F. (1966) A study of parotid salivation in the horse. *J Physiol* **184**:646–56.

Alexander F. (1977) The effect of diuretics on the faecal excretion of water and electrolytes in horses. *Br J Pharmacol* **60**:589–93.

Arieff A, Llach F, Massry SG. (1976) Neurological manifestations and morbidity of hyponatraemia: correlation with brain water and electrolytes. *Medicine* **55**:121–9.

Barr JM, Khan SA, McCullough SM, et al. (2004) Hypernatremia secondary to homemade play dough ingestion in dogs: a review of 14 cases from 1998 to 2001. *J Vet Emerg Crit Care* **3**:196–202.

Beck C, Dart AJ, McClintock SA, et al. (1996) Traumatic rupture of the urinary bladder in a horse. *Aust Vet J* **73**:154–5.

Behr MJ, Hackett RP, Bentinck-Smith J, et al. (1981) Metabolic abnormalities associated with rupture of the urinary bladder in neonatal foals. *J Am Vet Med Assoc* **178**:263–6.

Bello-Reuss E. (1980) Effect of catecholamines on fluid reabsorption by the isolated proximal convoluted tubule. *Am J Physiol* **238**:F347.

Berl T, Schrier RW. (2010) Disorders of water homeostasis. In: Schrier RW (ed.) *Renal and Electrolyte Disorders*, 6th edn. Philadelphia: Lippincott Williams & Wilkins; pp. 1–44.

Biswas M, Davies JS. (2007) Hyponatraemia in clinical practice. *Postgrad Med J* **83**:373–8.

Brewer BD, Clement SF, Lotz WS, et al. (1991) Renal clearance, urinary excretion of endogenous substances, and urinary diagnostic indices in healthy neonatal foals. *J Vet Intern Med* **5**:28–33.

Broughton Pipkin F, Ousey JC, Wallace CP, et al. (1984) Studies on equine prematurity 4: Effect of salt and water loss on the renin-angiotensin-aldosterone system in the newborn foal. *Equine Vet J* **16**:292–7.

Buchanan BR, Sommardahl CS, Rohrbach BW, et al. (2005) Effect of a 24-hour infusion of an isotonic electrolyte replacement fluid on the renal clearance of electrolytes in healthy neonatal foals. *J Am Vet Med Assoc* **227**:1123–9.

Burgess BA, Lohmann KL, Blakley BR. (2010) Excessive sulfate and poor water quality as a cause of sudden deaths and an outbreak of diarrhea in horses. *Can Vet J* **51**:277–82.

Clarke LL, Roberts MC, Grubb BR, et al. (1992) Short-term effect of aldosterone on Na-Cl transport across equine colon. *Am J Physiol* **262**:R939–46.

Couëtil LL, Hoffman AM. (1998) Adrenal insufficiency in a neonatal foal. *J Am Vet Med Assoc* **212**:1594–6.

Denton KM, Fennessy PA, Alcorn D, et al. (1992) Morphometric analysis of the actions of angiotensin II on renal arterioles and glomeruli. *Am J Physiol* **262**:F367–F372.

Dimeski G, Morgan TJ, Presneill JJ, et al. (2012) Disagreement between ion selective electrode direct and indirect sodium measurements: estimation of the problem in a tertiary referral hospital. *J Crit Care* **27**:326.e9–16.

Divers TJ, Whitlock RH, Byars TD, et al. (1987) Acute renal failure in six horses resulting from haemodynamic causes. *Equine Vet J* **19**:178–84.

Dowling PM, Williams MA, Clark TP. (1993) Adrenal insufficiency associated with long-term anabolic steroid administration in a horse. *J Am Vet Med Assoc* **203**:1166–9.

Dunkel B, Palmer JE, Olson KN, et al. (2005) Uroperitoneum in 32 foals: influence of intravenous fluid therapy, infection, and sepsis. *J Vet Intern Med* **19**:889–93.

Dunn FL, Brennan TJ, Nelson AE, et al. (1973) The role of blood osmolality and volume in regulating vasopressin secretion in the rat. *J Clin Invest* **52**:3212–19.

Ecke P, Hodgson DR, Rose RJ. (1998) Induced diarrhoea in horses. Part 1: Fluid and electrolyte balance. *Vet J* **155**:149–59.

Edelman IS, Leibman J, O'Meara MP, et al. (1958) Interrelations between serum sodium concentration, serum osmolarity and total exchangeable sodium, total exchangeable potassium and total body water. *J Clin Invest* **37**:1236–56.

el-Ashker MR. (2011) Acute kidney injury mediated by oxidative stress in Egyptian horses with exertional rhabdomyolysis. *Vet Res Commun* **35**:311–20.

Fielding CL, Magdesian KG, Carlson GP, et al. (2008) Application of the sodium dilution principle to calculate extracellular fluid volume changes in horses during dehydration and rehydration. *Am J Vet Res* **69**:1506–11.

Fielding CL, Magdesian KG, Rhodes DM, et al. (2009) Clinical and biochemical abnormalities in endurance horses eliminated from competition for medical complications and requiring emergency medical treatment: 30 cases (2005–2006). *J Vet Emerg Crit Care (San Antonio)* **19**:473–8.

Fielding CL, Magdesian KG. (2011) A comparison of hypertonic (7.2%) and isotonic (0.9%) saline for fluid resuscitation in horses: a randomized, double-blinded, clinical trial. *J Vet Intern Med* **25**:1138–43.

Fortgens P, Pillay TS. (2011) Pseudohyponatremia revisited: a modern-day pitfall. *Arch Pathol Lab* **135**:516–19.

Freestone JF, Gossett K, Carlson GP, et al. (1991) Exercise induced alterations in the serum muscle enzymes, erythrocyte potassium and plasma constituents following feed withdrawal or furosemide and sodium bicarbonate administration in the horse. *J Vet Intern Med* **5**:40–6.

Genetzky RM, Hagemoser WA. (1985) Physical and clinical pathological findings associated with experimentally induced rupture of the equine urinary bladder. *Can Vet J* **26**:391–5.

Geor RJ. (2007) Acute renal failure in horses. *Vet Clin Equine* **23**:577–91.

Giddings RF, Argenzio RA, Stevens CE. (1974) Sodium and chloride transport across the equine cecal mucosa. *Am J Vet Res* **35**:1511–14.

Gossett KA, French DD, Cleghorn B, et al. (1990) Blood biochemical response to sodium bicarbonate infusion during sublethal endotoxemia in ponies. *Am J Vet Res* **51**:1370–4.

Groenendyk S, English PB, Abetz I. (1988) External balance of water and electrolytes in the horse. *Equine Vet J* **20**:189–93.

Grossman BS, Brobst DF, Kramer JW, et al. (1982) Urinary indices for differentiation of prerenal azotemia and renal azotemia in horses. *J Am Vet Med Assoc* **180**:284–8.

Hartnoll G, Bétrémieux P, Modi N. (2000) Randomised controlled trial of postnatal sodium supplementation on body composition in 25 to 30 week gestational age infants. *Arch Dis Child Fetal Neonatal Ed* **82**:F24–8.

Heath SE, Peter AT, Janovitz EB, et al. (1995) Ependymoma of the neurohypophysis and hypernatremia in a horse. *J Am Vet Med Assoc* **207**:738–41.

Hijab S, Havalad S, Snyder AK. (2011) The role of organic osmolytes in the response of cultured astrocytes to hyperosmolarity. *Am J Ther* **18**:366–70.

Houpt KA, Thorton SN, Allen WR. (1989) Vasopressin in dehydrated and rehydrated ponies. *Physiol Behav* **45**:659–61.

Irvine CH, Alexander SL, Donald RA. (1989) Effect of an osmotic stimulus on the secretion of arginine vasopressin and adrenocorticotropin in the horse. *Endocrinology* **124**:3102–8.

Johnson JA, Davis JO, Witty RT. (1995) Effects of catecholamines and renal nerve stimulation on renin release in the nonfiltering kidney. *Hypertension* **25**:1021–4.

Jones NL, Houpt KA, Houpt TR. (1989) Stimuli of thirst in donkeys (Equus asinus). *Physiol Behav* **46**:661–5.

Karp BI, Laureno R. (1993) Pontine and extrapontine myelinolysis: a neurologic disorder following rapid correction of hyponatremia. *Medicine (Baltimore)* **72**:359–73.

Katsarou A, Singh S. (2010) Hyponatraemia associated rhabdomyolysis following water intoxication. *BMJ Case Rep* Sep 9; **pii**: bcr0220102720. doi: 10.1136/bcr.02.2010.2720.

Kingston JK, Geor RJ, McCutcheon LJ. (1997) Rate and composition of sweat fluid losses are unaltered by hypohydration during prolonged exercise in horses. *J Appl Physiol* **83**:1133–43.

Kurtz I, Nguyen MK. (2005) Evolving concepts in the quantitative analysis of the determinants of the plasma water sodium concentration and the pathophysiology and treatment of the dysnatremias. *Kidney Int* **68**:1982–93.

Lakritz J, Madigan J, Carlson GP. (1992) Hypovolemic hyponatremia and signs of neurologic disease associated with diarrhea in a foal. *J Am Vet Med Assoc* **200**:1114–16.

Latson KM, Nieto JE, Beldomenico PM, et al. (2005) Evaluation of peritoneal fluid lactate as a marker of intestinal ischaemia in equine colic. *Equine Vet J* **37**:342–6.

Lee JW. (2010) Fluid and electrolyte disturbances in critically ill patients. *Electrolyte Blood Press* **8**:72–81.

Liamis G, Rodenburg EM, Hofman A, et al. (2013) Electrolyte disorders in community subjects: prevalence and risk factors. Am J Med; doi:10.1016/j.amjmed.2012.06.037.

Lien YH, Shapiro JI, Chan L. (1990) Effects of hypernatremia on organic brain osmoles. *J Clin Invest* **85**:1427–35.

Lindinger MI, Ecker GL. (2013) Gastric emptying, intestinal absorption of electrolytes and exercise performance in electrolyte-supplemented horses. *Exp Physiol* **98**:193–206.

Lindner A. (1991) Comparison of clinical chemical variables in blood plasma and serum of horses. *Eur J Clin Chem Clin Biochem* **29**:837–40.

Lopes MA, White NA 2nd, Donaldson L, et al. (2004) Effects of enteral and intravenous fluid therapy, magnesium sulfate, and sodium sulfate on colonic contents and feces in horses. *Am J Vet Res* **65**:695–704.

Loutzenhiser R, Hayashi K, Epstein M. (1988) Atrial natriuretic peptide reverses afferent arteriolar vasoconstriction and potentiates efferent arteriolar vasoconstriction in the isolated perfused rat kidney. *J Pharmacol Exp Ther* **246**:522–8.

Magdesian KG, Hirsh DC, Jang SS, et al. (2002) Characterization of Clostridium difficile isolates from foals with diarrhea: 28 cases (1993–1997). *J Am Vet Med Assoc* **220**:67–73.

Mayhew IG, Whitlock RH, Tasker JB. (1977) Equine cerebrospinal fluid: reference values of normal horses. *Am J Vet Res* **38**:1271–4.

MohmandHK, Issa D, Ahmad Z, Cappuccio JD, Kouides RW, Sterns RH. (2007) Hypertonic saline for hyponatremia: risk of inadvertent overcorrection. *Clin J Am Soc Nephrol* **2**:1110–17.

Nguyen MK, Kurtz I. (2004) New insights into the pathophysiology of the dysnatremias: a qualitative analysis. *Am J Physiol Renal Physiol* **287**:F172–F180.

Perkins G, Valberg SJ, Madigan JM, et al. (1998) Electrolyte disturbances in foals with severe rhabdomyolysis. *J Vet Intern Med* **12**:173–7.

Peruzzo M, Milani GP, Garzoni L, et al. (2010) Body fluids and salt metabolism – part II. *Ital J Pediatr* **36**:78.

Quinn CT, Carmalt JL. (2012) Ruptured urinary bladder in a horse. *Vet Anaesth Analg* **39**:557–8.

Rawlings CA, Bisgard GE. (1975) Renal clearance and excretion of endogenous substances in the small pony. *Am J Vet Res* **36**:45–8.

Rivas LJ, Hinchcliff KW, Kohn CW, et al. (1997) Effect of sodium bicarbonate administration on blood constituents of horses. *Am J Vet Res* **58**:658–63.

Robert C, Goachet AG, Fraipont A, et al. (2010) Hydration and electrolyte balance in horses during an endurance season. *Equine Vet J Suppl* **38**:98–104.

Rose RJ, Arnold KS, Church S, et al. (1980) Plasma and sweat electrolyte concentrations in the horse during long distance exercise. *Equine Vet J* **12**:19–22.

Roussel AJ, Cohen ND, Ruoff WW, et al. (1993) Urinary indices of horses after intravenous administration of crystalloid solutions. *J Vet Intern Med* **7**:241–6.

Sakr Y, Rother S, Ferreira AM, et al. (2013) Fluctuations in serum sodium level are associated with an increased risk of death in surgical ICU patients. *Crit Care Med* **41**:133–42.

Sam R, Feizi I. (2012) Understanding hypernatremia. *Am J Nephrol* **36**:97–104.

Schott HC, Bayly WM, Reed SM, et al. (1993) Nephrogenic diabetes insipidus in sibling colts. *J Vet Intern Med* **7**:68–72.

Schott HC, Patterson KS, Fitzgerald SD, et al. (1997) *Chronic renal failure in 99 horses. In: Proceedings of the 43rd Annual Convention of the American Association of Equine Practitioners.* American Association of Equine Practitioners, pp. 345–6.

Seo W, Oh H. (2010) Alterations in serum osmolality, sodium, and potassium levels after repeated mannitol administration. *J Neurosci Nurs* **42**:201–7.

Sneddon JC, Van Der Walt J, Mitchell G, et al. (1993) Effects of dehydration and rehydration on plasma vasopressin and aldosterone in horses. *Physiol Behav* **54**:223–8.

Somero GN. (1986) Protons, osmolytes, and fitness of internal milieu for protein function. *Am J Physiol* **251**:R197–R213.

Sood L, Sterns RH, Hix JK, et al. (2012) Hypertonic saline and desmopressin: a simple strategy for safe correction of severe hyponatremia. *Am J Kidney Dis* **61**:571–8.

Spooner HS, Nielsen BD, Schott HC, et al. (2010) Sweat composition in Arabian horses performing endurance exercise on forage-based, low Na rations. *Equine Vet J Suppl* **38**:382–6.

Sterns RH, Riggs JE, Schochet SS. (1986) Osmotic demyelination syndrome following correction of hyponatremia. *N Engl J Med* **314**:1535–42.

Sterns RH. (1987) Severe symptomatic hyponatremia: Treatment and outcome. A study of 64 cases. *Ann Intern Med* **107**:656–64.

Sterns RH, Cappuccio JD, Silver SM, et al. (1994) Neurologic sequelae after treatment of severe hyponatremia: A multicenter perspective. *J Am Soc Nephrol* **4**:1522–30.

Stewart MC, Hodgson JL, Kim H, et al. (1995) Acute febrile diarrhoea in horses: 86 cases (1986–1991). *Aust Vet J* **72**:41–4.

Stick JA, Robinson NE, Krehbiel JD. (1981) Acid-base and electrolyte alterations associated with salivary loss in the pony. *Am J Vet Res* **42**:733–7.

Tasker JB. (1967a) Fluid and electrolyte studies in the horse III. Intake and output of water, sodium, and potassium in normal horses. *Cornell Vet* **57**:649–57.

Tasker JB. (1967b) Fluid and electrolyte studies in the horse V. The effects of diarrhea. *Cornell Vet* **57**:668–77.

Toribio RE, Kohn CW, Rourke KM, et al. (2007) Effects of hypercalcemia on serum concentrations of magnesium, potassium, and phosphate and urinary excretion of electrolytes in horses. *Am J Vet Res* **68**:543–54.

Tucker BJ, Mundy CA, Blantz RC. (1987) Adrenergic and angiotensin II influences on renal vascular tone in chronic sodium depletion. *Am J Physiol* **252**:F811–17.

Ullrey DE, Struthers RD, Hendricks DG, et al. (1966) Composition of mare's milk. *J Anim Sci* **25**:217–21.

Wang T, Chan YL. (1990) Mechanism of angiotensin II action on proximal tubular transport. *J Pharmacol Exp Ther* **252**:689–95.

Watson ZE, Steffey EP, VanHoogmoed LM, et al. (2002) Effect of general anesthesia and minor surgical trauma on urine and serum measurements in horses. *Am J Vet Res* **63**:1061–5.

Wong DM, Sponseller BT, Brockus C et al. (2007) Neurologic deficits associated with severe hyponatremia in 2 foals. *J Vet Emerg Crit Care* **17**:275–85.

Yancey PH, Clark ME, Hands SC, et al. (1982) Living with water stress: evolution of osmolyte systems. *Science* **217**:1214–22.

CHAPTER 3

Potassium homeostasis and derangements

C. Langdon Fielding

Loomis Basin Equine Medical Center Penryn, CA, USA

Introduction

While the majority of potassium ions (98%) reside within cells, clinical medicine is more often focused on the concentration of potassium in the extracellular fluid. More than most other ions, plasma potassium concentrations have a wide range, from nearly 1 mmol/L in cases of severe hypokalemia to 10 mmol/L in life-threatening hyperkalemia. Equine veterinarians have the tools available to make significant and rapid changes in plasma potassium concentration (easily doubling the concentration over the course of a few hours), but a comprehensive understanding of potassium physiology is important because of its multiple roles and potential for causing morbidity. The consequences of incorrectly manipulating a patient's plasma potassium concentration can be fatal. Table 3.1 shows the concentration of potassium in common biological fluids in the horse.

The maintenance requirement for potassium in horses has been reported to range from 30 to 48 mg/kg/day (Hintz & Schryver, 1976, Meyer et al., 1982). Horses typically are fed diets that provide potassium significantly in excess of this amount (10 times the daily requirement in some studies) (Tasker, 1967). The kidneys are the primary route for elimination of excess potassium; however, there may be increased fecal excretion with chronic potassium supplementation (>10 days) (Jansson et al., 1999). Significant quantities of potassium can be lost through high volumes of sweat in exercising horses (Figure 3.1).

Potassium intake

The gastrointestinal system is the primary route for potassium intake in horses. The apparent digestibility can reach as high as 95% if diets high in potassium are fed (Hintz & Schryver, 1976). Magnesium supplementation (0.8% of the diet) further increases the apparent digestibility of potassium (Hintz & Schryver, 1976). The majority of potassium absorption takes place passively in the small intestine but there have been few investigative studies in horses (Cehak et al., 2009; Lindinger & Ecker, 2013). Smaller amounts of potassium are absorbed in the large intestine and may be actively transported under the effects of aldosterone (Hintz & Schryver, 1976; Jansson et al., 2002). The high digestibility of potassium makes oral supplementation an effective means for treating hypokalemia in horses with a functioning gastrointestinal system.

Potassium excretion

Urinary excretion of potassium

The majority of potassium is eliminated from horses (and other species) through the kidneys (Tasker, 1967). Under normal circumstances, the kidney is the main control point for the potassium concentration in plasma (Figure 3.2). However, during renal failure (particularly chronic renal failure) active transport in the colon plays a larger role in potassium regulation thus protecting the body from dangerous hyperkalemia. The large amounts

Equine Fluid Therapy, First Edition. Edited by C. Langdon Fielding and K. Gary Magdesian.
© 2015 John Wiley & Sons, Inc. Published 2015 by John Wiley & Sons, Inc.

Table 3.1 Potassium concentrations in body fluids of the horse.

Fluid type	[K⁺] (mEq/L)	Reference
Serum	3.5±0.2 to 3.8±0.3	Watson et al. (2002), Groenendyk et al. (1988)
Urine	192±70 to 268±57	Rawlings et al. (1975), Morris et al. (1984)
Cerebrospinal fluid	3.0±0.1	Mayhew et al. (1977)
Sweat	46±3 to 99±50	Hejłasz et al. (1994), Spooner et al. (2010)
Peritoneal fluid	3.6±0.3	Latson et al. (2005)
Normal feces	221±16	Ecke et al. (1998)
Saliva	14–15	Alexander (1966)
Mare's milk	25	Ullrey et al. (1966)

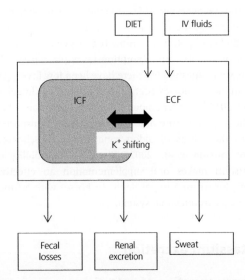

Figure 3.1 Potassium intake, distribution, and loss from the horse. ECF, extracellular fluid; ICF, intracellular fluid.

of potassium ingested daily by horses requires that a high percentage (anywhere from 50% to 80%) be eliminated by the kidneys (Groenendyk et al., 1988; Jansson et al., 1999; Tasker, 1967). The remaining potassium is lost in feces, sweat, or other insensible losses (Groenendyk et al., 1988; Tasker, 1967).

Potassium is freely filtered through the glomerulus and the majority is reabsorbed in the proximal tubule (Palmer & Dubose, 2010). While the specific amount that is absorbed in the horse is not known, values in other species have ranged from 55 to 70%. The reabsorption takes place primarily due to the concentration gradient of potassium created when water is reabsorbed (increasing the luminal concentration of potassium). There may also be absorption with water through the mechanism commonly referred to as "solvent drag". There is little specific regulation of potassium reabsorption in the proximal tubule, though it may be modified with chronic potassium depletion.

The thick ascending limb of the loop of Henle is the next major site of potassium reabsorption. The $Na^+/K^+/2Cl^-$ cotransporter is located on the luminal membrane and is responsible for moving potassium out of the lumen. As much as 25% of filtered potassium may be reabsorbed in this section of the kidney. This is an active transport mechanism and is affected by some of the common diuretics used in equine practice (i.e. furosemide).

The distal nephron is responsible for both additional reabsorption and secretion of potassium in the kidney (Palmer & Dubose, 2010). It represents the most significant control point in regulating the plasma potassium concentration, and the connecting tubule is particularly important in controlling the excretion of potassium. Normal control of potassium secretion in this segment is affected by three major factors (Box 3.1).

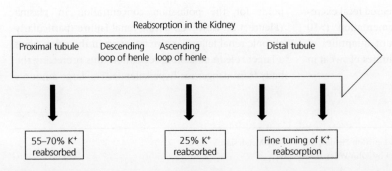

Figure 3.2 Potassium reabsorption in the kidney.

> **Box 3.1 Major factors affecting potassium excretion in the distal tubule.**
>
> - Plasma potassium concentration
> - Aldosterone concentration
> - Urine flow

> **Box 3.2 Summary of renal handling of potassium regulation.**
>
> - 90% of filtered potassium is reabsorbed in the proximal tubule and loop of Henle.
> - Potassium secretion is influenced in the distal nephron by the plasma potassium concentration, aldosterone, and the rate of urine flow.
> - Most horses excrete large amounts of potassium unless intake or losses are very abnormal.

Plasma potassium concentration

Increases in plasma potassium concentration result in uptake by the Na/K-ATPase pumps leading to an increased intracellular concentration of potassium (DiBartola & DeMorais, 2012). An increase in intracellular potassium concentration results in a gradient that favors potassium movement into the lumen and therefore increases potassium excretion. Conversely, a decrease in plasma potassium concentration results in a lower intracellular potassium concentration and a decreased concentration gradient into the lumen.

Aldosterone concentration

Aldosterone stimulates tubular potassium secretion by the principal cells (Palmer & Dubose, 2010). The cells in the adrenal cortex responsible for secreting aldosterone are sensitive to the extracellular concentration of potassium surrounding them. Increases in potassium concentration result in a increased secretion of aldosterone while decreases in potassium concentration have the opposite effect. In the kidney, aldosterone has the effect of increasing uptake of potassium into the cells (thus favoring a concentration gradient into the lumen), as well as increasing the permeability to potassium moving from the cells into the lumen (Palmer & Dubose, 2010). These combined effects result in an increase in the excretion of potassium. While aldosterone secretion is affected by potassium, it is also controlled by the renin-angiotensin system and specifically by angiotensin II. The effects of angiotensin II tend to outweigh the effects of plasma potassium concentration and therefore sodium balance is a more powerful regulator of aldosterone secretion than potassium balance.

Urine flow

Urine flow is another determinant of potassium secretion by the distal nephron (Palmer & Dubose, 2010). Increased urine flow increases potassium excretion by the kidney through a simple mechanism. Potassium is moved into the lumen in the distal nephron passively down its concentration gradient. The effect of the increased urine flow is to continually remove higher potassium fluid from the lumen and therefore create a favorable concentration gradient for potassium to continue to enter the lumen. The potassium excreting effect of increased urine flow is very important as it balances the effects of other factors controlling potassium. For example, a severely dehydrated patient will tend to have an increased aldosterone concentration due to the effects of the renin-angiotensin system. This increased aldosterone concentration could lead to a loss of potassium in urine. However, the decreased urine flow associated with a dehydrated patient (under normal circumstances) will help to minimize the loss of potassium caused by aldosterone (Box 3.2).

Other factors

While less significant, antidiuretic hormone (ADH) also has an effect by directly stimulating secretion of potassium. Similar to aldosterone, the effects of ADH tend to balance the effects of changes in urine flow on potassium excretion. For example, a dehydrated patient could have a higher level of ADH resulting in increased secretion of potassium. This would be counteracted by the low urine flow of a dehydrated patient with subsequent decreased potassium excretion.

Gastrointestinal secretion of potassium

Evidence in humans and small animals suggests that individuals with impaired renal function may increase the fecal elimination of potassium through the effects of aldosterone. This secretion takes place in the large intestine and can be significant in patients with renal failure (DiBartola & De Morais, 2011). Changes in fecal potassium content in horses have been shown to occur with the administration of aldosterone, certain diuretics (furosemide), and phenylbutazone (Alexander, 1977, 1982a,1982b; Jansson et al., 2002). It is unknown whether fecal potassium content in horses becomes altered in chronic renal failure, but it would be reasonable to expect that long-term hyperkalemia may have similar effects in horses as it does in other species.

External influence of potassium excretion

Diuretics can influence potassium excretion in the horse by increasing urine flow, which is one of the main mechanisms affecting potassium excretion in the distal nephron. They may also directly affect the $Na^+/K^+/2Cl^-$ pumps in the ascending limb of the loop of Henle resulting in decreased reabsorption of potassium. Furosemide (frusemide) is the most commonly used diuretic and its administration in horses has been associated with increased urinary losses of potassium and a resulting hypokalemia (Alexander, 1977; Freestone et al., 1989; Johansson et al., 2003). Continuous infusion of furosemide further increases the urinary losses of potassium as compared to intermittent administration (Johansson et al., 2003). Acetazolamide administration induces a decrease in serum potassium concentrations, which may be in part due to increased urinary losses (Rose et al., 1990). Other diuretics that have been described in horses include hydrochlorothiazide, ethacrynic acid, bumetanide, and spironolactone (Alexander, 1977, 1982b). Although these medications did not induce hypokalemia in horses, some have been shown to have this effect in other species. The common diuretics used in horses and their effects on potassium are given in Table 3.2.

Fluid diuresis due to intravenous fluid administration is another mechanism that can result in increased urinary potassium losses, specifically through the mechanism of increased urine flow. This effect has been observed in horses using different types of intravenous fluids (Bertone & Shoemaker, 1992; Carlson & Rumbaugh, 1983; Fielding et al., 2008). Based on the limited data available in horses combined with results from other species, it should be anticipated that intravenous fluid administration will be associated with the increased loss of urinary potassium and has the potential to contribute to hypokalemia.

The effects of other electrolytes have also been shown to play a role in the excretion of potassium from the kidney of the horse. Specifically, supplementation with intravenous calcium has increased urinary losses of potassium (Toribio et al., 2007). Changes in the dietary cation-anion balance (DCAB) also influence urinary potassium losses (McKenzie et al., 2002). More recently, the influence of magnesium on the loss of potassium from the kidney has been elucidated. While not well documented in the horse, hypomagnesemia has been described as a predisposing factor leading to hypokalemia (Stewart, 2011). Intracellular magnesium is a critical determinant of renal outer medullary potassium channel (ROMK)-mediated potassium secretion in the distal nephron (Huang & Kuo, 2007; Yang et al., 2010). ROMK is one of the channels responsible for basal potassium secretion and therefore hypomagnesemia can predispose to hypokalemia. Figure 3.3 is a simplified illustration of the effects of magnesium on the prevention of potassium loss into the urine.

Glucocorticoid administration also increases potassium excretion via the kidneys. The effect is predominantly due to an increased glomerular filtration rate (GFR) creating increased tubular flow. Hypokalemia was noted in one study involving steroid administration in horses (Picandet et al., 2003).

Acid–base balance can effect urinary excretion of potassium. Alkalosis favors potassium secretion/excretion from the kidney. This is primarily mediated through the effects of alkalosis on the Na^+/K^+-ATPase pumps in the cortical collecting ducts. Acidosis does not necessarily have the opposite effect.

Internal potassium balance: extracellular–intracellular shifting

Potassium functions as the major intracellular cation and aids in the maintenance of fluid balance between the intracellular and extracellular space. The majority of

Table 3.2 Anticipated effects of diuretics on potassium concentration.

Diuretic	Effect	Research in horses	Reference
Furosemide	Hypokalemia	Y	Johansson et al. (2003)
Mannitol	Hypokalemia	N	Seo and Oh (2010)
Hydrochlorothiazide	No change	Y	Alexander (1977)
Acetazolamide	Hypokalemia	Y	Rose et al. (1990)
Spironolactone	No change	Y	Alexander (1982b)

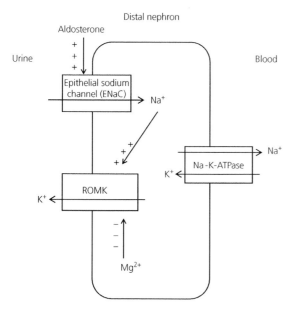

Figure 3.3 The ROMK channel secretes potassium into the luminal fluid of the distal nephron. Increased sodium reabsorption under the effects of aldosterone will increase this movement of potassium into the luminal fluid. Intracellular magnesium inhibits the movement of potassium through ROMK into the luminal fluid. When hypomagnesemia is present, increased amounts of potassium will be lost into the urine.

potassium ions are located within the intracellular compartment. An estimate of the intracellular potassium concentration in horses is approximately 93 mmol/L but it depends on the cell type (Johnson et al., 1991; Muylle et al., 1984a). This is much higher than reported normal plasma potassium concentrations of approximately 3.5 mmol/L (Johnson et al., 1991; Muylle et al., 1984a). Interestingly, there does not appear to be a consistent ratio between intracellular and extracellular potassium concentrations across different horses (Muylle et al., 1984a).

Significant shifts of potassium from the intracellular to extracellular fluid compartment can cause dramatic changes in plasma potassium concentration. The two major substances affecting the uptake of potassium by cells are insulin and catecholamines, and both are associated with effects on the Na^+/K^+-ATPase located on the plasma membrane of the cell (Palmer & Dubose, 2010). Insulin may be released in response to increased plasma glucose concentrations and therefore hyperglycemia can lead to a decrease in plasma potassium concentration.

Insulin can also be exogenously administered as part of treatment for hyperglycemia or it may be used to directly combat severe hyperkalemia. Epinephrine (adrenaline) may be released in a variety of situations including exercise, trauma, and stress. Beta-agonists (specifically β_2) can be administered exogenously to help combat hyperkalemia, but their use for this purpose is described more commonly in other species (Palmer & Dubose, 2010).

The effects of acid–base changes on intracellular–extracellular potassium balance are controversial and particularly difficult to evaluate in horses given the lack of available data. Acidosis is classically understood to shift potassium out of cells into the extracellular fluid space thereby increasing the plasma potassium concentration. Alkalosis is thought to have the opposite effect leading to hypokalemia. The usefulness of treating hyperkalemia with sodium bicarbonate or other alkalinizing agents is not completely understood at this time. Multiple studies in horses and calves have shown that the administration of sodium bicarbonate or other alkalinizing treatments results in a decrease in plasma potassium concentrations (Grünberg et al., 2011; Koch & Kaske, 2008; Pedrick et al., 1998; Rivas et al., 1997). However, possible mechanisms for the resulting drop in serum potassium concentrations include not only a transcellular shift, but also increased losses of urinary potassium and an increase in plasma volume (dilution of the remaining potassium ions).

While the kidney excretes the majority of potassium ingested by the horse, there is evidence that potassium excretion in feces is influenced by aldosterone as reported in other species (Jansson et al., 2002). This would allow for a mechanism whereby an increase in plasma potassium concentration would trigger the release of aldosterone and an increase in fecal elimination of potassium if the kidneys were not functioning normally. Box 3.3 summarizes all of the primary control points for the plasma potassium concentration.

Hypokalemia

Hypokalemia refers to a decrease in the plasma potassium concentration; this is not the same as a total body potassium deficit. Many clinical conditions may lead to total body losses of potassium without resulting in hypokalemia. Likewise, not all horses with hypokalemia

---

> **Box 3.3 Major controllers of plasma potassium concentration.**
>
> **Changes in potassium intake**
>
> - Oral administration
> - Intravenous administration
>
> **Changes in loss of potassium**
>
> - Renal influencers of potassium loss
>   - Plasma potassium concentration
>   - Urine flow
>   - Aldosterone
>   - Antidiuretic hormone
> - Gastrointestinal influencers of potassium loss
>   - Aldosterone
>   - Increased fluid loss (diarrhea)
> - Sweat loss
>
> **Factors causing intracellular/extracellular shifting of potassium**
>
> - Insulin
> - Beta-agonists
> - Aldosterone
> - Acid–base balance

> **Box 3.4 Main clinical points for hypokalemia.**
>
> **1** Decreased dietary intake of potassium has not been commonly described in clinical or experimental studies as a cause of hypokalemia in horses.
> **2** Loss of significant potassium from the gastrointestinal tract in horses with diarrhea is not a well described cause of hypokalemia.
> **3** Losses from sweat, kidneys, or internal potassium exchange (between ECF and ICF) are more widely described causes of hypokalemia in horses and should be considered first.

have low total body potassium as shifting can take place between the extracellular and intracellular fluid space (Box 3.4).

Decreased intake

Horses with a variety of medical conditions have been documented to have hypokalemia, and anorexia may be a contributing factor. While anorexia results in total body depletion of potassium, there is little research documenting that decreased feed intake alone contributes to a significant hypokalemia in horses. In fact, feed deprivation over a 72-hour period in one study did not result in a significant decrease in the plasma potassium concentration (Freestone et al., 1991). Horses experiencing significant losses of potassium through other routes (renal, sweat, diarrhea, etc.) may be more prone to hypokalemia if the intake of potassium is reduced. In other species, decreased dietary intake has been shown to produce hypokalemia, and further research in horses may reach the same conclusions. However, the observation of hypokalemia in clinically ill horses warrants a search for additional or contributing causes beyond anorexia.

Increased losses
Gastrointestinal

Similar to decreased intake, evidence is lacking that diarrhea causes a significant hypokalemia through fecal losses in horses. In one study with experimentally induced diarrhea, fecal dry matter potassium content changed very little as the severity of diarrhea increased. (Ecke et al., 1998). In this study, the primary route of potassium loss documented in horses developing diarrhea was through the kidneys (Ecke et al., 1998). Other studies describing diarrhea in horses have not consistently documented hypokalemia (Roberts et al., 1989; Staempfli et al., 1991; Stewart et al., 1995). Hypokalemia associated with clinical cases of colitis is more frequently described in other animal species (Andrejak et al., 1996; Cebra et al., 2007; Dennis et al., 1993).

Sweat

Horse sweat is hypertonic and contains 46–99 mmol/L of potassium, which is significantly higher than the plasma concentration (Hejłasz et al., 1994; Spooner et al., 2010). Prolonged exercise can result in significant potassium losses, and increased heat and humidity have been shown to accelerate this effect (Gottlieb-Vedi et al., 1996; McConaghy et al., 1995; McCutcheon & Geor, 1996). Clinical studies evaluating horses undergoing prolonged exercise identified decreases in plasma potassium concentration in healthy horses, with even more severe changes in horses eliminated for poor cardiovascular recovery (Fielding et al., 2009; Viu et al., 2010). Horses presented for emergency care following prolonged exercise should be suspected of hypokalemia and may require potassium supplementation (oral or intravenous).

Renal losses

The kidney represents the most likely route of potassium loss resulting in clinical hypokalemia in non-exercising horses. Increased renal losses of potassium have been reported with the administration of medications (most commonly diuretics), intravenous fluids, and with diseases causing renal tubular dysfunction. Newer research continues to elucidate the role of hypomagnesemia in exacerbating potassium loss from the kidneys resulting in refractory hypokalemia (Huang & Kuo, 2007).

Diuresis (diuretics, fluid therapy)

The administration of diuretics contributes to renal loss of potassium by a number of mechanisms. Specifically, these medications can (i) interfere with the active transport of potassium out of the urine in the ascending loop of Henle (loop diuretics), and (ii) increase urine flow leading to increased secretion of potassium in the more distal segments of the nephron. The majority of research in horses has focused on the effects of furosemide and has documented the hypokalemia that results following administration (Freestone et al., 1988, 1989). Other diuretics are less commonly used in horses but have also been shown to result in hypokalemia (Rose et al., 1990). This is similar to findings in other species where hypokalemia is a significant problem with the administration of these medications.

Fluid diuresis is another described cause of increased renal losses of potassium and resulting hypokalemia (Carlson & Rumbaugh, 1983; Freestone et al., 1989; Rumbaugh et al., 1981). This has been produced experimentally in horses and is particularly severe when combined with diuretic administration (Fielding et al., 2008; Freestone et al., 1989). The administration of intravenous fluids is common in equine intensive care units and during treatment in field situations. Clinicians should be aware of the increased renal losses of potassium from prolonged fluid administration. Monitoring of plasma or serum potassium status is important with prolonged fluid therapy particularly if the administered fluids do not contain potassium (e.g. 0.9% saline or sodium bicarbonate).

Renal dysfunction

Increased potassium loss from the kidneys due to renal dysfunction has been reported in other species (Dow et al., 1989), but does not appear to be a significant cause of hypokalemia in horses (Bayly et al., 1986;

Divers et al., 1987; Schott et al., 1997). The high potassium content of the diet in horses may be one reason why hypokalemia is not commonly observed with chronic renal disease. Tubular disorders leading to increased renal losses of potassium have been reported extensively in humans and include Fanconi syndrome, Gitelman syndrome, Barter syndrome, and other variations (Umami et al., 2011). These disorders have not been reported in horses; however, features similar to Fanconi syndrome were seen in one horse following toxicity with mercuric chloride (Roberts et al., 1982). Renal tubular acidosis has been reported in horses, but hypokalemia prior to treatment was an inconsistent feature of this syndrome (Aleman et al., 2001). Therapy with large volumes of sodium bicarbonate (treatment of renal tubular acidosis (RTA)), however, is likely to result in hypokalemia. Both intravenous and oral supplementation with potassium are often required (Grunberg et al., 2011; Koch & Kaske, 2008; Pedrick et al., 1998; Rivas et al., 1997).

Hypomagnesemia

Hypomagnesemia has been associated with refractory hypokalemia in humans, and its association has been noted in horses as well (Stewart, 2011). Recent research has more precisely described the mechanism by which hypomagnesemia can lead to hypokalemia (Huang & Kuo, 2007). Specifically, magnesium deficiency can increase potassium secretion by the distal nephron. A decrease in intracellular magnesium releases the magnesium-mediated inhibition of ROMK channels and increases potassium secretion as shown in Figure 3.2. Magnesium status should be evaluated in horses with unexplained hypokalemia or when hypokalemia is refractory to conventional therapy.

Transcellular shifting

A transcellular shift of potassium from the extracellular fluid volume (ECFV) to the intracellular fluid volume (ICFV) may be the most commonly identified cause of hypokalemia in critically ill equine patients in addition to fluid diuresis. As discussed previously, these shifts can occur due to insulin, catecholamines, or possibly alkalosis.

Insulin is likely to cause hypokalemia in horses, but there is little research to support this conclusion. More evidence is available in other species; however, most studies evaluated a combination of dextrose and insulin, making the effect of each specific treatment more difficult to interpret (Allon et al., 1993; Blumberg et al., 1988). Based on the available data, the administration of dextrose-containing fluids or exogenous insulin should be considered potential causes for hypokalemia in horses.

Stimulation of β_2 receptors increases cellular uptake of potassium. Activation of these receptors can be from endogenous catecholamines released as a normal physiologic response. However, medications affecting β_2 receptors (particularly β_2 agonists used in respiratory disease) will also cause the uptake of potassium into cells. Beta-agonist toxicity resulting in hypokalemia has been described in other species and could likely occur in horses (McCown et al., 2008). In cases of unexplained hypokalemia, a thorough history of medication administration is warranted.

The causal role of acid–base disturbances in hypokalemia remains controversial. It has been reported that hyperventilation leading to a respiratory alkalosis has a significant but clinically minimal effect on plasma potassium concentration (Li & Sun, 2004; Muir et al., 1990; Sanchez & Finlayson, 1978). In one study, the effects of acid–base abnormalities had an inconsistent effect on plasma potassium concentrations (Adrogué & Madias, 1981). Acid–base status should be evaluated in horses with hypokalemia but other causes should be considered before attributing the abnormality entirely to an alkalemia (Box 3.5).

Clinical effects of hypokalemia

The clinical effects of hypokalemia in horses are unclear and may be minimal. Hypokalemia has been described in cases of synchronous diaphragmatic flutter; however, other electrolyte abnormalities were also present (Mansmann et al., 1974). Hypokalemia has been noted as a feature of a number of clinical conditions including laminitis, liver disease, and heat exhaustion, but the decreased plasma potassium concentration is unlikely to be the cause of the clinical disease observed.

Muscle weakness is the most commonly reported complication of mild to moderate hypokalemia in humans (Riggs, 2002; Schaefer & Wolford, 2005). The electrocardiogram changes observed with hypokalemia include an increased P-wave amplitude, prolonged PR interval, and reduction in T-wave amplitude (Schaefer & Wolford, 2005). However, these changes are not correlated with the severity of hypokalemia (Schaefer &

Box 3.5 Diagnostic approach to hypokalemia.

1 Evaluate for causes of potassium shifting from the extracellular to intracellular fluid space:
   a Insulin
   b Catecholamines
2 Evaluate for potassium losses through the renal system:
   a Diuretic administration
   b Fluid diuresis
   c Hypomagnesemia
3 Evaluate for increased sweat losses.
4 Evaluate for contributing factors:
   a Anorexia
   b Diarrhea
   c Other medications

Wolford, 2005). It is interesting to note that some endurance horses will have plasma potassium concentrations less than 2.0 mmol/L and still continue to compete successfully; the author has observed these horses to have no apparent changes during clinical examinations by veterinarians at the time the blood was sampled. Before attributing clinical signs to hypokalemia, a thorough search for other potential causes should be completed.

Treatment of hypokalemia
Identify and treat the cause

The inciting cause and/or contributing factors associated with hypokalemia should be identified and corrected if possible. For example, if hypomagnesemia is documented then supplementation with magnesium-containing fluids should be initiated. If the cause cannot be identified or corrected, empiric supplementation with potassium should be initiated.

Potassium supplementation

Oral administration of KCl can be used at a dose of 0.1 g/kg as frequently as 2–4 times per day (Box 3.6). From a practical standpoint, this is often purchased in the form of Lite-Salt, which contains a combination of NaCl and KCl. However, KCl solution can also be given orally at the same dose. Electrolyte monitoring is important especially in patients with compromised renal function. If the gastrointestinal system is functioning, oral supplementation may be an effective way to increase total body potassium and the plasma potassium

---

Box 3.6 Guidelines for potassium supplementation to horses.

- Intravenous: maximum rate of 0.5 mEq/kg/h
- Oral: 0.1 g/kg orally 2–4 times per day

---

concentration (Freestone et al., 1989). When intravenous access is not already in place and the horse is in a stable condition, oral supplementation is commonly used. For example, the hypokalemia observed in some cases of renal tubular acidosis can be corrected with oral potassium supplementation.

Potassium chloride (2 mEq/mL) added to intravenous fluids (usually an isotonic crystalloid) is the typical form of intravenous potassium supplementation. A maximal rate of 0.5 mEq/kg/h should not be exceeded; however, this number has not been well evaluated in horses. Significantly higher rates were required to induce abnormalities of the electrocardiogram, and some authors have speculated that horses may be more tolerant to high potassium loads than other species (Glazier et al., 1982; Pourjafar et al., 2008). If potassium is being supplemented at high rates or to horses with renal insufficiency, frequent re-checking of plasma potassium concentration is very important. As discussed in the next section, clinical signs and effects of hyperkalemia are serious and frequently described in horses, whereas clinical signs of hypokalemia may be more theoretical and of unknown significance unless severe.

Hyperkalemia

Causes of hyperkalemia in horses

Box 3.7 summarizes the common causes of hyperkalemia in horses.

Increased intake

Excessive dietary intake of potassium rarely causes hyperkalemia in other species (Schaefer & Wolford, 2005) and is unlikely to do so in horses given their ability to handle the already high potassium content of their diet. While the majority of an increased oral potassium load is absorbed, the excess potassium can be redistributed intracellularly in the acute phase and then be excreted by the kidneys over time. There is

---

Box 3.7 Common causes of hyperkalemia in horses.

1 Transcellular shifting:
   a Rhabdomyolysis
   b Hemolysis
   c Hyperkalemic periodic paralysis
2 Urinary system dysfunction:
   a Renal failure
   b Ruptured bladder
3 Increased intake:
   a Rapid intravenous administration

Table 3.3 Potassium content of common intravenous fluids.

Intravenous fluid	Potassium concentration (mEq/L)
Normosol™-M	13
Normosol™-R	5
Plasma-Lyte® A or 148	5
Lactated Ringer's solution	4
0.9% NaCl	0
7.2% NaCl	0
5% Dextrose	0

some potential for increased secretion by the colon over longer periods of time. Increased intake may exacerbate pre-existing hyperkalemia if other factors are present (e.g., renal failure). Intravenous administration of potassium (typically potassium chloride) is unlikely to cause hyperkalemia unless the administration rate is rapid (Pourjafar et al., 2008) (Table 3.3). Potassium should not be bolused intravenously under most circumstances. Impaired renal function would also make intravenous potassium administration more likely to result in hyperkalemia.

Transcellular shifting

Traditionally, acidosis has been associated with an increased plasma potassium concentration. However, there is limited evidence supporting the view that respiratory or metabolic acidosis contributes significantly to marked hyperkalemia (Schaefer & Wolford, 2005). Hyperkalemia has been noted in studies with concurrent acidosis in horses (Datt & Usenik, 1975). It is not known if the observed hyperkalemia was directly related to the acidosis or a result of the underlying disease condition (i.e. intestinal volvulus). In evaluating an equine patient with hyperkalemia, an exhaustive search for other causes should be completed before concluding that the derangement is due to an acid–base disorder.

Rhabdomyolysis occurs in horses and can be associated with a massive destruction and lysis of cells resulting in the release of potassium (as well as other intracellular contents). This release of potassium could potentially result in severe hyperkalemia; many animals with rhabdomyolysis have concurrent renal failure due to the toxicity of myoglobin that is released. It is likely that a component of the observed hyperkalemia may be due to renal insufficiency in addition to the release of potassium from damaged muscle cells. In horses, hyperkalemia was a consistent feature of one study describing rhabdomyolysis in horses or foals (Perkins et al., 1998). However, two additional studies found no change in plasma potassium concentration in horses and identified only one horse (combined from both studies) with an increased plasma potassium concentration (El-Deeb & El-Bahr, 2010; Finno et al., 2006). If hyperkalemia is identified in horses with clinically significant rhabdomyolysis, renal function must be evaluated before concluding that the increased potassium concentration is primarily or solely due to cellular lysis.

Release of potassium during the destruction of red cells could potentially result in hyperkalemia, but this has not been described in horses. Red cell transfusions have been implicated as a cause of hyperkalemia in humans (Vraets et al., 2011). Hyperkalemia was also documented in a patient with hemolytic anemia (Farfel et al., 1990) and it is likely that similar mechanisms could exist in horses. If renal function is adequate, the amount of potassium released from hemolysis may not be large enough to result in hyperkalemia. As with rhabdomyolysis, renal function can be affected by a large-scale hemolytic event.

A well described clinical condition associated with hyperkalemia in horses is hyperkalemic periodic paralysis (HYPP) (Naylor et al., 1999; Spier et al., 1990). Horses with this condition have been documented with potassium concentrations as high as 9.0 mmol/L (Spier et al., 1990). A defect in the sodium channel (alpha subunit) has been identified as the mutation resulting in the clinical condition of HYPP in horses. It is a semi-dominant genetic disease associated with Quarter horses and related breeds (Naylor et al., 1999). Hyperkalemia in a horse with appropriate breeding (halter type Quarter horses) and clinical signs (weakness, sweating, muscle fasciculations, prolapse of the third eyelid) should be suspected of HYPP (Tryon et al., 2009). Genetic testing is available to confirm clinical cases.

Urinary system dysfunction

The inability of the affected animal to adequately excrete the potassium that is ingested in the diet is the underlying mechanism for hyperkalemia in most horses. As the kidney is the main excretory route for potassium, hyperkalemia is often caused by failure of the urinary system. Severe decreases in filtration or the inability to eliminate urine from the body (urethral obstruction, ruptured bladder) are the most commonly described causes in horses.

Anuric renal failure has the greatest potential for causing hyperkalemia. When urine no longer flows from the kidneys, the horse is unable to excrete the large potassium load that is normally ingested. In equine studies, hyperkalemia was identified in some, but not all, horses with acute renal insufficiency depending on the presence of anuria (Divers et al., 1987; Gallatin et al., 2005; Stewart et al., 1995). Interestingly, a retrospective study of horses with chronic renal failure demonstrated mild hyperkalemia as a consistent feature (Schott et al., 1997).

Foals or adult horses with ruptured bladders have been identified with hyperkalemia as a consistent finding (Behr et al., 1981; Butters, 2008; Kablack et al., 2000). Interestingly, foals diagnosed with ruptured bladders and receiving concurrent fluid support with balanced electrolyte solutions, did not develop the severe electrolyte derangements observed in foals without fluid support (Dunkel et al., 2005). Hyperkalemia was not a consistent finding in an equine study with experimentally induced bladder rupture (Genetzky & Hagemoser, 1985). Neonatal foals with hyperkalemia should be evaluated for both renal insufficiency and bladder rupture as these are two common diagnoses in critically ill foals.

Clinical signs of hyperkalemia

The clinical effects of hyperkalemia in horses are better documented than the effects of hypokalemia (Epstein, 1984; Glazier et al., 1982; Pourjafar et al., 2008). Neuromuscular weakness has been described in humans with hyperkalemia, but is more difficult to evaluate in horses (Schaefer & Wolford, 2005). The classic electrocardiogram changes associated with hyperkalemia

(Figure 3.4) appear to be similar in horses as in humans and include:

- tall or peaked T-waves;
- flattened P-waves;
- prolongation of the QRS complex;
- eventual asystole.

Initial changes could be detected at potassium concentrations as low as 6.2 mmol/L (Epstein, 1984) but abnormalities became more consistent as the concentration climbed above 7–8 mmol/L. Arrhythmias that have been reported in association with experimental hyperkalemia in horses include first degree A-V block, ventricular premature beats, sinus arrest, bradycardia and sinus tachycardia (Pourjafar et al., 2008). It is extremely important to remember that the observed ECG changes are not always correlated with the potassium concentration and other factors (hydration, concurrent electrolyte abnormalities) likely play a role. For this reason, the absence of ECG abnormalities should not be used to exclude the possibility of severe or life-threatening hyperkalemia. ECG changes were associated with plasma potassium concentrations in newborn foals (Escabias et al., 1990). However, the clinical significance of the changes is uncertain.

Pseudohyperkalemia

Leakage of potassium from the intracellular space of red or white blood cells and platelets can occur either during or after a blood sample is collected. This cause should be considered when hyperkalemia is observed in a previously normal patient with no clinical signs. Increased potassium concentration can be measured when analysis is performed from collection tubes containing K-EDTA (potassium ethylenediaminetetraacetic acid).

Treatment of hyperkalemia

Based on the results of experimentally induced hyperkalemia in horses, treatment for hyperkalemia should be initiated when the plasma potassium concentration has reached or exceeded 6.0 mmol/L. As with hypokalemia, the cause for hyperkalemia needs to be identified and addressed, as well as specific treatment for the increased potassium. A number of potential treatments have been described for hyperkalemia and are outlined below. See also Table 3.4 and Box 3.8.

Intravenous calcium administration

Intravenous calcium supplementation provides cardioprotection from the dangerous effects of hyperkalemia. It serves to help normalize the difference between

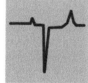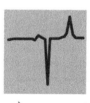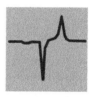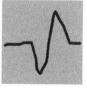

Increasing K$^+$ concentration

Figure 3.4 Characteristic ECG changes due to increasing serum potassium concentration.

Table 3.4 Emergency treatments for hyperkalemia in horses.

Treatment	Dose	Comments
Intravenous 23% calcium gluconate	0.5 mL/kg	Give over 20 minutes diluted in IV fluids
Intravenous 50% dextrose	10 mg/kg/min	Dilute in fluids to 3–5% dextrose and give over 30 minutes
Intravenous insulin (100 units/mL)	0.1 to 0.2 U/kg/h	Dilute in fluids and give over 30 minutes
Intravenous sodium bicarbonate	1–2 mEq/kg	Dilute in fluids (without calcium) and give over 30 minutes
Intravenous furosemide (50 mg/mL)	1–2 mg/kg	
Intravenous isotonic crystalloid	20 mL/kg	Fluids low in potassium may be preferable
Inhaled albuterol	2 µg/kg	Effectiveness and dose for hyperkalemia is unknown in horses
Sodium polystyrene enema	15 g/100 mL of 10% dextrose per 50 kg foal	Useful for foals with hyperkalemia; monitor sodium and potassium carefully

> **Box 3.8 Summary of treatment approach to hyperkalemia.**
>
> 1 Intravenous calcium administration provides protection from the myocardial effects of hyperkalemia but does not alter the plasma potassium concentration significantly.
> 2 Intravenous dextrose and insulin are probably two of the more effective treatments for hyperkalemia and should be given either concurrently with calcium or shortly following.
> 3 Additional treatments that can be used if calcium, dextrose, and insulin are ineffective include intravenous bicarbonate, beta-agonists (inhaled), furosemide, and intravenous fluid therapy.

resting and threshold potentials (by raising threshold potential) and thereby decreases the dangerous arrhythmogenic effects of hyperkalemia. This treatment is rapidly acting and should probably be initiated immediately in patients with severe hyperkalemia (>7.5 mmol/L) and particularly when abnormalities of the electrocardiogram are already present. Calcium borogluconate (23%) can be administered at a dose of 0.5 mL/kg over 15–20 minutes. It is safest to dilute the calcium in a 3–5 L bag of intravenous fluids and administer over 30–60 minutes. Rapid intravenous calcium administration can result in cardiac arrhythmias. Care should be taken not to mix calcium and bicarbonate solutions in the same bag of intravenous fluids. A rate of 0.5–1 mL/kg of 10% calcium gluconate has been recommended over 5–10 minutes in humans with hyperkalemia (Lehnhardt & Kemper, 2011).

Dextrose administration

The administration of intravenous dextrose will lead to the release of endogenous insulin and shift potassium from the extracellular to the intracellular fluid space. Typical rates of dextrose supplementation are 1–2 mg/kg/min in adult horses and 4–8 mg/kg/min in neonatal foals. In humans, rates of 8–16 mg/kg/min have been advocated when concurrent insulin is administered, and higher doses may be required in horses as well, especially if insulin is co-administered and as long as blood glucose is being serially monitored (Lehnhardt & Kemper, 2011). Excessive rates of dextrose administration may lead to unwanted diuresis and increased plasma lactate concentrations, and

might contribute to increased mortality in certain diseases. The optimal level of dextrose administration to provide the maximum shift of potassium from the extracellular to intracellular fluid space is not known and likely depends on concurrent disease conditions. A practical, but more aggressive, approach is to create a 5 L bag of intravenous fluids containing 3% dextrose for average-sized adult horses, and to administer this over approximately 30 minutes. It is easy to make as it simply requires adding 300 mL of 50% dextrose to a 5 L bag of 0.9% saline. This rate of dextrose administration is closer to 10 mg/kg/min for an average 500 kg horse.

Insulin administration

Exogenous insulin is often administered in conjunction with intravenous dextrose to provide further support to shift potassium from the extracellular to intracellular fluid space (Blumberg et al., 1988). Regular insulin can be administered at a rate of 0.005 IU/kg/h, but higher rates may provide a more effective treatment for hyperkalemia. In humans, rates of 0.1–0.2 IU/kg/h have been advocated when high levels of intravenous dextrose are administered concurrently (8–16 mg/kg/min of dextrose) (Lehnhardt & Kemper, 2011). These more aggressive rates may be warranted only when plasma potassium concentrations reach life-threatening levels. In the practical example described previously, 0.25 mL of regular insulin (100 units/mL) could be added to the 5 L bag of fluids and administered over 30 minutes. Insulin administration should be done very carefully; inadvertent bolus administration through fluid lines (while flushing) must be avoided. In addition, high doses of insulin must be used with caution in horses at risk for laminitis and only where the benefit outweighs the risk.

Sodium bicarbonate administration

The benefits of sodium bicarbonate administration for the treatment of hyperkalemia are equivocal (Blumberg et al., 1988). At a minimum, treatment with calcium, dextrose, and insulin should be a priority with bicarbonate treatment as a secondary consideration. Intravenous administration of sodium bicarbonate has been recommended by some authors for hyperkalemia and can be given at a rate of 1–2 mEq/kg over a 30–60 min period (Lehnhardt & Kemper, 2011). There is considerable evidence from horses and other animals to show that sodium bicarbonate administration will lower plasma potassium levels. However, this treatment may be less effective than other options (insulin and dextrose) and its effects may not be mediated through a transcellular shift (Grünberg et al., 2011; Koch & Kaske, 2008; Pedrick et al., 1998; Rivas et al., 1997).

Beta-agonist administration

The reduction in plasma potassium concentration associated with the administration of beta-agonists is described in other species, but its effectiveness is not universal (Blumberg et al., 1988; Bouyssou et al., 2010; Singh et al., 2002). Inhaled albuterol has been shown to effectively reduce extracellular potassium concentrations in humans of varying ages (Allon et al., 1989; Singh et al., 2002). It is likely that it would have a similar effect on plasma potassium concentration across species and therefore this is a potential treatment in horses. Inhaled albuterol has been administered to horses for respiratory disease at doses ranging from 180 to 900 μg depending on the study (Bailey et al., 1999; Bertin et al., 2011). In humans, a much higher dose by body weight was used to decrease plasma potassium concentrations as compared to the dose used for respiratory disease in horses (Singh et al., 2002).

Diuresis

If a functioning urinary system is present, diuresis is another potential means for lowering the plasma potassium concentration. However, the effects of this treatment may be less rapid as compared to dextrose and insulin administration. Commonly used diuretics in equine practice such as furosemide have been shown to decrease plasma potassium concentrations (Freestone et al., 1988, 1989). Additionally, increased urinary flow will improve the removal of potassium from the kidneys. For this reason, administering increased rates (3–5 mL/kg/h) of intravenous fluids (ideally with a low potassium concentration) may also help to decrease the plasma potassium concentration over time as long as urine is being produced. The ideal intravenous fluid for this purpose is controversial, with some authors advocating isotonic saline (0.9%) due to the lack of potassium. However, the acidifying effects of this fluid could have some theoretic disadvantages in patients with hyperkalemia. Recent research in other species has shown that lactated Ringer's solution (LRS) may be effective and has challenged the absolute recommendation for using normal saline solution (Cunha et al., 2010; Drobatz &

Cole, 2008). While not commercially available, it is possible that an isotonic bicarbonate solution (made by combining sterile water and sodium bicarbonate) might also be advantageous for the treatment of hyperkalemia. This fluid is alkalinizing, contains no potassium, replaces intravascular volume, and induces diuresis.

Selected tests for potassium disorders

Transtubular potassium gradient (TTKG)

The transtubular potassium gradient (TTKG) is used to evaluate the ability of the cortical collecting ducts to conserve potassium depending on the plasma potassium concentration. In some ways, it serves as a measure of the effects of aldosterone on potassium excretion. Baseline values were determined from foals in one study, which found a TTKG of approximately 24 (Buchanan et al., 2005). This value decreased dramatically with potassium wasting during the course of the study to a value of approximately 5 (Buchanan et al., 2005).

In humans, TTKG has been shown to be useful in evaluating the potential causes for hypokalemia in patients (Joo et al., 2000). Values of TTKG below 6 would suggest an inappropriate renal response to hyperkalemia, whereas values greater than 2 during hypokalemia point to renal losses of potassium (Choi & Ziyadeh, 2008; Ethier et al., 1990). More research is needed on this test in horses, but it could potentially be useful in determining the underlying cause for potassium abnormalities. The calculation for TTKG is:

$$TTKG = [(K^+ \text{concentration}_{urine})/(K^+ \text{concentration}_{blood})] \times [(Osmolality_{blood})/(Osmolality_{urine})]$$

$$(3.1)$$

Use of the TTKG requires that urine osmolality be greater than or equal to plasma osmolality and that urine sodium concentration is greater than 25 mmol/L (Choi & Ziyadeh, 2008).

Fractional excretion of potassium

The fractional excretion of potassium (FE_K) represents the amount of potassium that is filtered by the kidney that is then excreted in the urine. This calculation has been used to evaluate the effect of different diets, training programs, and overall potassium status in horses (Beech et al., 1993; McKenzie et al., 2002; Robert et al., 2010). However, it is altered by diet and by the administration of intravenous fluids making its interpretation in a clinical setting complex (Roussel et al., 1993).

Normal values for FE_K in horses have ranged from 23 to 75% (Kohn & Strasser, 1986; Morris et al., 1984). Values greater than normal could signify urinary losses of potassium but the larger normal range and variability of the diet (these values could be exceeded with high-potassium diets such as orchard grass or alfalfa hay) make the usefulness of this test unclear. Normal values reported in foals were $13 \pm 4\%$ as a baseline value in one study; however, another study found foals to have higher values at approximately 33% (Brewer et al., 1991; Buchanan et al., 2005). The fractional excretion of potassium by the kidneys is given by the equation:

$$\text{Fractional excretion of } K^+ = ([Cr_{plasma}]/[Cr_{urine}]) + ([K^+_{urine}]/[K^+_{plasma}]) \times 100$$

$$(3.2)$$

where Cr_{plasma} is the concentration of creatinine in the plasma, Cr_{urine} is the concentration of creatinine in the urine, K^+_{urine} is the concentration of potassium in the urine, and K^+_{plasma} is the concentration of potassium in the plasma.

Foals and potassium balance

In general, foals retain potassium for two reasons. First and perhaps most importantly, they are growing and therefore need to increase the total body potassium (i.e., net positive retention). This is in contrast to adults, who maintain a zero balance where they lose or eliminate all of the potassium that is ingested. Secondly, foals are born with a lower ICFV/ECFV ratio than adults (Fielding et al., 2011). As they get older, the size of the ICFV expands significantly (especially as compared to the ECFV). Since the vast majority of the potassium is located within the ICFV, it is very important for foals to retain enough potassium to account for the enlargement of this fluid space. Research in humans suggests that neonates, in order to retain enough potassium, increase potassium absorption in the gut, reduce potassium secretion by the kidney, and have a decreased ability to shift potassium from the intracellular to extracellular space, as compared to adults (Aizman et al., 1998). In foals in one study, the fractional excretion of potassium at 4 days of age was reported as $13 \pm 4\%$, which is lower than the rate observed for adults (Brewer et al., 1991).

Fortunately there is adequate potassium in mare's milk to achieve the net positive retention of potassium that is required. However, foals maintained on long-term intravenous fluids require significant potassium supplementation, especially if intolerant of milk feeding. Maintenance potassium supplementation can be provided to foals at 1–2 mEq/kg/day. On a typical fluid rate (3–5 mL/kg/h), however, the requirement for potassium is greater than is available in a typical isotonic replacement fluid (LRS, Normosol™-R). Most foals that receive long-term intravenous fluids without access to milk will require potassium supplementation (20–50 mEq/L) depending on the rate of fluid administration.

Premature foals, as compared to normal term foals, may have an even more complex potassium homeostasis based on the information available in humans. In premature human infants, there is an initial increase in plasma potassium concentration after birth due to a dramatic shift of potassium from the intracellular to extracellular fluid space (Lorenz et al., 1997; Mildenberger & Versmold, 2002). This is likely due to failure of the Na^+/K^+ pump controlling the transcellular movement of potassium (Stefano et al., 1993). Following this shift of potassium to the ECFV, there is an increase in the excretion of potassium that normalizes the plasma potassium concentration (Lorenz et al., 1997). Renal insufficiency would interfere with the clearance of this additional potassium potentially resulting in life-threatening hyperkalemia. While much less research is available in horses, premature foals do have a higher serum potassium concentration as compared to term foals (Broughton et al., 1984). It also appears that the distal convoluted tubule of the newborn foal is less responsive to the effects of aldosterone in maintaining potassium regulation (Broughton et al., 1984).

References

Adrogué HJ, Madias NE. (1981) Changes in plasma potassium concentration during acute acid-base disturbances. *Am J Med* **71**:456–67.

Aizman R, Grahnquist L, Celsi G. (1998) Potassium homeostasis: ontogenic aspects. *Acta Paediatr* **87**:609–17.

Aleman MR, Kuesis B, Schott HC, et al. (2001) Renal tubular acidosis in horses (1980–1999). *J Vet Intern Med* **15**:136–43.

Alexander F. (1966) A study of parotid salivation in the horse. *J Physiol* **184**:646–56.

Alexander F. (1977) The effect of diuretics on the faecal excretion of water and electrolytes in horses. *Br J Pharmacol* **60**:589–93.

Alexander F. (1982a) Effect of phenylbutazone on electrolyte metabolism in ponies. *Vet Rec* **110**:271–2.

Alexander F. (1982b) The effect of ethacrynic acid, bumetanide, frusemide, spironolactone and ADH on electrolyte excretion in ponies. *J Vet Pharmacol Ther* **5**:153–60.

Allon M, Dunlay R, Copkney C. (1989) Nebulized albuterol for acute hyperkalemia in patients on hemodialysis. *Ann Intern Med* **110**:426–9.

Allon M, Takeshian A, Shanklin N. (1993) Effect of insulin-plus-glucose infusion with or without epinephrine on fasting hyperkalemia. *Kidney Int* **43**:212–17.

Andrejak M, Lafon B, Decocq G, et al. (1996) Antibiotic-associated pseudomembranous colitis: retrospective study of 48 cases diagnosed by colonoscopy. *Therapie* **51**:81–6.

Bailey J, Colahan P, Kubilis P, et al. (1999) Effect of inhaled beta 2 adrenoceptor agonist, albuterol sulphate, on performance of horses. *Equine Vet J Suppl* **30**:575–80.

Bayly WM, Brobst DF, Elfers RS, et al. (1986) Serum and urinary biochemistry and enzyme changes in ponies with acute renal failure. *Cornell Vet* **76**:306–16.

Beech J, Lindborg S, Braund KG. (1993) Potassium concentrations in muscle, plasma and erythrocytes and urinary fractional excretion in normal horses and those with chronic intermittent exercise-associated rhabdomyolysis. *Res Vet Sci* **55**:43–51.

Behr MJ, Hackett RP, Bentinck-Smith J, et al. (1981) Metabolic abnormalities associated with rupture of the urinary bladder in neonatal foals. *J Am Vet Med Assoc* **178**:263–6.

Bertin FR, Ivester KM, Couëtil LL. (2011) Comparative efficacy of inhaled albuterol between two hand-held delivery devices in horses with recurrent airway obstruction. *Equine Vet J* **43**:393–8.

Bertone JJ, Shoemaker KE. (1992) Effect of hypertonic and isotonic saline solutions on plasma constituents of conscious horses. *Am J Vet Res* **53**:1844–9.

Blumberg A, Weidmann P, Shaw S, et al. (1988) Effect of various therapeutic approaches on plasma potassium and major regulating factors in terminal renal failure. *Am J Med* **85**:507–12.

Bouyssou T, Casarosa P, Naline E, et al. (2010) Pharmacological characterization of olodaterol, a novel inhaled beta2-adrenoceptor agonist exerting a 24-hour-long duration of action in preclinical models. *J Pharmacol Exp Ther* **334**:53–62.

Brewer BD, Clement SF, Lotz WS, et al. (1991) Renal clearance, urinary excretion of endogenous substances, and urinary diagnostic indices in healthy neonatal foals. *J Vet Intern Med* **5**:28–33.

Broughton Pipkin F, Ousey JC, Wallace CP, et al. (1984) Studies on equine prematurity 4: Effect of salt and water loss on the renin-angiotensin-aldosterone system in the newborn foal. *Equine Vet J* **16**:292–7.

Buchanan BR, Sommardahl CS, Rohrbach BW, et al. (2005) Effect of a 24-hour infusion of an isotonic electrolyte replacement fluid on the renal clearance of electrolytes in healthy neonatal foals. *J Am Vet Med Assoc* **227**:1123–9.

Butters A. (2008) Medical and surgical management of uroperitoneum in a foal. *Can Vet J* **49**:401–3.

Carlson GP, Rumbaugh GE. (1983) Response to saline solution of normally fed horses and horses dehydrated by fasting. *Am J Vet Res* **44**:964–8.

Cebra CK, Valentine BA, Schlipf JW, et al. (2007) Eimeria macusaniensis infection in 15 llamas and 34 alpacas. *J Am Vet Med Assoc* **230**:94–100.

Cehak A, Burmester M, Geburek F, et al. (2009) Electrophysiological characterization of electrolyte and nutrient transport across the small intestine in horses. *J Anim Physiol Anim Nutr (Berl)* **93**:287–94.

Chatzizisis YS, Misirli G, Hatzitolios AI, et al. (2008) The syndrome of rhabdomyolysis: complications and treatment. *Eur J Intern Med* **19**:568–74.

Choi MJ, Ziyadeh FN. (2008) The utility of the transtubular potassium gradient in the evaluation of hyperkalemia. *Am Soc Nephrol* **19**:424–6.

Cummings JH, Sladen GE, James OF, et al. (1974) Laxative-induced diarrhoea: a continuing clinical problem. *Br Med J* **i**:537–41.

Cunha MG, Freitas GC, Carregaro AB, et al. (2010) Renal and cardiorespiratory effects of treatment with lactated Ringer's solution or physiologic saline (0.9% NaCl) solution in cats with experimentally induced urethral obstruction. *Am J Vet Res* **71**:840–6.

Datt SC, Usenik EA. (1975) Intestinal obstruction in the horse. Physical signs and blood chemistry. *Cornell Vet* **65**:152–72.

Dennis JS, Kruger JM, Mullaney TP. (1993) Lymphocytic/plasmacytic colitis in cats: 14 cases (1985–1990). *J Am Vet Med Assoc* **202**:313–18.

DiBartola SP, De Morais HA. (2011) Disorders of potassium: hypokalemia and hyperkalemia. In: DiBartola SP (ed.) *Fluid, Electrolyte, and Acid–Base disorders in Small Animal Practice*, 4th edn. Saunders, pp. 92–119.

Divers TJ, Whitlock RH, Byars TD, et al. (1987) Acute renal failure in six horses resulting from haemodynamic causes. *Equine Vet J* **19**:178–84.

Dow SW, Fettman MJ, Curtis CR, et al. (1989) Hypokalemia in cats: 186 cases (1984–1987). *J Am Vet Med Assoc* **194**:1604–8.

Drobatz KJ, Cole SG. (2008) The influence of crystalloid type on acid base and electrolyte status of cats with urethral obstruction. *J Vet Emerg Crit Care* **18**:355–61.

Dunkel B, Palmer JE, Olson KN, et al. (2005) Uroperitoneum in 32 foals: influence of intravenous fluid therapy, infection, and sepsis. *J Vet Intern Med* **19**:889–93.

Ecke P, Hodgson DR, Rose RJ. (1998) Induced diarrhoea in horses. Part 1: Fluid and electrolyte balance. *Vet J* **155**:149–59.

Edwards DJ, Brownlow MA, Hutchins DR. (1990) Indices of renal function: values in eight normal foals from birth to 56 days. *Aust Vet J* **67**:251–4.

el-Ashker MR. (2011) Acute kidney injury mediated by oxidative stress in Egyptian horses with exertional rhabdomyolysis. *Vet Res Commun* **35**:311–20.

El-Deeb WM, El-Bahr SM. (2010) Investigation of selected biochemical indicators of equine rhabdomyolysis in Arabian horses: pro-inflammatory cytokines and oxidative stress markers. *Vet Res Commun* **34**:677–89.

Epstein V. (1984) Relationship between potassium administration, hyperkalaemia and the electrocardiogram: an experimental study. *Equine Vet J* **16**:453–6.

Escabias MI, Santisteban R, Rubio MD, et al. (1990) Relationship between plasmatic concentrations of K, Na and Ca, and ECG from foals during postnatal phase. *Nihon Juigaku Zasshi* **52**:257–63.

Ethier JH, Kamel KS, Magner PO, et al. (1990) The transtubular potassium concentration in patients with hypokalemia and hyperkalemia. *Am J Kidney Dis* **15**:309–15.

Farfel Z, Freimark D, Mayan H, et al. (1990) Spurious hypoglycemia, hyperkalemia and hypoxemia in chronic hemolytic anemia. *Isr J Med Sci* **26**:606–10.

Fielding CL, Magdesian KG, Carlson GP, et al. (2008) Application of the sodium dilution principle to calculate extracellular fluid volume changes in horses during dehydration and rehydration. *Am J Vet Res* **69**:1506–11.

Fielding CL, Magdesian KG, Rhodes DM, et al. (2009) Clinical and biochemical abnormalities in endurance horses eliminated from competition for medical complications and requiring emergency medical treatment: 30 cases (2005–2006). *J Vet Emerg Crit Care (San Antonio)* **19**:473–8.

Fielding CL, Magdesian KG, Edman JE. (2011) Determination of body water compartments in neonatal foals by use of indicator dilution techniques and multifrequency bioelectrical impedance analysis. *Am J Vet Res* **72**:1390–6.

Finno CJ, Valberg SJ, Wünschmann A, et al. (2006) Seasonal pasture myopathy in horses in the midwestern United States: 14 cases (1998–2005). *J Am Vet Med Assoc* **229**:1134–41.

Freestone JF, Carlson GP, Harrold DR, et al. (1988) Influence of furosemide treatment on fluid and electrolyte balance in horses. *Am J Vet Res* **49**:1899–902.

Freestone JF, Carlson GP, Harrold DR, et al. (1989) Furosemide and sodium bicarbonate-induced alkalosis in the horse and response to oral KCl or NaCl therapy. *Am J Vet Res* **50**:1334–9.

Freestone JF, Gossett K, Carlson GP, et al. (1991) Exercise induced alterations in the serum muscle enzymes, erythrocyte potassium and plasma constituents following feed withdrawal or furosemide and sodium bicarbonate administration in the horse. *J Vet Intern Med* **5**:40–6.

Gallatin LL, Couëtil LL, Ash SR. (2005) Use of continuous-flow peritoneal dialysis for the treatment of acute renal failure in an adult horse. *J Am Vet Med Assoc* **226**:756–9.

Genetzky RM, Hagemoser WA. (1985) Physical and clinical pathological findings associated with experimentally induced rupture of the equine urinary bladder. *Can Vet J* **26**:391–5.

Glazier DB, Littledike ET, Evans RD. (1982) Electrocardiographic changes in induced hyperkalemia in ponies. *Am J Vet Res* **43**:1934–7.

Gottlieb-Vedi M, Dahlborn K, Jansson A, et al. (1996) Elemental composition of muscle at rest and potassium levels in muscle,

plasma and sweat of horses exercising at 20 degrees C and 35 degrees C. *Equine Vet J Suppl* **22**:35–41.

Groenendyk S, English PB, Abetz I. (1988) External balance of water and electrolytes in the horse. *Equine Vet J* **20**:189–93.

Grünberg W, Hartmann H, Burfeind O, et al. (2011) Plasma potassium-lowering effect of oral glucose, sodium bicarbonate, and the combination thereof in healthy neonatal dairy calves. *J Dairy Sci* **94**:5646–55.

Hejłasz Z, Nicpoń J, Czerw P. (1994) The role of sweat in maintaining the stimulation of effort homeostasis in horses. *Arch Vet Pol* **34**:231–9.

Hintz HF, Schryver HF. (1976) Potassium metabolism in ponies. *J Anim Sci* **42**:637–43.

Huang CL, Kuo E. (2007) Mechanism of hypokalemia in magnesium deficiency. *J Am Soc Nephrol* **18**:2649–52.

Jansson A, Lindholm A, Lindberg JE, et al. (1999) Effects of potassium intake on potassium, sodium and fluid balance in exercising horses. *Equine Vet J Suppl* **30**:412–17.

Jansson A, Lindholm A, Dahlborn K. (2002) Effects of acute intravenous aldosterone administration on Na(+), K(+), and water excretion in the horse. *J Appl Physiol* **92**:135–41.

Johansson AM, Gardner SY, Levine JF, et al. (2003) Furosemide continuous rate infusion in the horse: evaluation of enhanced efficacy and reduced side effects. *J Vet Intern Med* **17**:887–95.

Johnson PJ, Goetz TE, Foreman JH, et al. (1991) Effect of whole-body potassium depletion on plasma, erythrocyte, and middle gluteal muscle potassium concentration of healthy, adult horses. *Am J Vet Res* **52**:1676–83.

Joo KW, Chang SH, Lee JG, et al. (2000) Transtubular potassium concentration gradient (TTKG) and urine ammonium in differential diagnosis of hypokalemia. *J Nephrol* **13**:120–5.

Kablack KA, Embertson RM, Bernard WV, et al. (2000) Uroperitoneum in the hospitalised equine neonate: retrospective study of 31 cases, 1988–1997. *Equine Vet J* **32**:505–8.

Kerr MG, Snow DH. (1983) Composition of sweat of the horse during prolonged epinephrine (adrenaline) infusion, heat exposure, and exercise. *Am J Vet Res* **44**:1571–7.

Kingston JK, Geor RJ, McCutcheon LJ. (1997) Rate and composition of sweat fluid losses are unaltered by hypohydration during prolonged exercise in horses. *J Appl Physiol* **83**:1133–43.

Koch A, Kaske M. (2008) Clinical efficacy of intravenous hypertonic saline solution or hypertonic bicarbonate solution in the treatment of inappetent calves with neonatal diarrhea. *J Vet Intern Med* **22**:202–11.

Kohn CW, Strasser SL. (1986) 24-hour renal clearance and excretion of endogenous substances in the mare. *Am J Vet Res* **47**:1332–7.

Latson KM, Nieto JE, Beldomenico PM, et al. (2005) Evaluation of peritoneal fluid lactate as a marker of intestinal ischaemia in equine colic. *Equine Vet J* **37**:342–6.

Lehnhardt A, Kemper MJ. (2011) Pathogenesis, diagnosis and management of hyperkalemia. *Pediatr Nephrol* **26**:377–84.

Li Y, Sun L. (2004) Effects of different respiratory rates on PaCO2 and plasma potassium concentration. *Sichuan Da Xue Xue Bao Yi Xue Ban* **35**:385–7.

Lindinger MI, Ecker GL. (2013) Gastric emptying, intestinal absorption of electrolytes and exercise performance in electrolyte-supplemented horses. *Exp Physiol* **98**:193–206.

Lorenz JM, Kleinman LI, Markarian K. (1997) Potassium metabolism in extremely low birth weight infants in the first week of life. *J Pediatr* **131**:81–6.

Mansmann RA, Carlson GP, White NA, et al. (1974) Synchronous diaphragmatic flutter in horses. *J Am Vet Med Assoc* **165**: 265–70.

Mayhew IG, Whitlock RH, Tasker JB. (1977) Equine cerebrospinal fluid: reference values of normal horses. *Am J Vet Res* **38**:1271–4.

McConaghy FF, Hodgson DR, Evans DL, et al. (1995) Equine sweat composition: effects of adrenaline infusion, exercise and training. *Equine Vet J Suppl* **20**:158–64.

McCown JL, Lechner ES, Cooke KL. (2008) Suspected albuterol toxicosis in a dog. *J Am Vet Med Assoc* **232**:1168–71.

McCutcheon LJ, Geor RJ. (1996) Sweat fluid and ion losses in horses during training and competition in cool vs. hot ambient conditions: implications for ion supplementation. *Equine Vet J Suppl* **22**:54–62.

McKenzie EC, Valberg SJ, Godden SM, et al. (2002) Plasma and urine electrolyte and mineral concentrations in Thoroughbred horses with recurrent exertional rhabdomyolysis after consumption of diets varying in cation-anion balance. *Am J Vet Res* **63**:1053–60.

Meyer H, Muuss H, Güldenhaupt V, et al. (1982) Intestinal water, sodium and potassium metabolism in the horse. *Fortschr Tierphysiol Tierernahr* **13**:52–60.

Mildenberger E, Versmold HT. (2002) Pathogenesis and therapy of non-oliguric hyperkalaemia of the premature infant. *Eur J Pediatr* **161**:415–22.

Morris DD, Divers TJ, Whitlock RH. (1984) Renal clearance and fractional excretion of electrolytes over a 24-hour period in horses. *Am J Vet Res* **45**:2431–5.

Muir WW, Wagner AE, Buchanan C. (1990) Effects of acute hyperventilation on serum potassium in the dog. *Vet Surg* **19**:83–7.

Muylle E, Van den Hende C, Nuytten J, et al. (1984a) Potassium concentration in equine red blood cells: normal values and correlation with potassium levels in plasma. *Equine Vet J* **16**:447–9.

Muylle E, Nuytten J, Van den Hende C, et al. (1984b) Determination of red blood cell potassium content in horses with diarrhoea: a practical approach for therapy. *Equine Vet J* **16**:450–2.

Naylor JM, Nickel DD, Trimino G, et al. (1999) Hyperkalaemic periodic paralysis in homozygous and heterozygous horses: a co-dominant genetic condition. *Equine Vet J* **31**:153–9.

Palmer BF, Dubose TD. (2010) Disorders of potassium metabolism. In: Schrier RW (ed.) *Renal and Electrolyte Disorders*, 7th edn. Lippincott Williams & Wilkins, pp. 137–65.

Pedrick TP, Moon PF, Ludders JW, et al. (1998) The effects of equivalent doses of tromethamine or sodium bicarbonate in healthy horses. *Vet Surg* **27**:284–91.

Perkins G, Valberg SJ, Madigan JM, et al. (1998) Electrolyte disturbances in foals with severe rhabdomyolysis. *J Vet Intern Med* **12**:173–7.

Picandet V, Léguillette R, Lavoie JP. (2003) Comparison of efficacy and tolerability of isoflupredone and dexamethasone in the treatment of horses affected with recurrent airway obstruction ('heaves'). *Equine Vet J* **35**:419–24.

Pourjafar M, Kojouri GH, Dehkordi AJ, et al. (2008) The relationship between KCl infusion and changes of ECG, electrolytes of plasma and K content of donkey's red blood cells. *Pak J Biol Sci* **11**:433–7.

Rawlings CA, Bisgard GE. (1975) Renal clearance and excretion of endogenous substances in the small pony. *Am J Vet Res* **36**:45–8.

Riggs JE. (2002) Neurologic manifestations of electrolyte disturbances. *Neurol Clin* **20**:227–39.

Rivas LJ, Hinchcliff KW, Kohn CW, et al. (1997) Effect of sodium bicarbonate administration on renal function of horses. *Am J Vet Res* **58**:664–71.

Robert C, Goachet AG, Fraipont A, et al. (2010) Hydration and electrolyte balance in horses during an endurance season. *Equine Vet J Suppl* **42**:98–104.

Roberts MC, Seawright AA, Ng JC, et al. (1982) Some effects of chronic mercuric chloride intoxication on renal function in a horse. *Vet Hum Toxicol* **24**:415–20.

Roberts MC, Clarke LL, Johnson CM. (1989) Castor-oil induced diarrhoea in ponies: a model for acute colitis. *Equine Vet J Suppl* **7**:60–7.

Rose RJ, Hodgson DR, Kelso TB, et al. (1990) Effects of acetazolamide on metabolic and respiratory responses to exercise at maximal O_2 uptake. *J Appl Physiol* **68**:617–26.

Roussel AJ, Cohen ND, Ruoff WW, et al. (1993) Urinary indices of horses after intravenous administration of crystalloid solutions. *J Vet Intern Med* **7**:241–6.

Rumbaugh GE, Carlson GP, Harrold D. (1981) Clinicopathologic effects of rapid infusion of 5% sodium bicarbonate in 5% dextrose in the horse. *J Am Vet Med Assoc* **178**:267–71.

Sanchez MG, Finlayson DC. (1978) Dynamics of serum potassium change during acute respiratory alkalosis. *Can Anaesth Soc J* **25**:495–8.

Schaefer TJ, Wolford RW. (2005) Disorders of potassium. *Emerg Med Clin N Am* **23**:723–47.

Schott HC, Patterson KS, Fitzerald SD, et al. (1997) Chronic renal failure in 99 horses. In: Proceedings of the 43rd Annual Convention of the American Association of Equine Practitioners, pp. 345–6.

Seo W, Oh H. (2010) Alterations in serum osmolality, sodium, and potassium levels after repeated mannitol administration. *J Neurosci Nurs* **42**:201–7.

Singh BS, Sadiq HF, Noguchi A, et al. (2002) Efficacy of albuterol inhalation in treatment of hyperkalemia in premature neonates. *J Pediatr* **141**:16–20.

Spier SJ, Carlson GP, Holliday TA, et al. (1990) Hyperkalemic periodic paralysis in horses. *J Am Vet Med Assoc* **197**: 1009–17.

Spooner HS, Nielsen BD, Schott HC, et al. (2010) Sweat composition in Arabian horses performing endurance exercise on forage-based, low Na rations. *Equine Vet J* **42**:382–6.

Staempfli HR, Townsend HG, Prescott JF. (1991) Prognostic features and clinical presentation of acute idiopathic enterocolitis in horses. *Can Vet J* **32**:232–7.

Stefano JL, Norman ME, Morales MC, et al. (1993) Decreased erythrocyte Na+,K(+)-ATPase activity associated with cellular potassium loss in extremely low birth weight infants with nonoliguric hyperkalemia. *J Pediatr* **122**:276–84.

Stewart AJ. (2011) Magnesium disorders in horses. *Vet Clin North Am Equine Pract* **27**:149–63.

Stewart MC, Hodgson JL, Kim H, et al. (1995) Acute febrile diarrhoea in horses: 86 cases (1986–1991). *Aust Vet J* **72**:41–4.

Tasker JB. (1967) Fluid and electrolyte studies in the horse III. Intake and output of water, sodium, and potassium in normal horses. *Cornell Vet* **57**:649–57.

Toribio RE, Kohn CW, Rourke KM, et al. (2007) Effects of hypercalcemia on serum concentrations of magnesium, potassium, and phosphate and urinary excretion of electrolytes in horses. *Am J Vet Res* **68**:543–54.

Tryon RC, Penedo MC, McCue ME, et al. (2009) Evaluation of allele frequencies of inherited disease genes in subgroups of American Quarter Horses. *J Am Vet Med Assoc* **234**:120–5.

Ullrey DE, Struthers RD, Hendricks DG, et al. (1966) Composition of mare's milk. *J Anim Sci* **25**:217–21.

Umami V, Oktavia D, Kunmartini S, et al. (2011) Diagnosis and clinical approach in Gitelman's syndrome. *Acta Med Indones* **43**:53–8.

Viu J, Jose-Cunilleras E, Armengou L, et al. (2010) Acid–base imbalances during a 120 km endurance race compared by traditional and simplified strong ion difference methods. *Equine Vet J Suppl* **42**:76–82.

Vraets A, Lin Y, Callum JL. (2011) Transfusion-associated hyperkalemia. *Transfus Med Rev* **25**:184–96.

Watson ZE, Steffey EP, VanHoogmoed LM, et al. (2002) Effect of general anesthesia and minor surgical trauma on urine and serum measurements in horses. *Am J Vet Res* **63**:1061–5.

Yang L, Frindt G, Palmer LG. (2010) Magnesium modulates ROMK channel-mediated potassium secretion. *J Am Soc Nephrol* **21**:2109–16.

CHAPTER 4

Chloride homeostasis and derangements

C. Langdon Fielding

Loomis Basin Equine Medical Center, Penryn, CA, USA

Introduction

Chloride is the predominant extracellular anion. Its importance is often overlooked though it plays a major role in osmolality and acid–base regulation. The role of chloride channels in normal physiology and disease is of growing interest and the regulation of chloride in different organ systems continues to be investigated.

In horses the majority of chloride is ingested in feed, where dietary intake was reported as 3008 mmol/day (Groenendyk et al., 1988). This varies considerably depending on the feed and supplements provided. Losses of chloride in urine and feces combined represented 84% of intake; however, the majority of the lost chloride was through the urine (Groenendyk et al., 1988). The remaining chloride is likely lost in sweat, where concentrations can be as high as 268 mmol/L (Hejłasz et al., 1994; Rose et al., 1980; Spooner et al., 2010). Respiratory secretions and other insensible losses also contain chloride.

Normal chloride concentrations for body fluids in the horse are shown in Table 4.1. Normal serum concentrations for chloride in horses have been reported to range from 95 ± 1 mmol/L (Watson et al., 2002) to 100 ± 2 mmol/L (Groenendyk et al., 1988). However, diet can have a significant effect on serum chloride concentration (McKenzie et al., 2002). Intracellular chloride concentrations are much lower than values in the extracellular fluid, but depend on the specific cell type. Abnormalities in serum or plasma chloride concentration typically result from derangements in normal intake or loss from the body. The gastrointestinal and renal systems are the primary regulators of chloride balance. Abnormalities of chloride transport in either system can lead to clinical derangements.

Chloride regulation in the gastrointestinal system

Chloride is handled by two major mechanisms throughout the gastrointestinal system:
1 Chloride undergoes electro-neutral absorption with sodium in most segments of the intestine.
2 Chloride is secreted and is the major mechanism driving fluid secretion.

There are only a small number of studies evaluating the movement of chloride (either absorption or secretion) in the gastrointestinal tract of horses (Alexander, 1962; Cehak et al., 2009; Giddings et al., 1974; Rikihisa et al., 1992). Chloride secretion was documented in the jejunum, although the transport mechanisms appear different to those in other species (Cehak et al., 2009). The equine cecum can provide net absorption or secretion of chloride depending on the electrolyte content of the fluid on the luminal surface (Giddings et al., 1974). The large colon was shown to absorb chloride along with sodium but the more proximal portion of the colon was capable of chloride secretion (Clarke & Argenzio, 1990). Similarly, chloride secretion was identified in the small colon (Clarke et al., 1992).

In disease, the colon may lose its ability to absorb chloride effectively (Rikihisa et al., 1992), which can result in clinically observed chloride imbalances. This has been observed in both experimental (Roberts et al., 1989) and clinical diarrhea in horses (Rikihisa et al.,

Equine Fluid Therapy, First Edition. Edited by C. Langdon Fielding and K. Gary Magdesian.
© 2015 John Wiley & Sons, Inc. Published 2015 by John Wiley & Sons, Inc.

1992). When chloride, sodium, and water are lost in similar proportions, observed changes in plasma electrolyte concentrations may be minimal. However, when losses of sodium, chloride, and water occur in different proportions as compared to plasma concentrations, acid–base and electrolyte derangements may be significant.

Chloride regulation in the renal system

The chloride ion is freely filterable in the glomerulus and therefore as much as 99% must be reabsorbed by the kidney. Chloride transport in the kidney can be conceptually simplified where energy is used to move chloride from the tubular lumen into the cell, and then the concentration gradient allows chloride to move from the cell into the interstitium (Planelles, 2004). Movement of chloride is generally considered in partnership with sodium to maintain electroneutrality, and it is often

Table 4.1 Chloride concentration in body fluids of the horse.

Fluid type	[Cl^-] (mEq/L)	Reference
Serum	95 ± 1 to 100 ± 2	Watson et al. (2002), Groenendyk et al. (1988)
Urine	29 ± 14 to 192 ± 47	Rawlings & Bisgard (1975), Morris et al. (1984)
Sweat	131 ± 6 to 269 ± 98	Hejłasz et al. (1994), Spooner et al. (2010)
Peritoneal fluid	105 ± 2	Latson et al. (2005)
Saliva	48–50	Alexander (1966)
Cerebrospinal fluid	109 ± 7	Mayhew et al. (1977)

considered to "follow" sodium. This classic view of the sodium–chloride relationship is, however, evolving and the increasing importance of the chloride ion is becoming better understood. A simplification of chloride reabsorption in the kidney is shown in Figure 4.1.

The majority of filtered chloride is reabsorbed in the proximal tubule. The exact amount has not been investigated in horses; based on other species it may be between 50 and 65%. Active chloride reabsorption in the proximal tubule is achieved by Cl^-/base exchangers that work in parallel with Na^+/H^+ exchangers (Planelles, 2004).

Chloride plays a particularly important role in the loop of Henle. The descending limb is not permeable to the chloride ion, but approximately 25% of the filtered chloride load is absorbed in the ascending limb. The main transport mechanism in this segment of the kidney is the NKCC2 isoform of the Na^+/K^+/$2Cl^-$ symporter. The chloride ion is the rate-limiting step for transport of sodium and potassium, as well as chloride, out of the lumen. This symporter is the target for furosemide, the most commonly used diuretic in equine practice (Carlson & Jones, 1999; Johansson et al., 2003).

In the distal tubule, chloride transport is linked to sodium through the Na^+/Cl^- symporter. This segment is typically responsible for reabsorption of approximately 5% of the filtered chloride ion. The Na^+/Cl^- symporter is the site of action for thiazide diuretics, which block its action. The use of thiazide diuretics has been described in horses, but they are not commonly used in equine clinical practice (Alexander, 1977).

Chloride reabsorption in the collecting ducts takes place primarily by the paracellular route. Approximately 4–5% of the filtered chloride load is reabsorbed in this segment of the kidney, and reabsorption here is linked to bicarbonate transport.

In normal horses or ponies the concentration of chloride in urine has been reported to range from 28.9 to

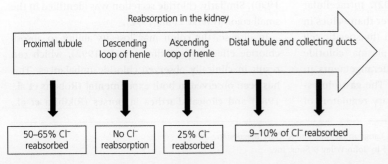

Figure 4.1 Chloride reabsorption in the kidney.

192 mEq/L (Morris et al., 1984; Rawlings & Bisgard, 1975; Rumbaugh et al., 1982; Watson et al., 2002). The fractional excretion of chloride in normal horses ranges from 0.60 to 1.9% (McKenzie et al., 2002; Morris et al., 1984; Toribio et al., 2007). These values vary with the dietary intake or fluid administration (McKenzie et al., 2002; Toribio et al., 2007). Administration of medications may also alter the excretion of chloride (Dyke et al., 1999).

Measurement of chloride

Numerous analyzers are now available for measurement of chloride concentration in serum, plasma, or whole blood. Serum is preferable when the samples will be stored for a significant length of time. While not all analyzers have been specifically validated for horses, point-of-care analyzers may be particularly useful in the intensive care or field setting (Grosenbaugh et al., 1998). The presence of bromide in plasma or serum, as occurs with sodium or potassium bromide administration, results in a false increase in the measured chloride concentration depending on the analyzer used (Fielding et al., 2003). Hyperlipemia may also have an effect on the measurement of chloride and result in a falsely lowered value, depending on the analyzer utilized.

Hypochloremia

Chloride concentrations that fall below the reference range can usually be placed in one of three categories described below and summarized in Box 4.1. The sample should be checked first for the presence of hyperlipemia as this could create a falsely low value. If lipemia is not

---

Box 4.1 Common causes of hypochloremia in horses.

- Increased loss of chloride:
  - Renal losses
  - Gastrointestinal losses
  - Sweat
- Decreased intake of chloride
- Dilution effect: increased extracellular fluid volume (ECFV) diluting remaining chloride ions.

---

present, the cause for the low chloride should be investigated. A finding of hypochloremia has been shown to have prognostic significance in equine medicine and can be associated with disease severity (Bristol, 1982; Clarke et al., 1982; Hjortkjaer & Svendsen, 1979; Koterba & Carlson, 1982; Reeves et al., 1989).

Increased chloride loss

Renal failure has been associated with hypochloremia in multiple studies in horses (Bayly et al., 1986; Brobst et al., 1977; Divers et al., 1987; Groover et al., 2006; Schott et al., 1997). In some cases, these horses had concurrent gastrointestinal disease making the true cause of the hypochloremia difficult to interpret. While fractional excretion of chloride may increase in renal failure, changes in the fractional excretion of electrolytes can be variable depending on electrolyte intake and should be interpreted in light of intake.

Chloride losses from the kidney may also increase in the absence of renal failure. Administration of fluids (particularly intravenous) has been shown to accelerate renal chloride losses (Rivas et al., 1997; Roussel et al., 1993; Rumbaugh et al., 1981), and specific medications (particularly diuretics) may also contribute (Carlson & Jones, 1999; Johansson et al., 2003; Toribio et al., 2007; Trim & Hanson, 1986). Perhaps most importantly, response to an acid–base abnormality (metabolic or respiratory acidosis) may result in a decrease in reabsorption of chloride and a resulting hypochloremia. It is important to recognize that this decrease in chloride concentration may be entirely appropriate and not require treatment. The role of chloride in acid–base balance is discussed more thoroughly in Chapter 8.

Gastrointestinal losses of chloride may occur due to decreased chloride absorption or increased chloride secretion. Chloride loss has been observed experimentally with increased salivary losses (Stick et al., 1981) and in a horse with esophageal obstruction (Brook & Schmidt, 1979). However, this is not a consistent feature of all horses with esophageal obstruction (Chiavaccini & Hassel, 2010). Increased volume of gastric reflux was speculated as a possible cause of hypochloremia in one study, but concurrent renal disease may have played a role as well (Groover et al., 2006). Colitis has also been associated with increased chloride losses, both clinically and experimentally (Ecke et al., 1998; Rikihisa et al., 1992; Roberts et al., 1989). Some medications may also increase chloride loss through the gastrointestinal system (Alexander, 1977).

Horse sweat has an increased chloride concentration relative to plasma; therefore prolonged exercise, particularly in hot climates, can produce hypochloremia (Barnes et al., 2010; Carlson et al., 1979; Deldar et al., 1982; Rose et al., 1980; Viu et al., 2010). Chloride losses in sweat may be attenuated by increased intake in the form of orally administered electrolytes. Oral electrolyte administration may explain the lack of hypochloremia observed in recent studies evaluating endurance horses (Fielding et al., 2009).

Decreased chloride intake

A large percentage of the chloride that is ingested daily by horses is eliminated in fecal output and urine (84% in one study: Groenendyk et al., 1988). Feed deprivation alone caused only a very mild hypochloremia (Freestone et al., 1991). In fact feed and water deprivation combined was shown to induce a hyperchloremia due to relative water deficit (Carlson et al., 1979; Carlson & Rumbaugh, 1983; Friend, 2000). Decreased chloride intake may exacerbate other causes of hypochloremia, but it should not necessarily be assumed as the primary cause in most clinical cases.

Dilution effect

The measured chloride concentration reflects the number of chloride ions divided by the volume of extracellular fluid. Hypochloremia can occur when the total number of chloride ions remains the same (i.e., there is no net loss of chloride ions) but the volume of fluid containing these ions increases (i.e., an expansion of the extracellular fluid volume (ECFV) with a low-chloride containing fluid).

A simple means for detecting this change is to correct the measured chloride concentration for expansion in the extracellular fluid volume. This can be done using the following equation:

$$Cl^-(corrected) = Cl^-(measured)$$
$$\times [Na^+(normal)/Na^+(measured)] \quad (4.1)$$

This equation relies on the principle that an expansion of the ECFV with water will have a similar effect on sodium and chloride and thus the corrected chloride will remain unchanged. One disadvantage is that this equation requires knowledge of one particular "normal"

serum sodium concentration for the specific animal on the given analyzer. This information is usually not available, but using an estimated normal can still provide a reasonable indication of the contribution of dilutional effects on the observed hypochloremia.

Hypochloremia resulting from the dilution effect is observed in clinical equine practice and can result when horses have access only to free water with no source of feed (Friend, 2000). Dilutional hypochloremia can also appear when intravenous fluids with minimal to no electrolytes (e.g., 5% dextrose in water) are administered. Dilution may also be a significant component of the hypochloremia observed in foals and horses with uroperitoneum (e.g., ruptured bladder) (Behr et al., 1981; Morley & Desnoyers, 1992; Richardson & Kohn, 1983). The urine in the peritoneal cavity represents an expansion of the ECFV with a fluid that is low in chloride.

Clinical approach to hypochloremia

When evaluating a horse with hypochloremia, the following stepwise evaluation can prove helpful:

1 Calculate the corrected chloride and determine if there is a dilutional effect. If the corrected chloride is normal, evaluate for causes of free water expansion of the ECF volume.

2 If the corrected chloride is decreased, evaluate for increased losses of chloride:

   (a) *Renal system:* Complete blood biochemistry panel and urinalysis (fractional excretion of chloride is not usually necessary). Evaluate specifically for renal disease and acid–base disturbances.

   (b) *Gastrointestinal system:* Evaluate for gastric reflux or signs of diarrhea.

   (c) *Sweat:* Evaluate for a history of prolonged exercise and excessive sweating or hyperhidrosis.

Clinical signs of hypochloremia

Hypochloremia is unlikely to be the cause of abnormal clinical examination findings in an equine patient. Its effects on acid–base balance may be associated with an alkalosis (see Chapter 8), which could manifest as observable clinical abnormalities. Hypochloremia can contribute to contraction of the ECFV (Garella et al., 1991) and could theoretically potentiate dehydration. Hypochloremia is often an important sign of ongoing acid–base or metabolic abnormalities in the patient, such as compensation for acidosis, and rapid correction may be unnecessary.

Treatment of hypochloremia

In many cases of hypochloremia, no specific treatment is required. If the low chloride concentration is providing normalization of an acid–base abnormality, correction of the hypochloremia could prove detrimental.

If it is deemed necessary to correct a hypochloremia, such as that associated with metabolic alkalosis, it can be corrected through intravenous or oral routes. Typically, intravenous treatment with a balanced electrolyte solution (e.g., Normosol™-R) that contains chloride in a concentration similar to equine plasma is sufficient to correct mild hypochloremia. In mild cases, oral supplementation with electrolytes or even just the normal diet may be enough to return chloride concentrations to normal.

As a general rule, treatment with a high-chloride-containing fluid (e.g., 0.9% saline) should be reserved for horses with a clinically significant metabolic alkalosis and concurrent hypochloremia. This is most likely to occur in horses that have lost large amounts of chloride through excessive sweating (i.e., endurance horses) or prolonged gastrointestinal losses (long-term esophageal obstruction or ongoing production of gastric reflux). If a metabolic alkalosis is not present with the hypochloremia, careful thought should be given to whether correction is necessary before administering fluids with a high chloride concentration (Box 4.2).

Hyperchloremia

Chloride concentrations that rise above the reference range can usually be attributed to one of three main causal categories as summarized in Box 4.3 and described below. A history of bromide administration should be ruled out as this can result in falsely elevated

> **Box 4.2 Important consideration for treating hypochloremia.**
>
> - If metabolic alkalosis is present, consider treatment with an intravenous fluid that has a high chloride concentration relative to plasma (e.g., 0.9% NaCl).
> - If metabolic alkalosis is not present, consider whether treatment is needed. A more balanced electrolyte solution (Normosol-R) may be appropriate.

> **Box 4.3 Common causes of hyperchloremia in horses.**
>
> - Retention of chloride:
>   - Renal dysfunction
> - Increased intake of chloride
> - Contraction effect: decreased extracellular fluid volume (ECFV) concentrating remaining chloride ions.

values. A finding of hyperchloremia has not been described as a significant feature of most diseases in equine practice. Unlike hypochloremia, it does not carry the same prognostic association in horses. However, given recent research findings describing an association of hyperchloremia with mortality in humans, this electrolyte abnormality should still be monitored carefully (Boniatti et al., 2011).

Retention of chloride

Renal dysfunction resulting in hyperchloremia is primarily described in cases of renal tubular acidosis (RTA). There are numerous reports in horses of this condition but the prevalence in equine practice is unknown (Aleman et al., 2001; MacLeay & Wilson, 1998; Trotter et al., 1986; van der Kolk 1994; van der Kolk & Kalsbeek, 1993; van der Kolk et al., 2007; Ziemer et al., 1987). It is possible that some mild cases may go undiagnosed and resolve without treatment.

Two types of RTA have been described in horses. They both result in a hyperchloremic metabolic acidosis and clinical signs of depression and anorexia. Tachypnea may also be present due to the compensatory mechanisms for metabolic acidosis (Aleman et al., 2001). Type I RTA occurs with distal tubular dysfunction and is classically described as a failure to excrete hydrogen ions. A strong ion approach to the mechanism of type I RTA would suggest that there is insufficient urinary NH_4^+ to remove adequate amounts of chloride in the urine. In type II RTA, the proximal tubule fails to resorb adequate bicarbonate. A strong ion approach to type II RTA would be consistent with an inappropriate reabsorption of chloride. Evaluation of urine pH has been proposed as a means for distinguishing between the two types of RTA in horses, but this may be more complicated given the normally alkaline urine of horses (Aleman et al., 2001). Type I RTA would be associated with more alkaline urine, and type II RTA with relatively more acidic urine.

An ammonium chloride challenge test was used to achieve a diagnosis in one study (Ziemer et al., 1987).

Renal retention of chloride may be appropriate in cases of respiratory alkalosis. Though not well documented in horses, this has been described in other species (Gennari et al., 1972). This is part of the normal response to an acid–base imbalance and the hyperchloremia does not require treatment. Diagnosis and management of the primary disease is warranted. The administration of diuretics including spironolactone and acetazolamide lead to renal retention of chloride and may result in hyperchloremia (Alexander, 1982a; Rose et al., 1990).

Increased intake of chloride

Changes in diet have been shown to alter plasma chloride concentrations in horses (McKenzie et al., 2002). Specifically, feeding a diet with a low dietary cation-anion balance (DCAB) resulted in a higher plasma chloride concentration as compared to a higher DCAB diet. The clinical significance of these changes is unclear, but likely has an effect on acid–base balance.

Administration of intravenous fluids containing chloride in concentrations above the normal plasma level has been shown to induce hyperchloremia in horses (Carlson & Rumbaugh, 1983; Fielding et al., 2008; Fielding & Magdesian, 2011). Figure 4.2 shows the changes in serum chloride concentration resulting from the administration of 0.9% NaCl in horses. Common intravenous fluids used in horses can have chloride concentrations as low as 0 mEq/L (5% dextrose), and as high as 1248 mEq/L (7.2% hypertonic

saline). If hyperchloremia develops in a horse receiving continuous intravenous fluids, careful assessment of the animal's fluid and electrolyte status as compared to the administered fluid should be performed. Even "balanced" fluids such as lactated Ringers' solution contain concentrations of chloride (109 mEq/L) that are higher than the plasma of many horses. Fluids supplemented with KCl will have even higher chloride concentrations and this additional chloride needs to be considered in the fluid plan. The change in chloride concentration may be particularly significant in cases where horses do not have access to free water (e.g., a horse with gastric reflux).

Administration of parenteral nutrition has been associated with hyperchloremia in foals (Myers et al., 2009). This may be due to the presence of amino acids that release chloride and generate hydrogen ions; alternatively, some amino acid solutions contain electrolytes with a relative excess of chloride and thus contribute to hyperchloremia; for example, Aminosyn II 8.5% with electrolytes (Hospira Inc., Lake Forest, Il) contains the following: $Na = 78$, $Cl = 86$, $K = 66$, $Mg = 10$, $P = 30$, acetate $= 61$ mEq/L. Horses receiving total parenteral nutrition (TPN) should be monitored carefully and fluids with a lower chloride concentration (i.e., Normosol-R) may be preferred as the concurrently administered fluid.

Contraction effect

The measured chloride concentration reflects the number of chloride ions divided by the volume of extracellular fluid. Hyperchloremia can occur when the total

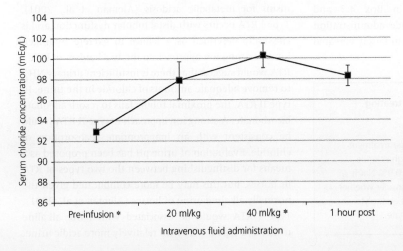

Figure 4.2 The effects of 0.9% NaCl administration on the serum chloride in dehydrated horses (n = 6). Based on C.L. Fielding and K.G. Magdesian, unpublished data.

number of chloride ions remains the same (i.e., there is no net loss of chloride ions) but the volume of fluid containing those ions decreases (i.e., a contraction of the ECFV, as in the case of water deprivation).

A simple means for detecting this change is to correct the measured chloride concentration for contraction of the extracellular fluid volume. This can be done using Equation 4.1. Hyperchloremia from the contraction effect is observed clinically when free water is unavailable to horses (Carlson et al., 1979; Friend, 2000).

Clinical approach to hyperchloremia

When evaluating a horse with hyperchloremia, the following stepwise evaluation can prove helpful:

1 Calculate the corrected chloride and determine if there is a contraction effect. If the corrected chloride is normal, evaluate for causes of a free water contraction of the ECFV.
2 If the corrected chloride is increased, evaluate for retention of chloride:
   (a) *Renal system:* Complete blood panel and urinalysis (including evaluation of urinary pH). Evaluate specifically for renal disease and acid–base disturbances.
   (b) *Medications:* Evaluate any medications that the animal is receiving.
   (c) *Gastrointestinal system:* Evaluate for secretory diarrhea (sodium bicarbonate loss).
3 Evaluate the fluid therapy plan and make sure that excessive chloride is not being administered (e.g., 0.9% sodium chloride).

Clinical signs of hyperchloremia

Hyperchloremia is unlikely to be the sole cause of abnormal clinical exam findings in an equine patient. Its effects on acid–base balance may be associated with an acidosis (see Chapter 8), and this may manifest as depression, anorexia, mild colic, or increased respiratory rate. The underlying disease is more likely to be the cause of any observed clinical abnormalities.

Treatment of hyperchloremia

Hyperchloremia should always be evaluated in conjunction with the acid–base status of the animal. Identification and treatment of the underlying cause should be the first priority unless a significant acidemia (pH < 7.2) is present. Treatment with sodium bicarbonate can be initiated and has been shown to

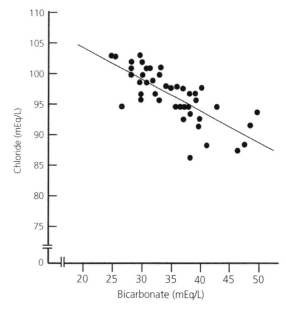

Figure 4.3 The inverse linear relationship of plasma chloride to plasma [HCO_3^-]. From Rumbaugh GE, Carlson GP, Harrold D. Clinicopathologic effects of rapid infusion of 5% sodium bicarbonate in 5% dextrose in the horse. *J Am Vet Med Assoc* 1981;**178**:267–71. Reproduced with permission.

reduce plasma chloride concentration in horses, as shown in Figure 4.3 (Rumbaugh et al., 1981). Sodium bicarbonate can be administered orally or intravenously. Calculation of the "required amount" of bicarbonate (using the base excess and ECFV) to correct hyperchloremic acidosis is commonly inaccurate due to ongoing losses. Beginning treatment with an intravenous isotonic sodium bicarbonate solution (made to a concentration of 140 mEq/L of sodium) at a rate of 2–4 mL/kg/h may be more useful. Monitoring of electrolytes every 6–12 hours is important. Adding sodium bicarbonate to a "balanced" electrolyte solution is less ideal as chloride ions would continue to be administered to the patient (as part of the balanced electrolyte solution).

Administration of oral sodium bicarbonate can be effective in patients with a functioning gastrointestinal system. In cases of severe renal tubular acidosis, intravenous sodium bicarbonate alone may be unsuccessful in resolving the hyperchloremic metabolic acidosis. Oral sodium bicarbonate can be administered in 100 g doses 2–4 times per day, but the dose can often be reduced in 24–48 hours or when the base deficit and pH are corrected. Some horses with RTA will require long-term oral sodium bicarbonate administration.

Foals

Available data suggest that plasma chloride concentrations and urinary fractional excretion rates are lower in healthy newborn foals as compared to adults (Edwards et al., 1990). This is consistent with a low chloride intake as through a primary milk diet in the newborn. In other species, there is evidence that newborn animals, as compared to adults, have altered chloride transport in the proximal tubule (Baum, 2008). Specifically, the neonatal proximal tubule is much less permeable to chloride as compared to adults (Baum, 2008). No specific research is available in foals.

The causes of hypochloremia in foals are similar to those in adult horses, but much less research is available. Loss of chloride can potentially occur with renal failure, as was described in one foal with renal dysplasia (Zicker et al., 1990). Hypochloremia can also be a normal compensatory response to an acidosis. Losses from the gastrointestinal system may occur with enteritis. Sweat losses are an unlikely cause of hypochloremia in foals because of reduced sweating ability in foals as compared to adults. Decreased intake of chloride may contribute to hypochloremia, but it is unlikely to be the sole cause. The dilution effect with free water can be observed in foals when there are mixing errors in milk replacers, and this problem has been identified in neonates in other species (Felder et al., 1987). Foals with access only to free water can show similar abnormalities (along with hyponatremia).

Hypochloremia was documented in some foals derived from somatic cell nuclear transfer (Johnson et al., 2010), but it was not a consistent feature of all animals. Hypochloremia was not associated with survival in foals in a large retrospective study utilizing a probability model (Rohrbach et al., 2006) or in a retrospective study evaluating foals with diarrhea (Magdesian et al., 2002). In the author's experience, hypochloremia can be observed in some sick newborn foals without an obvious etiology; there is no research in foals available to elucidate the cause.

Hyperchloremia can be observed in foals as a compensatory response to an alkalosis. There are no scientific reports of RTA in foals; however, some hospitalized foals develop hyperchloremia that has not been described in the scientific literature. Administration of parenteral nutrition (Myers et al., 2009) has been associated with hyperchloremia in foals. Continuous infusion of an isotonic crystalloid in healthy foals mildly increased serum chloride concentrations (Buchanan et al., 2005), but foals were able to increase their renal elimination of chloride in response to the infusion. Similarly, a bolus administration of 0.9% isotonic saline to newborn foals resulted in mild increases in chloride concentration similar to adults (C.L. Fielding & K.G. Magdesian, unpublished data).

References

Aleman MR, Kuesis B, Schott HC, et al. (2001) Renal tubular acidosis in horses (1980–1999). *J Vet Intern Med* **15**:136–43.

Alexander F. (1962) The concentration of certain electrolytes in the digestive tract of the horse and pig. *Res Vet Sci* **3**:78–84.

Alexander F. (1966) A study of parotid salivation in the horse. *J. Physiol* **184**:646–56.

Alexander F. (1977) The effect of diuretics on the faecal excretion of water and electrolytes in horses. *Br J Pharmacol* **60**:589–93.

Alexander F. (1982a) The effect of ethacrynic acid, bumetanide, frusemide, spironolactone and ADH on electrolyte excretion in ponies. *J Vet Pharmacol Ther* **5**:153–60.

Alexander F. (1982b) Effect of phenylbutazone on electrolyte metabolism in ponies. *Vet Rec* **110**:271–2.

Barnes A, Kingston J, Beetson S, et al. (2010) Endurance veterinarians detect physiologically compromised horses in a 160 km ride. *Equine Vet J Suppl* **38**:6–11.

Baum M. (2008) Developmental changes in proximal tubule NaCl transport. *Pediatr Nephrol* **23**:185–94.

Bayly WM, Brobst DF, Elfers RS, et al. (1986) Serum and urinary biochemistry and enzyme changes in ponies with acute renal failure. *Cornell Vet* **76**:306–16.

Behr MJ, Hackett RP, Bentinck-Smith J, et al. (1981) Metabolic abnormalities associated with rupture of the urinary bladder in neonatal foals. *J Am Vet Med Assoc* **178**:263–6.

Boniatti MM, Cardoso PR, Castilho RK, et al. (2011) Is hyperchloremia associated with mortality in critically ill patients? A prospective cohort study. *J Crit Care* **26**:175–9.

Bristol DG. (1982) The anion gap as a prognostic indicator in horses with abdominal pain. *J Am Vet Med Assoc* **181**:63–5.

Brobst DF, Grant BD, Hilbert BJ, et al. (1977) Blood biochemical changes in horses with prerenal and renal disease. *J Eq Med Surg* **1**:171–7.

Brook D, Schmidt GR. (1979) Pre-renal azotaemia in a pony with an oesophageal obstruction. *Equine Vet J* **11**:53–5.

Buchanan BR, Sommardahl CS, Rohrbach BW, et al. (2005) Effect of a 24-hour infusion of an isotonic electrolyte replacement fluid on the renal clearance of electrolytes in healthy neonatal foals. *J Am Vet Med Assoc* **227**:1123–9.

Carlson GP, Ocen PO, Harrold D. (1976) Clinicopathologic alterations in normal and exhausted endurance horses. *Theriogenology* **6**:93–104.

Carlson GP, Rumbaugh GE, Harrold D. (1979) Physiologic alterations in the horse produced by food and water deprivation during periods of high environmental temperatures. *Am J Vet Res* **40**:982–5.

Carlson GP, Rumbaugh GE. (1983) Response to saline solution of normally fed horses and horses dehydrated by fasting. *Am J Vet Res* **44**:964–8.

Carlson GP, Jones JH. (1999) Effects of frusemide on electrolyte and acid–base balance during exercise. *Equine Vet J Suppl* **30**:370–4.

Cehak A, Burmester M, Geburek F, et al. (2009) Electrophysiological characterization of electrolyte and nutrient transport across the small intestine in horses. *J Anim Physiol Anim Nutr (Berl)* **93**:287–94.

Chiavaccini L, Hassel DM. (2010) Clinical features and prognostic variables in 109 horses with esophageal obstruction (1992–2009). *J Vet Intern Med* **24**:1147–52.

Clarke LL, Garner HE, Hatfield D. (1982) Plasma volume, electrolyte, and endocrine changes during onset of laminitis hypertension in horses. *Am J Vet Res* **43**:1551–5.

Clarke LL, Argenzio RA. (1990) NaCl transport across equine proximal colon and the effect of endogenous prostanoids. *Am J Physiol* **259**:G62–9.

Clarke LL, Roberts MC, Grubb BR, et al. (1992) Short-term effect of aldosterone on Na-Cl transport across equine colon. *Am J Physiol* **262**:R939–46.

Deldar A, Fregin FG, Bloom JC, et al. (1982) Changes in selected biochemical constituents of blood collected from horses participating in a 50-mile endurance ride. *Am J Vet Res* **43**:2239–43.

Divers TJ, Whitlock RH, Byars TD, et al. (1987) Acute renal failure in six horses resulting from haemodynamic causes. *Equine Vet J* **19**:178–84.

Dyke TM, Hinchcliff KW, Sams RA. (1999) Attenuation by phenylbutazone of the renal effects and excretion of frusemide in horses. *Equine Vet J* **31**:289–95.

Ecke P, Hodgson DR, Rose RJ. (1998) Induced diarrhoea in horses. Part 1: Fluid and electrolyte balance. *Vet J* **155**:149–59.

Edwards DJ, Brownlow MA, Hutchins DR. (1990) Indices of renal function: values in eight normal foals from birth to 56 days. *Aust Vet J* **67**:251–4.

Felder CC, Robillard JE, Roy S 3rd, et al. (1987) Severe chloride deficiency in the neonate: the canine puppy as an animal model. *Pediatr Res* **21**:497–501.

Fielding CL, Magdesian KG. (2011) A comparison of hypertonic (7.2%) and isotonic (0.9%) saline for fluid resuscitation in horses: a randomized, double-blinded, clinical trial. *J Vet Intern Med* **25**:1138–43.

Fielding CL, Magdesian KG, Elliott DA, et al. (2003) Pharmacokinetics and clinical utility of sodium bromide

(NaBr) as an estimator of extracellular fluid volume in horses. *J Vet Intern Med* **17**:213–17.

Fielding CL, Magdesian KG, Carlson GP, et al. (2008) Application of the sodium dilution principle to calculate extracellular fluid volume changes in horses during dehydration and rehydration. *Am J Vet Res* **69**:1506–11.

Fielding CL, Magdesian KG, Rhodes DM, et al. (2009) Clinical and biochemical abnormalities in endurance horses eliminated from competition for medical complications and requiring emergency medical treatment: 30 cases (2005–2006). *J Vet Emerg Crit Care (San Antonio)* **19**:473–8.

Freestone JF, Carlson GP, Harrold DR, et al. (1989) Furosemide and sodium bicarbonate-induced alkalosis in the horse and response to oral KCl or NaCl therapy. *Am J Vet Res* **50**:1334–9.

Freestone JF, Gossett K, Carlson GP, et al. (1991) Exercise induced alterations in the serum muscle enzymes, erythrocyte potassium and plasma constituents following feed withdrawal or furosemide and sodium bicarbonate administration in the horse. *J Vet Intern Med* **5**:40–6.

Friend TH. (2000) Dehydration, stress, and water consumption of horses during long-distance commercial transport. *J Anim Sci* **78**:2568–80.

Garella S, Cohen JJ, Northrup TE. (1991) Chloride-depletion metabolic alkalosis induces ECF volume depletion via internal fluid shifts in nephrectomized dogs. *Eur J Clin Invest* **21**:273–9.

Gennari FJ, Goldstein MB, Schwartz WB. (1972) The nature of the renal adaptation to chronic hypocapnia. *J Clin Invest* **51**:1722–30.

Giddings RF, Argenzio RA, Stevens CE. (1974) Sodium and chloride transport across the equine cecal mucosa. *Am J Vet Res* **35**:1511–14.

Groenendyk S, English PB, Abetz I. (1988) External balance of water and electrolytes in the horse. *Equine Vet J* **20**:189–93.

Groover ES, Woolums AR, Cole DJ, et al. (2006) Risk factors associated with renal insufficiency in horses with primary gastrointestinal disease: 26 cases (2000–2003). *J Am Vet Med Assoc* **228**:572–7.

Grosenbaugh DA, Gadawski JE, Muir WW. (1998) Evaluation of a portable clinical analyzer in a veterinary hospital setting. *J Am Vet Med Assoc* **213**:691–4.

Hejłasz Z, Nicpoń J, Czerw P. (1994) The role of sweat in maintaining the stimulation of effort homeostasis in horses. *Arch Vet Pol* **34**:231–9.

Hjortkjaer RK, Svendsen CK. (1979) Simulated small intestinal volvulus in the anesthetized horse. *Nord Vet Med* **31**:466–83.

Johansson AM, Gardner SY, Levine JF, et al. (2003) Furosemide continuous rate infusion in the horse: evaluation of enhanced efficacy and reduced side effects. *J Vet Intern Med* **17**:887–95.

Johnson AK, Clark-Price SC, Choi YH, et al. (2010) Physical and clinicopathologic findings in foals derived by use of somatic cell nuclear transfer: 14 cases (2004–2008). *J Am Vet Med Assoc* **236**:983–90.

Kingston JK, Geor RJ, McCutcheon LJ. (1997) Rate and composition of sweat fluid losses are unaltered by hypohydration during prolonged exercise in horses. *J Appl Physiol* **83**:1133–43.

Koterba A, Carlson GP. (1982) Acid-base and electrolyte alterations in horses with exertional rhabdomyolysis. *J Am Vet Med Assoc* **180**:303–6.

Latson KM, Nieto JE, Beldomenico PM, et al. (2005) Evaluation of peritoneal fluid lactate as a marker of intestinal ischaemia in equine colic. *Equine Vet J* **37**:342–6.

MacLeay JM, Wilson JH. (1998) Type-II renal tubular acidosis and ventricular tachycardia in a horse. *J Am Vet Med Assoc* **212**:1597–9.

Magdesian KG, Hirsh DC, Jang SS, et al. (2002) Characterization of Clostridium difficile isolates from foals with diarrhea: 28 cases (1993–1997). *J Am Vet Med Assoc* **220**:67–73.

Mayhew IG, Whitlock RH, Tasker JB. (1977) Equine cerebrospinal fluid: reference values of normal horses. *Am J Vet Res* **38**:1271–4.

McKenzie EC, Valberg SJ, Godden SM, et al. (2002) Plasma and urine electrolyte and mineral concentrations in Thoroughbred horses with recurrent exertional rhabdomyolysis after consumption of diets varying in cation-anion balance. *Am J Vet Res* **63**:1053–60.

Morley PS, Desnoyers M. (1992) Diagnosis of ruptured urinary bladder in a foal by the identification of calcium carbonate crystals in the peritoneal fluid. *J Am Vet Med Assoc* **200**:1515–17.

Morris DD, Divers TJ, Whitlock RH. (1984) Renal clearance and fractional excretion of electrolytes over a 24-hour period in horses. *Am J Vet Res* **45**:2431–5.

Myers CJ, Magdesian KG, Kass PH, et al. (2009) Parenteral nutrition in neonatal foals: clinical description, complications and outcome in 53 foals (1995–2005). *Vet J* **181**:137–44.

Planelles G. (2004) Chloride transport in the renal proximal tubule. *Pflugers Arch* **448**:561–70.

Rawlings CA, Bisgard GE. (1975) Renal clearance and excretion of endogenous substances in the small pony. *Am J Vet Res* **36**:45–8.

Reeves MJ, Curtis CR, Salman MD, et al. (1989) Prognosis in equine colic patients using multivariable analysis. *Can J Vet Res* **53**:87–94.

Richardson DW, Kohn CW. (1983) Uroperitoneum in the foal. *J Am Vet Med Assoc* **182**:267–71.

Rikihisa Y, Johnson GC, Wang YZ, et al. (1992) Loss of absorptive capacity for sodium and chloride in the colon causes diarrhoea in Potomac horse fever. *Res Vet Sci* **52**:353–62.

Rivas LJ, Hinchcliff KW, Kohn CW, et al. (1997) Effect of sodium bicarbonate administration on renal function of horses. *Am J Vet Res* **58**:664–71.

Roberts MC, Clarke LL, Johnson CM. (1989) Castor-oil induced diarrhoea in ponies: a model for acute colitis. *Equine Vet J Suppl* **7**:60–7.

Rohrbach BW, Buchanan BR, Drake JM, et al. (2006) Use of a multivariable model to estimate the probability of discharge in hospitalized foals that are 7 days of age or less. *J Am Vet Med Assoc* **228**:1748–56.

Rose RJ, Arnold KS, Church S, et al. (1980) Plasma and sweat electrolyte concentrations in the horse during long distance exercise. *Equine Vet J* **12**:19–22.

Roussel AJ, Cohen ND, Ruoff WW, et al. (1993) Urinary indices of horses after intravenous administration of crystalloid solutions. *J Vet Intern Med* **7**:241–6.

Rumbaugh GE, Carlson GP, Harrold D. (1981) Clinicopathologic effects of rapid infusion of 5% sodium bicarbonate in 5% dextrose in the horse. *J Am Vet Med Assoc* **178**:267–71.

Rumbaugh GE, Carlson GP, Harrold D. (1982) Urinary production in the healthy horse and in horses deprived of feed and water. *Am J Vet Res* **43**:735–7.

Schott HC, Patterson KS, Fitzgerald SD, et al. (1997) Chronic renal failure in 99 horses. In: Proceedings of the 43rd Annual Convention of the American Association of Equine Practitioners, pp. 345–6.

Schott HC, Marlin DJ, Geor RJ, et al. (2006) Changes in selected physiological and laboratory measurements in elite horses competing in a 160 km endurance ride. *Equine Vet J Suppl* **36**:37–42.

Spooner HS, Nielsen BD, Schott HC, et al. (2010) Sweat composition in Arabian horses performing endurance exercise on forage-based, low Na rations. *Equine Vet J Suppl* **42**:382–6.

Stick JA, Robinson NE, Krehbiel JD. (1981) Acid-base and electrolyte alterations associated with salivary loss in the pony. *Am J Vet Res* **42**:733–7.

Toribio RE, Kohn CW, Rourke KM, et al. (2007) Effects of hypercalcemia on serum concentrations of magnesium, potassium, and phosphate and urinary excretion of electrolytes in horses. *Am J Vet Res* **68**:543–54.

Trim CM, Hanson RR. (1986) Effects of xylazine on renal function and plasma glucose in ponies. *Vet Rec* **118**:65–7.

Trotter GW, Miller D, Parks A, et al. (1986) Type II renal tubular acidosis in a mare. *J Am Vet Med Assoc* **188**:1050–1.

van der Kolk JH. (1994) Renal tubular acidosis (type 2) in a Friesian mare. *Tijdschr Diergeneeskd* **119**:675–6.

van der Kolk JH, Kalsbeek HC. (1993) Renal tubular acidosis in a mare. *Vet Rec* **133**:43–4.

van der Kolk JH, de Graaf-Roelfsema E, Joles JA, et al. (2007) Mixed proximal and distal renal tubular acidosis without aminoaciduria in a mare. *J Vet Intern Med* **21**:1121–5.

Viu J, Jose-Cunilleras E, Armengou L, et al. (2010) Acid–base imbalances during a 120 km endurance race compared by traditional and simplified strong ion difference methods. *Equine Vet J Suppl* **38**:76–82.

Watson ZE, Steffey EP, VanHoogmoed LM, et al. (2002) Effect of general anesthesia and minor surgical trauma on urine and serum measurements in horses. *Am J Vet Res* **63**:1061–5.

Zicker SC, Marty GD, Carlson GP, et al. (1990) Bilateral renal dysplasia with nephron hypoplasia in a foal. *J Am Vet Med Assoc* **196**:2001–5.

Ziemer EL, Parker HR, Carlson GP, et al. (1987) Renal tubular acidosis in two horses: diagnostic studies. *J Am Vet Med Assoc* **190**:289–93.

CHAPTER 5

Calcium homeostasis and derangements

Escolástico Aguilera-Tejero

Dept. Medicina y Cirugía Animal Universidad de Córdoba, Spain

Physiology of calcium homeostasis

Calcium is an important mineral in all vertebrates. Even though the vast majority of calcium is located in the skeleton for structural purposes, calcium also has major functions in a variety of key physiologic processes like muscle contraction, blood coagulation, and cardiovascular function, among others.

The body distribution of calcium in horses is shown in Figure 5.1. Skeletal calcium accounts for more than 99% of the total body calcium content and represents a store of calcium that, to a certain limit, can be mobilized when necessary. In contrast, the intracellular calcium concentration in soft tissues is very low. The relationship between extracellular and intracellular calcium is of several orders of magnitude (millimolar vs nanomolar, respectively). Thus although intracellular calcium is a key secondary messenger for a wide variety of cellular processes, rarely will it be compromised by pathologic changes in extracellular calcium. In addition to its role as an intracellular messenger, calcium has marked influence on resting and threshold membrane potentials. Movement of calcium across the cell membrane, through calcium channels, is very important in the function of muscle and nerve cells.

From a clinical point of view, extracellular calcium concentration is the most relevant. Changes in extracellular calcium are responsible for clinical disorders – hypercalcemia and hypocalcemia – and fluid therapy is aimed at correcting abnormalities in extracellular calcium. Extracellular calcium includes the calcium contained in the interstitial fluid and plasma, the latter being the only one that can be readily sampled and thus monitored.

In plasma, calcium is found in three fractions: protein-bound calcium, ionized calcium, and complexed calcium. The protein-bound calcium is non-diffusible in contrast to ionized and complexed calcium, which represent what is also called ultrafilterable calcium. The sum of these three fractions is total calcium (Figure 5.1). Total plasma calcium concentration in horses is relatively high when compared with most mammals. The normal concentration of total calcium in equine plasma is approximately 12 mg/dL, which is approximately 20% more than in other species such as many carnivores, ruminants, or humans. About 50% of plasma calcium is bound to proteins, primarily albumin, and this calcium fraction is inactive because it cannot interact with calcium receptors. However, since the protein-bound calcium can be displaced to form ionized calcium, it represents a blood store of calcium that is more accessible than the calcium contained in bone. Ionized calcium is the active fraction of calcium and represents roughly the other half of total blood calcium. In reality both protein-bound and ionized calcium represent slightly less than 50% each, because 3–5% of calcium is complexed to different anions: citrate, bicarbonate, phosphate, and lactate (Lopez et al., 2006a). The physiologic dogma considers that only ionized calcium is active since it is the only form able to bind the calcium-sensing receptor; however, there is evidence suggesting that complexed calcium may also have some biological activity.

In the interstitial fluid, calcium is present in the non-protein-bound fractions, ionized and complexed calcium,

---

Equine Fluid Therapy, First Edition. Edited by C. Langdon Fielding and K. Gary Magdesian.

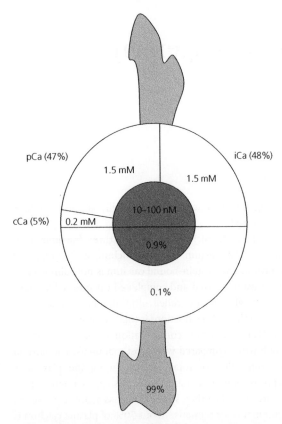

pCa (47%)

iCa (48%)

1.5 mM

1.5 mM

10–100 nM

cCa (5%)   0.2 mM

0.9%

0.1%

99%

Figure 5.1 Body distribution of calcium in horses. Calcium is located in three main compartments: intracellular (inner circle), extracellular (outer circle), and the skeleton. cCa, complexed calcium; iCa, ionized calcium; pCa, protein-bound calcium.

at the same concentration as in plasma. From a physiologic point of view it makes sense to consider the ultrafilterable calcium pool, in plasma and interstitial fluid, as a single compartment of biologically active calcium (i.e., the ultrafilterable calcium pool of the extracellular fluid compartment).

Extracellular calcium concentration is regulated by a complex hormonal mechanism that modulates the intestinal absorption of calcium, its urinary excretion, and the osseous storage or disposition. The calcium-sensing receptor (CaSR) is central in this system because it senses extracellular calcium concentration and signals the secretion of calciotropic hormones. The CaSR is a G-protein-coupled cell surface receptor with three structural domains (extracellular, transmembrane, and cytoplasmic) that represents the molecular mechanism by which many cell types perceive calcium changes in

blood. The extracellular domain interacts with ionized calcium, triggering several intracellular mechanisms involved in the cell response to changes in calcium. The CaSR is located in all cell types that secrete calciotropic hormones including parathyroid cells and thyroid C-cells, and also in cells that regulate calcium transport (e.g., intestinal and renal cells). The CaSR is not calcium-specific and can be activated by other divalent cations (e.g. Mg^{2+}), trivalent cations (Gd^{3+}), and polycations (neomycin) (Brown et al., 1993).

The main hormones involved in calcium homeostasis are: parathyroid hormone, vitamin D, and calcitonin (Figure 5.2).

Parathyroid hormone (PTH) is secreted by the chief cells of the parathyroid glands in response to decreased levels of blood ionized calcium. Anatomically, parathyroid glands are quite different in horses when compared with better studied species (humans, carnivores, rodents). As in other ungulates, in addition to the external and internal glands adjacent to the thyroid, accessory parathyroid glands located more caudally, along the trachea, may be found in horses. Despite the anatomic difference in the glands, the actions of PTH in horses are very similar to those in carnivores, rodents, and humans. PTH is the main hormone involved in the acute regulation of extracellular calcium concentration; the PTH response to changes in calcium concentrations is almost instantaneous. When a decrease in blood ionized calcium concentration is sensed by the CaSR located in the parathyroid cells, PTH synthesis and secretion increase. The PTH response is best described by a sigmoidal curve: the PTH–calcium curve. The PTH–calcium curve in horses is similar to that in other mammals, although due to the higher baseline calcium values, the set-point of the curve (serum calcium corresponding to 50% of maximal PTH secretion) is also higher in horses. Hysteresis of the PTH–calcium curve (lower PTH values during recovery from hypocalcemia than during induction of hypocalcemia) has been documented in horses (Toribio et al., 2003c). When extracellular calcium is low, the increased PTH concentration will act at two target organs, bone and kidney, where PTH interacts with its receptor. There are two PTH receptors but most of the physiologic PTH actions are due to interaction with what is known as the "classical" PTH receptor (PTHR1). It is interesting to note that even though PTH promotes bone resorption to shift calcium from bone to the extracellular compartment, osteoclasts do

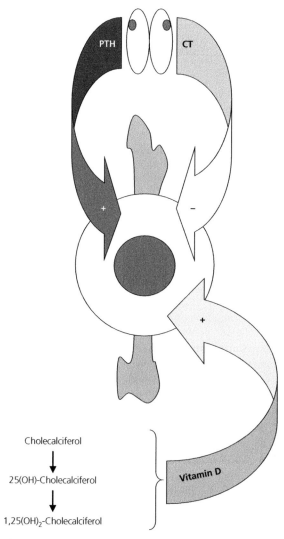

Cholecalciferol

$\downarrow$

25(OH)-Cholecalciferol

$\downarrow$

1,25(OH)$_2$-Cholecalciferol

Figure 5.2 Hormonal influences on extracellular calcium. Both parathyroid hormone (PTH) and vitamin D have hypercalcemic actions while calcitonin (CT) has a hypocalcemic effect.

Vitamin D is ingested with the diet as a provitamin: vitamin D$_2$ (of vegetal origin) or vitamin D$_3$ (of animal origin). Vitamin D$_3$ can also be synthesized in the skin exposed to sunlight from 7-dehydrocholesterol. Vitamin D must be metabolized to attain biological activity. In most species this involves hepatic hydroxylation to form 25-hydroxyvitamin D (also known as calcidiol), with little biological activity, and a second renal hydroxylation that originates 1,25-dihydroxyvitamin D (also named calcitriol), which is the active form of vitamin D. In addition, other metabolites with variable vitamin D activity (e.g. 24,25-dihydroxyvitamin D) can be measured in blood. In horses vitamin D metabolism seems to be complex, and contradictory reports can be found in the literature. It has been suggested that horses lack 1-α-hydroxylase (the renal enzyme that converts calcidiol to calcitriol) and that calcitriol would not be the main active vitamin D metabolite in this species (Breidenbach et al., 1998). However, many authors have reported consistent measurements of calcitriol in horse plasma. Although quite variable, calcitriol levels tend to be lower in horses than in most mammals (Estepa et al., 2006; Harmeyer & Schlumbohm, 2004). Whether this means that vitamin D is less important in horses than in other species or that vitamin D metabolites other than calcitriol are mainly responsible for vitamin D actions remains to be elucidated. Vitamin D interacts with the vitamin D receptor (VDR), a nuclear receptor that is widely distributed in the body. Calcium metabolism is regulated by VDRs located in the intestine, the kidney, and the parathyroid glands. At the intestinal level vitamin D promotes calcium absorption. An equine peculiarity is a low level of VDR expression in the small intestine (Rourke et al., 2010), and this could explain why in horses intestinal absorption of calcium seems to be somewhat independent of vitamin D. The interaction of vitamin D with bone VDR results in movement of calcium from bone to extracellular fluid and, based on the studies in which high doses of vitamin D have been administered to horses, the main calcemic actions of vitamin D seem to be skeletal (Harmeyer & Schlumbohm, 2004). Thus, although vitamin D also inhibits PTH synthesis and secretion by acting on VDRs located in the parathyroid glands, the combined effect of vitamin D at intestinal and osseous levels is hypercalcemic. It is also important to note that, in contrast with PTH, vitamin D does not participate in the acute regulation of extracellular calcium; its effects are more delayed and influence longer term calcium balance.

not express PTH receptors. In bone the PTH receptors are located in osteoblasts, thus some kind of paracrine signaling is necessary to activate osteoclasts in response to elevated PTH. The second target organ is the kidney and here PTH has two distinct actions: (i) decreasing urinary excretion of calcium; and (ii) increasing the production of active vitamin D metabolites. Both renal actions will have a common result – an increase in extracellular calcium.

Calcitonin is a hypocalcemic hormone secreted by thyroid C-cells in response to hypercalcemia. Calcitonin interacts with its receptor and promotes hypocalcemia primarily by decreasing osteoclastic bone resorption. In addition, calcitonin also has some positive influence on renal calcium excretion and in the long term may impair intestinal calcium absorption. The sequence of the calcitonin gene has been recently elucidated in horses and its homology with human calcitonin has been determined to be around 90% (Toribio et al., 2003b). In most mammals, and probably horses as well, calcitonin has a minor role in the homeostatic mechanisms that control extracellular calcium concentration.

Calcium balance results from the equilibrium between calcium intake and calcium excretion (Figure 5.3). Calcium enters the body by the digestive system and is excreted in feces, urine, sweat, and milk. Since horses have obligatory losses of calcium that approach 2.5 g of calcium per 100 kg of body weight, this would be the minimum daily requirement of calcium. However, absorption of ingested calcium ranges between 50 and 66%, thus it would be necessary to provide at least 5 g of calcium per 100 kg of body weight to assure correct daily intake (Schryver et al., 1970). The calcium

Table 5.1 Calcium content of common equine foods. It should be noted that vegetal food may be subject to substantial variations in calcium content.

Food	% Calcium
Alfalfa hay	1–2
Beet pulp	0.7–1.1
Grass hay[a]	0.2–0.5
Cereal grain[b]	0.05–0.1

[a] Bermuda, timothy, orchard-grass, etc.
[b] Oats, barley, corn (maize), etc.

contained in most equine foods is readily available, although there are large differences in calcium content of feedstuffs (Table 5.1).

Intestinal absorption of calcium, which takes place preferentially in the upper half of the small intestine, is directly correlated with dietary calcium intake. Two mechanisms are involved in intestinal calcium transport: paracellular (passive, concentration dependent) and transcellular (active, regulated by hormones) transportation. Paracellular calcium transport seems to be more important in horses than in other species. In horses the main genes involved in transcellular calcium transport are the transient receptor potential vanilloid member 5 (TRPV5) and calbinding D9k (CB9) (Rourke et al., 2010). Excretion of fecal calcium has two components: endogenous fecal calcium excretion, which is somewhat independent of calcium intake; and unabsorbed fecal excretion, which depends on the calcium content of the diet. Renal calcium excretion is very important in horses and is directly related to calcium intake. In the kidney, most of the filtered calcium (around 60%) is reabsorbed passively in the proximal tubules. In the distal nephron an additional 30–35% of the filtered calcium is actively reabsorbed. The remaining 5–10% is excreted in urine. The high fractional excretion of calcium seems to be coupled to intestinal absorption. Since horses absorb great quantities of calcium in the intestine, they also must be able to excrete large amounts of calcium in urine. Calcium losses by sweat, which may be substantial (up to 500 mg of calcium per hour), are not part of the normal calcium homeostatic system but rather an epiphenomenon derived from thermoregulatory needs (Schryver et al., 1978). An additional source of calcium loss is milk in lactating mares. Mare's milk contains close to 1 g of calcium per liter. Thus, lactation represents an

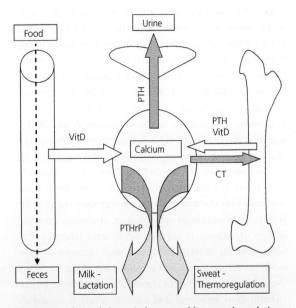

Figure 5.3 Calcium balance in horses and hormonal regulation of calcium transport. White arrows indicate calcium influx and gray arrows calcium efflux. CT, calcitonin; PTH, parathyroid hormone; PTHrP, parathyroid hormone-related peptide; VitD, vitamin D.

Table 5.2 Reference values for parameters of calcium metabolism in horses. Ranges reported in the table have been kept fairly narrow on purpose, to facilitate practical application. Thus small deviations from these values may not have clinical significance.

	tCa	iCa	I-PTH	Calcidiol	Calcitriol	Calcitonin
Conventional units	11–14 mg/dL	5.5–7.0 mg/dL	10–60 pg/mL	2–12 ng/mL	10–35 pg/mL	5–30 pg/mL
International (SI) units	2.8–3.3 mmol/L	1.4–1.6 mmol/L	1.1–6.3 pmol/L[a]	5–30 nmol/L	25–85 pmol/L	5–30 ng/L

tCa, total calcium; iCa, ionized calcium; I-PTH, intact PTH.
[a] Since PTH is measured with a heterologous assay, perfect conversion to SI units is not possible; the conversion factor has been based on the molecular weight of human PTH.

important source of calcium loss. When horses are in positive calcium balance, calcium is stored in bone. Skeletal calcium storage in horses on high-calcium diets is achieved primarily by decreasing calcium removal from bone rather than by increasing calcium deposition in bone (Schryver et al., 1974).

Calcium metabolism has not been well studied in foals. Parathyroid hormone related peptide (PTHrP) plays a major role in fetal calcium metabolism and may also be important in young foals since this hormone is present in high concentrations in milk (Care et al., 1997). As with all growing animals, foals have increased requirements for dietary calcium and calcium losses are minimized to facilitate bone growth.

Measurement of calcium and related parameters

This chapter is focused on the diagnosis and treatment of hyper- and hypocalcemia in horses. Thus, it is interesting to review the parameters that are useful for diagnosing and monitoring these disorders and their normal ranges in horses (Table 5.2).

Calcium measurement
Total calcium

Total calcium (tCa) is the most frequently reported measurement of extracellular calcium. Quantification of tCa is included in most biochemical profiles. It can be measured in plasma or in serum and samples do not have special requirements for storage. In fact plasma/serum calcium is quite stable. If plasma is going to be used, it is essential not to employ an EDTA-based anticoagulant (heparinized plasma is acceptable). Traditionally, tCa is reported as mg/dL and the normal range in horses is 11–14 mg/dL (slight interlab variation).

Ionized calcium

Ionized calcium (iCa or Ca^{2+}) is the active calcium fraction and, therefore, the one with the most clinical interest. Ionized calcium can be measured in whole blood, plasma, or serum. The preferred sample is whole blood, thus iCa is often referred to as "blood iCa". The sample should be taken in anaerobic conditions and processed as soon as possible because, since the equilibrium between ionized calcium and protein-bound calcium is pH dependent, changes in pH will alter iCa: acidemia increases iCa and alkalemia decreases iCa. If immediate measurement cannot be performed samples should be refrigerated until measurement. Ionized calcium can also be quantified in plasma or serum; the main problem associated with these measurements is the difficulty in avoiding air exposure of the sample and thus changes in sample pH are often found. Ionized calcium is measured by selective electrodes or dry chemistry techniques and most measurement machines provide the actual values in the sample and values corrected to a standard pH (7.4). An equation has been specifically developed for pH correction of iCa values in horses (van der Kolk et al., 2002) but other studies reported a poor predictability in the correction of iCa values from pH (Kohn & Brooks, 1990). On the other hand it is important to keep in mind that the "real" iCa of the patient is the calcium at the measured pH and not what would be at a standard pH. Several formulae permit calculation of iCa from tCa by taking into account the albumin or total protein concentrations. However, since a poor correlation between albumin and calcium has been reported in horses (Bienzle et al., 1993), the use of these equations should be viewed with caution. In conclusion, although possible, it is not very reliable to use equations for calculation of iCa and whenever feasible iCa should be measured. It is common to report iCa as mmol/L and the normal range in horses is 1.4–1.6 mmol/L.

Measurement of calciotropic hormones

In the investigation of hyper- and hypocalcemia it is often necessary to measure calciotropic hormones. In the next sections, the measurements that are available and have been validated for use in horses are briefly reviewed.

Parathyroid hormone

Parathyroid hormone is measured mainly by immuno-radiometric (IRMA) techniques. No homologous assay is currently available for measurement of equine PTH, thus heterologous assays (assays incorporating antibodies against the PTH molecule of other species) are used. Assays using antibodies against both rat and human PTH have been validated in horses (Estepa et al., 1998). Most laboratories will use human assays. The immnunochemical behavior of equine PTH suggests that this hormone possesses a 1–34 aminoterminal portion, that is responsible for its biological activity, very similar to human PTH (Raulais et al., 1981). In human medicine there are second-generation assays that measure "intact" PTH, and third-generation assays for measurement of "whole" PTH. Both of these have been validated in horses (Estepa et al., 2003). Although the third-generation assays theoretically have better diagnostic sensitivity, due to limited availability most laboratories utilize assays for measurement of "intact" human PTH. Parathyroid hormone can be measured in plasma or serum samples, and no special handling requirements are necessary. Samples can be safely refrigerated for 24 h and can be frozen for more than 2 months. Conventional units for PTH are pg/mL and "intact" PTH values in normal horses range between 10 and 60 pg/mL (although some inter-laboratory variation may be present).

Vitamin D metabolites

As discussed above, knowledge about vitamin D metabolites in horses is incomplete. From a practical point of view, the clinician must rely on the measurements available in diagnostic laboratories. Although not routine analytes, calcitriol (1,25-dihydroxyvitamin D) and calcidiol (25-hydroxyvitamin D) can be measured by most human and some veterinary laboratories. Both are measured in plasma or serum, are very stable (although sunlight exposure should be avoided), and provide information on the vitamin D status of the animal. The units in which they are conventionally reported are pg/mL for calcitriol, and ng/mL for calcidiol. Normal values of calcitriol and calcidiol in horses are not well established. The ranges considered normal in the author's laboratory are shown in Table 5.2.

Calcitonin

A human radioimmunoassay has been recently reported to be useful for measurement of equine calcitonin (Rourke et al., 2009). This assay detected increases in calcitonin after induction of hypercalcemia in research horses. Normal values of calcitonin in horses reported in that study were approximately 15 pg/mL. However, in some horses very low calcitonin concentrations are measured. This is not surprising because calcitonin concentrations may be undetectable in other species in which calcitonin is better studied (e.g., humans). This or similar assays could prove useful in the future for the investigation of hypercalcemia in horses. However, at present the limited information that is available makes such assays more valuable for research purposes. Similar to other calciotropic hormones, calcitonin can be measured either in plasma or serum. It is fairly stable and is usually reported as pg/mL.

Foals and other equines

Although serum parameters of calcium metabolism are less studied in foals than in adult horses, no major differences related to age have been described. Both tCa and iCa values have been reported to be slightly lower in foals than in adults (Berlin & Aroch, 2009) but in general they are within the reference ranges for adult horses. Parathyroid hormone in foals aged 7–90 days has been reported to be similar to adult horses (Estepa et al., 2003). The few studies that have measured vitamin D levels in foals have not found differences with adult horses in either calcidiol or calcitriol (Estepa et al., 2006; Maenpaa et al., 1988).

Serum parameters of calcium metabolism in donkeys also fall within reference ranges for horses, although a tendency towards increased iCa and calcitriol and lower PTH has been reported (Lopez et al., 2006b).

Urinalysis

Urinary excretion of calcium, in most circumstances measured as fractional excretion (FE_{Ca}), is a routine test in the investigation of calcium disorders. Basically, calcium excretion by urine is influenced by three factors: (i) dietary calcium intake; (ii) calciotropic hormone activity (mainly PTH activity); and (iii) renal function. Thus, in the face of normal renal function, urinary calcium excretion would be determined by calcium intake and PTH activity. Urinary calcium excretion has been traditionally viewed as a substitute for PTH quantification, but such use has limited applications and may lead to misunderstandings. For instance, in horses with nutritional hyperparathyroidism a decreased calcium excretion in urine has been considered an important diagnostic criterion. However, it must be emphasized that the decrease in urinary excretion of calcium will be present whenever calcium intake is low and it does not reflect the degree of PTH stimulation and skeletal involvement, which are the clinically relevant factors. Both a healthy horse temporarily placed on a low-calcium diet and a horse with nutritional hyperparathyroidism will decrease urinary calcium excretion. However, in the first case PTH levels will be normal or slightly increased while in the second case PTH will be extremely high, indicating increased bone resorption. In conclusion, urinary calcium excretion has limited diagnostic value since: (i) it can be influenced by renal function; (ii) it often reflects calcium intake; and (iii) it is not a reliable indicator of PTH activity (which can be directly measured for better accuracy).

When evaluating urinary excretion of calcium it is important to consider that some of the calcium present in horse urine is precipitated and thus it is necessary to dissolve the precipitates, usually by adding acid. Normal ranges of FE_{Ca} in horses lie between 2 and 10%.

Hypercalcemia

Horses in general are very tolerant of hypercalcemia. In fact, the concentrations of extracellular calcium normally found in healthy horses would cause serious clinical signs in other species. Thus, hypercalcemia is often a subclinical laboratory finding in horses. In most situations clinical signs are due to the primary disease that causes the elevation in calcium rather than to the hypercalcemia itself. In very severe cases, clinical signs of hypercalcemia including central nervous system changes, muscle weakness, constipation, and polyuria may appear. Although clinical signs are less evident with hypercalcemia than with hypocalcemia, in general equine hypercalcemic diseases carry a poorer prognosis than hypocalcemic disorders.

> **Box 5.1 Main diseases that cause hypercalcemia in horses.**
>
> - Renal failure
> - Hypercalcemia of malignancy
> - Vitamin D toxicosis
> - Primary hyperparathyroidism

Clinical conditions

The main conditions associated with hypercalcemia in adult horses are listed in Box 5.1.

Renal failure

Horses affected by both acute and chronic renal failure may show hypercalcemia (Elfers et al., 1986; Tennant et al., 1982). This is interesting because in most species renal failure is associated with hypocalcemia. The pathophysiology of hypercalcemia secondary to renal failure in horses is not well understood. The simplest explanation is that calcium metabolism in healthy horses involves a high degree of calcium absorption from the intestine and that the excess calcium is subsequently excreted by the urine. When renal function is compromised, the ability of the diseased kidney to excrete calcium decreases and then calcium accumulates in blood. Hypercalcemia is not only a particular finding but also a central phenomenon that determines all the mineral metabolism of the horse with renal failure. Hypercalcemia is usually accompanied by hypophosphatemia, which is also the opposite of what happens in most mammals with renal failure. Moreover, it has been shown that the high blood calcium concentration inhibits PTH secretion leading to hypoparathyroidism (Aguilera-Tejero et al., 2000) in lieu of the hyperparathyroidism typical of uremic humans, carnivores, and rodents. In these horses clinical signs are predominantly those of decreased renal function, either acute (depression, oliguria, azotemia) or, most commonly, chronic (weight loss, polyuria, anemia, azotemia). The biochemical profile of the horse with renal failure includes: hypercalcemia, hypophosphatemia, decreased PTH, and, possibly, decreased calcitriol due to diminished renal production (although this contention is not well supported by scientific evidence). It is important to highlight the fact that many horses with renal failure also suffer from hypoalbuminemia, which may mask hypercalcemia if only tCa is measured (Brewer, 1982).

Hypercalcemia of malignancy

Some neoplasms (e.g., squamous cell carcinoma, lymphosarcoma, and ameloblastoma) have been associated with hypercalcemia in horses (Karcher et al., 1990; Marr et al., 1989). Hypercalcemia of malignancy, also known as pseudohyperparathyroidism, is a well studied paraneoplastic syndrome in humans and other species. Its pathophysiology is based on the secretion by neoplastic cells of humoral factors with hypercalcemic activity. The best known protein associated with hypercalcemia of malignancy is parathyroid hormone related peptide (PTHrP). This hormone is secreted by many normal tissues but in healthy individuals only exerts a paracrine action and is present at very low concentrations in blood. When neoplastic cells synthesize large quantities of PTHrP, the blood concentration of this peptide increases. This PTHrP interacts with the PTH receptor (PTHR1), thereby eliciting most of its PTH actions, including induction of hypercalcemia. In addition to PTHrP, neoplasms may secrete other humoral factors that also cause hypercalcemia by promoting bone resorption. As a result of the increased extracellular calcium concentrations, the secretion of PTH is inhibited. The clinical picture in these horses is dominated by the clinical signs associated with malignant neoplasia. When clinical signs are subtle, the finding of unexplained hypercalcemia may direct the clinician towards a thorough search for the tumor. The biochemical profile of the horse with pseudohyperparathyroidism is characterized by elevated calcium, normal to low phosphate, and decreased PTH. In most cases circulating concentrations of PTHrP are high. Calcitriol has been reported to be decreased in a horse with hypercalcemia associated with an ameloblastoma (Rosol et al., 1994).

Vitamin D toxicosis

Vitamin D poisoning can be the consequence of excessive ingestion of vitamin D-containing plants, for example Solanum spp, *Cestrum diurnum* (Krook et al., 1975) and *Trisetum flavescens* (Grabner et al., 1985). It can also be iatrogenic, as a result of the administration of high doses of vitamin D. A particular form of vitamin D toxicosis is systemic granulomatous disease in which hypercalcemia is due to excessive and unregulated production of calcitriol by activated macrophages. In horses, granulomatous disorders are rare and do not seem to be strongly associated with hypercalcemia (Sellers et al., 2001). Although, as already discussed, the physiology of vitamin D and its metabolites in horses is not completely understood, it is well documented that the administration of high doses of vitamin D results in hypercalcemia. In fact, horses seem to be more sensitive than many other species to vitamin D poisoning and substantial extraosseous calcifications can occur with relatively low doses of vitamin D. The pathophysiology of hypercalcemia secondary to vitamin D intoxication is not well known. Calcium movement from bone to extracellular fluid probably plays an important role since, in the limited balance studies that have been reported after vitamin D administration, calcium uptake did not increase and there was a significant increase in the renal excretion of calcium (Harmeyer & Schlumbohm, 2004). Clinical signs in these horses are often vague and include anorexia, limb stiffness, weakness, and recumbency. It is interesting to note that horses affected by vitamin D toxicosis have very high plasma phosphate levels. Thus the biochemical profile of the horse with vitamin D intoxication includes: hypercalcemia, hyperphosphatemia, elevated vitamin D metabolites, and very low PTH concentrations, which are suppressed both by hypercalcemia and high vitamin D. When investigating vitamin D metabolites for the diagnosis of vitamin D poisoning, it is preferable to measure calcidiol over calcitriol, since larger increases have been reported in the former after experimental administration of vitamin D (Harrington & Page, 1983).

Primary hyperparathyroidism

Equine primary hyperparathyroidism is a rare condition resulting from hyperplastic or neoplastic (parathyroid adenoma) proliferation of PTH-secreting cells. The pathophysiology of the disease is based on the fact that high PTH leads to an increase in extracellular calcium by increasing calcium extraction from bone and decreasing renal excretion of calcium. In addition, although this has not been proven in horses, high PTH should stimulate calcitriol production in the kidney and increase intestinal absorption of calcium. Moreover, the hyperplastic or neoplastic parathyroid tissue fails to reduce PTH secretion in response to hypercalcemia. In the cases that have been reported in the literature, affected horses showed clinical signs that ranged from vague and nonspecific signs (anorexia, weight loss) to severe bone remodeling (osteodystrophia of the facial bones) (Frank et al., 1989; Peauroi et al., 1989). The clinical chemistry abnormalities of these horses include hypercalcemia, hypophosphatemia, and high PTH concentrations.

Inappropriate fluid therapy

It is unusual to induce hypercalcemia by inappropriate fluid therapy because most fluid solutions have lower calcium concentrations than the extracellular fluid of horses. However, because it is common practice to supplement fluids with calcium, especially in horses with gastrointestinal disorders, errors in which excessive calcium is incorporated in the fluid solution may occur. Rapid administration of a solution containing a high concentration of calcium leads to changes in the electrolyte profile (hypercalcemia, hyperphosphatemia, hypomagnesemia, and hypokalemia), promotes diuresis, and induces volume depletion (Toribio et al., 2007).

Hypercalcemia in foals

In foals, hypercalcemia may be related to the same problems already discussed for adult horses, but is rare in this age group. In addition, a syndrome of neonatal hypercalcemia and asphyxia has been reported. Although not well documented this syndrome could be associated with placental insufficiency and excessive production of PTHrP (Toribio, 2011).

Differential diagnosis of hypercalcemia in horses

From a practical point of view, in most situations the clinician will be faced with a horse presented for a variety of clinical signs as a result of the underlying disorders. These signs can be very obvious (e.g., neoplasia), but in some cases may be subclinical or mild and thus a detailed clinical exam is always warranted. In the absence of signs derived from the primary disease, since horses usually do not show clinical signs of hypercalcemia, the latter will often be an incidental finding after a routine blood analysis. The steps to follow in the investigation of hypercalcemia include:

1 Re-check: repeat tCa determination and measure iCa (if not previously tested).
2 Evaluate renal function.
3 Measure plasma/serum phosphate concentration.
4 Measure plasma/serum PTH concentration.
5 Measure vitamin D metabolites in plasma/serum.

The algorithm for differential diagnosis of hypercalcemia is presented in Figure 5.4. When hypercalcemia has been proven to be consistent (i.e., confirmed by at least two measurements), the clinician should:

- First, determine if there is a discrepancy between tCa and iCa values. If only tCa is increased, conditions that would increase the protein-bound calcium fraction should be considered (e.g., hyperproteinemia). This is very unusual.
- Once iCa has been concluded to be consistently increased as well, renal function should be evaluated. In cases where azotemia is present, the likely cause of hypercalcemia is renal failure.
- Next, plasma phosphate should be evaluated because hypophosphatemia is common in horses with hypercalcemia associated with renal failure. If plasma phosphorus is increased, vitamin D toxicity with secondary renal damage due to nephrocalcinosis should be included in the differential diagnosis. Further investigations (measurement of vitamin D metabolites in blood) should be undertaken.
- If renal function is normal and plasma phosphate is increased in the face of hypercalcemia, the primary clinical suspicion should be vitamin D toxicosis, and confirmation should be obtained by measurement of vitamin D metabolites. Most cases of vitamin D toxicity are not in renal failure.
- If plasma phosphate concentration is low in a horse with hypercalcemia and no indicators of renal dysfunction, then an abnormally increased PTH activity should be suspected and plasma PTH should be measured. An increase in plasma PTH activity in a hypercalcemic horse would indicate primary hyperparathyroidism. If on the contrary plasma PTH is abnormally low, the suspicion would be a paraneoplastic syndrome that results in hypercalcemia of malignancy. Measurement of PTHrP activity could be supportive in these cases. It is important to note than when interpreting PTH concentrations they should be evaluated together with the plasma calcium concentration. For example, a hypercalcemic horse should have a low PTH concentration; if PTH is not decreased this should be interpreted as an inappropriately high PTH.

Treatment of hypercalcemia

From a mechanistic point of view treatment of hypercalcemia can be approached in three ways:

1 Reducing intestinal absorption of calcium.
2 Increasing renal calcium excretion.
3 Mobilizing calcium from the extracellular compartment to bone or reducing mobilization of calcium from bone.

The reduction in intestinal absorption of calcium is achieved primarily by decreasing the calcium content in the diet. Although this measure alone will rarely correct

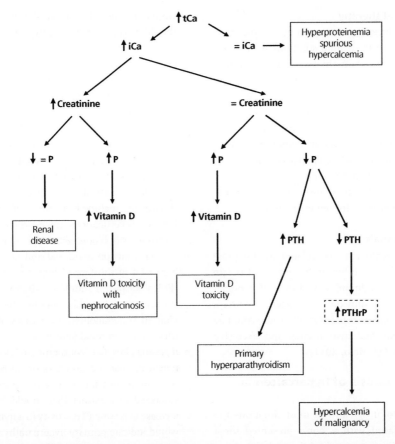

Figure 5.4 Algorithm for diagnosis of hypercalcemia in horses. iCa, ionized calcium; tCa, total calcium; P, phosphorus; PTH, parathyroid hormone; PTHrP, parathyroid hormone-related peptide.

hypercalcemia, it should always be considered as an adjunctive therapy. This therapeutic measure is particularly indicated in horses with long-standing hypercalcemia, for example, renal failure, and involves providing feeds with low calcium content (see Table 5.1). However, it is important not to be overly aggressive in the calcium reduction of the diet. Experimental evidence in animals with calcium metabolism similar to horses has shown that when they are in renal failure, if the diet has a low Ca/P ratio, they may develop secondary hyper-parathyroidism. This is far more deleterious than the hypercalcemia with low PTH levels normally found in horses with renal failure (Bas et al., 2004).

The most effective treatment for acute hypercalcemia (Box 5.2) is to increase renal calcium excretion through the use of fluid therapy. In horses with hypercalcemia, fluid therapy is aimed at diluting plasma calcium

---

Box 5.2 Guidelines for fluid therapy in hypercalcemic horses.

Severe hypercalcemia (tCa >16 mg/dL)

- 0.9% NaCl, Plasma-Lyte® A or Normosol™-R (10 mL/kg/h)
- Furosemide: loading dose (1–2 mg/kg) + continuous infusion (0.12 mg/kg/h)

Moderate hypercalcemia (tCa =14–16 mg/dL)

- 0.9% NaCl, Plasma-Lyte® A or Normosol™-R (5–10 mL/kg/h)
- Furosemide: 1 mg/kg/8 hours

Minor hypercalcemia (tCa =12–14 mg/dL)

- Plasma-Lyte® A, Normosol™-R or Ringer's lactate (5 mL/kg/h)

concentration, as a result of volume expansion, and to increase calcium excretion by promoting glomerular filtration of calcium. In addition, the diuresis of low-density urine (i.e., more dilute urine) will help to prevent calcium precipitation in the kidney. The fluid used to decrease plasma calcium should have an extracellular distribution and be calcium free. Therefore, saline (0.9% NaCl) is frequently recommended as the fluid of choice. However, some precautions should be taken when using 0.9% NaCl. First it is important to consider that 0.9% NaCl has a sodium and chloride concentration in excess of the normal values of equine plasma. This could result in fluid or electrolyte imbalances in patients with renal failure. Second, 0.9% NaCl will result in a decrease in blood pH and this could cause a further increase in the ionized fraction of calcium, which could aggravate hypercalcemia. Therefore, if fluid therapy is going to be extended, a more physiologic fluid like Plasma-Lyte® A (Baxter Healthcare Corp., Deerfield, IL) or Normosol™-R (Abbott Laboratories, North Chicago, IL) should be used. If these fluids are not accessible or their use is impractical (in some countries 5-liter bags are not available) lactated Ringer's solution (LRS) can also be considered as an alternative. Although LRS contains calcium, its calcium concentration is lower than that in the normal equine plasma. Thus LRS will dilute plasma calcium and at the same time promote diuresis. The rate of fluid administration is variable and depends on the severity of hypercalcemia. Rates of 5–10 mL/kg/h are commonly used. Care should be taken to avoid fluid overload when using high infusion rates, particularly in patients with renal failure.

In addition to fluid therapy, renal excretion of calcium can be increased by diuretics. Diuretics should only be used when the extracellular volume is adequate or, preferably, after being moderately expanded by fluid therapy. Furosemide is the most commonly used drug to promote diuresis in horses with hypercalcemia. In addition to its diuretic action, furosemide has some calcium-wasting properties (inhibition of distal tubular calcium reabsorption), which make it particularly useful for the treatment of hypercalcemia. Furosemide in horses has poor oral bioavailability and thus should be administered parenterally (IM or IV) at doses ranging from 1 to 2 mg/kg every 8 hours. In cases in which intensive treatment is warranted, a continuous rate infusion of furosemide should be considered. A continuous infusion of furosemide preceded by a loading dose has been shown to be superior to intermittent administration both in its diuretic effect and in promoting urinary calcium excretion (Johansson et al., 2003). During treatment with furosemide, it is necessary to monitor plasma sodium, potassium, and magnesium concentrations and to replace them according to losses.

In most practical situations it is not feasible to increase calcium transport from plasma to bone. However, many hypercalcemic horses would benefit from reducing calcium movement from bone to extracellular fluid. Drugs that act to inhibit bone resorption (biphosphonates) are the treatment of choice in other species to limit calcium transfer from bone to the extracellular fluid. In horses, information about the hypocalcemic effect of biphosphonates is minimal. Although a biphosphonate (tiludronate) is currently used for the treatment of musculoskeletal problems in horses, there is little information regarding its hypocalcemic effect. Unpublished data from the author's laboratory do not support a consistent hypocalcemic action of tiludronate at the doses (0.1 mg/kg) recommended for treatment of skeletal diseases in horses.

Glucocorticoids are frequently used for the treatment of hypercalcemia in humans and small animals, and appear to be more effective in treatment of hypercalcemia associated with excessive vitamin D. The mechanism of action seems to be multifactorial: glucocorticoids decrease intestinal absorption of calcium, increase urinary calcium excretion, and reduce bone resorption. Studies in ponies treated with dexamethasone indicate that its effect is more pronounced at the skeletal level (Glade et al., 1982). In clinical cases dexamethasone may be administered at conventional anti-inflammatory doses (0.04 mg/kg/day). Other glucocorticoids (e.g., prednisolone) should have similar actions and may be used at equivalent doses. Dosage should be adjusted depending on the severity of hypercalcemia and the risk factors of the individual patient for treatment with glucocorticoids (obesity, pituitary dysfunction, history of laminitis, etc.). Glucocorticoids should be used for the treatment of long-standing hypercalcemia since their short-time effects are small.

Hypocalcemia

Hypocalcemia in horses is more frequently associated with clinical signs than hypercalcemia. Reported clinical signs in hypocalcemic horses include depression, tachycardia, tachypnea, inability to chew and swallow, profuse sweating, muscle fasciculations, involuntary movements of the tongue and lips, altered behavior, instability and recumbency, and opisthotonos or seizures in more severely affected animals (Brewer, 1982). Synchronous diaphragmatic flutter is also a clinical sign frequently associated with hypocalcemia, especially in horses with severe hypocalcemia or in horses that develop hypocalcemia after exercising. It is often associated with hypochloremic metabolic alkalosis and hypokalemia. This problem, characterized by rhythmic contractions of the diaphragm and abdominal musculature ("thumps") that are synchronized with the heartbeat, is a manifestation of neuromuscular irritability that results in stimulation of the phrenic nerve by atrial depolarization.

It is interesting to note that in the author's experience, horses with experimentally induced hypocalcemia show very few clinical signs, even when hypocalcemia is quite severe. This may reflect the fact that the hypocalcemia has been of short duration in these research horses (although it would be expected that horses would better tolerate chronic hypocalcemia than acute hypocalcemia). However, it is also possible that some of the clinical signs classically attributed to hypocalcemia may be due to additional concurrent electrolyte imbalances present in hypocalcemic horses. This would apply particularly to neuromuscular signs; a combination of factors, including alterations in other electrolytes (e.g., magnesium and potassium) and pH, are known to influence the changes in membrane excitability responsible for neuromuscular irritability (Jose-Cunilleras, 2004).

During experimentally induced hypocalcemia, electromyographic measurements in horses have demonstrated spontaneous muscular activity indicative of nerve hyperirritability even in the absence of clinical signs (Wijnberg et al., 2002). Although the classic neuromuscular clinical signs may appear late in the course of hypocalcemia or only when hypocalcemia is severe, it is important to note that hypocalcemia has a negative influence on smooth muscle contraction. Therefore, ileus may be a serious complication in hypocalcemic horses.

Clinical conditions

The more common causes of hypocalcemia in horses are listed in Box 5.3.

Gastrointestinal disorders

Decreased ionized calcium concentrations are a consistent feature in horses with colic and may represent an important pathophysiologic complication due to their

> **Box 5.3 Main diseases that cause hypocalcemia in horses.**
>
> - Colic
> - Acute diarrhea
> - Septicemia
> - Lactation tetany
> - Secondary hyperparathyroidism of nutritional origin
> - Primary hypoparathyroidism
> - Exhaustion syndrome in exercising horses
> - Cantharidin toxicosis

influence on intestinal motility. In these horses, the reduced plasma calcium concentration may be a reflection of sequestration of calcium-containing fluids within the intestinal lumen. Other factors may be involved as horses with strangulating intestinal lesions have been reported to suffer more severe hypocalcemia (Dart et al., 1992, Garcia-Lopez et al., 2001). Thus both gastrointestinal mechanisms and factors related to severity of illness seem to influence hypocalcemia. Hypocalcemia is a prognostic parameter in the colic patient with regards to both the probability of developing ileus during hospitalization and survival (Delesalle et al., 2005). Horses with diarrhea also tend to develop hypocalcemia as a consequence of increased fecal losses of calcium (Toribio et al., 2001; van der Kolk et al., 2002). Endotoxemia is an important complicating factor in both colic and acute diarrhea and may play a major role in the hypocalcemia observed in horses with gastrointestinal disease. Experimental induction of endotoxemia in healthy horses results in hypocalcemia (Toribio et al., 2005), which may develop from several mechanisms. Endotoxemia can impair PTH function – interleukins have been shown to negatively affect parathyroid secretion *in vitro* (Toribio et al., 2003a). Endotoxemia also interferes with PTH effects and promotes peripheral resistance to PTH action since the induction of hypocalcemia in endotoxic horses results in higher PTH values than does induction of hypocalcemia in control horses (Estepa et al., 2007). The clinical chemistry profile of the horse with colic or acute diarrhea shows hypocalcemia, hypomagnesemia, hyperphosphatemia, and, in most cases, elevated PTH concentrations. When evaluating hypocalcemia in horses with acute gastrointestinal disorders, an important consideration is that they are often acidotic and the decrease in blood pH in these patients will artificially increase the ionized calcium fraction.

Hypocalcemia in post-parturient and lactating mares

Lactation tetany should be suspected in any lactating mare with clinical signs of hypocalcemia. Compared to other species, mares are not very prone to develop hypocalcemia post-partum but lactation tetany may be seen occasionally (Baird, 1971; Meijer, 1982). This usually happens during the first week of lactation, although it may appear in a time frame that ranges from before parturition through weaning. Serum calcium normally decreases in post-parturient mares, reaching a nadir 2 days after giving birth. This is accompanied by an increase in PTH (Martin et al., 1996). Although poorly documented in horses, lactation tetany potentially would be the consequence of increased losses of calcium through milk or inadequate PTH response to compensate for hypocalcemia. It is interesting to note that hypocalcemia has also been incriminated as a causative factor of retained placenta in mares (Sevinga et al., 2002).

Nutritional imbalances in the Ca/P content of the diet

A low Ca/P ratio in the diet, due to low calcium and/or high phosphorus, leads to the development of nutritional secondary hyperparathyroidism. This nutritional problem may result from a poorly formulated diet or from the ingestion of plants containing high levels of oxalates that will impair the intestinal absorption of calcium (Joyce et al., 1971; McKenzie, 1988). The pathophysiology of the disease involves an increase in PTH secretion in response to the decreased plasma calcium and the increased phosphate concentrations. Parathyroid hormone will be increased in an effort to compensate for the electrolyte abnormalities by extracting calcium from bone and promoting urinary excretion of phosphate. In severe cases these horses often show skeletal abnormalities: bone deformations secondary to osteodystrophia fibrosa affecting preferentially the head ("big head") that facilitate the diagnosis (Clarke et al., 1996; Ronen et al., 1992); however, in some cases clinical signs are too vague to allow for a correct diagnosis (Little et al., 2000). Horses with nutritional secondary hyperparathyroidism may be normo- or hypocalcemic depending on the severity of the condition (Denny, 1985). Mild cases do not show marked hypocalcemia because the elevation in

PTH is able to maintain blood calcium within physiologic limits. However, in severe cases hypocalcemia is a consistent finding. The blood picture of these horses includes hypocalcemia, hyperphosphatemia, and high PTH concentrations. A decrease in the urinary excretion of calcium, together with increased urinary excretion of phosphate, is considered a test for diagnosis of nutritional hyperparathyroidism. However, it is important to keep in mind that these changes will be a reflection of the Ca/P content of the diet and do not provide information on PTH concentrations and degree of bone resorption, which are key features in this syndrome.

Primary hypoparathyroidism

Primary hypoparathyroidism is a rare condition in horses. Four cases have been described in the literature (Couetil et al., 1998; Durie et al., 2010; Hudson et al., 1999). The exact cause was not determined. In one case, the authors suggested functional hypoparathyroidism secondary to persistent hypomagnesemia (Couetil et al., 1998). In other species hypoparathyroidism may be congenital or the consequence of autoimmune or neoplastic disorders. The pathophysiology of the condition involves a decrease in PTH secretion leading to low circulating calcium concentrations. This may be due to reduced bone resorption, decreased intestinal absorption (probably mediated by low vitamin D concentrations), and increased renal excretion of calcium. It is interesting to note that hypocalcemia is usually severe and all horses with hypoparathyroidism have been reported to show classical signs of hypocalcemia. The biochemical profile of affected horses includes severe hypocalcemia, hypomagnesemia, hyperphosphatemia, and very low to undetectable PTH levels. As already mentioned, PTH values should always be interpreted in conjunction with calcium levels: A normal PTH concentration in a horse with severe hypocalcemia must be considered inappropriately low and suggestive of hypoparathyroidism. In the author's experience, hypoparathyroidism in horses may be transient (i.e., hypocalcemic horses with very low or undetectable PTH concentrations that normalize after correction of hypocalcemia and resumption of regular PTH production). Thus symptomatic treatment to correct hypocalcemia is warranted in all cases. Concomitant electrolyte alterations need to be addressed and this would be especially important in horses with severe hypomagnesemia, since magnesium is necessary for PTH secretion.

Exercise-associated hypocalcemia

Although exercise-associated hypocalcemia is a consistent feature even after mild exercise, for example, show-jumping (Aguilera-Tejero et al., 1998), the condition is only clinically relevant in horses performing prolonged and strenuous exercise, such as endurance races. Endurance horses may develop hypocalcemia due to calcium losses in sweat and compartmental redistribution of calcium. In addition, the injudicious use of calcium supplements during training may impair the PTH response to hypocalcemia during competition. Moreover, since metabolic alkalosis is a frequent acid–base disorder in these horses, the increase in pH will favor a reduction in the ionized fraction of calcium. Hypocalcemia is one of the pathophysiologic factors that influence exhaustion syndrome and contribute to the development of synchronous diaphragmatic flutter. Horses with exercise-associated hypocalcemia have a clinical chemistry profile that includes: hypocalcemia, hyperphosphatemia, and elevated PTH concentrations. However, a lack of PTH increase in response to hypocalcemia has been identified in some endurance horses (Aguilera-Tejero et al., 2001).

Cantharidin toxicosis

Cantharidin toxicosis occurs in horses as a consequence of the ingestion of beetles belonging to the *Epicauta* genus (blister beetles). The beetles that contain the toxic product (cantharidin) are accidentally ingested by the horse after being entrapped in hay, usually alfalfa hay, during harvest. Clinical signs are variable and depend on the amount of toxin ingested. In addition to signs of general illness (anorexia, depression) frequently reported clinical signs are primarily gastrointestinal and neurologic. Synchronous diaphragmatic flutter has been reported in some horses, and signs of shock may also be present in severely ill animals (Helman & Edwards, 1997). Hypocalcemia is a consistent finding in horses with cantharidin toxicosis; it has been argued that hypocalcemia is often due to a decrease in total calcium in these cases and related to hypoproteinemia while ionized calcium is not as consistently decreased (Schmitz, 1989). The biochemical profile of these horses with regards to mineral metabolism is characterized by hypocalcemia, more accentuated when total calcium is considered, and hypomagnesemia (Shawley & Rolf, 1984).

Box 5.4 Drugs that can produce hyper- and hypocalcemia.

Hypercalcemia
- Vitamin D
- Calcium salts

Hypocalcemia
- Furosemide
- Tetracyclines
- Citrate transfusions
- Bicarbonate
- Magnesium salts
- Biphosphonates

Drug-induced hypocalcemia

A variety of drugs can result in hypocalcemia (Box 5.4). The mechanisms by which these drugs decrease plasma calcium are diverse and include chelation (tetracycline, citrate), displacement of ionized calcium as a consequence of alkalosis (sodium bicarbonate), increased renal calcium excretion (furosemide), or reduction in bone resorption (biphosphonates). The decrease in ionized calcium associated with drug administration is usually moderate and without clinical significance. From a practical point of view two clinically relevant situations should be considered: acute cases in which clinical signs of hypocalcemia may be evident during or immediately after drug (e.g., oxytetracycline) administration, and chronic cases in which drugs (e.g., furosemide) may be responsible for an abnormally low calcium value detected in the biochemical profile of a horse that does not show clinical signs of hypocalcemia.

Hypocalcemia in foals

In foals hypocalcemia may be related to nutritional problems, diseases that cause electrolyte disturbances, and a syndrome of idiopathic hypocalcemia (described in neonatal foals) (Beyer et al., 1997). However, the most important cause of hypocalcemia in foals is sepsis. Although they usually do not present with clinical signs of hypocalcemia, critically ill septic foals have decreased iCa levels and increased plasma PTH concentrations. A number of mechanisms including increased calcium losses, calcium shifts, and dysregulation of calciotropic hormones have been proposed to explain septicemic hypocalcemia. Reduced ionized calcium concentrations in foals are strongly associated with sepsis but not with survival. However, increased PTH concentrations are associated with non-survival in septic foals (Hurcombe et al., 2009). This would indicate that, in addition to the PTH response to hypocalcemia, PTH is stimulated by other mechanisms related to the severity of illness (e.g., increased catecholamines) in critically ill foals.

Miscellaneous causes of hypocalcemia

Hypocalcemia has been reported in adult horses and foals associated with a variety of diseases that are not directly related to calcium metabolism; in most cases the etiopathogenesis is not known. This category of diseases includes rhabdomyolysis (Perkins et al., 1998), hepatic failure (Scarrat et al., 1991), and pleuropneumonia (Toribio, 2011).

Differential diagnosis of hypocalcemia in horses

Horses with hypocalcemia may present classical clinical signs, such as neuromuscular manifestations, or signs related to an underlying mineral disorder (e.g., bone deformations) that could indicate or suggest a diagnosis. In some horses, clinical signs may be highly suggestive

of the underlying electrolyte disorder, for example, diaphragmatic flutter. In other cases, hypocalcemia will be discovered after a routine blood analysis in hospitalized horses or in horses with severe or acute disease. The diagnostic steps to follow in the investigation of hypocalcemia of horses would include the following:

1 Re-check: repeat calcium determination and if it was not done before, measure serum albumin concentration. A low serum albumin concentration is a common cause of spurious decreases in tCa; because hypoalbuminemia is a common complication of many equine diseases (malabsorption syndromes, diarrhea, hepatic and renal failure, etc.) it is critical to evaluate tCa concentration in the context of albumin levels.

2 Measure iCa.

3 Evaluate clinical signs.

4 Measure plasma PTH concentration.

The algorithm for differential diagnosis of hypocalcemia is presented in Figure 5.5 and includes the following steps.

Once ionized hypocalcemia has been confirmed, evaluation of clinical signs is important. Thus, a careful and detailed physical exam is warranted. Based on the

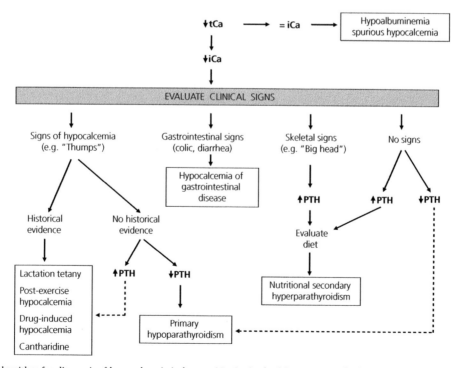

Figure 5.5 Algorithm for diagnosis of hypocalcemia in horses. iCa, ionized calcium; tCa, total calcium; PTH, parathyroid hormone.

clinical picture horses can be distributed into four categories:

1 *Horses with clinical signs of hypocalcemia:* In these horses additional clinical evidence as to the underlying etiology can often be found (e.g., lactating mares or post-exercising horses). In the absence of such clinical evidence, the possibilities related to drug administration or toxicosis should be thoroughly investigated through clinical history. If no apparent cause can be found for the hypocalcemia, a primary disorder of the parathyroid glands should be suspected and PTH should be measured. An inadequately low PTH concentration in a hypocalcemic horse is highly suggestive of primary hypoparathyroidism. If PTH is increased, clinical signs and history should be reassessed.

2 *Horses with gastrointestinal clinical signs:* When hypocalcemia is detected in a horse suffering a serious gastrointestinal disorder, especially colic or diarrhea, the diagnosis is fairly straightforward. Further diagnostic steps in these animals should include a complete plasma electrolyte profile. It is particularly important to check magnesium and potassium concentrations. Although the acute clinical course of the disease combined with the turnaround time necessary for PTH measurements does not make it practical in many situations, determination of PTH concentration is helpful to evaluate the degree of skeletal resistance to the calcemic action of PTH, which provides important prognostic information.

3 *Horses with skeletal clinical signs:* Skeletal signs may be very noticeable and in some cases are the primary reason for veterinary consultation, for example, "big head" associated with secondary nutritional hyperparathyroidism. In other cases bone changes are subtle and may require a detailed clinical examination to be identified. In any hypocalcemic horse with skeletal signs, hyperparathyroidism should be suspected and PTH should be measured. Elevated PTH concentrations in a hypocalcemic horse would indicate secondary hyperparathyroidism. These horses will generally show a decrease in urinary FE_{Ca} and an increase in the fractional excretion of phosphorus (FE_p). The next step should be a dietary evaluation to confirm the nutritional origin of hyperparathyroidism.

4 *Horses with vague or absent clinical signs:* By definition, in these cases hypocalcemia is an incidental laboratory finding in the course of the investigation or may be detected in a routine blood panel (wellness assessment). There is usually not a well-defined problem in such cases. Most commonly these horses will have either a nutritional or primary parathyroid problem, thus measurement of PTH would be the diagnostic step to differentiate these.

Treatment of hypocalcemia

Fluid therapy is the main approach for treatment of hypocalcemia in horses. This will be especially relevant in horses with acute hypocalcemia and/or horses with clinical signs of hypocalcemia (Box 5.5).

Due to the volume required and the complications that extravascular administration may cause, the route of choice to deliver calcium solutions to horses is intravenous. Several calcium salts can be used (calcium gluconate, calcium borogluconate, calcium chloride, etc.). At equal concentrations, calcium chloride provides more calcium per unit volume than calcium gluconate and thus may be more useful for the rapid treatment of severe hypocalcemia. However, calcium chloride is very irritating and extreme care should be taken to avoid perivascular infusion. Since many hypocalcemic horses are also hypomagnesemic, it is common practice to employ supplements that contain both calcium and magnesium, many of which are designed for use in

---

Box 5.5 Guidelines for fluid therapy in hypocalcemic horses.

Severe hypocalcemia (tCa <8 mg/dL + clinical signs)

- Bolus dose: 200 mL of 23% calcium gluconate in 1 L Ringer's lactate administered in 15–30 minutes
- Loading dose: 200 mL of 23% calcium gluconate in 5 L Ringer's lactate administered in 2–4 h

Moderate hypocalcemia (tCa <8 mg/dL without clinical signs)

- Loading dose: 300–400 mL of 23% calcium gluconate in 5 L Ringer's lactate administered in 4 h

Minor hypocalcemia (tCa = 8–12 mg/dL)

- Sustained dose: 200 mL of 23% calcium gluconate in 5 L Ringer's lactate administering each bag in 4 h[a]

[a]When neces.sary, the sustained dose should be adjusted to compensate additional losses and anorexia.

cows. If instead of commercial preparations, magnesium sulfate is added to fluid therapy, it is important not to mix it in the same intravenous line with calcium solutions. This will avoid the formation of calcium sulfate, which can precipitate. In addition, none of the calcium salts should be mixed with sodium bicarbonate-containing solutions because of the possibility of precipitation.

As with any other electrolyte, calcium needs are calculated considering calcium deficit plus additional (pathologic) losses and obligatory (physiologic) losses.

It is not easy to calculate the calcium deficit in a hypocalcemic patient. Calcium is different from other electrolytes because the skeleton contains an abundant source of calcium that, in theory, would be sufficient to compensate the needs of a hypocalcemic horse. However, in the hypocalcemic patient this calcium is not readily available either because there is not enough PTH to compensate for calcium losses or because there is peripheral resistance to PTH action. When calculating calcium deficit it is practical to consider a "closed" pool of available calcium by assuming that the measured blood calcium level is reflective of the calcium concentration in the extracellular space (plasma + interstitial fluid) and that no calcium fluxes from bone are expected. Thus in a standard-size (450 kg) horse, in which the extracellular fluid would be approximately 100 liters, the calcium deficit can be calculated by the following equation:

$$Ca\,deficit\,(mg)\,in\,450\text{-}kg\,horse = [12 - measured\,plasma$$
$$tCa\,(mg/dL)] \times 1000$$

$$(5.1)$$

where 12 is used as the target calcium concentration (12 mg/dL) and 1000 represents the extracellular fluid volume converted to dL units (in this case 1000 dL = 100 L, or 22% of body weight) of extracellular fluid. This would be valid for a standard-size horse but for large horses, ponies, or foals the extracellular volume should be adjusted according to body weight. For example, in a normal sized (i.e. 450 kg) horse with a 50% decrease in plasma calcium (tCa = 6 mg/dL) the calcium deficit would be 12 − 6 x 1000 = 6000 mg.

The large variety of combinations of calcium salts available (gluconate, borogluconate, heptonate, etc.) may be a source of misunderstanding when translating the calcium needs to the volume of calcium solution required. Also, the different units in which calcium is expressed add further confusion when making calculations. It is important to keep in mind that: 2 mEq Ca = 1 mmol Ca = 40 mg Ca. Most commercial solutions include 20–25% (w/v) of gluconate-related calcium salts (e.g., 23% calcium gluconate) and will provide around 20 mg of calcium/mL (1 mEq Ca/mL).

In the above example the horse would need 300 mL of 23% calcium solution to provide 6000 g of calcium. Rapid administration of this amount of calcium should in fact increase plasma calcium above the target level because calcium is not immediately transferred to interstitial fluid. This contention is supported by experiments in which calcium has been administered to healthy horses to induce hypercalcemia (Rourke et al., 2009). It is also important to note that Equation 5.1 tends to overestimate the calcium deficit, since in the interstitial fluid, where protein-bound calcium is not present, calcium concentration is lower than 12 mg/dL. However, most published protocols for treatment of severe acute hypocalcemia in horses recommend higher volumes of calcium solutions (up 500 mL). Actually, although the available data are sparse and difficult to interpret, clinical evidence seems to support this need for or benefit of higher volumes of calcium supplementation. This may reflect the fact that most hypocalcemic horses have ongoing calcium losses that are difficult to account for or quantify: calcium sequestration within the gastrointestinal tract, excessive urinary calcium loss, changes in pH that reduce iCa, etc.

In addition to replacing deficits, any accountable loss of calcium (gastrointestinal reflux, diarrhea, polyuria, sweat, etc.) should be considered when calculating calcium requirements. A conservative practical approach is to assume that the fluid being lost has the same calcium concentration as equine plasma; thus 120 mg of calcium should be added for every liter of fluid lost. At the same time, obligatory calcium losses need to be replaced, particularly if the horse is not eating. In an adult horse (450 kg) obligatory calcium losses (maintenance calcium) would represent approximately 500 mg of calcium per hour (approximately 25 mL of 23% calcium gluconate/h).

The above calculations can also be used in foals, factoring for body weight. However, since extracellular volume as well as calcium needs are higher in foals it is safe to multiply the resulting volume of calcium solution by 2 (doubling the calcium dose).

Because the calculation of calcium requirements for fluid therapy is subjected to many variables, some of which are difficult to account for, frequent monitoring of plasma calcium concentration is essential.

Another important consideration when providing intravenous calcium supplementation is that calcium has profound cardiovascular effects and may produce fatal arrhythmias. Therefore, when administering substantial amounts of calcium as in the treatment of severe hypocalcemia, it is recommended to continuously auscultate the patient or to monitor using an ECG. In cases where arrhythmias are detected, calcium infusion should be immediately stopped. Because of these potential adverse effects, calcium should be administered dilute in fluids and at a slow rate except when life-threatening hypocalcemia is present.

In addition to fluid therapy, in more chronic situations of hypocalcemia, calcium balance can be adjusted to increase extracellular fluid (ECF) calcium concentrations. From a mechanistic point of view modification of calcium balance for treatment of chronic hypocalcemia can be approached in three ways:

1 Increasing intestinal absorption of calcium.
2 Decreasing renal calcium excretion.
3 Mobilizing calcium from bone to the extracellular fluid compartment.

Dietary management to increase calcium intake is essential in all horses with long-standing hypocalcemia. Dietary adjustments imply not only providing adequate calcium intake but also a balanced diet with normal Ca/P ratio. In normal horses the Ca/P ratio of the diet should range between 2/1 and 1/1. However, in horses with hypocalcemia higher ratios (3/1 to 4/1) should be used. Diet formulation may be very different depending on the local availability of feedstuffs but the purpose is to provide a calcium-rich diet, combining feeds to create a balanced diet. A diet with low cation-anion difference would be preferable for its acidifying effect since it will increase the ionized calcium fraction. When the high calcium requirements needed in a hypocalcemic horse cannot be met by the use of regular feedstuffs, calcium supplements (e.g., calcium carbonate, 100–300 g/horse/day) are indicated (Toribio, 2011). In cases of nutritional secondary hyperparathyroidism, diet adjustment is an etiologic treatment. However, a diet with high calcium and low phosphate content is important in many other hypocalcemic diseases, as with primary hypoparathyroidism. Although scientific evidence in horses is very limited, from what is known in other species many hypoparathyroid animals can be maintained without clinical signs and lead a nearly normal life

provided that calcium intake is adequate. Theoretically, intestinal calcium absorption would be favored by increasing the vitamin D content of the diet; however, in horses in particular, increasing dietary vitamin D supplementation is not very important because vitamin D is likely to have little effect at the intestinal level.

In cases of hypocalcemia, if no renal damage is present, renal excretion of calcium is already decreased because low plasma calcium results in a reduction of filtered calcium. In addition, as previously stated, most horses with renal failure tend to retain calcium rather than waste it. However, some horses with acute renal failure may be hypocalcemic. In these horses, in order to promote diuresis without causing additional urinary calcium loss, a calcium-sparing diuretic (e.g., chlorthiazide) should be preferred to calcium-wasting diuretics (e.g., furosemide).

The most effective means to promote calcium movement from bone to the extracellular fluid is through the use of vitamin D. In contrast to its modest effect on calcium absorption at the level of the intestine, vitamin D has a marked effect of mobilizing calcium from bone. However, vitamin D should be used with extreme care because of the high risk of promoting soft-tissue calcifications. Although there is evidence of a direct calcifying effect of vitamin D, most of the soft tissue mineralizing effect is secondary to the increase in the serum Ca × P product. It is interesting to note that, in horses, vitamin D is much more likely to increase phosphorus than calcium concentrations in the blood. Therefore, since many hypocalcemic horses are also hyperphosphatemic, vitamin D would aggravate hyperphosphatemia rather than alleviate hypocalcemia.

In conclusion, the optimal means to treat hypocalcemia in horses is by providing calcium either parenterally (when an acute correction is needed) or enterally (in most chronic situations). Although this may seem obvious it should be underscored because the alternative treatments (e.g., vitamin D) are likely to be more deleterious than helpful.

References

Aguilera-Tejero E, Garfia B, Estepa JC, Lopez I, Mayer-Valor R, Rodriguez M. (1998) Effects of exercise and EDTA administration on blood ionized calcium and parathyroid hormone in horses. *Am J Vet Res* **59**:1605–7.

Aguilera-Tejero E, Estepa JC, Lopez I, Bas S, Rodriguez M. (2000) Polycystic kidneys as a cause of chronic renal failure and secondary hypoparathyroidism in a horse. *Equine Vet J* **32**:167–9.

Aguilera-Tejero E, Estepa JC, Lopez I, Bas S, Garfia B, Rodriguez M. (2001) Plasma ionized calcium and parathyroid hormone concentrations in horses after endurance rides. *J Am Vet Med Assoc* **219**:488–90.

Baird TG. (1971) Lactation tetany (eclampsia) in a Shetland pony mare. *Aust Vet J* **47**:402–4.

Bas S, Bas A, Estepa JC, Mayer-Valor R, Rodriguez M, Aguilera-Tejero E. (2004) Parathyroid gland function in the uremic rabbit. *Domest Anim Endocrinol* **26**:99–110.

Berlin D, Aroch I. (2009) Concentrations of ionized and total magnesium and calcium in healthy horses: effects of age, pregnancy, lactation, pH and sample type. *Vet J* **181**: 305–11.

Beyer MJ, Freestone JF, Reimer J, Bernard WV, Rueve ER. (1997) Idiopathic hypocalcemia in foals. *J Vet Intern Med* **11**: 356–60.

Bienzle D, Jacobs RM, Lumsden JH. (1993) Relationship of serum total calcium to serum albumin in dogs, cats, horses and cattle. *Can Vet J* **34**:360–4.

Breidenbach A, Shlumbohm C, Harmeyer J. (1998) Peculiarities of vitamin D and of the calcium and phosphate homeostatic system in horses. *Vet Res* **29**:173–86.

Brewer BD. (1982) Disorders of equine calcium metabolism. *Comp Cont Educ Pract Vet* **4**:S244–S252.

Brown EM, Gamba G, Riccardi D, et al. (1993) Cloning and characterization of an extracellular Ca2+ sensing receptor from bovine parathyroid. *Nature* **366**:575–80.

Care AD, Abbas SK, Ousey J, Johnson L. (1997) The relationship between the concentration of ionised calcium and parathyroid hormone-related protein (PTHrP[1-34]) in the milk of mares. *Equine Vet J* **29**:186–9.

Clarke CJ, Roeder PL, Dixon PM. (1996) Nasal obstruction caused by nutritional osteodystrophia fibrosa in a group of Ethiopian horses. *Vet Rec* **138**:568–70.

Couetil LL, Sojka JE, Nachreiner RF. (1998) Primary hypoparathyroidism in a horse. *J Vet Intern Med* **12**:45–9.

Dart AJ, Snyder JR, Spier SJ, Sullivan KE. (1992) Ionized calcium concentration in horses with surgically managed gastrointestinal disease: 147 cases (1988–1990). *J Am Vet Med Assoc* **201**:1244–8.

Delesalle C, Dewulf J, Lefebvre RA, Schuurkes JA, Van Vlierbergen B, Deprez P. (2005) Use of plasma ionized calcium levels and Ca2+ substitution response as prognostic parameters for ileus and survival in colic horses. *Vet Quart* **27**:157–72.

Denny JE. (1985) Equine blood serum calcium and phosphorus concentrations in progressive nutritional hyperparathyroidism. *J S Afr Vet Assoc* **56**:123–5.

Durie I, van Loon G, Hesta M, Bauwens C, Deprez P. (2010) Hypocalcemia caused by primary hypoparathyroidism in a 3-month-old filly. *J Vet Intern Med* **24**:439–42.

Elfers RS, Bayly WM, Brobst DF, et al. (1986) Alterations in calcium, phosphorus and C-terminal parathyroid hormone levels in acute renal disease. *Cornell Vet* **76**:317–29.

Estepa JC, Aguilera-Tejero E, Mayer-Valor R, Almaden Y, Felsenfeld AJ, Rodriguez M. (1998) Measurement of parathyroid hormone in horses. *Equine Vet J* **30**:476–81.

Estepa JC, Garfia B, Gao P, Cantor T, Rodriguez M, Aguilera-Tejero E. (2003) Validation and clinical utility of a novel immunoradiometric assay exclusively for biologically active whole parathyroid hormone in the horse. *Equine Vet J* **35**:291–5.

Estepa JC, Aguilera-Tejero E, Zafra R, Mayer-Valor R, Rodriguez M, Perez J. (2006) An unusual case of generalized soft-tissue mineralization in a suckling foal. *Vet Pathol* **43**:64–7.

Estepa JC, Mendoza FJ, Cañadillas S, Guerrero F, Lopez I, Aguilera-Tejero E. (2007) Parathyroid gland response to hypocalcemia in horses with experimentally induced endotoxemia. *J Vet Intern Med* **21**:881.

Frank N, Hawkins JF, Couetil LL, Raymond JT. (1989) Primary hyperparathyroidism with osteodystrophia fibrosa of the facial bones in a pony. *J Am Vet Med Assoc* **212**:84–6.

Garcia-Lopez JM, Provost PJ, Rush JE, Zicker SC, Burmaster H, Freeman LM. (2001) Prevalence and prognostic importance of hypomagnesemia and hypocalcemia in horses that have colic surgery. *Am J Vet Res* **62**:7–12.

Glade MJ, Krook L, Schryver HF, Hintz HF. (1982) Calcium metabolism in glucocorticoid-treated pony foals. *J Nutr* **112**:77–86.

Grabner A, Kraft W, Essich G, Hanichen T. (1985) Enzootic calcinosis in the horse. *Tierarztliche Praxis* **1**:84–93.

Harmeyer J, Schlumbohm C.(2004) Effects of pharmacological doses of vitamin D3 on mineral balance and profiles of plasma vitamin D3 metabolites in horses. *J Steroid Biochem Mol Biol* **89–90**:595–600.

Harrington DD, Page EH. (1983) Acute vitamin D3 toxicosis in horses: case reports and experimental studies of the comparative toxicity of vitamins D2 and D3. *J Am Vet Med Assoc* **182**:1358–69.

Helman RG, Edwards WC. (1997) Clinical features of blister beetle poisoning in equids: 70 cases (1983–1996). *J Am Vet Med Assoc* **211**:1018–21.

Hudson NP, Church DB, Trevena J, Nielsen IL, Major D, Hodgson DR. (1999) Primary hypoparathyroidism in two horses. *Aust Vet J* **77**:504–8.

Hurcombe SDA, Toribio RE, Slovis NM, et al. (2009) Calcium regulating hormones and serum calcium and magnesium concentrations in septic and critically ill foals and their association with survival. *J Vet Intern Med* **23**:335–43.

Johansson AM, Gardner SY, Levine JF, et al. (2003) Furosemide continuous rate infusion in the horse: evaluation of enhanced efficacy and reduced side effects. *J Vet Intern Med* **17**:887–95.

Jose-Cunilleras E. (2004) Abnormalities of body fluids and electrolytes in athletic horses. In: Hinchcliff KW, Kaneps AJ, Geor RJ (eds) *Equine Sports Medicine and Surgery*. Edinburgh: Saunders, pp 898–918.

Joyce JR, Pierce KR, Romane WM, Baker JM. (1971) Clinical study of nutritional secondary hyperparathyroidism in horses. *J Am Vet Med Assoc* **158**:2033–42.

Karcher LF, Le Net J-L, Turner BF, Reimers TJ, Tennant BC. (1990) Pseudohyperparathyroidism in a mare associated with squamous cell carcinoma of the vulva. *Cornell Vet* **80**:153–62.

Kohn CW, Brooks CL. (1990) Failure of pH to predict ionized calcium percentage in healthy horses. *Am J Vet Res* **51**: 1206–10.

Krook L, Wasserman RH, Shively JN, Tashjian AH, Brokken TD, Morton JF. (1975) Hypercalcemia and calcinosis in Florida horses: implication of the shrub, Cestrum diurnum, as the causative agent. *Cornell Vet* **65**:26–56.

Little D, Redding WR, Spaulding KA, Dupree SH, Jones SL. (2000) Unusual presentation of nutritional secondary hyperparathyroidism in a Paint colt. *Equine Vet Educ* **2**:388–94.

Lopez I, Estepa JC, Mendoza FJ, Mayer-Valor R, Aguilera-Tejero E. (2006a) Fractionation of calcium and magnesium in equine serum. *Am J Vet Res* **67**:463–6.

Lopez I, Estepa JC, Mendoza FJ, Rodriguez M, Aguilera-Tejero E. (2006b) Serum concentrations of calcium, phosphorus, magnesium and calciotropic hormones in donkeys. *Am J Vet Res* **67**:1333–6.

Maenpaa PH, Koskinen T, Koskinen E. (1988) Serum profiles of vitamins A, E and D in mares and foals during different seasons. *J Anim Sci* **66**:1418–23.

Marr CM, Love S, Pirie HM. (1989) Clinical, ultrasonographic and pathological findings in a horse with splenic lymphosarcoma and pseudohyperparathyroidism. *Equine Vet J* **21**:221–6.

Martin KL, Hoffman RM, Kronfeld DS, Ley WB, Warnick LD. (1996) Calcium decreases and parathyroid hormone increases in serum of periparturient mares. *J Anim Sci* **74**:834–9.

McKenzie RA. (1988) Purple pigeon grass (Setaria incrassata): a potential cause of nutritional secondary hyperparathyroidism of grazing horses. *Aust Vet J* **65**:329–30.

Meijer P. (1982) Two cases of tetany in the horse. *Tijdschrift von Diegeneeskunde* **107**:329–32.

Peauroi JR, Fisher DJ, Mohr C, Vivrette SL. (1989) Primary hyperparathyroidism caused by a functional parathyroid adenoma in a horse. *J AmVet Med Assoc* **212**:1915–18.

Perkins G, Valberg SJ, Madigan JM, Carlson GP, Jones SL. (1998) Electrolyte disturbances in foals with severe rhabdomyolisis. *J Vet Intern Med* **12**:173–7.

Raulais D, Desplan C, Monet J-D, Boccard B, Milhaud G. (1981) Immunochemical and biological properties of horse parathyroid hormone. *Proc Soc Exp Biol Med* **167**:542–6.

Ronen N, van Heerden J, van Amstel SR. (1992) Clinical and biochemistry findings, and parathyroid hormone concentrations in three horses with secondary hyperparathyroidism. *J S Afr Vet Assoc* **63**:134–6.

Rosol TJ, Nagode LA, Robertson JT, Leeth BD, Steinmeyer CL, Allen CM. (1994) Humoral hypercalcemia of malignancy associated with ameloblastoma in a horse. *J Am Vet Med Assoc* **204**:1930–3.

Rourke KM, Kohn CW, Levine AL, Rosol TJ, Toribio RE. (2009) Rapid calcitonin response to experimental hypercalcemia in healthy horses. *Domest Anim Endocrinol* **36**:197–201.

Rourke KM, Coe S, Kohn CW, Rosol TJ, Mendoza FJ, Toribio RE. (2010) Cloning, comparative sequence analysis and mRNA expression of calcium-transporting genes in horses. *Gen Comp Endocrinol* **167**:6–10.

Scarrat WK, Furr MO, Robertson JL. (1991) Hepatoencephalopathy and hypocalcemia in a miniature horse mare. *J Am Vet Med Assoc* **199**:1754–6.

Schmitz DG. (1989) Cantharidin toxicosis in horses. *J Vet Intern Med* **3**:208–15.

Schryver HF, Craig PH, Hintz HF. (1970) Calcium metabolism in ponies fed varying levels of calcium. *J Nutr* **100**:955–64.

Schryver HF, Hintz HF, Lowe JE. (1974) Calcium and phosphorus in the nutrition of the horse. *Cornell Vet* **64**:493–515.

Schryver HF, Hintz HF, Lowe JE. (1978) Calcium metabolism, body composition, and sweat losses of exercised horses. *Am J Vet Res* **39**:245–8.

Sellers RS, Toribio RE, Blomme EAG. (2001) Idiopathic systemic granulomatous disease and macrophage expression of PTHrP in a miniature pony. *J Comp Pathol* **125**:214–18.

Sevinga M, Barkema HW, Hesselink JW. (2002) Serum calcium and magnesium concentrations and the use of a calcium-magnesium-borogluconate solution in the treatment of Friesian mares with retained placenta. *Theriogenology* **57**:941–7.

Shawley RV, Rolf LL. (1984) Experimental cantharidiasis in the horse. *Am J Vet Res* **45**:2261–6.

Tennant B, Bettleheim P, Kaneko JJ. (1982) Paradoxic hypercalcemia and hypophosphatemia associated with chronic renal failure in horses. *J Am Vet Med Assoc* **180**:630–4.

Toribio RE. (2011) Disorders of calcium and phosphate metabolism in horses. *Vet Clin N Am-Equine* **27**:129–47.

Toribio RE, Kohn CW, Chew DJ, Sams RA, Rosol TJ. (2001) Comparison of serum parathyroid hormone and ionized calcium and magnesium concentrations and fractional urinary clearance of calcium and phosphorus in healthy horses and horses with enterocolitis. *Am J Vet Res* **62**:938–47.

Toribio RE, Kohn CW, Capen CC, Rosol TJ. (2003a) Parathyroid hormone (PTH) secretion, PTH mRNA and calcium-sensing receptor mRNA expression in equine parathyroid cells, and effects of interleukin (IL)-1, IL-6, and tumor necrosis factor-α on equine parathyroid cell function. *J Mol Endocrinol* **31**:609–20.

Toribio RE, Kohn CW, Leone GW, Capen CC, Rosol TJ. (2003b) Molecular cloning and expression of equine calcitonin, calcitonin gene-related peptide-I, and calcitonin gene-related peptide-II. *Mol Cell Endocrinol* **199**:119–28.

Toribio RE, Kohn CW, Sams RA, Capen CC, Rosol TJ. (2003c) Hysteresis and calcium set-point for the calcium parathyroid hormone relationship in healthy horses. *Gen Comp Endocrinol* **130**:279–88.

Toribio RE, Kohn CW, Hardy J, Rosol TJ. (2005) Alterations in serum parathyroid hormone and electrolyte concentrations and urinary excretion of electrolytes in horses with induced endotoxemia. *J Vet Intern Med* **19**:223–31.

Toribio RE, Kohn CW, Rourke KM, Levine AL, Rosol TJ. (2007) Effects of hypercalcemia on serum concentrations of magnesium, potassium, and phosphate and urinary excretion of electrolytes in horses. *Am J Vet Res* **68**:543–54.

van der Kolk JH, Nachreiner RF, Refsal KR, Brouillet D, Wensing Th. (2002) Heparinised blood ionised calcium concentrations in horses with colic or diarrhoea compared to normal subjects. *Equine Vet J* **34**:528–31.

Wijnberg ID, van der Kolk JH, Franssen H, Breukink HJ. (2002) Electromyographic changes of motor unit activity in horses with induced hypocalcemia and hypomagnesemia. *Am J Vet Res* **63**:849–56.

CHAPTER 6

Magnesium homeostasis and derangements

Allison Jean Stewart

Professor of Equine Medicine, Auburn University, Auburn, AL, USA

Magnesium (Mg) often receives little attention in the formation of fluid therapy plans. If an animal is eating or the duration of intravenous fluid administration is short then inadequate Mg supplementation is probably of little consequence. Homeostatic mechanisms normally maintain intracellular and extracellular concentrations within narrow limits. However, during severe illness such homeostatic mechanisms may fail and magnesium supplementation may be warranted, especially if ongoing losses from reflux or diarrhea are present.

Magnesium is an essential macroelement that is important in several physiologic processes. It is required for cellular energy-dependent reactions involving ATP including glycolysis, oxidative phosphorylation, nucleic acid and protein synthesis, and ion pump function. Magnesium is involved in the regulation of calcium channel function and therefore neurotransmitter release, neuronal excitation, vasomotor tone, cardiac excitability, and skeletal muscle contraction. Severe Mg deficiency results in neuromuscular disturbances, but clinical signs are rarely documented in horses. In contrast, subclinical hypomagnesemia is common in critically ill patients, including horses. Subclinical hypomagnesemia can lead to ileus, cardiac arrhythmias, refractory hypokalemia, and hypocalcemia. It has also been shown to increase the severity of the systemic inflammatory response syndrome (SIRS) and worsens the systemic response to endotoxin.

Chemistry

The atomic weight of magnesium is 24.3 and its valence is 2^+, therefore 1 mEq (0.5 mmol) = 12.156 mg. Conversion factors are:

$mg/dL = 2.43 \times mmol/L$

$mmol/L = mg/dL \times 0.411$

$mmol/L = mEq/L \times 0.5$

$mg/dL = mEq/L$

Dietary Mg is reported in g/kg of feed, parts per million (ppm) = mg/kg = g/kg × 1000, or as a percentage by dividing by 10. Magnesium oxide (MgO; MagOx™), which contains 60.25% elemental Mg, is most commonly used for oral supplementation. Magnesium carbonate ($MgCO_3$) and magnesium sulfate ($MgSO_4$) can also be fed. Magnesium sulfate for intravenous injection is commercially available as $MgSO_4 \cdot 7H_2O$ in a 50% solution. Although the $MgSO_4$ compound is 20.2% elemental Mg, the $MgSO_4 \cdot 7H_2O$ solution contains only 9.9% elemental Mg. Each mL of 50% $MgSO_4 \cdot 7H_2O$ solution contains 99 mg (8 mEq = 4 mmol) of elemental Mg. The 50% solution (500 mg/mL = 4 mEq/mL) has an osmolarity of 4000 mOsm/L, and is therefore hypertonic, and

Equine Fluid Therapy, First Edition. Edited by C. Langdon Fielding and K. Gary Magdesian.
© 2015 John Wiley & Sons, Inc. Published 2015 by John Wiley & Sons, Inc.

should be diluted to at least a 10% solution prior to intravenous administration.

Distribution of magnesium within the body

Magnesium is the second most abundant intracellular cation after potassium. It is the fourth most abundant cation in the body of domestic animals, making up 0.05% of the total body weight. Total body Mg is distributed between bone (60%), soft tissues (38%), and extracellular fluids (1–2%). Only 30% of bone Mg is readily exchangeable and therefore available as a reservoir to maintain extracellular Mg concentrations. The remaining 70% of bone Mg has structural functions and is held within the hydroxyapatite lattice, and can be released only during active bone resorption. Although most soft tissue Mg is in the intracellular compartment, intracellular and extracellular ionized Mg (Mg^{2+}) concentrations are similar with only a very small transmembrane gradient compared to Ca^{2+}. Intracellular Mg^{2+} concentrations are variable, being proportional to the metabolic activity of the cell.

Less than 1% of the total body Mg is contained in the extracellular fluid; therefore, similar to potassium, serum Mg concentration may not adequately reflect total body Mg stores. In equine serum 30% of Mg is protein bound, 10% is complexed to weak acids, and the remaining 60% is in the ionized form (Mg^{2+}) (Lopez et al., 2006; Stewart, 2004). It is the ionized form that is biologically active, therefore it is preferable to measure serum ionized rather than total Mg (tMg) concentrations. Red blood cells contain approximately three times the concentration of Mg in serum; therefore hemolysis can elevate measured serum Mg concentrations. Delayed separation of serum from red blood cells can lead to elevations in serum Mg concentrations.

Serum tMg concentration depends on protein concentration, whereas Mg^{2+} concentration depends on acid–base status. Acidosis increases Mg^{2+} while alkalosis reduces Mg^{2+}. During alkalosis there are fewer hydrogen ions to bind to the negative charges on proteins, which increases subsequent protein binding of cations such as Ca^{2+} and Mg^{2+}. This is clinically important when treating alkalotic conditions such as exercise-associated hypochloremic metabolic alkalosis in endurance horses, nasogastric reflux associated with small intestinal obstruction or duodenitis/jejunitis, and respiratory alkalosis with hyperventilation, or when administering significant amounts of sodium bicarbonate. Clinical signs of hypomagnesemia can develop due to low Mg^{2+} despite normal tMg concentrations. Feeding an acidic diet with a low dietary cation–anion balance (DCAB) will increase the percentage of Mg^{2+} (Stewart, 2004).

Magnesium physiology

Magnesium serves as an essential cofactor for more than 300 enzymatic reactions involving ATP, such as transcription and translation of genetic information, and in the cellular energy-dependent reactions of glycolysis and oxidative phosphorylation (Elin, 1988; Wacker & Parisi, 1968). Magnesium is necessary for nerve conduction, membrane stabilization, ion transportation, regulation of calcium channel activity, and for normal function of the sodium-potassium activated ATP (Na^+/K^+-ATPase) pump (Rude & Oldham, 1990). This pump maintains the Na^+/K^+ gradient across all membranes, as well as regulating intracellular K^+ balance. Calcium (Ca) ATPase and proton pumps also require Mg as a cofactor. Defective function of ATPase pumps and ion channels may result in interference with the electrochemical gradient, alteration in resting membrane potential, and disturbances in repolarization, resulting in neuromuscular and cardiovascular abnormalities (Elin, 1988; Marino, 1995; McLean, 1994; White & Hartzell, 1989). Magnesium's role in the regulation of movement of calcium into the myocyte gives it a pivotal role in cardiac contractile strength, visceral peristalsis, and peripheral vascular tone (White & Hartzell, 1989).

Gastrointestinal absorption of magnesium

The magnesium ion is absorbed by saturable transcellular active transport and passive, non-saturable, and concentration-dependent paracellular diffusion. Magnesium digestibility is higher in foals than in adult horses (Harrington & Walsh, 1980). In adult horses, 25% of ingested Mg is absorbed in the proximal half of the small intestine, 35% from the distal small intestine, and only 5% from the cecum and large and small colons (Hintz & Schryver, 1972). Intestinal Mg absorption increases in proportion to the amount supplied in the diet, but the absorptive efficiency decreases as dietary Mg content increases until a plateau is reached (Hintz & Schryver, 1973). Average absorption of Mg from feed by horses is 49.5% (30–60%), which is higher than in ruminants (Hintz & Schryver, 1972; Rook 1969). Alfalfa has the highest Mg digestibility of 50%; for clover and meadow hay it is 31%, and for hay and grain 38% (Martens & Schweigel, 2000). Diet type does not affect the site of Mg absorption (Hintz & Schryver, 1972). Oral MgO, $MgSO_4$, and $MgCO_3$ have equivalent digestibilities (50–70%) with absorption rates higher than from organic sources. Excessive amounts of fiber, oxalates, phosphates, and fatty acids decrease Mg absorption in horses, whereas phytates, calcium, and aluminum content have little effect (Hintz & Schryver, 1972). Increased dietary Mg leads to increases in bone, tissue, erythrocyte, and serum Mg concentrations.

Renal excretion and reabsorption of magnesium

Magnesium is primarily excreted through the gastrointestinal tract and kidneys. During pregnancy there are losses to the developing fetus and to milk during lactation. In heavily exercising horses there is significant loss of Mg in sweat.

Renal excretion of Mg varies directly with dietary changes in order to regulate Mg balance and maintain stable serum Mg concentrations. With low Mg intake, the kidney avidly conserves Mg and virtually no Mg is excreted into the urine. Conversely, when excess Mg is ingested, it is rapidly excreted into the urine because of diminished renal tubular reabsorption. Ionized and anion-bound fractions of Mg are filtered by the glomerulus (ultrafilterable), while protein-bound Mg passes directly through the renal efferent arteriole without passing into the glomerular filtrate. Approximately 70% of blood Mg is filtered by the glomeruli, with 70–90% reabsorbed in different segments of the nephron. The proximal tubule reabsorbs 5–15%, the thick ascending limb of the loop of Henle 70–80%, and the distal convoluted tubule absorbs ~10% of the Mg filtered by the glomerulus (Quamme & Dirks, 1983). There is minimal absorption beyond the distal tubule, and it is this segment that is responsible for determining the final urinary Mg excretion.

Magnesium requirements of horses

Obligatory urinary and fecal Mg loss in horses has been estimated at 2.8 mg/kg (BW)/day and 1.8 mg/kg BW/day, respectively (Hintz & Schryver, 1972). Maintenance Mg requirement for horses is estimated at 13 mg/kg (BW)/day, and can be provided by a diet containing 0.16% Mg (1600 ppm of feed) (Hintz & Schryver, 1972, 1973). Growing, lactating, and exercising animals have a higher requirement of dietary Mg. The mammary gland actively secretes 3–6 mg/kg (BW)/day of Mg into the milk. During the first week of lactation milk Mg concentration is 120–300 mg/L, then it decreases to 50–70 mg/L for the next 2 to 3 months (Grace et al., 1999). During lactation mares require 15 to 30 mg/kg dietary intake of Mg (Burkitt et al., 2007). Hypomagnesemia is more likely to occur in high-producing mares, especially if transported long distances without feed. Substantial amounts of Mg can also be lost in sweat. The Mg intake should be increased 1.5–2 times maintenance for horses undergoing moderate to intense exercise.

Dietary magnesium deficiency in horses is unlikely unless extreme conditions combine to result in decreased consumption and increased demand, such as long-distance transportation of unfed lactating mares or prolonged administration of enteral or parenteral fluid or nutrition solutions deficient in Mg.

Magnesium homeostasis

Although the extracellular concentration of Mg depends on gastrointestinal absorption, renal excretion, and bone exchange, there is no precise homeostatic regulating system for Mg (Kayne & Lee, 1993). However, parathyroid hormone (PTH), PTH-related peptide (PTHrP), arginine vasopressin (AVP, antidiuretic hormone), insulin, aldosterone, and beta-adrenergic agonists all increase renal reabsorption of Mg (Toribio, 2010). *In vitro* and *in vivo* studies have demonstrated that insulin may modulate the shift of Mg^{2+} from the extracellular to intracellular space. Activation of the calcium-sensing receptor in the thick ascending loop of Henle by hypercalcemia increases urinary Ca^{2+} and Mg^{2+} excretion (Toribio et al., 2007). Reabsorption of Mg^{2+} is impaired with osmotic diuresis (volume expansion), hyperglycemia, hypercalcemia, hypercalciuria, hypermagnesemia, hypokalemia, hypophosphatemia, tubular acidosis, metabolic acidosis, and toxicities due to amphotericin B or aminoglycosides (Toribio, 2010). Administration of furosemide and induction of hypercalcemia causes reduction in serum tMg and Mg^{2+} concentrations in healthy horses by inhibition of the $Na^+/K^+/2Cl^-$ transporter. This reduces the transepithelial voltage gradient and directly decreases the reabsorption of Ca and Mg (Toribio et al., 2001). PTH indirectly increases Mg^{2+} release from bone during bone resorption. PTH, vitamin D, calcitonin, glucagon, AVP, and calcium concentrations influence Mg absorption and excretion to some degree.

Parathyroid hormone acts on the renal tubules to increase Mg reabsorption (Rasmussen & Bordier, 1974). Micropuncture studies have shown that PTH changes the potential difference of the cortical thick ascending limb of the loop of Henle, which increases the transepithelial voltage gradient to enhance paracellular Mg reabsorption (de Rouffignac et al., 1993; Quamme & Dirks 1983).

Pathophysiology of hypomagnesemia and inflammation

Magnesium has a role in protection against cardiotoxicity, neurotoxicity, inflammation, and free radical damage (Freedman et al., 1990; Kramer et al., 1994; Mak et al., 1994; Salem et al., 1995). Hypomagnesemia is associated with increased cytokine production and systemic inflammation (Malpuech-Brugere et al., 1999; Weglicki et al., 1992). Subclinical hypomagnesemia is common in the intensive care unit and is associated with increased risk of death. Experimental endotoxin administration in horses results in acute decreases in tMg and Mg^{2+} concentrations (Toribio et al., 2005). While endotoxemia can induce acute hypomagnesemia, it appears that Mg administration may be protective in hypomagnesemic endotoxemic patients. Endotoxemic humans with concurrent hypomagnesemia have a worse outcome compared to normomagnesemic patients (Salem et al., 1995). Considering that approximately 40% of horses with colic are endotoxic, and that free radical injury is an important mechanism in intestinal ischemia-reperfusion injury, the role of Mg and its therapeutic importance in equine disease warrants investigation.

Hypomagnesemic equine patients: incidence and outcome

Hypomagnesemia is commonly observed in critically ill patients, but it is unknown if it contributes to mortality, or whether it is merely associated with severe disease. A retrospective study found that 48.7% (401/823) of hospitalized horses had tMg values below the reference range (Johansson et al., 2003). Hypomagnesemia was associated with gastrointestinal disease, infectious respiratory disease, and multi-organ system disease (Johansson et al., 2003). Although no association with mortality was detected, the length of hospitalization was longer for horses with hypomagnesemia (Johansson et al., 2003). In equine surgical colic patients 54% had low serum Mg^{2+} and 17% had low tMg concentrations. Horses with ionized hypomagnesemia had a significantly greater prevalence of postoperative ileus than normomagnesemic equine surgical colic patients (Garcia-Lopez et al., 2001). Surgical colic patients that were euthanized at the time of surgery (7/35) had significantly lower preoperative serum concentrations of Mg^{2+} compared with horses that survived, but serum Mg concentration did not predict hospitalization time or survival (Garcia-Lopez et al., 2001). Low Mg^{2+} was documented in 78% (50/64) of horses with enterocolitis (Toribio et al., 2001). In other species a clear association has been made between hypomagnesemia, severity of disease, and mortality, but larger studies in severely ill horses may be required to determine if similar associations exist in horses. Although 15% of critically ill foals were found to have low serum Mg^{2+} concentrations no association between hypomagnesemia and mortality was detected (Henninger & Horst, 1997). Hypomagnesemia is also commonly seen in blister beetle toxicosis and horses with synchronous diaphragmatic flutter (SDF) (Helman & Edwards, 1997).

Sepsis-induced hypocalcemia and hypomagnesemia may be associated with intracellular ionic shift, hemodilution, or sequestration. Magnesium may function as a Ca antagonist, and low Mg may enhance intracellular entry of Ca in sepsis and endotoxemia (Salem et al., 1995). It is undetermined if Mg administration to acutely hypomagnesemic patients is beneficial in reducing mortality or length of hospitalization. It seems reasonable to therapeutically maintain serum concentrations within reference ranges during times of severe illness when physiologic homeostatic mechanisms are overwhelmed.

Association of hypomagnesemia with hypokalemia

Hypomagnesemia is frequently associated with hypokalemia and kaliuresis in other species (Martin et al., 1994; Reinhart & Desbiens, 1985; Ryzen, 1989; Whang et al., 1984, 1992). Magnesium deficiency has been associated with loss of cellular potassium stores, and as is the case in hypocalcemic patients, it may be difficult to restore normokalemia until the concurrent Mg deficiency is corrected (al-Ghamdi et al., 1994). Hypomagnesemia affects the ability of Mg to act as a coenzyme for the Na^+/K^+-ATPase pump, resulting in decreased intracellular K and increased intracellular Na concentrations, which lower the resting membrane potential. This predisposes cells to spontaneous depolarization and impaired transmission of electrical impulses. Hypomagnesemia can result in the blockade of voltage-gated K channels, which interferes with electrical repolarization and the propagation of the action potential (Roden & Iansmith, 1987). Hypomagnesemia can also lead to increased Purkinje fiber excitability, which predisposes to arrhythmia generation (Tobey et al., 1992). Clinically, concurrent hypomagnesemia and hypokalemia leads to hyperexcitability, cardiac arrhythmias, seizures, muscle fasciculations, and weakness.

Association of hypomagnesemia with hypocalcemia

Hypocalcemia and hypomagnesemia are concurrently observed in horses with blister beetle poisoning, endotoxemia, enterocolitis, intestinal strangulation, ileus, and SDF (Garcia-Lopez et al., 2001; Helman & Edwards, 1997; Toribio et al., 2001, 2005). Hypocalcemic patients with concurrent hypomagnesemia are often refractory to Ca therapy unless the low serum Mg concentrations are identified and corrected (Fatemi et al., 1991; Leicht et al., 1992; Ryzen et al., 1985; Shah et al., 1994). Although the mechanisms by which hypomagnesemia results in hypocalcemia are not completely understood, low serum Mg can impair PTH synthesis and secretion and induce target tissue resistance to PTH. This affects renal resorption of Ca^{2+} and Mg^{2+}, decreases bone resorption, and reduces renal synthesis of 1,25-dihydroxyvitamin D_3 (Abbot & Rude, 1993). Consequently, parallel determination of Mg, Ca, and PTH concentrations is important in the investigation of Mg and Ca homeostasis.

Mg is considered nature's physiological calcium blocker, as it reduces the release of calcium from and into the sarcoplasmic reticulum and protects the cell against calcium overload under conditions of ischemia (Dacey, 2001). These Ca-channel-blocking effects of magnesium appear to be decreased in the hypomagnesemic state with a subsequent increase in intracellular Ca concentration, leading to enhanced cellular sensitivity to cardiotoxic drugs or ischemic events.

Association of magnesium and endotoxemia

Hypocalcemia and hypomagnesemia are common in horses with sepsis and endotoxemia (Garcia-Lopez et al., 2001; Johansson et al., 2003; Toribio et al., 2001). Experimental endotoxin infusion in horses resulted in electrolyte abnormalities that included hypomagnesemia, hypocalcemia, hypokalemia, hypophosphatemia, and increased serum PTH and insulin concentrations, but no changes in serum sodium or chloride (Toribio et al., 2005). Correction of electrolyte abnormalities is well recognized as part of the care of the critically ill equine patient, and it appears that correction of serum Mg^{2+} concentrations is warranted. Experimental rodent studies have implicated Mg in cell messaging and cytokine production. Hypomagnesemic rats exhibit increased circulating cytokine concentrations – interleukin-1 (IL-1), IL-6, tumor necrosis factor (TNF) – indicative of a generalized inflammatory state (Malpuech-Brugere et al., 1999; Weglicki et al., 1992). Hypomagnesemic rats are acutely sensitive to the effects of experimentally administered endotoxin, and this vulnerability is correlated with higher plasma TNF concentrations (Malpuech-Brugere et al., 1999). In a rodent model, progressive Mg deficiency led to increasing mortality rates from the effects of endotoxin administration, while Mg supplementation reduced the endotoxin-induced mortality (Salem et al., 1995). Hypomagnesemia also predisposed animals to free radical-associated injury, leading to the formation of cardiomyopathic lesions and altered vascular tone (Freedman et al., 1990, 1991; Kramer et al., 1994; Mak et al., 1994). These rodent studies were performed after chronic dietary-induced hypomagnesemia, and care must be taken when extrapolating this information to critically ill patients, which have redistribution of serum and cellular Mg rather than a state of whole body Mg depletion.

Association of magnesium and insulin resistance

There are anecdotal reports that Mg supplementation can help in the treatment of metabolic syndrome in horses, but there is no research to support this conclusion. Extrapolation from human medicine may not be relevant due to dietary differences between horses and humans.

A great deal of controversy exists about the role of Mg in human diabetes. There have been epidemiologic studies linking low Mg status with insulin-dependent and non-insulin-dependent diabetes mellitus (Nielsen, 2010). Intracellular Mg^{2+} concentrations modulate the action of insulin, and there is an increased incidence of low intracellular Mg^{2+} concentrations in human patients with non-insulin-dependent diabetes mellitus (Barbagallo et al., 2003). There have been suggestions that this may result in defective tyrosine-kinase activity at the insulin receptor level resulting in increased intracellular Ca^{2+} concentrations, which can contribute to worsening insulin resistance (Barbagallo et al., 2003; Nielsen, 2010). Daily oral Mg supplementation to human patients with non-insulin-dependent diabetes mellitus has resulted in restoration of intracellular Mg^{2+} concentrations and improved insulin-mediated glucose uptake (Nielsen, 2010).

Care should be taken when making inferences from humans to horses as human epidemiologic data are often confounded with poor dietary intake and alcoholism. There has been some discussion as to the usefulness of Mg supplementation to horses with insulin resistance with either equine metabolic syndrome or pituitary pars intermedia dysfunction. However, it seems unlikely that horses would develop chronic whole-body Mg deficiency; efforts to induce Mg depletion have required long-term feeding of severely Mg-depleted artificial diets in young, growing animals (Hintz & Schryver, 1972, 1973; Stewart, 2004). It is therefore the author's opinion that dietary Mg supplementation for horses is infrequently required when a normal diet is fed.

Experimental manipulation of dietary magnesium in horses

Hypomagnesemia was induced in mature ponies by feeding 5–6 mg/kg (BW)/day of Mg (using a 370 ppm diet), whereas 20 mg/kg (BW)/day met Mg requirements (Meyer & Ahlswede, 1977). A deficiency state can be more readily induced in growing animals because of their higher dietary requirement for Mg. Foals fed an extremely Mg-deficient diet (7–8 ppm or 0.0007%) developed severe mineralization of the aorta, with severe clinical signs of hypomagnesemia becoming apparent after 90 days in 2 of 11 foals (Harrington, 1974).

Urinary excretion of electrolytes is useful for assessing dietary supply of minerals. The urinary Mg concentration decreased from a baseline of 30 mg/dL to 4 mg/dL after 6 days on a Mg-deficient diet (370 ppm) and increased to over 300 mg/dL on a high-Mg diet supplemented with 36 g of MgO/day (Meyer & Ahlswede, 1977). Increasing the Mg content of a diet from 3100 ppm to 8600 ppm increased Mg digestibility, retention, and excretion in urine and feces and increased serum concentrations from 2.21 mg/dL to 3.39 mg/dL (Hintz & Schryver, 1973). In foals fed a severely Mg-deficient diet (7–8 ppm), serum Mg concentration decreased rapidly from a baseline of 0.78 mmol/L to 0.53 mmol/L after 7 days and then decreased steadily to 0.26 mmol/L after 150 days. The slower rate of reduction in serum Mg concentrations was presumed to be due to mobilization of Mg from bone. Bone magnesium content decreased in response to Mg depletion, but, surprisingly, there was no effect on tissue (brain, liver, kidney, spleen, lung, cardiac, or skeletal muscle) concentrations of Mg, Ca, or P after 71–180 days (Harrington, 1975).

Clinical signs and consequences of magnesium deficiency

In comparison to cattle, clinical signs of hypomagnesemia are rarely reported in horses. The signs include weakness, muscle fasciculations, ventricular arrhythmias, seizures, ataxia, and coma. Hypocalcemic tetany complicated by hypomagnesemia was reported in Welsh mountain ponies after prolonged transportation (Green et al., 1935). Similar signs were experimentally induced after 90 days in 2/11 foals fed an extremely

Mg-deficient diet (7–8 ppm). Signs of hypomagnesemic tetany were precipitated by loud noises, with foals initially exhibiting nervousness, muscular tremors and ataxia, followed by collapse, with profuse sweating, hyperpnea, and convulsions. One foal died during its third seizure on day 150 of the deficiency trial (Harrington, 1974).

Concurrent hypocalcemic and hypomagnesemic tetany was reported in two thoroughbred broodmares that had been transported for breeding. The mares were nursing foals that were 4 and 7 weeks old. The serum tCa was 4.0 mg/dL and 5.4 mg/dL while the tMg was 1.0 mg/dL and 1.9 mg/dL, respectively. The mares responded to intravenous calcium borogluconate and magnesium chloride (Meijer, 1982).

Severe hypomagnesemia can lead to ventricular arrhythmias, supraventricular tachycardia, or atrial fibrillation. Characteristic findings on electrocardiogram (ECG) include prolongation of the P–R interval, widening of the QRS complex, ST segment depression, and peaked T waves (Marr, 2004).

Hypomagnesemia and hypocalcemia are common perioperatively in horses requiring exploratory celiotomy for colic, particularly in horses with strangulating intestinal lesions and ileus. Significantly lower serum concentrations of Mg^{2+} occurred in horses that developed postoperative ileus (Garcia-Lopez et al., 2001). Horses with strangulating lesions were more likely to be hypomagnesemic and hypocalcemic, and have ECG changes than horses with non-strangulating lesions (Garcia-Lopez et al., 2001). There are probably multiple factors that contribute to the observed ECG disturbances, but the routine detection and correction of the electrolyte abnormalities (including Mg^{2+} and Ca^{2+}) is recommended.

Synchronous diaphragmatic flutter is associated with hypomagnesemia and hypocalcemia. Horses with dehydration, electrolyte derangements, and especially hypochloremic metabolic alkalosis associated with prolonged endurance exercise, gastric outflow obstruction, and sometimes after inappropriate bicarbonate administration are predisposed. Irritation of the phrenic nerve causes unilateral or bilateral contraction of the diaphragm synchronously with the heartbeat. Prolonged sweating or reflux of gastric origin can result in massive chloride and hydrogen ion loss. The resulting metabolic alkalosis can expose the negative charges on serum protein molecules. These negative charges can bind calcium

and magnesium ions and result in a relative ionized hypocalcemia and hypomagnesemia. Sodium bicarbonate administration in large amounts can have a similar effect. Measurement of total Ca and Mg may be normal but Mg^{2+} and Ca^{2+} will be low. The condition may resolve spontaneously after resolution of the primary cause or after the correction of electrolyte and acid–base imbalance and rehydration. Intravenous administration of calcium gluconate and magnesium sulfate diluted in fluids often speeds recovery.

Brain injury and magnesium

Magnesium is involved in the regulation of neuroexcitation by blockage of signal transmission through inhibition of Ca^{2+}-dependent presynaptic excitation-secretion coupling (Hoenderop & Bindels, 2005). Depletion of Mg contributes to tetany by increasing acetylcholine release from the neuromuscular junction and delaying degradation by acetylcholinesterase. Magnesium infusions have been advocated in the treatment of human brain and spinal trauma patients, but the efficacy of such treatments is still uncertain (Hoenderop & Bindels, 2005; Wilkins, 2001; Zhang et al., 1996). Based upon evidence from human medicine, Mg infusions have also been used in the empirical treatment of hypoxic ischemic encephalopathy (HIE) in neonatal foals (Wilkins, 2001).

Cerebral hypoxia impairs maintenance of ionic gradients across cell membranes, resulting in an influx of calcium and glutamate. Intracellular calcium and glutamate overload results in neuronal cell death. Traumatic brain injury induces the activation of the N-methyl-D-aspartate (NMDA) subtype of the glutamate receptor, and has been implicated in the pathophysiology of HIE (Thordstein et al., 1993; Zhang et al., 1996). Magnesium is important in the voltage-dependent blockade of NMDA calcium channels, preventing calcium entry into the cell and decreasing neurotransmitter release. Magnesium also blocks the entry of calcium through the voltage-gated calcium channels in the presynaptic membrane (Leonard & Kirby, 2002). Normal blood brain vessel vasodilation is also dependent on Mg (Seelig et al., 1983). Lower Mg concentrations increase vascular smooth muscle tone potentiating vasospasm with reduction of oxygen and substrate delivery to tissues. Focal traumatic brain and spinal cord injury in rats can reduce free brain Mg concentrations by as much as 60%, with the reduction proportional to the extent of the injury (Leonard & Kirby, 2002). Therefore, brain injury reduces brain Mg concentrations; this results in the loss of Mg's protective role and potentiation of further brain injury.

The reduction in the voltage-dependent Mg^{2+} blockade of the NMDA current in mechanically injured neurons can be restored by increasing the extracellular Mg concentration. Administration of magnesium sulfate has been shown to dramatically improve the immediate recovery of rats from hypoxia and improve the motor outcome in rats treated after severe traumatic axonal brain injury (Heath & Voink, 1999; Seimkowicz, 1997). Magnesium sulfate has also been shown to protect the fetal brain during severe maternal hypoxia (Hallak et al., 2000). The available experimental literature and reasoning suggest that in most cases Mg therapy may be advantageous in the treatment of HIE in foals and traumatic brain injury in horses, but further evidence is still required before the benefits, if any, can be proven (Wilkins, 2001; Zhang et al., 1996).

Diagnostic testing

Clinical laboratory evaluation of Mg status is generally limited to measurement of serum and urine tMg or Mg^{2+} concentrations, 24-hour urinary excretion, and percent retention following parenteral Mg loading. However, results for these tests do not necessarily correlate with intracellular ionized concentrations. There is no universally accepted, validated, and readily available test to determine intracellular/total body magnesium status.

Measurement of serum tMg or Mg^{2+} concentrations is the easiest way to assess Mg status. Serum Mg^{2+} is more useful than tMg as it is the active form and is minimally affected by serum protein concentrations. Hypoalbuminemia results in a low measured serum tMg concentration (pseudohypomagnesemia) and does not require Mg supplementation if the serum Mg^{2+} concentration is normal. Formulas to correct tMg concentration based on adjustment for protein concentrations are not accurate, and Mg^{2+} concentration should be measured. Plasma pH can affect the availability of serum Mg and the percent in the active ionized form. Similar to calcium, Mg binds to anionic (negatively charged) protein binding sites, with the binding affinity

dependent on pH. During acidosis, the increased hydrogen ion concentration displaces Ca^{2+} and Mg^{2+} from their protein binding sites, increasing the percent of these cations in the ionized form. This displacement results in increased serum Ca^{2+} and Mg^{2+} concentrations. In animals with respiratory or metabolic alkalosis (often observed after prolonged strenuous endurance exercise), Ca^{2+} and Mg^{2+} concentrations may be low, due to increased protein binding. As Mg^{2+} is the physiologically active component, supplementation is recommended to treat ionized hypomagnesemia, especially if clinical signs of synchronous diaphragmatic flutter (thumps), ileus, or, rarely, muscle fasciculations, ataxia, or tetany are observed.

Although not likely to be of consequence in an animal with adequate renal function, resolution of the alkalosis may result in increases in serum Mg^{2+} concentration. In contrast, animals with metabolic acidosis secondary to sepsis, SIRS, and severe gastrointestinal disease rarely have serum ionized hypermagnesemia. Serum Mg^{2+} concentration tends to be low from altered Mg homeostasis, cellular or third space redistribution, gastrointestinal loss of Mg, or from diuresis secondary to aggressive fluid therapy with intravenous fluids not supplemented with Mg.

Renal excretion of Mg may be used to evaluate Mg balance. With low dietary Mg intake, urinary Mg excretion falls to negligible levels (Stewart, 2004). Renal Mg excretion is measured in urine collected over 24 hours (mg/kg/day). The fractional clearance of Mg (FMg) can be determined by expressing the renal Mg clearance relative to the creatinine clearance. FMg in healthy horses fed grass hay ranges from 15 to 35%, and values less than 6% indicate inadequate dietary Mg intake (Stewart, 2004; Toribio et al., 2005). The Mg retention test to assess total body status has been evaluated in horses receiving Mg-deficient diets, using 10 mg/kg IV of elemental Mg (100 mg/kg of $MgSO_4$ of the 50% solution, diluted to 10%) administered over 60 minutes. Percent retention (%Ret) is calculated as:

$$\% \, Ret = (1 - [Mg \, excretion \, in \, 24 \, h] / [Mg \, infused]) \times 100 \quad (6.1)$$

However, in the study validating the Mg retention test in horses, the 24-hour excretion of Mg was found to be a more sensitive indicator of reduced Mg intake than the Mg retention test. The spot FMg reflected the 24-h excretion of Mg, providing a simple method to assess Mg status in horses (Stewart, 2004).

Muscle Mg content has been used as an estimate of total body Mg stores in horses (Grace et al., 1999; Stewart, 2004). In horses fed a moderately Mg-deficient diet, no differences were found in muscle Mg content compared to controls, but intracellular Mg^{2+} concentrations were lower in Mg-deficient horses (Stewart, 2004).

Treatment for hypomagnesemia

Intravenous magnesium

When supplementing intravenous solutions with Mg it is important to determine whether the dose reported is for elemental Mg or for the particular salt. For $MgSO_4$ solution (9.7% Mg), a dose of 100 mg/kg provides 9.7 mg/kg of elemental Mg, whereas for $MgCl_2$ (25.5%) a dose of 100 mg/kg provides 25.5 mg/kg of elemental Mg. Confusion and subsequent overdose may be fatal.

Dose rates for $MgSO_4$ that can be recommended in adult horses range from 25 to 150 mg/kg/day (0.05 to 0.3 mL/kg of a 50% solution) diluted to a 5% solution in normal saline, dextrose, or a polyionic isotonic solution and given by slow intravenous infusion. A constant rate infusion (CRI) with 150 mg/kg/day IV of $MgSO_4$ solution (0.3 mL/kg/day of the 50% solution) would provide the horse's daily requirements (Mogg, 2001). Practically speaking, for a 500-kg horse receiving 30 L/d of IV fluids, add 25 mL of 50% $MgSO_4$ solution to each 5-L bag, and for a horse receiving 60 L/d add 12 mL of

$MgSO_4$ solution per 5-L bag). Such therapy should be considered in horses with postoperative ileus, diarrhea, and SDF.

Plasma-Lyte®-A and Normosol™-R contain 3 mEq/L (3.6 mg/dL) of elemental Mg. If a horse received 60 mL/kg/day of the replacement fluid, it would receive 2.16 mg/kg/day of elemental Mg (equivalent to 20 mg/kg of $MgSO_4$). Additional Mg is therefore required for long-term fluid support of an inappetent animal.

Magnesium sulfate is also used to treat refractory ventricular arrhythmias including those caused by idiosyncratic quinidine reactions (especially torsades de pointes). For ventricular arrhythmias, small repeated doses of 2–6 mg/kg/min of $MgSO_4$ IV (1.8–5.4 mL of 50% $MgSO_4$/450-kg horse/min) to effect are recommended. Some authors recommend a maximum dose of 25 g (56 mg/kg) of $MgSO_4$, but studies in normal horses indicate that 100 mg/kg of $MgSO_4$ can be safely administered over 60 minutes, with mild sedation being occasionally noted (Stewart, 2004). Experimental administration of 100 mg/kg of magnesium sulfate solution over 30 minutes induced rapid decreases in serum calcium concentration, with subsequent elevations in plasma PTH concentrations, followed by subsequent rebound in calcium concentrations (A. Stewart, unpublished data; see Figure 6.1).

For the treatment of HIE in neonatal foals, a CRI of $MgSO_4$ at an initial dose of 50 mg/kg/h IV for 1 hour, followed by 25 mg/kg/h CRI for 24 hours can be used (Wilkins, 2001). For a 50-kg foal, add 62 mL of 50% $MgSO_4$ solution to a 1-liter bag of isotonic fluids and

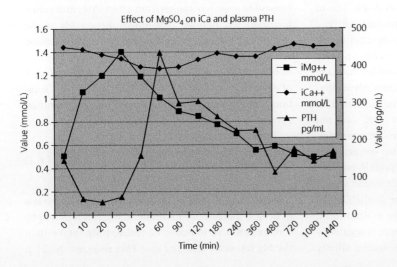

Figure 6.1 Experimental administration of 100 mg/kg of magnesium sulfate solution over 30 minutes. The infusion produces rapid decreases in serum calcium concentration, with subsequent elevations in plasma parathyroid hormone (PTH) concentrations, followed by subsequent rebound in calcium concentrations. iCa++, ionized calcium; iMg++, ionized magnesium.

run at 85 mL/h for 1 hour then decrease to 42 mL/h. This dose provides 600 mg/kg/day of $MgSO_4$ and is much higher than required for maintenance. Therapy has been continued for up to 3 days without visible detrimental effects other than possible trembling (Wilkins, 2001). Magnesium sulfate has also been recommended as a muscle relaxant as an adjunctive treatment for tetanus. Magnesium sulfate can be infused with a high therapeutic safety index, with the safety dependent on the dose and the infusion rate, but is contraindicated with undiagnosed disturbances in cardiac conduction, renal failure, or elevated serum Mg concentration. Early anesthetic regimens consisted of chloral hydrate and large dosages $MgSO_4$. Large volumes of concentrated $MgSO_4$ can be lethal and should never be administered.

Oral magnesium supplementation

The typical equine herbivore diet contains sufficient Mg for maintenance, with supplementation rarely required. Magnesium supplementation is, however, important when formulating oral replacement fluids for inappetent horses. If necessary, oral Mg can be provided with inorganic MgO, $MgSO_4$, or $MgCO_3$, which have equivalent digestibilities of approximately 70%. The maintenance requirement of 13 mg/kg/day of elemental Mg could be provided by 31 mg/kg/day of MgO, 93 mg/kg/day of $MgSO_4$, or 64 mg/kg/day of $MgCO_3$. Dolomite – $CaMg(CO_3)_2$ – is another inorganic salt containing calcium and magnesium in a 2:1 ratio and is commonly used as fertilizer for increasing the calcium and magnesium contents of deficient soils. Magnesium gluconate and magnesium aspartate are organic forms of magnesium and tend to be much more expensive, and have little benefit over inorganic forms for oral administration.

Magnesium sulfate (Epsom salt) is commonly used as an osmotic cathartic in the treatment of large colon impactions. A dose of 0.5–1.0 g/kg of $MgSO_4$ in 6–8 L of water can be administered by stomach tube when the horse is metabolically stable. A second dose can be administered 24–36 hours later in severe cases only if serum Mg concentrations have returned to normal. A side effect of $MgSO_4$ administration is mild sedation, which can be useful in a painful horse with a large intestinal impaction. Repeated smaller doses can be used as fecal softeners in mares prior to repair of third-degree perineal lacerations. Care must be taken with the total dose administered as hypermagnesemic, hypocalcemic neuromuscular paralysis has been reported following administration of $MgSO_4$ enterally to horses (Henninger & Horst, 1997; Nancy Aronoff, personal communication, 2009).

Hypermagnesemia

Hypermagnesemia is rare in all species and is commonly the result of iatrogenic Mg overdose, or excessive supplementation to a patient in renal failure. Serum hypermagnesemia (with hyperkalemia and hyperphosphatemia) occurs after severe cellular damage (rhabdomyolysis, hemolysis, severe sepsis, tumor lysis syndrome).

Hypermagnesemia was reported in two horses given excessive Epsom salt ($MgSO_4$) in addition to dioctyl sodium sulfosuccinate (DSS) for the treatment of large colon impaction (Henninger & Horst, 1997). The 450-kg and 500-kg horses were reportedly given 750 g and 1000 g of $MgSO_4$, respectively. The horses showed signs of agitation, sweating, and muscle tremors followed by recumbency and flaccid paralysis 4–6 hours after the $MgSO_4$ overdose. Tachycardia and tachypnea developed, peripheral pulses were undetectable and capillary refill time was prolonged at 4 seconds. Serum tMg concentrations rose to five times the reported reference range. The horses were treated with 250 mL of a 23% solution of calcium gluconate (diluted in 1 L of 0.9% NaCl) administered slowly IV. Intravenous fluids were given to induce diuresis. One horse was able to stand 10 minutes after the completion of the calcium infusion. A second calcium infusion was required when muscle tremors recurred 1 hour later in this horse. The second horse remained weak for several hours, being able to stand only for short periods. These two horses were given $MgSO_4$ at 1.5–2 times the recommended maximum dose, but it is unlikely that this dose of Epsom salt alone would normally be able to induce such severe clinical signs.

The authors suggested that the concurrently administered DSS may have increased intestinal permeability and increased the Mg absorption, with exacerbation of the signs of hypermagnesemia due to the concurrent low serum calcium concentration. Epsom salt should only be given to treat large colon impactions after correction of dehydration and metabolic imbalances.

Simultaneous administration of excessive doses of Epsom salt with DSS should be avoided (Henninger & Horst, 1997).

References

Abbot L, Rude R. (1993) Clinical manifestations of magnesium deficiency. *Miner Electrolyte Metab* **19**:314–22.

al-Ghamdi SM, Cameron EC, Sutton RA. (1994) Magnesium deficiency: pathophysiologic and clinical overview. *Am J Kidney Dis* **24**:737–52.

Barbagallo M, Dominguez LJ, Galiato A, et al. (2003) Role of magnesium in insulin action, diabetes and cardio-metabolic syndrome X. *Mol Aspects Med* **24**:39–52.

Burkitt JM, Sturges BK, Jandrey KE, et al. (2007) Risk factors associated with outcome in dogs with tetanus: 38 cases (1987–2005). *J Am Vet Med Assoc* **230**:76–83.

Chameroy KA, Frank N, Elliott SB, et al. (2011) Effects of a supplement containing chromium and magnesium on morphometric measurements, resting glucose, insulin concentrations and insulin sensitivity in laminitic obese horses. *Equine Vet J* **43**:494–9.

Dacey MJ. (2001) Hypomagnesemic disorders. *Crit Care Clin* **17**:155–73.

de Rouffignac C, Mandon B, Wittner M, et al. (1993) Hormonal control of renal magnesium handling. *Miner Electrolyte Metab* **19**:226–31.

Elin RJ. (1988) Magnesium metabolism in health and disease. *Dis-Mon* **34**:161–218.

Fatemi S, Ryzen E, Flores J, et al. (1991) Effect of experimental human magnesium depletion on parathyroid hormone secretion. *Endocrinol Metab* **73**:1067–72.

Freedman A, Atrakchi A, Cassidy M, et al. (1990) Magnesium deficiency-induced cardiomyopathy: Protection by vitamin E. *Biochem Biophys Res Comm* **170**:1102–6.

Freedman A, Cassidy M, Weglacki W. (1991) Captopril protects against myocardial injury induced by magnesium deficiency. *Hypertension* **18**:142–7.

Garcia-Lopez JM, Provost PJ, Rush JE, et al. (2001) Prevalence and prognostic importance of hypomagnesemia and hypocalcemia in horses that have colic surgery. *Am J Vet Res* **62**:7–12.

Grace N, Pearce S, Firth E, Fennessy P. (1999) Content and distribution of macro- and micro-elements in the body of pasture fed horses. *Aus Vet J* **77**:172–6.

Green HH, Allcroft WM, Montgomerie RF. (1935) Hypomagnesaemia in equine transit therapy. *J Comp Path Ther* **48**:74.

Hallak M, Hotra JW, Kupsky WJ. (2000) Magnesium sulfate protection of fetal rat brain from severe maternal hypoxia. *Obstet Gynecol* **96**:124–8.

Harrington D. (1974) Pathological features of magnesium deficiency in young horses fed purified rations. *Am J Vet Res* **35**:503.

Harrington D. (1975) Influence of magnesium deficiency on horse foal tissue concentrations of magnesium, calcium and phosphorus. *Brit J Nutr* **34**:45.

Harrington D, Walsh J. (1980) Equine magnesium supplements: Evaluation of magnesium oxide, magnesium sulphate and magnesium carbonate in foals fed purified diets. *Equine Vet J.* **12**:32–3.

Heath DL, Voink R. (1999) Pretreatment with magnesium sulfate protects against hypoxic-ischemic brain injury but postasphyxial treatment worsens brain injury in 7-day old rats. *Am J Obstet Gynecol* **180**:725–30.

Helman R, Edwards W. (1997) Clinical features of blister beetle poisoning in equids: 70 cases (1983–1996). *J Am Vet Med Assoc* **211**:1018–21.

Henninger RW, Horst J. (1997) Magnesium toxicosis in two horses. *J Am Vet Med Assoc* **211**:82–5.

Hintz H, Schryver H. (1972) Magnesium metabolism in the horse. *J Anim Sci* **35**:755.

Hintz F, Schryver H. (1973) Magnesium, calcium and phosphorus metabolism in ponies fed varying levels of magnesium. *J Anim Sci* **37**:927–30.

Hoenderop JG, Bindels RJ. (2005) Epithelial Ca2+ and Mg2+ channels in health and disease. *J Am Soc Nephrol* **16**:15–26.

Johansson AM, Gardner SY, Jones SL, et al. (2003) Hypomagnesemia in hospitalized horses. *J Vet Int Med* **17**:860–7.

Kayne L, Lee D. (1993) Intestinal magnesium absorption. *Minor Electrolyte Metab* **19**:210–17.

Kramer J, Misik V, Weglecki W. (1994) Magnesium-deficiency potentiates free radical production associated with postischemic injury to rat hearts: vitamin E affords protection. *Free Radic Biol Med* **16**:713–23.

Leicht E, Schmidt-Gayk H, Langer HJ. (1992) Hypomagnesemia induced hypocalcemia: Concentrations of parathyroid hormone, prolactin and 1,25-dihydroxyvitamin D during magnesium replenishment. *Magnes Res* **5**:33–6.

Leonard SE, Kirby R. (2002) The role of glutamate, calcium and magnesium in secondary brain injury. *J Vet Emerg Crit Care* **12**:17–32.

Lopez I, Estepa JC, Mendoza FJ, et al. (2006) Fractionation of calcium and magnesium in equine serum. *Am J Vet Res* **67**:463–6.

Mak I, Stafford R, Weglecki W. (1994) Loss of red cell glutathione during Mg deficiency: prevention by vitamin E, D-propranolol, and chloroquine. *Am J Physiol* **267**:C1366–C1370.

Malpuech-Brugere C, Nowacki W, Rock E, et al. (1999) Enhanced tumour necrosis factor-alpha production following endotoxin challenge in rats is an early event during magnesium deficiency. *Acta Biochem Biophys* **1453**:35–40.

Marino P. (1995) Calcium and magnesium in critical illness: a practical approach. In: Sivak E, Higgins T, Seiver A (eds) *The High Risk Patient: Management of the Critically Ill.* Baltimore: Williams & Wilkins, pp. 1183–95.

Marr CM. (2004) Cardiac emergencies and problems of the critical care patient. *Vet Clin North Am-Equine Pract* **20**:217–30.

Martens H, Schweigel M. (2000) Pathophysiology of grass tetany and other hypomagnesemias – Implications for clinical management. *Vet Clin North Am–Food Animal Pract* **16**:339–68.

Martin L, Matteson V, Wingfield W. (1994) Abnormalities of serum magnesium in critically ill dogs: incidence and implications. *J Vet Emerg Crit Care* **1**:15–20.

McLean R. (1994) Magnesium and its therapeutic uses: a review. *Am J Med* **96**:63–76.

Meijer P. (1982) Two cases of tetany in the horse. *Tijdschr Diergeneeskd* **107**:329–32.

Meyer H, Ahlswede L. (1977) Untersuchungen zum Mg-Stofwechsel des pferdes. *Zentrabl Veterinarinacrmed* **24**:128–39.

Mogg TD. (2001) Magnesium disorders – their role in equine medicine. In: *Proceedings of the 19th Annual Veterinary Medical Forum*. American College of Veterinary Internal Medicine, pp. 229–31.

Nielsen FH. (2010) Magnesium, inflammation, and obesity in chronic disease. *Nutr Rev* **68**:333–40.

Quamme GA, Dirks JH. (1983) Renal magnesium transport. *Rev Physiol Biochem Pharmacol* **265**:H281–H288.

Rasmussen H, Bordier P. (1974) *The Physiological and Cellular Basis of Metabolic Bone Disease*. Baltimore: Williams & Wilkins.

Reinhart RA, Desbiens NA. (1985) Hypomagnesemia in patients entering the ICU. *Crit Care Med* **13**:506–7.

Roden DM, Iansmith DH. (1987) Effects of low potassium or magnesium concentrations on isolated cardiac tissue. *Am J Med* **82**:18–23.

Rook J. (1969) Spontaneous and induced magnesium deficiency in ruminants. *Ann NY Acad Sci* **162**: 727–731.

Rude RK, Oldham S. (1990) Disorders of magnesium metabolism. In: Bohen RD (ed.) *The Metabolic and Molecular Basis of Acquired Disease*. London: Ballière-Tindall, pp. 1124–48.

Ryzen E. (1989) Magnesium homeostasis in critically ill patients. *Magnesium* **8**:201–12.

Ryzen E, Wagners P, Singer F, et al. (1985) Magnesium deficiency in a medical ICU population. *Crit Care Med* **13**:19–21.

Salem M, Kasinski N, Munoz R, et al. (1995) Progressive magnesium deficiency increases mortality from endotoxin challenge: protective effects of acute magnesium therapy. *Crit Care Med* **23**:108–18.

Seelig JM, Wei EP, Kontos HA, et al. (1983) Effect of changes in magnesium ion concentration on cat cerebral arterioles. *Am J Physiol* **245**:H22–H26.

Seimkowicz E. (1997) Pretreatment with magnesium sulfate protects against hypoxic-ischemic brain injury but post-asphyxial treatment worsens brain injury in 7-day old rats. *Resuscitation* **35**:53–9.

Shah B, Santucci M, Finberg L. (1994) Magnesium deficiency as a cause of hypocalcemia in the CHARGE association. *Arch Pediatr Adolesc Med* **148**:486–9.

Stewart AJ. (2004) Magnesium disorders. In: Reed SM, Bayly WM, Sellon DC (eds) *Equine Internal Medicine*, 2nd edn. St Louis: Saunders, pp. 1365–79.

Thordstein M, Bagenholm R, Thiringer K, et al. (1993) Scavengers of free oxygen radicals in combination with magnesium ameliorate perinatal hypoxic-ischemic brain damage in the rat. *Pediatr Res* **34**:23–6.

Tobey RC, Birnbaum GA, Allegra JR, et al. (1992) Successful resuscitation and neurologic recovery from refractory ventricular fibrillation after magnesium sulfate administration. *Ann Emerg Med* **21**:92–6.

Toribio RE. (2010) Magnesium and disease. In: Reed SM, Bayley WM, Sellon DC (eds) *Equine Internal Medicine*, 3rd edn. St Louis: Saunders, pp. 1291–5.

Toribio RE, Kohn CW, Chew DJ, et al. (2001) Comparison of serum parathyroid hormone and ionized calcium and magnesium concentrations and fractional urinary clearance of calcium and phosphorus in healthy horses and horses with enterocolitis. *Am J Vet Res* **62**:938–47.

Toribio RE, Kohn CW, Hardy J, et al. (2005) Alterations in serum parathyroid hormone and electrolyte concentrations and urinary excretion of electrolytes in horses with induced endotoxemia. *J Vet Intern Med* **19**:223–31.

Toribio RE, Kohn CW, Rourke KM, et al. (2007) Effects of hypercalcemia on serum concentrations of magnesium, potassium, and phosphate and urinary excretion of electrolytes in horses. *Am J Vet Research* **68**:543–54.

Wacker WEC, Parisi AF. (1968) Magnesium metabolism. *N Engl J Med* **278**:658–63, 712–17, 772–6.

Whang R, Oei TO, Aikawa JK, et al. (1984) Predictors of clinical hypomagnesemia. Hypokalemia, hypophosphatemia, hyponatremia, and hypocalcemia. *Arch Intern Med* **144**:1794–6.

Whang R, Whand D, Ryan M. (1992) Refractory potassium repletion: A consequence of magnesium deficiency. *Arch Intern Med* **152**:40–5.

White R, Hartzell H. (1989) Magnesium ions in cardiac function. *Biochem Pharmacol* **38**:859–67.

Weglicki W, Phillips T, Freedman A, et al. (1992) Magnesium-deficiency elevates circulating levels of inflammatory cytokines and endothelin. *Mol Cell Biochem* **110**:169–73.

Wilkins PA. (2001) Magnesium infusion in hypoxic ischemic encephalopathy. In: *Proceedings of the 19th Annual Veterinary Medical Forum*. American College of Veterinary Internal Medicine, pp. 242–4.

Zhang L, Rzigalinski BA, Ellis EF, et al. (1996) Reduction of voltage-dependent Mg2+ blockade of NMDA current in mechanically injured neurons. *Science* **274**:1921–3.

CHAPTER 7

Phosphorus homeostasis and derangements

Ramiro E. Toribio

Associate Professor, The Ohio State University, College of Veterinary Medicine, Columbus, OH, USA

Introduction

In the assessment of the critically ill equine patient, a routine approach is to focus on the fluid, acid–base, and electrolyte disturbances. Within electrolytes, attention is directed towards sodium, potassium, chloride, and calcium. However, a number of conditions are associated with dysregulation of other essential ions, including phosphorus and magnesium. Relevant to intensive care medicine, phosphate is required for cell integrity and function, and abnormal phosphorus concentrations in sick patients can have devastating consequences. Phosphorus is reported in most equine biochemical profiles; however, the clinical implications of hypophosphatemia or hyperphosphatemia are often underappreciated, with even less attention placed on therapies to directly correct phosphorus.

Phosphorus distribution

Phosphorus has structural (skeletal) and regulatory (metabolic) functions. Approximately 1% of the body weight in horses comprises phosphorus, with most of it (85%) located in the bone mineralized matrix as hydroxyapatite crystals. Approximately 15% of phosphorus is located within blood and soft tissues, with less than 0.1% in the extracellular fluid (Tenenhouse, 2005). In the extracellular fluid, phosphorus exists as organic and inorganic phosphates. Organic phosphate consists of phosphate esters (phospholipids) bound to proteins and blood cells, and represents most of the phosphorus in circulation (70%); however, only inorganic phosphate (P_i) is measured.

In blood, P_i is found as ionized phosphate (~50%), complexed with cations (Na^+, Ca^{2+}, Mg^{2+}; ~35%), and bound to proteins (~15%). Four forms of P_i exist in biological fluids: H_3PO_4, $H_2PO_4^-$, HPO_4^{2-}, and PO_3^{2-}; however, at physiological pH only divalent (HPO_4^{2-}) and monovalent ($H_2PO_4^-$) forms of inorganic phosphate are present at significant concentrations (Tenenhouse, 2005). At pH 7.4, HPO_4^{2-} and $H_2PO_4^-$ are in a 4:1 ratio. In the presence of acidosis this ratio is 1:1 and it can be as high as 9:1 during alkalosis (Endres & Rude, 2006). This results in an average valence for serum P_i of –1.8 at pH 7.4, giving a milliequivalency of 1.8 mEq/L per 1 mmol/L of P_i.

Phosphate is the primary intracellular anion, existing in organic – phospholipids, nucleic acids, phosphoproteins, creatine phosphate, ATP, cAMP, $NADP^+$, 2,3-diphosphoglycerate (2,3-DPG) – and inorganic forms. Inorganic phosphate concentrations in the intracellular compartment are 20–40-fold higher than in the extracellular fluid. The cytosolic free P_i concentration is very low, and most intracellular P_i is in the mitochondria.

Most methods to determine serum P_i concentrations are based on the reaction between P_i with ammonium molybdate to form an orthophosphate (phosphomolybdate) complex that is measured by colorimetric methods or spectrophotometry (Endres & Rude, 2006). Hemolysis, hyperproteinemia, hyperbilirubinemia, and lipemia spuriously increase serum Pi concentrations.

Equine Fluid Therapy, First Edition. Edited by C. Langdon Fielding and K. Gary Magdesian.

The atomic weight of phosphorus is 31; therefore:

1 mmol/L = 3.1 mg/dL (31 mg/L) of phosphorus (or phosphate)

mg/dL × 0.32 = mmol/L

1 mg/dL = 0.32 mmol/L

1 mg = 0.032 mmol

1 mmol/L = 1.8 mEq/L

Unlike Ca^{2+}, blood P_i has more fluctuations that are influenced by age, physiologic status, activity, dietary phosphate content, diurnal variations, disease, glycemia, hormones, acid–base status, and quality of sample (pH, hemolysis, hyperlipemia, hyperproteinemia, and gammopathies). In adult horses, serum P_i ranges from 3.0 to 5.0 mg/dL (0.96–1.6 mmol/L), while concentrations in healthy foals are greater (5.0–9.0 mg/dL; 1.6–2.6 mmol/L). Similar to K^+ and Mg^{2+}, serum P_i is an unreliable indicator of body stores. Rapid movement of P_i between the intracellular and extracellular compartments can change serum P_i concentrations within short periods of time.

In young animals, high serum P_i concentrations are the result of increased intestinal absorption and renal reabsorption of P_i to supply the growing skeleton as well as other tissues. Similarly, alkaline phosphatase activity, likely from the intestine and bone, is increased in young animals. These processes are in part regulated by growth hormone (through insulin-like growth factor 1 (IGF-1)) (Denis et al., 1994).

Blood P_i concentrations are more indicative of the dietary phosphorus intake and status than serum Ca^{2+} is of dietary calcium intake because P_i homeostasis is not as precise as that of Ca^{2+} (Toribio, 2011). Concentrations of P_i are primarily controlled by intestinal absorption and renal reabsorption. In monogastric animals, the kidneys are the major regulators of serum P_i concentrations (Rosol & Capen, 1996). Parathyroid hormone, vitamin D, and phosphatonins are the main hormonal factors involved with P_i homeostasis (see "Phosphate homeostasis" below).

Phosphate functions

As part of the bone mineralized matrix in the form of hydroxyapatite crystals ($[Ca_{10}(PO_4)_6(OH)_2]$) phosphorus has important structural functions. As a regulatory ion, phosphate plays essential roles in processes such as muscle contraction, neurologic function, cell proliferation and differentiation, cell membrane integrity, enzyme activity, electrolyte transport, oxygen transport, gene transcription, and in the intermediary metabolism of proteins, carbohydrates, and fats (Endres & Rude, 2006; Toribio, 2011). The functions of P_i are closely linked with other ions, in particular Mg^{2+}, K^+, Na^+, and Ca^{2+}. For example, several proteins and enzymes involved in the transmembrane movement of these ions (e.g., plasma membrane calcium ATPase, Na^+/K^+-ATPase) indirectly require P_i because these are ATP-dependent processes. This movement also involves Mg^{2+} because ATP is associated with Mg^{2+} ($Mg \cdot ATP$) within the cell. It is not unusual for an animal with hypophosphatemia to have concurrent hypokalemia and hypomagnesemia. Unfortunately, these abnormalities often go unnoticed in critically ill equine patients.

Phosphate requirements, absorption, and excretion

Requirements

Phosphorus requirements depend on age, physiological status, work, exercise, and diseases (Table 7.1). Requirements are greater in growing animals, pregnant and lactating mares, and exercising horses. Similarly, physical activity and diseases leading to P_i redistribution, P_i waste, hypophosphatemia, or increased energy expenditure increase the P_i needs.

Absorption

Phosphate absorption occurs by passive diffusion and active mechanisms, using Na^+-dependent P_i cotransporters (Na^+/P_i) (Berndt & Kumar, 2007; Murer et al., 2001). Increased luminal content of Na^+ enhances P_i transport. Passive paracellular diffusion is important when luminal P_i concentrations are high, while active transcellular transport is more important at low dietary P_i content. Phosphatonins directly and indirectly decrease P_i absorption: directly by inhibiting Na^+/P_i function and indirectly by decreasing renal 1-α-hydroxylase activity and synthesis of 1,25-dihydroxyvitamin D3 (calcitriol; $1,25(OH)_2D_3$) (Bergwitz & Juppner, 2010; Fukumoto, 2008). There is evidence that intestinal Na^+/P_i can adapt to low dietary P_i independent of $1,25(OH)_2D_3$ (Amanzadeh & Reilly, 2006).

In the horse, P_i absorption occurs in the small and large intestines, and ranges from 30 to 55% (Barlet et al., 1995; NRC, 2007; Schryver, 1975). Most P_i absorption

Table 7.1 Requirements of calcium (Ca) and phosphorus (P) in horses (500-kg adult weight).

	% in the diet		Daily (grams)	
	Ca	P	Ca	P
Foals (<6 months)	0.80	0.55	39	22
Weanlings	0.60	0.45	38	22
Yearlings	0.50	0.35	37	21
Two-year-olds	0.40	0.30	35	20
Late pregnancy[a]	0.50	0.45	36	27
Early lactation[b]	0.50	0.45	60	38
Exercising horse[c]	0.40	0.30	35	21
Mature horses	0.30	0.20	20	14

Adapted from Argenzio et al. (1974), Hintz and Meakim (1981), NRC Committee on Nutrient Requirements of Horses (2007), Schryver et al. (1974), Schryver (1975), and Toribio (2011).
[a]Tenth month of pregnancy.
[b]First month of lactation.
[c]Moderate exercise.

occurs in the small intestine where hormonal regulation is minimal under physiological conditions (Barlet et al., 1995). Similar to P_i requirements, P_i absorption depends on breed, age, physiological status, physical activity, dietary content, diseases, and interfering substances (Schryver et al., 1972, 1974). The dietary source of phosphorus affects its absorption. Inorganic sources of phosphorus and bonemeals have high bioavailability while most phosphorus in concentrates is in the organic form of phytate, which is poorly utilized by monogastric animals (NRC, 2007). High dietary contents of oxalate and phytate reduce P_i absorption (NRC, 2007).

Unlike in other species, excess dietary aluminum or magnesium does not appear to interfere with P_i absorption in horses (Hintz et al., 1973; Hintz & Schryver, 1973; Roose et al., 2001). Phytase activity in the equine large colon can enhance P_i and calcium absorption (Hintz et al., 1973). A high calcium content has minimal effect on phosphorus absorption (Schryver et al., 1971).

Excretion

The kidneys are the major regulators of serum P_i concentrations (Tenenhouse, 2005; Toribio, 2011). Renal excretion is determined by the glomerular filtration rate (GFR) and tubular reabsorption rate. The proximal convoluted tubules reabsorb 60–80% of the filtered P_i, while 15–20%

is reabsorbed in the proximal straight tubules, and a small percentage in the distal nephron (Tenenhouse, 2005; Toribio, 2011). Most renal P_i reabsorption is transcellular. In the proximal tubules P_i transport is unidirectional, in three steps: (i) uptake at the apical brush border; (ii) transcellular translocation; and (iii) basolateral efflux (Bergwitz & Juppner, 2010; Tenenhouse, 2005). Proximal tubular uptake is the rate-limiting step in reabsorption and is the main site for P_i regulation. Uptake is mediated by the Na^+/P_i cotransporter whose activity depends on the gradient created by the basolateral Na^+/K^+-ATPase. Therefore, P_i reabsorption is indirectly an energy-dependent process (Bergwitz & Juppner, 2010; Biber et al., 2009; Tenenhouse, 2005).

Little is known about the transcellular and basolateral steps of P_i transport. Renal P_i reabsorption is increased with growth, lactation, pregnancy, and low-phosphate diets; it is decreased during slow growth, renal failure, excess dietary phosphate, and hyperparathyroidism (DiBartola & Willard, 2005; Rosol & Capen, 1996; Toribio, 2011). Horses have low urinary excretion of P_i (<0.5%) (Toribio et al., 2001).

Phosphate homeostasis

Organs involved in P_i absorption (intestine), excretion (kidney, intestine), and storage (bone) are under the direct control of extracellular P_i concentrations, as well as various endocrine systems. Humoral factors involved in P_i homeostasis include parathyroid hormone (PTH), $1,25(OH)_2D_3$ (calcitriol, active vitamin D), calcitonin, insulin, and phosphatonins (fibroblast growth factor 23 (FGF-23)/klotho axis) (Toribio, 2011). Under normal conditions the endocrine control of intestinal P_i absorption is minimal; however, during P_i deficiency, hormones such as $1,25(OH)_2D_3$ enhance P_i absorption. Once absorbed, P_i is incorporated into various organic forms (proteins, energy compounds, nucleic acids), stored in bone (hydroxyapatite), and transferred to the fetus and milk. Excess phosphorus is eliminated by the kidneys.

P_i homeostasis is primarily regulated by renal tubular transport (Bergwitz & Juppner, 2010; Berndt & Kumar, 2009; Blaine et al., 2011). The primary hormonal regulators of P_i reabsorption are PTH and the FGF-23/klotho axis (Bergwitz & Juppner, 2010; Blaine et al., 2011; Kuro-o, 2006). Although no specific receptor for P_i has been described, it is well documented that P_i interacts with cell membrane and cytoplasmic proteins. This interaction modifies cell function and homeostasis, especially during P_i deficiency or excess (Bergwitz & Juppner, 2011).

Low-P_i diets, insulin, growth hormone, IGF-1, $1,25(OH)_2D_3$, thyroid hormone, metabolic alkalosis, high-calcium diets, and high-K^+ diets stimulate P_i reabsorption (Levi & Popovtzer, 1999). In contrast, high-P_i diets, PTH, PTH-related protein (PTHrP), metabolic acidosis, calcitonin, epidermal growth factor, glucocorticoids, hypokalemia, diuretics, atrial natriuretic peptide (ANP), and phosphatonins inhibit renal P_i reabsorption (Bacic et al., 2004; Bergwitz & Juppner, 2010; Berndt & Kumar, 2009; Biber et al., 2009; Tenenhouse, 2005). PTH, $1,25(OH)_2D_3$, phosphorus intake, and FGF-23 are considered the main regulators of Na^+-dependent P_i reabsorption. Low P_i induces an upregulation of renal 1-α-hydroxylase activity and $1,25(OH)_2D_3$ synthesis. In turn, $1,25(OH)_2D_3$ increases the synthesis of Na^+/P_i cotransporters to enhance P_i reabsorption (Tenenhouse, 2005). In addition, increased $1,25(OH)_2D_3$ inhibits PTH synthesis to further promote P_i reabsorption. Phosphorus homeostasis is presented in conjunction with calcium homeostasis (see below).

Parathyroid hormone (PTH)

Hypocalcemia or hyperphosphatemia stimulates PTH release from the parathyroid glands. PTH enhances renal calcium absorption and $1,25(OH)_2D_3$ synthesis, and P_i excretion. PTH increases P_i excretion by inducing internalization of Na^+/P_i cotransporters in the proximal tubules (Biber et al., 2009; Pfister et al., 1998; Tenenhouse, 2005). In bone, PTH promotes osteoclastic bone resorption.

1,25-Dihydroxyvitamin D₃ (1,25(OH)₂D₃)

1,25-Dihydroxyvitamin D_3 increases intestinal absorption and renal reabsorption of Ca^{2+} and P_i. Vitamin D increases bone formation and resorption (remodeling). Vitamin D and its receptor (VDR) translocate to the nucleus to regulate the transcription of a number of genes involved in the transcellular movement of calcium (calbindins) and P_i (Na^+/P_i) (Razzaque, 2009; Toribio, 2011). Both hypocalcemia and hypophosphatemia stimulate $1,25(OH)_2D_3$ synthesis. PTH stimulates and FGF-23, klotho, and $1,25(OH)_2D_3$

inhibit renal 1-α-hydroxylase activity and $1,25(OH)_2D_3$ synthesis.

Calcitonin

Calcitonin is released in response to hypercalcemia in order to decrease serum calcium concentrations in a number of species, including horses (Rourke et al., 2009). The main function of calcitonin is to protect the skeleton from excessive bone loss by inhibiting osteoclastic activity (Woodrow et al., 2006). Calcitonin also inhibits the renal reabsorption of P_i (Berndt & Knox, 1984; Carney, 1997). There is some evidence, at least in other species, that calcitonin inhibits intestinal absorption of P_i (Matsui et al., 1983).

Parathyroid hormone-related protein (PTHrP)

Parathyroid hormone-related protein is a pleiotropic protein that activates the PTH receptor, thereby increasing the renal reabsorption of calcium and excretion of P_i. Parathyroid hormone-related protein has minimal calcium-regulating functions in adult animals, but it is important for fetal Ca^{2+} homeostasis (Wysolmerski & Stewart, 1998). Concentrations of PTHrP are increased in various equine malignancies, often associated with hypercalcemia and hypophosphatemia (Toribio, 2011).

Insulin

Insulin increases P_i movement from the extracellular to the intracellular compartment (Xie et al., 2000). It promotes P_i utilization through carbohydrate metabolism and energy-dependent electrolyte transport. Contrary to PTH, insulin stimulates the activity of the Na^+/P_i cotransporter in the renal proximal tubules (Amanzadeh & Reilly, 2006).

Insulin-like growth factor 1 (IGF-1; and growth hormone)

The effects of growth hormone on P_i transport and other functions are mediated by IGF-1 (Quigley & Baum, 1991). Renal tubular transport of P_i is increased by IGF-1 by stimulating Na^+/P_i cotransporter activity (Amanzadeh & Reilly, 2006; Blaine et al., 2011).

Glucocorticoids

Glucocorticoids inhibit renal P_i uptake, thereby promoting its excretion (Blaine et al., 2011).

Catecholamines

Beta-adrenergic stimulation is not considered to be important in P_i homeostasis; however, increases in blood catecholamine concentrations from pathologic conditions or use of beta-receptor agonists (e.g., albuterol, clenbuterol) can increase P_i movement into cells. Dopamine increases the urinary excretion of P_i (Cunningham et al., 2009).

Thyroid hormones

Thyroid hormones increase renal reabsorption of P_i (Amanzadeh & Reilly, 2006).

Atrial natriuretic peptide (ANP)

Similar to PTH, ANP induces internalization and degradation of Na^+/P_i cotransporters, resulting in natriuresis and phosphaturia (Bacic et al., 2004).

Phosphatonins and the FGF-23/klotho axis

Phosphatonin is a term that refers to a group of factors that induce hypophosphatemia, inhibit renal 1-α-hydroxylase (vitamin D synthesis), increase urinary P_i excretion, and decrease intestinal P_i absorption. Fibroblast growth factor-23 (FGF-23), secreted frizzled related protein 4 (sFRP-4), and matrix extracellular phosphoglycoprotein (MEPE) are examples of phosphatonins (Berndt et al., 2005). Phosphatonins cause internalization of Na^+/P_i cotransporters on renal epithelial cells (Berndt & Kumar, 2007; Murer et al., 2001). Both FGF-23 and sFRP4 are detectable in healthy individuals. Fibroblast growth factor -23 and klotho are part of the skeletal-renal axis that regulates $1,25(OH)_2D_3$ synthesis (Kiela & Ghishan, 2009). Phosphatonins are also secreted by some tumors, leading to a condition known as "tumor-induced hypophosphatemic osteomalacia" (Berndt et al., 2005). Information on phosphatonins in the horse is lacking; however, equine clinicians should be aware that there are other factors such as phosphatonins that can affect the P_i status in the critically ill patient.

Phosphate disorders

Disorders of P_i homeostasis are acute and chronic, leading to hypophosphatemia or hyperphosphatemia. In critically ill horses hypophosphatemia occurs with more frequency than hyperphosphatemia; however, in septic foals hyperphosphatemia seems to be a more common finding

(R. Toribio, personal communication). When acute hyperphosphatemia is present in these animals, it is usually associated with cell lysis or iatrogenesis. Genetic disorders that result in either hypo or hyperphosphatemia are poorly documented in domestic animals.

Hypophosphatemia

Pathogenesis

The development of hypophosphatemia occurs by three mechanisms: (i) decreased intestinal P_i absorption; (ii) increased urinary P_i excretion; and (iii) intracellular shift of P_i (redistribution). Acute hypophosphatemia could reflect a redistribution of P_i between compartments and not necessarily imply body depletion of P_i (Ritz et al., 2003). However, P_i depletion is often associated with hypophosphatemia. In the author's experience, hypophosphatemia occurs more commonly in miniature horses, ponies, and donkeys than in horses, often associated with hyperlipemia. It is also a common finding in animals receiving parenteral nutrition.

Absorption

Intestinal absorption of P_i is decreased by gastrointestinal diseases (diarrhea, inflammatory bowel disease, enteritis), hypovitaminosis D, diets deficient in P_i, and interfering substances (Table 7.2). Hypovitaminosis D can result in hypophosphatemia for various reasons. Vitamin D promotes intestinal absorption and renal reabsorption of calcium and P_i. A decrease in $1,25(OH)_2D_3$ results in hypocalcemia, which in turn increases PTH secretion, enhancing urinary P_i excretion. Low vitamin D concentrations also exacerbate PTH secretion because $1,25(OH)_2D_3$ is a negative regulator of PTH secretion. Parathyroid hormone also increases osteoclastic activity and bone demineralization.

Excretion

The urinary excretion of P_i is increased with hyperparathyroidism, low vitamin D, tumors, renal failure, and a number of drugs (aminoglycosides, diuretics). Hyperparathyroidism (primary and secondary) has been documented in horses (Benders et al., 2001; Frank et al., 1998; Peauroi et al., 1998). A hypocalcemic state, as occurs in critically ill horses and foals (Hurcombe et al., 2009; Toribio et al., 2001), can also lead to hypophosphatemia from increased PTH release.

Table 7.2 Causes of hypophosphatemia and hyperphosphatemia.

Causes of hypophosphatemia	Causes of hyperphosphatemia
Decreased absorption	**Increased absorption**
Decreased intake	Dietary excess
Malabsorption	Intravenous infusion
Malnutrition	Oral supplementation
Phosphate binders (small animals)	Vitamin D intoxication
Vitamin D deficiency	Phosphate-containing enemas
Redistribution	**Redistribution**
Diabetes	Rhabdomyolysis
Insulin administration	Hemolysis
Carbohydrate overload/ infusion	Tumor lysis syndrome
Hyperglycemia	Chemotherapy
Hyperlipemia	Metabolic acidosis (ketoacidosis,
Parenteral nutrition	lactic acidosis)
Refeeding syndrome	Respiratory acidosis
Catecholamines, xanthines	Crush injuries
Respiratory alkalosis	
Sepsis	
Increased excretion	**Decreased excretion**
Diuretics, overhydration	Hypoparathyroidism
Primary	Renal failure
hyperparathyroidism	Vitamin D intoxication
Increased PTHrP	Biphosphonate therapy
(malignancies)	Magnesium deficiency
Vitamin D deficiency	Multiple myeloma
Tumor-induced osteomalacia	Addison disease
(phosphatonins)	
Fanconi syndrome (other species)	
Chronic renal failure	
Other	**Other**
Laboratory error	Pseudohyperphosphatemia
Mannitol	(hyperproteinemia, bilirubin,
(pseudohypophosphatemia)	hyperlipemia, hemolysis)
	Physiologic hyperphosphatemia
	in growing animals

Adapted from different species (Bates, 2008; DiBartola & Willard, 2005; Endres & Rude, 2006; Geerse et al., 2010; Levi & Popovtzer, 1999; O'Brien & Coberly, 2003; Toribio, 2010, 2011).

Hypophosphatemia from cancer is well documented in humans and is primarily the result of increased urinary P_i excretion (see "Phosphatonins and the FGF-23/klotho axis" earlier). Cancer-induced hypophosphatemia occurs by two mechanisms: (i) phosphaturia from increased PTHrP concentrations (humoral hypercalcemia of malignancy; HHM) (Toribio, 2011; Wysolmerski & Stewart, 1998), and (ii) phosphatonin-mediated phosphaturia (Berndt & Kumar, 2007, 2009).

Humoral hypercalcemia of malignancy has been documented in horses with a number of malignancies (Barton et al., 2004; McCoy & Beasley, 1986; Toribio, 2011). These tumors secrete PTHrP, which interacts with PTH receptors to decrease renal P_i reabsorption. These animals also have hypercalcemia. Information on phosphatonin-mediated hypophosphatemia is lacking in domestic animals.

Genetic phosphaturic disorders such as X-linked hypophosphatemic rickets (XLH) and autosomal dominant hypophosphatemic rickets (ADHR) are well documented in people but not in domestic animals.

Hyperphosphatemia and hypocalcemia are the hallmarks of acute renal failure, while chronic renal failure is characterized by hypercalcemia and hypophosphatemia (Tennant et al., 1982; Toribio, 2011). Diuretics increase the urinary excretion of P_i, with those acting in the proximal tubules (carbonic anhydrase inhibitors) having the most phosphaturic effects because this is the main site for P_i reabsorption (DiBartola & Willard, 2005; Liamis et al., 2010). Neurogenic and nephrogenic diabetes insipidus may be associated with hypophosphatemia from renal loss as well. In other species, renal distal tubular acidosis, metabolic acidosis, and Fanconi syndrome can result in hypophosphatemia as additional causes of decreased renal reabsorption of P_i (DiBartola & Willard, 2005; Krapf et al., 1992).

Redistribution

Phosphate redistribution is due to several factors and is the main cause of hypophosphatemia in critically ill human patients (Amanzadeh & Reilly, 2006; Gaasbeek & Meinders, 2005; Geerse et al., 2010). Redistribution is also likely to be important in the development of hypophosphatemia in critically ill foals and horses. Specific causes of P_i redistribution include insulin-mediated P_i shift, elevation in catecholamine concentrations, and respiratory alkalosis (Amanzadeh & Reilly, 2006; Gaasbeek & Meinders, 2005; Geerse et al., 2010) (see Table 7.2). Sepsis, high-carbohydrate diets, hyperglycemia, insulin administration, starvation, refeeding syndrome, hyperlipemia, and parenteral nutrition (hyperglycemia, hyperinsulinemia) all decrease serum

P_i due to insulin-mediated intracellular shift of P_i and enhanced glycolysis. Hypophosphatemia from these disorders is well documented in critically ill humans and small animals (DiBartola & Willard, 2005). Clinical experience indicates that hypophosphatemia is associated with similar conditions in acutely ill equine patients (R.E. Toribio, personal communication). Catecholamines, similar to insulin, stimulate the activity of the Na^+/K^+-ATPase and the requirements for P_i. In respiratory alkalosis, as blood and intracellular CO_2 decrease, the pH rises. Alkalosis stimulates phospho-fructokinase activity (glycolysis) and the need for P_i increases to synthesize ATP. As a result, P_i from the extracellular compartment moves into the cells, leading to hypophosphatemia (O'Brien & Coberly, 2003; Shor et al., 2006). Hyperventilation (respiratory alkalosis) is considered the main cause of hypophosphatemia in human intensive care units (Amanzadeh & Reilly, 2006; O'Brien & Coberly, 2003). Even though diabetes mellitus is rare in horses (Durham et al., 2009), it has been linked with hypophosphatemia in other species (DiBartola & Willard, 2005). Diabetic animals develop hypophosphatemia from decreased insulin con-centrations (type 1 diabetes), insulin resistance (type 2 diabetes), and polyuria with phosphaturia, ultimately leading to body depletion of P_i. The mechanism for the development of hypophosphatemia from insulin's inability to move or maintain P_i into the cell (P_i waste) is different from that of increased insulin concentrations shifting P_i into the intracellular compartment (P_i redis-tribution), as previously described. Insulin admini-stration can worsen hypophosphatemia, an important consideration when treating equine patients with multiple metabolic derangements. An example of this would be the pony with hyperlipemia that is treated with insulin. Ketoacidosis is not a common problem in equine practice; however, ketoacidotic dogs and cats may develop hypophosphatemia from insulin therapy (DiBartola & Willard, 2005). Ketoacidosis *per se* is a cause of hyperphosphatemia.

In horses with a history of malnutrition, close moni-toring of serum P_i concentrations is indicated. After caloric intake is increased, these horses may develop abnormalities consistent with refeeding syndrome (Witham & Stull, 1998). In this condition, there is a shift from a catabolic to an anabolic state, increasing the intracellular needs for P_i. Insulin secretion leads to an intracellular redistribution of P_i during refeeding.

Other causes of hypophosphatemia

Hypophosphatemia can be spurious due to laboratory error. Large doses of mannitol can cause pseudohypo-phosphatemia because it binds to molybdate in the colorimetric reaction to measure P_i (Liamis et al., 2010).

Clinical signs of hypophosphatemia

Signs of acute hypophosphatemia are the result of skeletal, smooth muscle, and neurological dysfunction, while signs of chronic hypophosphatemia primarily involve the skeleton. Hypophosphatemia can be classified according to serum P_i concentrations as severe (< 1.0 mg/dL; < 0.32 mmol/L), moderate (1.0-2.0 mg/dL; 0.32-0.64 mmol/L), and mild (2.1-2.5 mg/dL; 0.67-0.8 mmol/L).

Acute hypophosphatemia

Clinical signs of hypophosphatemia in horses manifest when serum P_i concentrations are below 1.0 mg/dL, although often they go unnoticed. Horses with mild or moderate hypophosphatemia rarely show clinical signs. The signs of acute hypophosphatemia relate to P_i regulatory functions for ion transport, energy metabo-lism, and cell membrane stability. These include neu-romuscular irritability, muscle weakness, muscle fasciculations, arrhythmias, decreased gastrointestinal motility, and cell membrane fragility and lysis (hemo-lysis, rhabdomyolysis) from abnormal cell membrane potential, impaired glucose use, and decreased ATP synthesis (Amanzadeh & Reilly, 2006; DiBartola & Willard, 2005; Toribio, 2010). Hypophosphatemia can also lead to tissue hypo-oxygenation due to decreased erythrocyte concentrations of 2,3-bisphosphoglycerate (2,3-BPG; or 2,3-diphosphoglycerate (2,3-DPG)), shift-ing the hemoglobin dissociation curve to the left and impairing oxygen release, thus contributing to cell dysfunction. In humans, small animals, and ruminants, hypophosphatemia has been associated with muscle weakness, rhabdomyolysis, myocardial dysfunction, arrhythmias, seizures, pontine myelinolysis, and hemolysis (DiBartola & Willard, 2005; Geerse et al., 2010; Jubb et al., 1990). Hypophosphatemia also pre-disposes to infections due to impaired leukocyte che-motaxis and phagocytosis from low ATP production (Amanzadeh & Reilly, 2006). It has been proposed that hyperalimentation might predispose to sepsis due to reduced leukocyte phagocytosis from hypophosphate-mia (Amanzadeh & Reilly, 2006).

Chronic hypophosphatemia

Chronic hypophosphatemia is uncommon in horses and manifests as weight loss, weakness, pica (depraved appetite), bone mineral loss, lameness, developmental orthopedic diseases, rickets, and hemolysis (Toribio, 2011). Rickets from P_i deficiency is poorly documented in growing horses. Additional information on equine hypophosphatemia is provided elsewhere (NRC, 2007; Toribio, 2010, 2011).

Clinical pathology

Laboratory abnormalities associated with hypophosphatemia include hyperglycemia, hyperinsulinemia, hypokalemia, and hypomagnesemia. Hemolysis has been reported in small and large animals and humans (Adams et al., 1993; Amanzadeh & Reilly, 2006; Jubb et al., 1990; Ogawa et al., 1989; Willard et al., 1987). Muscle enzymes may be increased. Other abnormalities may be non-specific.

Treatment of hypophosphatemia

Compared to the amount of information available on therapeutic approaches to hypophosphatemia in other species, data in horses are scarce. In fact, critically ill horses and foals are rarely treated for hypophosphatemia. Due to the implications that P_i deficiency can have for numerous cellular processes (cell integrity, respiration, energy generation), in many instances therapy is warranted. Factors to consider in replacement therapy include serum P_i concentrations, energy balance (e.g., malnutrition), type of diet, caloric intake (enteral/parenteral), enteral P_i intake, metabolic status, type of disease, duration of condition, current treatments, hormone treatment, renal disease, fluid therapy, calcium concentrations, and calcium administration. Hypokalemia and hypomagnesemia are frequent findings in horses with hypophosphatemia and should be assessed during phosphate supplementation.

Similar to K^+ and Mg^{2+}, most P_i in the body is intracellular and deficit calculations from serum values do not represent the total body phosphorus status. The P_i deficit is calculated from standard electrolyte formulas and this amount should be overestimated, particularly with persistent hypophosphatemia, because cell depletion is likely to be present in these animals. Overestimation may not be necessary in animals with acute hypophosphatemia or hypophosphatemia from redistribution. Hypophosphatemia from respiratory alkalosis in general

improves without P_i supplementation, at least in humans (O'Brien & Coberly, 2003).

There are no approved products to treat hypophosphatemia in horses. However, injectable and oral products formulated for other species can be used (R.E. Toribio, personal communication). The author prefers potassium phosphate as a parenteral solution for the treatment of acute hypophosphatemia, although sodium phosphate is a good alternative (Table 7.3). The advantage of potassium phosphate is that it provides potassium, which often is concurrently low in these animals. Sodium phosphate would be a better option for horses with normokalemia. Unfortunately these salts are not readily accessible to the equine clinician, or are unavailable in sufficient volumes to treat an adult horse with severe hypophosphatemia. In the author's experience, sick horses can also be supplemented via nasogastric intubation with chemical grade potassium or sodium phosphate salts (Table 7.4). Additional information on bioavailability of these products is provided elsewhere. (NRC, 2007; Toribio, 2010, 2011).

Alternative compounds, formulated for other species, should be considered when sodium or potassium phosphate is not accessible (Tables 7.3 to 7.5). A number of products formulated for cattle also contain calcium, magnesium, and potassium. Oral products used in humans and small animals may be impractical in large equine patients (Table 7.5). Sodium phosphate enemas, which contain monobasic and dibasic sodium phosphate, are often used intravenously in ruminants to treat hypophosphatemia. There are anecdotal reports that they are occasionally used in horses.

The rate of phosphate administration is determined by the duration and severity of the hypophosphatemia (deficit, depletion), and the presence of clinical signs. Mild hypophosphatemia may not require treatment or can be treated with oral supplementation. Phosphate can be replaced within a short period of time (hours), particularly in animals showing clinical signs. Slower rates or continuous rate infusions (CRI) are considered better because there is less renal waste and more time for P_i to distribute. Limited data are available on enteral or parenteral rates of P_i administration for horses with acute hypophosphatemia. In small animals, rates of 0.01–0.06 mmol/kg/h are considered safe (DiBartola & Willard, 2005). For humans, rates of 0.08–0.16 mmol/kg/h are typically recommended (Amanzadeh & Reilly, 2006). However, in recent years the trend is to use

Table 7.3 Products used for parenteral supplementation of phosphate.

Product	Composition/mL	Phosphorus/mL	Potassium/mL	Sodium/mL	Presentation	Company
Potassium phosphate[a]	236 mg of K_2HPO_4 224 mg of KH_2PO_4	3 mM or 93 mg	4.4 mM or 170 mg	0	5, 15, 50 mL	American Reagents, Inc.
Sodium phosphate[a]	142 mg of Na_2HPO_4 276 mg of NaH_2PO_4	3 mM or 93 mg	0	4 mM or 92 mg	5, 15, 50 mL	American Reagents, Inc. Hospira, Inc.
Phosphaid[b,c]	200 mg of NaH_2PO_2	2 mM or 60 mg	0	2 mM or 46 mg	100 mL	Vedco, Inc.
Phos-Aid[b,c]	200 mg of NaH_2PO_2	2 mM or 60 mg	0	2 mM or 46 mg	100 mL	Neogen, Inc.
Phos P 200[b,c]	200 mg of NaH_2PO_2	2 mM or 60 mg	0	2 mM or 46 mg	100 mL	Phoenix, Inc.
CMPK[b,d]	5 mg of NaH_2PO_2 16 mg of KCl	0.05 mM or 1.5 mg	0.4 mM or 16 mg	0.05 mM or 1.1 mg	500 mL	Vedco, Inc.

[a] For human use.
[b] Approved for cattle. Contains phosphinic acid (hypophosphorous acid [H_3PO_2]; sodium hypophosphite [NaH_2PO_2]).
[c] Dose for adult cattle ranges from 1 mL/25–50 kg (50–100 lb) of body weight.
[d] To treat hypocalcemia and hypomagnesemia in cattle. Suggested dose for adult cattle is 500 mL/360–450 kg (800–1000 lb) of body weight.
Also contains magnesium, calcium, and potassium.
Other formulations that contain phosphorus include Cal-Phos (Vedco, Inc.) and Norcalciphos (Zoetis, Inc.).
K_2HPO_4 = dibasic potassium phosphate; KH_2PO_4 = monobasic potassium phosphate; Na_2HPO_4 = dibasic sodium phosphate;
NaH_2PO_4 = monobasic sodium phosphate.

Table 7.4 Calcium (Ca) and phosphorus (P) content in equine mineral supplements[a].

	Ca (%)	P (%)
Bone meal	30	13
Calcium carbonate	39	0
Defluorinated phosphate	32	18
Dicalcium phosphate	22	19
Ground limestone	34	0
Monocalcium phosphate	16 .	22
Monobasic sodium phosphate[b]	0	23
Dibasic sodium phosphate[b]	0	22
Monobasic potassium phosphate[b]	0	23
Dibasic potassium phosphate[b]	0	18

Adapted from Argenzio et al. (1974), Hintz and Meakim (1981), NRC Committee on Nutrient Requirements of Horses (2007), Schryver et al. (1974), Schryver (1975), and Toribio (2011).
[a] Phosphorus bioavailability for these supplements is 40–50%.
[b] Phosphorus content based on chemical grade anhydrous salts.
Sodium phosphate enemas contain monobasic and dibasic sodium phosphate.

higher doses (0.2–0.6 mmol/kg/h) for patients with severe hypophosphatemia (Charron et al., 2003; Clark et al., 1995; Geerse et al., 2010). Doses of phosphate of 40 mmol (1240 mg), at an infusion rate of up to 20 mmol (620 mg)/h are considered safe in humans with severe hypophosphatemia (Geerse et al., 2010). Recumbent

cows with severe hypophosphatemia can be treated with 50 g of phosphate administered as a drench (200 g of sodium phosphate) or with 6 g of phosphate (23 g of sodium phosphate) intravenously in saline solution (Goff, 2009). There is some evidence that rapid correction of hypophosphatemia may be beneficial to humans with cardiovascular dysfunction and septic shock (Bollaert et al., 1995).

It is important to monitor serum P_i and calcium concentrations during aggressive treatment as miscalculations or high P_i doses can result in hyperphosphatemia and acute hypocalcemia.

Depending on the type of salt used, phosphorus is generally administered (Tables 7.3 and 7.4) two to four times daily. For oral administration, phosphate bioavailability should be taken into consideration (Table 7.4), but most mineral supplements have an approximate bioavailability of 40–50% in horses (Barlet et al., 1995; Hintz et al., 1973; NRC, 2007; Schryver, 1975). The calculated deficit is for the extracellular fluid (ECF) only and does not reflect total body or intracellular P_i deficit or depletion, as P_i concentrations are more than 20-fold higher in the intracellular compartment. For this reason, repeated P_i administrations may be required, particularly when hypophosphatemia does not improve within 24 hours, suggesting total body P_i depletion or ongoing losses.

Table 7.5 Products used for enteral supplementation of phosphate in humans and small animals[a].

Product	Phosphorus/mL	Potassium/mL	Sodium/mL	Presentation	Company
Neutra-Phos	250 mg (8.1 mM)	278 mg (7.1 mM)	164 mg (7.1 mM)	Per tablet or 75 mL solution	Baker Norton
Neutra-Phos-K	250 mg (8.1 mM)	566 mg (14.2 mM)	0	Per tablet or 75 mL solution	Baker Norton
K-Phos-Neutral	250 mg (8.1 mM)	45 mg (1.1 mM)	298 mg (13 mM)	Per tablet	Beach
Fleet Phospho-soda[b]	129 mg (4.15 mM)	0	110 mg (4.8 mM)	Per 45 mL	Fleet
Fleet Enema[b,c]	49 mg (1.58 mM)	0	46 mg (2 mM)	Per 118 mL	Fleet

Other formulations of similar composition are available.

[a] Chemical grade sodium and potassium phosphate salts can be used via nasogastric intubation in horses.

[b] Adult enema containing monobasic (19) and dibasic (7 g) sodium phosphate in 118 mL.

[c] Fleet enemas are often used intravenously in ruminants to treat hypophosphatemia. There are anecdotal reports that they are also used in horses.

Box 7.1 Clinical example

A 6-year-old, 220-kg pony mare was presented with a 3-day history of diarrhea, anorexia, and hyperlipemia. Serum chemistry abnormalities included:

- mild hypokalemia (1.8 mmol/L; normal 3.5–4.6 mmol/L)
- hypertriglyceridemia (1550 mg/dL; normal <80 mg/dL)
- severe hypophosphatemia ($P_i = 1.0$ mg/dL; normal 3.0–5.0 mg/dL).

Initial treatment consisted of lactated Ringer's solution, 5% dextrose, and KCl. After 24 hours of treatment, serum K^+ concentrations increased (2.3 mmol/L) and hypophosphatemia persisted ($P_i = 0.8$ mg/dL). The animal developed signs consistent with hypophosphatemia, including muscle fasciculations and ileus (serum Na^+ and Ca^{2+} concentrations were normal). A decision to treat the hypophosphatemia was made.

The extracellular P_i deficit was calculated, assuming an ECF volume of 0.3. This resulted in a deficit of 2112 mg:

$$220 \text{ kg} \times (4.0 - 0.8 \text{ mg/dL}) \times 10 \text{ [conversion from dL to L]} \times 0.3 \text{ ECF} = 2112 \text{ mg}$$

Initial therapy consisted of 2000 mg (65 mmol) of injectable phosphate as potassium phosphate (see Table 7.3) over a 1-hour period, in saline solution. Treatment was repeated every 8 h. The pony was also supplemented with sodium phosphate through nasogastric intubation (4 g, PO, Q 6 h, in 500 mL of water). Potassium phosphate could have been another option.

After 1 day of treatment, serum P_i concentrations increased (2.0 mg/dL). Parenteral phosphate supplementation was discontinued but the pony was maintained with enteral supplementation for another day, when serum P_i was in the normal range (3.4 mg/dL).

A number of critically ill horses and foals develop concurrent hypophosphatemia and hypocalcemia. Calcium and phosphate salts should not be mixed in the same parenteral solution to avoid precipitation. Instead, alternate timing or different IV lines should be used. Commercial solutions formulated for cattle containing calcium borogluconate and sodium hypophosphite may be an alternative (Table 7.3).

Parenteral treatment may not be necessary in horses with chronic hypophosphatemia unless clinical signs are present. Instead, enteral supplementation may be a more practical and economical approach. Several products with and without calcium can be used for this purpose (Table 7.4).

Hyperphosphatemia

Hyperphosphatemia (serum P_i concentrations >5.0 mg/dL in horses; >8.5 mg/dL in foals (age dependent)) occurs due to increased P_i absorption, renal failure, hypoparathyroidism, vitamin D intoxication, metabolic acidosis, conditions that result in cell lysis (hemolysis, rhabdomyolysis, tumor necrosis), or iatrogenic causes (DiBartola & Willard, 2005; Toribio, 2011) (Table 7.2). Ketoacidosis and lactic acidosis may cause hyperphosphatemia by inducing a P_i shift to the extracellular compartment. Metabolic acidosis and high ATP levels inhibit phosphofructokinase, a key enzyme in glycolysis. In newborn foals, overuse of phosphate-based enemas is a common cause of hyperphosphatemia.

Before making a decision on the diagnosis and treatment of hyperphosphatemia, it is important to address sample quality, as improper handling can result in spuriously high P_i values, often associated with high K^+ concentrations. Hemolysis, hyperbilirubinemia, hyperlipemia, and hyperproteinemia can falsely increase P_i concentrations. Diseases such as multiple myeloma can result in pseudohyperphosphatemia due to the interference of the high concentrations of immunoglobulins with P_i determination (Barutcuoglu et al., 2003; Larner, 1995). Correct measurement of P_i in these samples requires serum deproteinization.

Acute hyperphosphatemia may result in hypocalcemia due to the interaction between P_i and Ca^{2+} (mass law) and decreased renal synthesis of $1,25(OH)_2D_3$. Hyperphosphatemia and a serum $calcium \times P_i$ product greater than 70 are risk factors for soft tissue mineralization in other species (Caudarella et al., 2007; DiBartola & Willard, 2005); however, there is minimal evidence that this is the case for horses, except for those with hypervitaminosis D (Harrington, 1982). Horses with a $calcium \times P_i$ product greater than 90 could develop soft tissue mineralization (R. Toribio, personal communication). Soft tissue calcification and hyperphosphatemia were documented in horses with a number of diseases, including enterocolitis, respiratory distress, and muscle necrosis (Tan et al., 2010). The definitive cause of calcinosis in these animals remains unclear, however. There are reports of humans developing hyperphosphatemia from bisphosphonate therapy, and this should be monitored for in horses undergoing similar treatment (Walton et al., 1975).

Clinical signs

The signs of acute hyperphosphatemia are those of acute hypocalcemia and include tetany, hyperexcitability, muscle fasciculations, colic, and arrhythmias. Chronic hyperphosphatemia results in signs consistent with calcium deficiency including lameness, abnormal cartilage and bone development, fractures, and osteodystrophia fibrosa (nutritional secondary hyperparathyroidism) (Toribio, 2010). Developmental orthopedic diseases can be a problem in growing animals. There can be soft tissue mineralization (calcinosis), but it is rare.

Treatment of hyperphosphatemia

Depending on the primary pathology and duration (acute or chronic), direct therapy to reduce serum P_i may not be necessary. If acute-onset hyperphosphatemia is the result of acute cell lysis (e.g., rhabdomyolysis) or iatrogenic causes (e.g., phosphate enemas), fluid

therapy and diuretics are the treatment of choice. Diuretics, in addition to decreasing the deleterious effects of pigment nephropathy, also increase P_i excretion.

In humans and small animals, chronic renal failure is the most common cause of hyperphosphatemia, while in horses this is rarely the case. The goal in patients with chronic hyperphosphatemia is to normalize serum P_i concentrations. Dietary phosphate restriction is one of the first measures employed when treating chronic hyperphosphatemia. Dialysis and the use of phosphate binders and other products to reduce serum P_i are in general impractical or very expensive in horses. In addition, equine conditions that are associated with prolonged hyperphosphatemia carry a poor prognosis. Calcium carbonate is a cheap and safe phosphate binder, which also provides calcium supplementation for horses that are in a negative calcium balance. Calcium acetate is even more effective than calcium carbonate. Since calcium-based compounds can potentially increase the $calcium \times P_i$ product and the risk for soft tissue calcification, they are being replaced by aluminum, magnesium, and lanthanum-based products. Phosphate-binding polymers (sevelamer) are considered the most effective in treating chronic hyperphosphatemia. Most of this information is from humans and small animals, and data in horses are lacking.

References

Adams LG, Hardy RM, Weiss DJ, Bartges JW. (1993) Hypophosphatemia and hemolytic anemia associated with diabetes mellitus and hepatic lipidosis in cats. *J Vet Intern Med* **7**, 266–71.

Amanzadeh J, Reilly RF Jr. (2006) Hypophosphatemia: an evidence-based approach to its clinical consequences and management. *Nat Clin Pract Nephrol* **2**:136–48.

Argenzio RA, Lowe JE, Hintz HF, Schryver HF. (1974) Calcium and phosphorus homeostasis in horses. *J Nutr* **104**:18–27.

Bacic D, Wagner CA, Hernando N, Kaissling B, Biber J, Murer H. (2004) Novel aspects in regulated expression of the renal type IIa Na/Pi-cotransporter. *Kidney Int Suppl* **66**:S5–S12.

Barlet JP, Davicco MJ, Coxam V. (1995) Physiology of intestinal absorption of phosphorus in animals [in French]. *Reprod Nutr Dev* **35**:475–89.

Barton MH, Sharma P, LeRoy BE, Howerth EW. (2004) Hypercalcemia and high serum parathyroid hormone-related protein concentration in a horse with multiple myeloma. *J Am Vet Med Assoc* **225**:409–13, 376.

Barutcuoglu B, Parildar Z, Mutaf I, Habif S, Bayindir O. (2003) Spuriously elevated inorganic phosphate level in a multiple myeloma patient. *Clin Lab Haematol* **25**:271–4.

Bates JA. (2008) Phosphorus: a quick reference. *Vet Clin North Am Small Anim Pract* **38**:471–5, viii.

Benders NA, Junker K, Wensing T, van den Ingh TS, van der Kolk JH. (2001) Diagnosis of secondary hyperparathyroidism in a pony using intact parathyroid hormone radioimmuno-assay. *Vet Rec* **149**:185–7.

Bergwitz C, Juppner H. (2010) Regulation of phosphate homeostasis by PTH, vitamin D, and FGF23. *Annu Rev Med* **61**:91–104.

Bergwitz C, Juppner H. (2011) Phosphate sensing. *Adv Chronic Kidney Dis* **18**:132–44.

Berndt TJ, Knox FG. (1984) Proximal tubule site of inhibition of phosphate reabsorption by calcitonin. *Am J Physiol* **246**:F927–F930.

Berndt T, Kumar R. (2007) Phosphatonins and the regulation of phosphate homeostasis. *Annu Rev Physiol* **69**:341–59.

Berndt T, Kumar R. (2009) Novel mechanisms in the regulation of phosphorus homeostasis. *Physiology (Bethesda)* **24**:17–25.

Berndt TJ, Schiavi S, Kumar R. (2005) "Phosphatonins" and the regulation of phosphorus homeostasis. *Am J Physiol Renal Physiol* **289**:F1170–F1182.

Biber J, Hernando N, Forster I, Murer H. (2009) Regulation of phosphate transport in proximal tubules. *Pflugers Arch* **458**:39–52.

Blaine J, Weinman EJ, Cunningham R. (2011) The regulation of renal phosphate transport. *Adv Chronic Kidney Dis* **18**:77–84.

Bollaert PE, Levy B, Nace L, Laterre PF, Larcan A. (1995) Hemodynamic and metabolic effects of rapid correction of hypophosphatemia in patients with septic shock. *Chest* **107**:1698–701.

Carney SL. (1997) Calcitonin and human renal calcium and electrolyte transport. *Miner Electrolyte Metab* **23**:43–7.

Caudarella R, Vescini F, Buffa A, Francucci CM. (2007) Hyperphosphatemia: effects on bone metabolism and cardio-vascular risk. *J Endocrinol Invest* **30**:29–34.

Charron T, Bernard F, Skrobik Y, Simoneau N, Gagnon N, Leblanc M. (2003) Intravenous phosphate in the intensive care unit: more aggressive repletion regimens for moderate and severe hypophosphatemia. *Intensive Care Med* **29**:1273–8.

Clark CL, Sacks GS, Dickerson RN, Kudsk KA, Brown RO. (1995) Treatment of hypophosphatemia in patients receiving special-ized nutrition support using a graduated dosing scheme: results from a prospective clinical trial. *Crit Care Med* **23**:1504–11.

Cunningham R, Biswas R, Brazie M, Steplock D, Shenolikar S, Weinman EJ. (2009) Signaling pathways utilized by PTH and dopamine to inhibit phosphate transport in mouse renal proximal tubule cells. *Am J Physiol Renal Physiol* **296**:F355–F361.

Denis I, Thomasset M, Pointillart A. (1994) Influence of exoge-nous porcine growth hormone on vitamin D metabolism and calcium and phosphorus absorption in intact pigs. *Calcif Tissue Int* **54**:489–92.

DiBartola SP, Willard MD. (2005) Disorders of phosphorus: hypophosphatemia and hyperphosphatemia. In: *Fluid, Electrolyte and Acid-Base Disorders in Small Animal Practice.* Philadelphia, PA: Elsevier Saunders, pp. 195–209.

Durham AE, Hughes KJ, Cottle HJ, Rendle DI, Boston RC. (2009) Type 2 diabetes mellitus with pancreatic beta cell dysfunction in 3 horses confirmed with minimal model anal-ysis. *Equine Vet J* **41**:924–9.

Endres DB, Rude RK. (2006) Mineral and bone metabolism. In: Burtis CA, Ashwood ER, Bruns DE (eds) *Tietz Textbook of Clinical Chemistry and Molecular Diagnostics.* St Louis, MO: Elsevier Saunders, pp. 1891–963.

Frank N, Hawkins JF, Couetil LL, Raymond JT. (1998) Primary hyperparathyroidism with osteodystrophia fibrosa of the facial bones in a pony. *J Am Vet Med Assoc* **212**:84–6.

Fukumoto S. (2008) Physiological regulation and disorders of phosphate metabolism – pivotal role of fibroblast growth factor 23. *Intern Med* **47**:337–43.

Gaasbeek A, Meinders AE. (2005) Hypophosphatemia: an update on its etiology and treatment. *Am J Med* **118**: 1094–101.

Geerse DA, Bindels AJ, Kuiper MA, Roos AN, Spronk PE, Schultz MJ. (2010) Treatment of hypophosphatemia in the intensive care unit: a review. *Crit Care* **14**:R147.

Goff JP. (2009) Calcium, magnesium, and phosphorus. In: Smith BP (ed.) *Large Animal Internal Medicine.* St Louis, MO: Mosby, pp. 1369–77.

Harrington DD. (1982) Acute vitamin D2 (ergocalciferol) toxi-cosis in horses: case report and experimental studies. *J Am Vet Med Assoc* **180**:867–73.

Hintz HF, Meakim DW. (1981) A comparison of the 1978 National Research Council's recommendations of nutrient requirements of horses with recent studies. *Equine Vet J* **13**:187–91.

Hintz HF, Schryver HF. (1973) Magnesium, calcium and phos-phorus metabolism in ponies fed varying levels of magnesium. *J Anim Sci* **37**:927–30.

Hintz HF, Williams AJ, Rogoff J, Schryver HF. (1973) Availability of phosphorus in wheatbran when fed to ponies. *J Anim Sci* **36**:522–5.

Hurcombe SD, Toribio RE, Slovis NM, et al. (2009) Calcium reg-ulating hormones and serum calcium and magnesium con-centrations in septic and critically ill foals and their association with survival. *J Vet Intern Med* **23**:335–43.

Jubb TF, Jerrett IV, Browning JW, Thomas KW. (1990) Haemoglobinuria and hypophosphataemia in postparturient dairy cows without dietary deficiency of phosphorus. *Aust Vet J* **67**:86–9.

Kiela PR, Ghishan FK. (2009) Recent advances in the renal-skeletal-gut axis that controls phosphate homeostasis. *Lab Invest* **89**:7–14.

Krapf R, Vetsch R, Vetsch W, Hulter HN. (1992) Chronic metabolic acidosis increases the serum concentration of 1,25-dihydroxyvitamin D in humans by stimulating its production rate. Critical role of acidosis-induced renal hypophosphatemia. *J Clin Invest* **90**:2456–63.

Kuro-o M. (2006) Klotho as a regulator of fibroblast growth factor signaling and phosphate/calcium metabolism. *Curr Opin Nephrol Hypertens* **15**:437–41.

Larner AJ. (1995) Pseudohyperphosphatemia. *Clin Biochem* **28**:391–3.

Levi M, Popovtzer M. (1999) Disorders of phosphate balance. In: Schrier RW (ed.) *Atlas of Diseases of the Kidney*. Philadelphia: Current Medicine, pp. 1–14.

Liamis G, Milionis HJ, Elisaf M. (2010) Medication-induced hypophosphatemia: a review. *Q J Med* **103**:449–59.

Matsui T, Kuramitsu N, Yano H, Kawashima R. (1983) Suppressive effect of calcitonin on intestinal absorption of calcium and phosphorus in sheep. *Endocrinol Jpn* **30**:485–90.

McCoy DJ, Beasley R. (1986) Hypercalcemia associated with malignancy in a horse. *J Am Vet Med Assoc* **189**:87–9.

Murer H, Hernando N, Forster L, Biber J. (2001) Molecular mechanisms in proximal tubular and small intestinal phosphate reabsorption (plenary lecture). *Mol Membr Biol* **18**:3–11.

NRC (2007) Minerals. In: *National Research Council (U.S.), Committee on Nutrient Requirements of Horses* (eds) Nutrient Requirements of Horses. Washington, DC: National Academies Press, pp. 69–108.

NRC Committee on Nutrient Requirements of Horses (2007) *Nutrient Requirements of Horses*, 6th rev. edn. Washington, DC: National Academies Press.

O'Brien TM, Coberly L. (2003) Severe hypophosphatemia in respiratory alkalosis. *Adv Stud Med* **3**:345–8.

Ogawa E, Kobayashi K, Yoshiura N, Mukai J. (1989) Hemolytic anemia and red blood cell metabolic disorder attributable to low phosphorus intake in cows. *Am J Vet Res* **50**:388–92.

Peauroi JR, Fisher DJ, Mohr FC, Vivrette SL. (1998) Primary hyperparathyroidism caused by a functional parathyroid adenoma in a horse. *J Am Vet Med Assoc* **212**:1915–18.

Pfister MF, Ruf I, Stange G, et al. (1998) Parathyroid hormone leads to the lysosomal degradation of the renal type II Na/Pi cotransporter. *Proc Natl Acad Sci USA* **95**:1909–14.

Quigley R, Baum M. (1991) Effects of growth hormone and insulin-like growth factor I on rabbit proximal convoluted tubule transport. *J Clin Invest* **88**:368–74.

Razzaque MS. (2009) The FGF23-Klotho axis: endocrine regulation of phosphate homeostasis. *Nat Rev Endocrinol* **5**:611–19.

Ritz E, Haxsen V, Zeier M. (2003) Disorders of phosphate metabolism – pathomechanisms and management of hypophosphataemic disorders. *Best Pract Res Clin Endocrinol Metab* **17**:547–58.

Roose KA, Hoekstra KE, Pagan JD, Geor RJ. (2001) Effect of an aluminum supplement on nutrient digestibility and mineral metabolism in Thoroughbred horses. In: *Proceedings of the 17th Equine Nutrition and Physiology Society Symposium*, The University of Kentucky, Lexington, 31 May–2 June 2001, pp. 364–9.

Rosol TJ, Capen CC. (1996) Pathophysiology of calcium, phosphorus, and magnesium metabolism in animals. *Vet Clin North Am Small Anim Pract* **26**:1155–84.

Rourke KM, Kohn CW, Levine AL, Rosol TJ, Toribio RE. (2009) Rapid calcitonin response to experimental hypercalcemia in healthy horses. *Domest Anim Endocrinol* **36**:197–201.

Schryver HF. (1975) Intestinal absorption of calcium and phosphorus by horses. *J S Afr Vet Assoc* **46**:39–45.

Schryver HF, Hintz HF, Lowe JE. (1971) Calcium and phosphorus inter-relationships in horse nutrition. *Equine Vet J* **3**:102–9.

Schryver HF, Hintz HF, Craig PH, Hogue DE, Lowe JE. (1972) Site of phosphorus absorption from the intestine of the horse. *J Nutr* **102**:143–7.

Schryver HF, Hintz HF, Lowe JE. (1974) Calcium and phosphorus in the nutrition of the horse. *Cornell Vet* **64**:493–515.

Shor R, Halabe A, Rishver S, et al. (2006) Severe hypophosphatemia in sepsis as a mortality predictor. *Ann Clin Lab Sci* **36**:67–72.

Tan JY, Valberg SJ, Sebastian MM, et al. (2010) Suspected systemic calcinosis and calciphylaxis in 5 horses. *Can Vet J* **51**:993–9.

Tenenhouse HS. (2005) Regulation of phosphorus homeostasis by the type iia Na/phosphate cotransporter. *Annu Rev Nutr* **25**:197–214.

Tennant B, Bettleheim P, Kaneko JJ. (1982) Paradoxic hypercalcemia and hypophosphatemia associated with chronic renal failure in horses. *J Am Vet Med Assoc* **180**:630–4.

Toribio RE. (2010) Disorders of calcium and phosphorus. In: Reed SM, Bayly WM, Sellon DC (eds) *Equine Internal Medicine*. St Louis, MO: Saunders/Elsevier, pp. 1277–91.

Toribio RE. (2011) Disorders of calcium and phosphate metabolism in horses. *Vet Clin North Am Equine Pract* **27**:129–47.

Toribio RE, Kohn CW, Chew DJ, Sams RA, Rosol TJ. (2001) Comparison of serum parathyroid hormone and ionized calcium and magnesium concentrations and fractional urinary clearance of calcium and phosphorus in healthy horses and horses with enterocolitis. *Am J Vet Res* **62**:938–47.

Walton RJ, Russell RG, Smith R. (1975) Changes in the renal and extrarenal handling of phosphate induced by disodium etidronate (EHDP) in man. *Clin Sci Mol Med* **49**:45–56.

Willard MD, Zerbe CA, Schall WD, Johnson C, Crow SE, Jones R. (1987) Severe hypophosphatemia associated with diabetes mellitus in six dogs and one cat. *J Am Vet Med Assoc* **190**:1007–10.

Witham CL, Stull CL. (1998) Metabolic responses of chronically starved horses to refeeding with three isoenergetic diets. *J Am Vet Med Assoc* **212**:691–6.

Woodrow JP, Sharpe CJ, Fudge NJ, Hoff AO, Gagel RF, Kovacs CS. (2006) Calcitonin plays a critical role in regulating skeletal mineral metabolism during lactation. *Endocrinology* **147**:4010–21.

Wysolmerski JJ, Stewart AF. (1998) The physiology of parathyroid hormone-related protein: an emerging role as a developmental factor. *Annu Rev Physiol* **60**:431–60.

Xie Z, Li H, Liu L, Kahn BB, Najjar SM, Shah W. (2000) Metabolic regulation of Na(+)/P(i)-cotransporter-1 gene expression in H4IIE cells. *Am J Physiol Endocrinol Metab* **278**: E648–E655.

CHAPTER 8

Acid–base homeostasis and derangements

Jon Palmer

Director of Perinatology/Neonatology Programs, Chief, Neonatal Intensive Care Service, Graham French Neonatal Section, Connelly Intensive Care Unit, New Bolton Center, University of Pennsylvania, USA

Acid–base abnormalities are common in horses requiring fluid therapy. Carefully characterizing the acid–base abnormality can point to the underlying disruption of the horse's physiology and give important clues to the underlying disease process that is responsible for the need for fluid therapy. There are multiple clinical approaches used to evaluate acid–base abnormalities. Which technique is used is more a matter of style than being correct or incorrect. The goal of all of these approaches is an understanding of the components of the acid–base abnormality, which will aid in formulating a rational approach to therapy.

Physiology of acid–base balance

Regulation of acid–base homeostasis

Blood pH is very tightly regulated. Hydrogen ion concentration [H^+] is extremely low, averaging 0.00004 mEq/L (Collings, 2010). In contrast, the interstitial fluid concentration of sodium is 3.5 million times higher than this value. The normal variation in H^+ concentration in extracellular fluid is only about one millionth as great as the normal variation in sodium ion concentration. This precision in H^+ regulation is vital because of the effect of pH on protein configurations, enzyme activity, transcellular ion transport mechanisms, and other vital cellular functions. It is also important in drug distribution, binding, and activity. Thus tight H^+ concentration regulation is very important in maintaining the health of the patient and the effectiveness of therapeutic interventions.

The mechanisms in place to maintain H^+ homeostasis are well coordinated. The acid–base balance is controlled by the lungs, kidneys, and a buffer system distributed between the blood, interstitial fluid, cells, and bone. All of these systems interact and respond to physiologic changes. The first line of defense responding to acid–base changes is the buffering system. This buffering system is composed of a variety of weak acids that are also components of the most basic cellular physiology. These buffers, by virtue of being within and surrounding the cells, protect the cellular metabolism from the negative effects of acid–base disturbances. The most important participants in this buffering system include the bicarbonate/carbonic acid buffer, intracellular and extracellular proteins (such as albumin, globulins, and hemoglobin), inorganic ions (such as phosphate and sulfate), and bone (which contains a large reservoir of bicarbonate and phosphate, which can actively buffer a significant acute acid load) (Collings, 2010).

Acid is a major by-product of normal metabolism that needs to be buffered and excreted efficiently, in order to avoid acidosis. Oxidation of carbon-containing fuels produces carbon dioxide (CO_2), resulting in the generation of 15,000 to 20,000 mEq of H^+ daily, which is excreted by respiration (DuBose, 2012; Kellum, 2005). In contrast, only 0.3–1 mEq/kg of anions are excreted through the kidney each day (DuBose, 2012). Hemoglobin is the major buffer of volatile acid. Deoxyhemoglobin is an active base. Within the erythrocyte CO_2 combines with H_2O, under the influence of carbonic anhydrase, to form H_2CO_3. This ionizes to hydrogen and bicarbonate. Hydrogen ions bind to

Equine Fluid Therapy, First Edition. Edited by C. Langdon Fielding and K. Gary Magdesian.
© 2015 John Wiley & Sons, Inc. Published 2015 by John Wiley & Sons, Inc.

histidine residues on deoxyhemoglobin (the "Haldane" effect), and bicarbonate is actively pumped from cells. Chloride moves inward to maintain electroneutrality (chloride shift) and to ensure the continued production of carbonic acid.

Carbon dioxide is also buffered directly by combining with hemoglobin (carbaminohemoglobin) and plasma proteins (carbamino proteins). The CO_2 added to venous blood is usually distributed as follows: 65% as HCO_3^- and H^+ bound to hemoglobin, 27% as carbaminohemoglobin (CO_2 bound to hemoglobin), and 8% dissolved. When respiratory failure occurs, the principal CO_2 buffering system, hemoglobin, becomes overwhelmed. This leads to the rapid development of acidosis. Severe anemia may decrease this buffering capacity (DuBose, 2011; Kellum, 2005).

Under resting conditions, P_{CO_2} is maintained within a narrow range by a negative feedback regulator involving two sets of chemoreceptors that sense $[H^+]$, one in the brain (central chemoreceptors) and one in the carotid bodies (peripheral chemoreceptors). When these chemoreceptors sense an increase in $[H^+]$, breathing is stimulated. This chemoreflex control system also protects against asphyxia by increasing the sensitivity of the peripheral chemoreceptors to $[H^+]$ under conditions of hypoxia. CO_2 concentration can be adjusted rapidly and precisely by the respiratory center in defense of arterial and body pH. Conversely, alterations in P_{CO_2} due to changes in alveolar ventilation can be the primary cause of abnormalities in pH.

In addition to the production of CO_2 metabolism generates a daily load of other acids (lactate, citrate, acetate, and pyruvate), which must be removed by other metabolic reactions. In general these are products that are further metabolized to CO_2. Organic acids are derived from intermediary metabolites formed by partial combustion of dietary carbohydrates, fats, and proteins as well as from nucleic acids (uric acid). The organic acid generated contributes to net endogenous acid production when the conjugate bases are excreted in the urine as organic anions. If full oxidation of these acids can occur, however, H^+ is reclaimed and eliminated as CO_2 and water. The complete combustion of carbon involves the intermediate generation and metabolism of 2000 to 3000 mmol of relatively strong organic acids, such as lactic acid, tricarboxylic acids, ketoacids, or other acids, depending on the type of fuel consumed. These organic acids do not accumulate in the body under most

circumstances, with concentrations remaining in the low millimolar range. If production and consumption rates become mismatched, however, these organic acids can accumulate causing significant metabolic acidosis (e.g., lactic acid accumulation in septic shock or with muscle activity) (DuBose, 2012).

Although temporary relief from changes in the pH of extracellular fluid may be derived from buffering or respiratory compensation, the ultimate defense against addition of non-volatile acid or of alkali resides is the kidneys. The metabolism of some body constituents such as proteins, nucleic acids, and small fractions of lipids and certain carbohydrates generates specific organic acids that cannot be burned to CO_2 (e.g., uric, oxalic, glucuronic, hippuric acids). In addition, the inorganic acids H_2SO_4 (derived from oxidation of methionine and cysteine) and H_3PO_4 (derived from organophosphates), must be excreted by the kidneys or the gastrointestinal tract (DuBose, 2012). The major effect of the kidney on acid–base balance relates to the ability to excrete non-volatile acids and bases, and maintain and modify strong ion concentrations. Because dietary intake of sodium and chloride is roughly equal, the kidney excretes a net Cl^- load with NH_4^+, a weak cation, to balance the charge in the urine. The control of excretion of Cl^- and NH_4^+ is the essence of metabolic (renal) compensation for acid–base abnormalities.

Each of these three acid–base-regulating systems dynamically responds to small changes in acid–base balance allowing for the precise physiologic control that is required for normal cellular function. Consequently, disorders of kidneys, lungs, and physiologic buffers can result in acid–base abnormalities. Physiologic insults such as gastric reflux, diarrhea, respiratory failure, kidney dysfunction, toxic ingestions, among others can result in life-threatening acid–base crises.

Consequences of acid–base abnormalities

Although acid–base abnormalities are an important sign of underlying disease, except in the most severe cases they are usually clinically silent being overshadowed by the signs produced by the primary problem. Patients with mild metabolic acidosis are often subclinical and the compensatory hyperventilation is usually not clinically evident. Initial respiratory compensation usually takes the form of less frequent but deeper breaths increasing alveolar ventilation by effectively decreasing dead space minute ventilation. This change often escapes detection on clinical examination. Metabolic alkalosis is frequently overlooked until it is evident on laboratory evaluation. If hypoventilation resulting in respiratory acidosis is caused by neuromuscular or mechanical problems, the patient will be dyspneic and tachypneic. But if the respiratory center is impaired, as commonly occurs in neonatal encephalopathy, ventilation may be reduced without any sense of dyspnea.

When symptomatic or clinical, only the most extreme derangements of acid–base balance are fatal. Alterations in the relative concentrations of hydrogen ions are generally less important than the pathologic abnormalities causing them. The primary underlying disease process resulting in the acid–base abnormality is usually the direct cause of mortality in the patient before the acid–base derangement becomes extreme enough to be fatal. However, when extreme acid–base derangements occur or changes in the acid–base balance develop quickly, dangerous disruption to the normal physiologic responses may occur leading to organ dysfunction. When the acid–base abnormality is superimposed on the primary pathologic process, it can significantly contribute to serious morbidity and mortality. The type of acidosis is also important. Mortality is highest when lactate accumulation is the cause of acidosis (Gunnerson et al., 2006; Kellum, 2005).

Less extreme derangements can sometimes produce harm because of the patient's response to the abnormality. For example, a patient with metabolic acidosis will attempt to compensate by increasing minute ventilation. The workload that is imposed by increasing minute ventilation can lead to respiratory muscle fatigue with respiratory failure or diversion of blood flow from vital organs to the respiratory muscles resulting in organ injury. Acidemia will cause increased adrenergic tone, which can, in turn, promote the development of cardiac dysrhythmias and increase myocardial oxygen demand especially in patients that already have significant ischemia (Effros & Swenson, 2010; Greenbaum, 2011; Kellum, 2005; Shannon, 2007,).

Acidemia, especially when caused by metabolic acidosis, may have direct cardiovascular consequences. Initially acidosis will result in a positive inotropic effect secondary to the adrenergic response. However, as the pH falls to less than 7.2 there can be a negative inotropic effect caused by impaired myocardial contractility. Initially the heart rate increases but as the pH declines to less than 7.1, the heart rate may fall as well. With

acidemia, there may be a decrease in the cardiovascular response to catecholamines, potentially exacerbating hypotension in cases with volume depletion or shock. It also decreases the effectiveness of exogenous therapeutic adrenergic drugs when treating shock. Acidemia will also predispose to ventricular arrhythmias especially in the presence of high endogenous adrenergic tone or exogenous adrenergic drug therapy.

Arterial vasodilation and venoconstriction may also occur in the acidemic patient. Pulmonary hypertension may develop as a result of acidemia, which in the neonate can lead to retention of or reversion to fetal circulation. The negative inotropic effects of acidemia, along with fluid shifts to central circulation caused by the venoconstriction, may lead to pulmonary edema. These cardiovascular effects of acidosis can lead to a vicious cycle of decreased myocardial contractility that produces hypoperfusion, which in turn increases lactic acidosis, further impairing myocardial contractility and adrenergic responsiveness leading to refractory shock (Effros & Swenson, 2010; Greenbaum, 2011; Shannon, 2007).

The acid–base balance has direct effects on gas exchange. Patients with a respiratory acidosis breathing room air will always have hypoxemia (Effros & Swenson, 2010; Ijland et al., 2010). As predicted by the Bohr effect, acidemia produces a rightward shift of the oxyhemoglobin dissociation curve, decreasing the affinity for oxygen. This results in less efficient oxygen loading of hemoglobin in the lungs but enhanced unloading in the tissues. Alkalosis shifts the oxyhemoglobin dissociation curve to the left resulting in reduced oxygen delivery to tissues (Effros & Swenson, 2010; Ijland et al., 2010; Shannon 2007).

Both acidemia and alkalemia may cause neurologic signs in part due to their effects on cerebral blood flow. Acidemia, especially caused by hypoventilation, will increase cerebral blood flow and cerebrospinal fluid pressure. Carbon dioxide is thought to have a direct CNS depressant effect (CO_2 narcosis). Respiratory acidosis tends to have a greater effect than metabolic acidosis on responsiveness and the effect is most marked when onset of hypercapnia is abrupt (Greenbaum, 2011; Shannon, 2007). Various central signs such as abnormal ventilatory patterns, abnormal responsiveness, depression, and loss of consciousness may be seen. These signs are more likely to occur when acidemia is secondary to respiratory acidosis (Effros & Swenson, 2010). With slow onset of hypercapnia the resulting acidemia may be tolerated with few signs. Severe acidemia is also thought to impair brain metabolism (Greenbaum, 2011). New evidence also points to acidosis causing neurologic injury; this is mediated by acid-sensing ion channels leading to a variety of effects including delayed ischemic neuronal death (Wang & Xu, 2011).

Alkalemia caused by hyperventilation can produce a marked (although transient) decrease in cerebral blood flow. Syncope cause by hyperventilation resulting in hypocapnia is due to the resulting reduction in cerebral blood flow. The reduction in cerebral blood flow is the rationale for using hyperventilation to treat increased intracranial pressure; however, it is now recognized that such therapy results in decreased oxygen delivery, making forced hyperventilation contraindicated in most cases. Acute respiratory alkalosis may also cause neuromuscular irritability, tetany, seizures and loss of consciousness (Greenbaum, 2011; Shannon, 2007).

There are other miscellaneous effects of acid–base imbalance. Acute metabolic acidemia can result in insulin resistance, increased protein degradation, and reduced ATP synthesis. Chronic metabolic acidosis can cause failure to thrive in neonates (Greenbaum, 2011). Emerging evidence suggests that changes in acid–base balance influence immune effector cell function. Thus, avoiding acid–base derangements can be important in the management of critically ill patients (Curley et al., 2010; Ijland et al., 2010; Kellum, 2005).

Although the strong ion balance is one determinant of acid–base balance, plasma concentrations of some electrolytes are affected by the acid–base balance. Acidemia causes potassium to move from the intracellular space to the extracellular space, thereby increasing the serum potassium concentration (Effros & Swenson, 2010). Alkalemia causes the opposite movement of potassium. The renal loss of potassium is also increased in alkalemia and decreased in acidemia. However, changes in serum potassium levels depend on the form of the acidosis (metabolic or respiratory). The specific types of metabolic acidosis, as well as several other factors, including changes in serum osmolality, changes in plasma insulin, aldosterone, and catecholamine levels all affect plasma potassium concentration (Shannon, 2007). Therefore, changes in plasma potassium concentrations are not a sensitive predictor of changes in acid–base status (Effros & Swenson, 2010; Greenbaum, 2011).

Acidemia results in an increase in plasma total and ionized calcium concentrations. Acid buffering in the bone causes mobilization of skeletal calcium, leading to this increase (Shannon, 2007). Likewise acid buffering by albumin displaces bound calcium resulting in an increase in ionized calcium levels. In the author's experience, hypercalcemia is most marked in subacute to chronic respiratory acidosis. During alkalemia, the opposite occurs; the ionized calcium concentration decreases as a result of increased binding of calcium to albumin (Greenbaum, 2011). Also alkalemia enhances calcium deposition into bone. When there are rapid changes, the resulting decrease in ionized calcium concentration has been thought to cause the clinical signs of tetany, and seizure in humans (Greenbaum, 2011). Hypomagnesemia and hypophosphatemia have also been associated with alkalemia (Effros & Swenson, 2010; Shannon, 2007).

Although the above discussion has listed a wide variety of possible clinical signs that can be attributed to alterations of acid–base balance, it is frequently impossible to determine which signs are a direct result of acidemia or alkalemia and which are the result of the underlying disease problem leading to the acid–base imbalance. Facilitating the return of blood pH toward normal values will have a positive effect on the patient, both physiologically and clinically. Moderating the abnormality by appropriate therapeutic intervention may allow the patient to redirect resources used by compensating mechanisms to support other vital areas. However , there may be some advantage to not completely normalizing the pH. Normalizing the patient's blood work does not necessarily make the patient normal, and may in fact be harmful. For more than a decade it has been recognized that permissive acidosis results in lower mortality in humans with acute respiratory distress syndrome, in part because of the immune-modulating effects of hypercapnic acidosis. This has led to the concept of therapeutic acidosis in which the administration of CO_2 is used to induce hypercapnic acidosis for its beneficial effect (Curley et al., 2010; Ijland et al., 2010). In the face of sepsis the situation is more complicated, with hypercapnic acidosis having both positive and negative influences (Curley et al., 2010).

Interpretation of the acid–base balance

Appropriate interpretation of acid–base abnormalities requires simultaneous measurement of plasma electrolytes and arterial blood gases, as well as an appreciation

Table 8.1 Comparison of arterial and venous blood gases drawn simultaneously from a patient.

Source	Venous blood	Arterial blood
pH	7.162	7.347
P_{CO_2}	59.8 mmHg	28.5 mmHg
P_{O_2}	28.4 mmHg	92.8 mmHg
BE	−7.3 mEq/L	−7.8 mEq/L
HCO_3	21.5 mEq/L	15.7 mEq/L
Glucose	18 mg/dL	50 mg/dL

BE, base excess.
Metatarsal artery and associated venous samples drawn within 2 minutes of each other in a foal with septic shock.

by the clinician of the physiologic adaptations and compensatory responses that occur with specific acid–base disturbances (DuBose, 2012). Although venous blood gases are often used as a surrogate for arterial values, this can be misleading. Venous pH reflects the regional metabolism of the tissues drained by the vein used whereas the arterial pH reflects respiratory compensation. With severe illness these may be very different (see Table 8.1). Interpretation of acid–base disturbances may be misleading without accurate measurements of the clinical chemistry components. Normal values for the laboratory and instruments used for the analysis also need to be considered. Because of the variation in measurements, when serial samples are analyzed, the same instruments should be used. Finally, it should be understood that although normal ranges are established for populations, the individual tends to maintain values with less variation within this normal range. This is especially true for pH values because of the strict control.

Traditional versus alternative approaches

Critically ill patients rarely have a single acid–base disorder. These patients typically manifest mixed acid–base physiology with multiple, often conflicting metabolic derangements superimposed on respiratory disease or compensation. A number of approaches are used on clinical cases first to diagnose the acid–base abnormality and then to try to understand the underlying pathologic origin of the abnormality. This section will review some of the analytical tools available to explore acid–base abnormalities and discuss their interrelationship, usefulness, and limitations. No matter which approach is used by a clinician to detect the presence of an acid–base imbalance, all methods will point out the presence of an abnormality making the choice of approach more a matter of style than acknowledging that one approach is superior to another. However, because of the nature of the analysis, different approaches may point to different underpinnings of the problem and lead to somewhat different approaches to therapy. No matter which approach is used to try to understand the underlying pathophysiology leading to a patient's acid–base status, no method will completely explain all derangements. The complex acid–base interactions of the various influences may even cancel each other's effects.

All approaches recognize the contribution of volatile acid (CO_2), usually referred to as the respiratory component and volatile base (HCO_3^-) considered part of the metabolic component. All approaches also recognize the contribution of non-volatile acids and bases to the metabolic component but traditional approaches rely on their presence being reflected in changes in HCO_3^- instead of measuring them independently. The non-volatile components include strong ions, inorganic weak acid buffers (e.g., PO_4, SO_4), organic weak acid buffers (e.g., albumin), and other organic metabolites (e.g., lactate). The inorganic and organic weak acid buffers are often referred to collectively as the buffer base and abbreviated as "A^-". There are three major methods of quantifying (describing) acid–base disorders, but each differs only in assessment of the "metabolic" component. These three methods quantify the metabolic component by using HCO_3, standard base excess (SBE) or strong ion difference (SID), and buffer base. Although there has been significant debate about the accuracy and usefulness of each method compared with the others, all three yield identical qualitative results when used to evaluate the acid–base status of a given blood sample. However, there are differences between these three approaches in the conceptual understanding of the underlying mechanism causing the acid–base imbalance and the relative quantitative importance of the components of the acid–base disturbance (Kellum, 2005).

History of the traditional approach (see Table 8.2)

In order to understand the evolution of the traditional approach, a historical perspective is helpful. It was O'Shaughnessy who first identified the loss of HCO_3^- from the blood as an important finding in patients dying of cholera in the London epidemic of 1831–2 (O'Shaughnessy, 1831). Thomas Latta was the first to

Table 8.2 Historical summary of acid–base analysis tools.

Analysis tool	Definition	Date proposed	Reference
Henderson equation	$[H^+] = K_i \times [CO_2]/[HCO_3]$	1907	Henderson (1907)
Henderson–Hasselbalch equation	$pH = pK_i + \log[HCO3]/(Sco_2 \times Pco_2)$	1916	Hasselbalch (1916)
Van Slyke's "buffer curve"	$\log Pco_2 = -pH + \log[HCO3]/K_i \times Sco_2$	1921	Van Slyke (1921)
Standard bicarbonate	Concentration of bicarbonate corrected for respiratory effects	1928	Van Slyke (1928)
Buffer base	Sum of the buffer anions HCO3, PO_4 and the protein anions	1948	Singer and Hastings (1948)
Base excess	Number of milliequivalents (mEq) of acid or base that are needed to titrate 1 liter of blood to pH 7.40 at 37 °C while the Pco$_2$ is held constant at 40 mmHg	1963	Siggaard-Andersen (1963)
Standard base excess	Base excess corrected for hemoglobin	1977	Siggaard-Andersen (1977)
Anion gap	(Na + K)–(Cl + HCO3)	1977	Emmett and Narins (1977)
SID (strong ion difference)	$(Na + K + Ca^{2+} + Mg^{2+})-Cl^-$	1981	Stewart (1981)
A_{tot}	Protein anions + phosphate anions	1981	Stewart (1981)
Simplified equine SIDe	2.25 [albumin] (g/dL) + 1.40 [globulin] (g/dL) + 0.59 [phosphate] (mg/dL)	1997	Constable (1997)

embrace O'Shaughnessy's findings when he began treating cholera victims with intravenous HCO_3^- in that epidemic in 1832 (Latta, 1832). But it wasn't until 1907 that Henderson coined the term "acid–base balance" and defined this process by his famous equation showing CO_2 and HCO_3 as the key elements (Henderson, 1907). In 1916 Hasselbalch reformulated the equation using negative logarithmic pH notation and the Pco$_2$ term (Hasselbalch, 1916). The Henderson–Hasselbalch equation attempted to characterize acid–base disturbances by suggesting that changes in Pco$_2$ only reflected respiratory influences whereas changes in HCO_3^- only reflected metabolic influences. However, the Henderson–Hasselbalch equation failed to account for the influence of non-bicarbonate buffers and serum electrolytes on acid–base interpretation (Rastegar, 2009). More importantly, it suggested that Pco$_2$ and HCO_3^- are independent predictors of pH when, in fact, these variables are interdependent. Specifically, HCO_3^- will change as a result of changes in Pco$_2$ and vice versa. This is the danger when clinical assessment of the metabolic acid–base balance relies solely on this traditional Henderson–Hasselbalch concept. Bicarbonate levels, or their common surrogate total CO_2 as used on many clinical chemistry screens, will not accurately reflect the metabolic acid–base status when there are respiratory abnormalities.

Due to this interdependency, other measurements of metabolic acid–base balance independent of Pco$_2$ were

suggested such as standard bicarbonate (Jorgensen & Astrup, 1957) or the more useful base excess (BE) (Astrup et al., 1960). Both of these parameters were standardized for a Pco$_2$ of 40 mmHg and fully saturated blood. Siggaard-Andersen defined base deficit/excess as the amount of strong acid or base required to return 1 liter of whole blood to pH 7.4, assuming a Pco$_2$ of 40 mmHg, full oxygen saturation, and temperature of 37 °C (Siggaard-Andersen, 1963). The influence of all buffers (bicarbonate and non-bicarbonate buffers – primarily albumin and inorganic phosphate) referred to as the "buffer base" (Singer & Hastings, 1948) was also recognized. The BE was developed to measure the change in buffer base to define the metabolic component. Although BE helped separate metabolic acid–base abnormalities from respiratory influences, it could not differentiate among the various possible sources of non-respiratory acid–base disturbances. In fact, complex situations may arise resulting in multiple metabolic influences cancelling each other and resulting in a normal BE despite significant acid–base abnormalities.

Standard base excess

Because of the pitfalls of using HCO_3 to detect metabolic acid–base abnormalities, standard base excess (SBE) is a traditional clinical tool commonly used in evaluating the metabolic status of clinical patients (Figure 8.1). Originally BE values were derived by

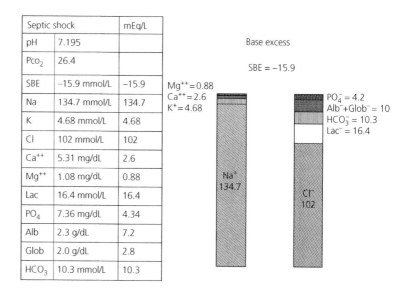

Septic shock		mEq/L
pH	7.195	
Pco₂	26.4	
SBE	−15.9 mmol/L	−15.9
Na	134.7 mmol/L	134.7
K	4.68 mmol/L	4.68
Cl	102 mmol/L	102
Ca⁺⁺	5.31 mg/dL	2.6
Mg⁺⁺	1.08 mg/dL	0.88
Lac	16.4 mmol/L	16.4
PO₄	7.36 mg/dL	4.34
Alb	2.3 g/dL	7.2
Glob	2.0 g/dL	2.8
HCO₃	10.3 mmol/L	10.3

Figure 8.1 Example of standard base excess (SBE). These blood values were taken from a foal in septic shock. Notice that the SBE approximates the lactate level.

in vitro experiments on whole blood. Although the BE calculation is accurate *in vitro*, inaccuracy exists when applied *in vivo*. This is because acute acid buffering occurs not only in blood but also throughout the whole extracellular fluid compartment, in the whole intracellular compartment (not just in the blood), and even in the bone matrix. As a result, BE becomes less accurate as acidosis increases and when there are changes in the buffer space as may occur in critical illness. When this limitation of the original BE equations was realized, the equations were modified to take into account that at least two-thirds of the extracellular fluid space that participates in buffering does not contain hemoglobin. So instead of using a normal hemoglobin value, one-third of that value was used in the formulas. The resulting value was termed the SBE. Modern blood gas machines often measure hemoglobin in the sample to use the patient's own value in the formula. When using this derived value, it is important for the clinician to know if the patient's current hemoglobin is used; both anemia and polycythemia from hemoconcentration may make the SBE value less useful if this is not taken into account. The clinician needs to realize that changes in the intravascular to interstitial fluid ratio will also decrease the value's usefulness (Kellum, 2005). These algorithms have been developed using human hemoglobin, which may lead to minor inaccuracies when used to evaluate horse acid–base status. This formula assumes a normal A_{TOT} (i.e., the total non-volatile weak acid buffer, also referred to as the buffer base), which is frequently

absent in critical patients. Wooten (2003; Kellum, 2005) developed a corrected formula (SBE_{corr}) that attempts to overcome this latter problem. It should be noted that this formula was derived using the buffering characteristics of human albumin, which are not identical to horse albumin. The equations for BE, SBE, and SBE_{corr} given here are from Kellum (2005):

$$BE = \{HCO_3^- - 24.4 + [2.3 \times (Hb \times 1.6) + 7.7] \times (pH - 7.4)\}$$
$$\times [1 - 0.023 \times (Hb \times 1.6)]$$

(8.1)

$$SBE = 0.9287 \times [HCO_3^- - 24.4 + 14.83 \times (pH - 7.4)] \quad (8.2)$$

$$SBE_{corr} = (HCO_3^- - 24.4) + [(8.3 \times Alb \times 0.15)$$
$$+ (0.29 \times PO_4 \times 0.32)] \times (pH - 7.4)$$

(8.3)

where Hb = hemoglobin (g/dL), HCO_3^- = bicarbonate (mEq/L), and PO_4 = phosphate (mg/dL).

Changes in SBE and HCO_3 frequently correlate closely, but not always. Traditionally, the difference has been ascribed to the effects of "buffering", the argument being that strong acids (or bases), quantified by SBE, are "buffered" by plasma proteins, hemoglobin, HCO_3, and even bone. The resulting changes in HCO_3 and pH are a result of this buffering process. As explained by Stewart and confirmed experimentally by others, the fundamental physical-chemical properties of biologic solutions dictate much of this so-called "buffering".

Beyond the traditional approach

Analysis beyond the traditional Henderson–Hasselbalch approach involves consideration of the roles of strong ions and the buffer base (Figure 8.2). Changes in both strong ions and buffer base will be reflected in changes in the Henderson–Hasselbalch equation (having effects on HCO_3^- levels); however, examining the changes themselves, rather than their reflection in changes in HCO_3^-, lends understanding to the underlying causes of the acid–base abnormality. In addition, this approach helps to explain complex situations where concurrent acidifying and alkalizing influences occur simultaneously, which cannot be detected using the traditional approach. In attempts to explain these more complex acid–base problems, methods have been developed based on a theoretical foundation of the principles of electroneutrality and recognizing the role of strong ions and plasma weak acids. These include the "anion gap" (AG), introduced by Emmet and Narins (1977) and identifying unmeasured anions, and concepts introduced by Stewart (1981) and Fencl and Leith (1993) including strong ion difference (SID) and strong ion gap (SIG).

Strong ions

Strong ions are ions that exist in solution in a completely dissociated state, maintaining their electrical charge. The degree of dissociation of substances in water determines whether they are strong acids or strong bases. Lactic acid, which has an ion dissociation constant

(pK_a) of 3.4, is virtually completely dissociated at physiologic pH and is a strong acid. Conversely, carbonic acid, which has a pK_a of 6.4, is incompletely dissociated and is a weak acid (weak ion). Similarly, ions such as Na^+, K^+ and Cl^- that do not easily bind other molecules are considered strong ions as they exist free in solution. Major strong ions in normal extracellular fluid include Na^+, Cl^-, K^+, SO_4^{2-}, Ca^{2+}, and Mg^{2+}. Their contribution to a solution's electrical charge must remain balanced by other strong or weak anions or cations. H^+ is a weak cation whose concentration changes as SID changes in order to maintain electrical neutrality. This is the basis forming the connection between SID and pH. Plasma ions such as Cu^{2+}, Fe^{2+}, Fe^{3+}, Zn^{2+}, Co^{2+}, and Mn^{2+}, which do not behave as simple ions, are assumed to be quantitatively unimportant because of their low plasma concentrations.

Electrical neutrality must always hold. Consequently, the accumulation of strong anions (Cl^-, lactate, ketones, sulfate, etc.) is the "footprint" or "ghost" left by a strong acid. When a strong acid such as lactate (Lac^-H^+) is produced, much of the H^+ is buffered (combining with a weak base) thus the electrical neutrality is preserved as anionic buffering sites are neutralized by combining with H^+ allowing the accumulation of Lac^- without changing the electrical neutrality. A small amount of unbuffered H^+ lowers the pH. The accumulation of strong anion is a reflection of the amount of acid added to the system as it is produced. We measure the

Neonatal Encephalopathy		mEq/L
pH	7.295	
Pco$_2$	52.7	
SBE	1.2	1.2
Na	140 mmol/L	140
K	3.51 mmol/L	3.51
Cl	103 mmol/L	103
Ca^{++}	6 mg/dL	3
Mg^{++}	1.1 mg/dL	0.9
Lac	7.1 mmol/L	7.1
PO$_4$	6.22 mg/dL	3.7
Alb	2.18 g/dL	4.9
Glob	1.62 g/dL	2.3
HCO$_3$	25.9 mmol/L	25.9

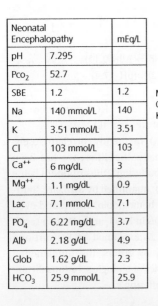
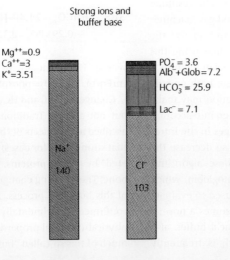

Figure 8.2 Gamblegram showing relative ratios of strong ions and components of the buffer base. Blood values from a foal with neonatal encephalopathy. SBE, standard base excess.

Lac⁻ level to determine the acid load introduced by lactate production even though it itself is a base.

Buffer base (non-volatile weak acids, A_{TOT})

There are a number of substances in the body that, because of their pK_a, act as buffers. In plasma, where pH is measured, there are only two substances that act as non-volatile weak acid buffers and have concentrations great enough to produce significant acid–base disturbances when abnormal: inorganic phosphate (PO_4) and plasma protein (especially serum albumin (Alb)). Albumin, because of its multiple buffering sites available at the physiologic (and pathophysiologic) pH range, can act as a non-volatile weak acid buffer. The charge makeup of albumin is quite complex. Specifically, human albumin contains 99 residues with fixed negative charges (mainly aspartate, and glutamate) and 77 fixed positive charges (lysine and arginine) that are independent of pH in the physiologic and pathophysiologic range. Therefore each molecule of albumin has a fixed negative charge of 22 mEq/L, no matter what the plasma pH is. In addition, albumin has 16 histidine residues that react with H^+ depending on the pH (Kurtz et al., 2008). These are the buffering sites. Therefore, albumin always has a net negative charge (−22 to −38 depending on buffering state). Normal serum globulins carry a smaller net electrical charge at pH values prevailing in plasma, which has been ignored by some investigators (Morgan et al., 2007).

The anionic contribution of albumin, globulin, and phosphate is dependent on their plasma concentrations and the pH. As they are good buffers with appropriate pK_a values and multiple buffer sites, changes in blood pH have a small effect until the pH reaches extremes. This allows calculation of the contribution of the total anionic charge of these buffers without consideration of pH, resulting in only a small error until the pH value begins to become extreme.

The following formulas have been proposed using data from humans and are useful in horses:

$$Alb^-[mEq/L] = (Alb[g/dL]\times 10)\times((0.123\times pH)-0.631)$$

(8.4a) (Figge et al., 1992)

Or shortcut without pH (assumes pH = 7.40):
$$Alb^-[mEq/L] = 2.8\times Alb[g/dL]$$

(Corey, 2003)

Note: at pH 7.0, then 2.3 × Alb; at pH 7.6, then 3.0 × Alb (Kellum, 2007a,b).

$$PO_4[mEq/L] = (PO_4[mg/dL]\times 0.323)\times((0.309\times pH)-0.469)$$

(8.4b) Figge et al., 1992)

Or shortcut without pH (assumes pH = 7.40): $PO_4^- = 0.58\times PO_4[mg/dL]$

(Corey, 2003)

Note: at pH 7.0, then 0.55 × PO_4; at pH 7.6, then 0.61 × PO_4 (Kellum, 2007a,b).

The following formula was derived using data from horses:

$$A^-[mEq/L]=(2.25\times Alb[g/dL])+(1.40\times Glob[g/dL])+(0.59\times PO_4[mg/dL])$$

(8.5) (Constable, 1997)

Anion gap (AG)

The anion gap (AG) was developed to estimate the accumulation of unmeasured anions as strong acids are produced (Emmett & Narins, 1977). The associated H^+ combines with and thus decreases the buffer base leaving behind an unmeasured anion producing the anion gap. These strong organic acids may accumulate because of increased production such as with lactate or ketoacids, toxic ingestion, decreased renal excretion, or errors of metabolism.

$$AG=(Na+K)-(Cl+HCO_3)$$

(8.6) (Emmett & Nairns, 1977)

As the underlying principle of AG is electrical neutrality AG represents the sum of charges of electrolytes not included in the equation, usually referred to as "unidentified" anions (UA) and cations (UC). In reality AG = UA − UC. UA are primarily albumin, PO_4 and organic anions (e.g., lactate) plus minor amounts OH^-, SO_4^{2-}, and CO_3^{2-}. Unidentified cations (UC) are Mg^{2+}, Ca^{2+}, and a large number of organic cations such as amines (epinephrine, dopamine, etc.), many drugs (about 40% of all conventional drugs) plus very small amounts of H^+. Usually UC are a minor contributor (but not always) and can be ignored. Normal AG is

Birth asphyxia		mEq/L
pH	7.009	
Pco$_2$	62.4	
AG	22.8mmol/L	
Na	131 mmol/L	131
K	4.8 mmol/L	4.8
Cl	98 mmol/L	98
Ca^{++}	6.58 mg/dL	3.3
Mg^{++}	1.3 mg/dL	1.1
Lac	14.5 mmol/L	14.5
PO$_4$	4.99 mg/dL	2.9
Alb	2.78 g/dL	6.3
Glob	1.92 g/dL	2.7
HCO$_3$	15.9 mmol/L	15.9
SBE	−13.3	13.3

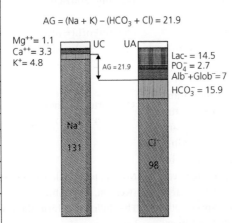

Anion gap

$$AG = (Na + K) - (HCO_3 + Cl) = 21.9$$

Mg^{++}= 1.1
Ca^{++}= 3.3
K^{+}= 4.8

UC   UA

AG = 21.9

Lac- = 14.5
PO$_4^-$ = 2.7
Alb$^-$+Glob$^-$=7
HCO$_3^-$ = 15.9

Na$^+$
131

Cl$^-$
98

Figure 8.3 Gamblegram showing the relationship of the anion gap (AG) to components of the buffer base and strong ions. Blood values taken from a foal with birth asphyxia. SBE, standard base excess; UA, unidentified anions; UC, unidentified cations.

A$^-$ (albumin, PO$_4$) plus small amounts of UA (lactate, sulfates, etc.), which are offset by excluded cations (Ca, Mg). An increased AG indicates an increase in UA, generally expected to be lactate in the horse but also possibly ketones, toxins, or other anions. AG was developed before measurement of lactate levels was easily achieved, primarily as a clinical aid to detect the presence and magnitude of lactic acidosis. Even though L-lactate levels are now easily measured, AG is still a valuable aid in detecting the presence and estimating the changing concentrations of other difficult to measure anions such as D-lactate, ketones, and toxins. This simple formula utilizing readily available laboratory data can be quite useful clinically. As variations in analysis techniques can cause different Cl$^-$ values, normal ranges are often considered laboratory specific (Figure 8.3).

Detecting abnormalities with AG is dependent on having a normal A$^-$, which is uncommon in critically ill patients. Errors in AG can come from variations in UC and UA, which are not of interest. It is unusual for UC to change significantly. Conversely UA, especially low albumin and low PO$_4$, can have a large effect on AG, which could mask the appearance of an organic acid of interest. High levels of PO$_4$, as are often found in neonates and can occur in renal failure, add to the AG; this falsely suggests the presence of other unidentified organic acids. The almost universal occurrence of hypoalbuminemia in critical patients has led to the development of a corrected AG (Figure 8.4).

$$AG_{Corr} = AG + 2.5 \times (Alb_{ref} - Alb_{measured}) \qquad (8.7)$$

In neonatal foals, the almost universally low albumin (relative to adults) and variable blood PO$_4$ levels are problematic. Normal neonatal foals usually have a PO$_4$ level higher than adults, which may counterbalance the usually low albumin level in the formula. Critically ill foals can have extremely high PO$_4$ or occasionally very low concentrations. Without correcting for both the albumin level and PO$_4$ level, AG can be misleading in foals. A "corrected AG" (cAG) has been utilized to take into account the patient's albumin and PO$_4$ levels, and if the lactate value is added the normal cAG is zero (this formula is designed for an acid pH):

$$cAG = ((Na + K) - (HCO_3 + Cl)) - ((2 \times Alb[g/dL])$$
$$+ (0.5 \times PO_4[mg/dL])) - Lac[mmol/L] = 0$$
$$(8.8) \ (Kellum, 2007a)$$

The AG method does not identify acid–base abnormalities that are due to alterations in plasma free water. Additionally, the AG method does not account for the correction of chloride concentration in the setting of altered plasma free water. As a result, a hyperchloremic acidosis in the setting of a dilutional alkalosis would not be identified with an analysis using the AG method. In general AG analysis is well suited to detect the rapid increase of UA in a patient that was previously normal but is suffering from an emergent problem such as hypovolemic shock with resulting lactic acidosis. However, the AG can fail in more complex, chronic situations.

Another problem with AG is its reliance on HCO$_3^-$. It does not account for changes associated with changes in

Foal after a dystocia		mEq/L
pH	7.390	
Pco$_2$	42.6	
AG	13.5 mmol/L	
Na	132 mmol/L	132
K	3.4 mmol/L	3.4
Cl	96 mmol/L	96
Ca^{++}	6.13 mg/dL	3
Mg^{++}	1.4 mg/dL	1
Lac	7 mmol/L	7
PO$_4$	4.19 mg/dL	2.5
Alb	1.28 g/dL	2.9
Glob	1.52 g/dL	2.1
HCO$_3$	26 mmol/L	26
SBE	1.3	1.3

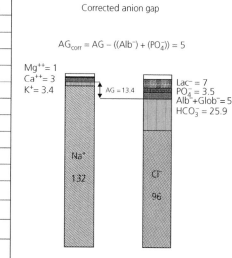

Corrected anion gap

$$AG_{corr} = AG - ((Alb^-) + (PO_4^-)) = 5$$

Figure 8.4 Gamblegram showing the value of the corrected anion gap (AG$_{corr}$). Blood values taken from a foal delivered from a dystocia at the time of birth. Note the calculated anion gap of 13.4 would be considered normal in many laboratories but is clearly abnormal when compared to the calculated corrected normal value of 5 in this foal. SBE, standard base excess.

Pco$_2$. To address this problem, the concept of "the delta-delta" was developed. Delta AG$_{Corr}$ (ΔAG$_{Corr}$) is the difference between the calculated AG$_{Corr}$ and the reference AG. Delta HCO$_3^-$ (ΔHCO$_3^-$) is defined as the difference between the reference HCO$_3^-$ and the measured HCO$_3^-$. The incremental increase in AG$_{Corr}$ should be mirrored by the same incremental decrease in HCO$_3^-$ so ΔAG$_{Corr}$ should equal ΔHCO$_3^-$ if the AG is only a result of metabolic acidosis. But this 1:1 ratio of ΔAG$_{Corr}$ to ΔHCO$_3^-$ fails to consider the role of non-bicarbonate buffers, assumes the same volume of distribution for both the conjugate base and the proton, and disregards the duration of acidosis. Taking these three conditions into account, the actual ratio is variable depending on the acid that is present and ranges from 0.8:1 to 1.8:1 for lactate and from 0.8:1 to 1:1 for ketoacids. The range of 1–1.6:1 has been used in delta–delta calculations. This range hides subtle confounding abnormalities.

AG will increase steadily as Pco$_2$ falls and pH rises, ultimately almost doubling. The AG increase with pH has been attributed to altered albumin and phosphate dissociation (Morgan et al., 2007). Therefore, AG is only useful in acidosis and has a number of confounding influences, which are largely eliminated with the Stewart–Fencl approach.

Strong ion difference (SID)

Peter Stewart based his approach on principles of physical chemistry keeping true to electrical neutrality, dissociation equilibriums, and mass conservation.

Although his original analysis is too cumbersome for routine use, his ideas have led to the derivation of clinically useful tools helpful in understanding the underlying cause of acid–base disturbances (Rastegar, 2009).

This approach recognizes only three independent variables: SID, concentration of weak acids (buffer base, A$_{TOT}$), and Pco$_2$. This analysis approach recognizes that all acid–base disturbances are a result of changes of these three variables, which are then reflected in changes in the dependent variables H$^+$ and HCO$_3^-$. These variables determine the pH, rather than merely being correlated (Kellum, 2005). Changes in Pco$_2$ are called respiratory acid–base disturbances, and changes in SID and/or A$_{TOT}$ are metabolic acid–base disturbances. A$_{TOT}$ is defined as the total amount of weak acid species in both the dissociated and the non-dissociated form, which is an independent variable whereas the amount dissociated is dependent on the pH (number of H$^+$ that need buffering) and the amount of weak acid present.

The SID can be calculated as the difference of the major strong cations and strong anions: SID$_A$ = (Na$^+$ + K$^+$)−(Cl$^-$ + Lac$^-$). When the levels of Ca^{2+} and Mg^{2+} are known they can be included to increase the accuracy of the result. In normal horses the SID is approximately 40 ± 2 (Figure 8.5). Changes in the SID will reflect the contribution of the strong ions to the acid–base balance. These changes can be quantified identifying not only whether the strong ion balance has an alkalizing or acidifying effect, but also the magnitude of the effect. This is especially useful when there is a hyponatremia

FIRS, sepsis		mEq/L
pH	7.46	
Pco$_2$	39.8	
SID	38	
Na	137 mmol/L	137
K	3.8 mmol/L	3.8
Cl	102 mmol/L	102
Ca^{++}	5.11 mg/dL	2.56
Mg^{++}	1.28 mg/dL	1.05
Lac	4.8 mmol/L	4.8
PO$_4$	4.14 mg/dL	2.4
Alb	4.9 g/dL	11
Glob	0.76 g/dL	1.1
HCO$_3$	28.6 mmol/L	28.6
SBE	4.7	4.7

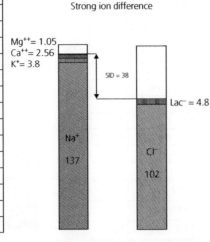

Figure 8.5 Gamblegram showing the apparent strong ion difference (SID$_A$). Blood values taken from a foal with FIRS (fetal inflammatory response syndrome) and sepsis. SBE, standard base excess.

and hypochloremia. In this situation, there may be a *relative* hyperchloremia (relative to sodium) despite a low chloride concentration resulting in a decreased SID. This would have an acidifying effect that might not be evident otherwise. The opposite may also be true.

Strong ion gap (SIG)

Strong ion difference can be calculated two different ways. Apparent SID (SID$_A$) is the difference between the identified strong cations and the identified strong anions as noted above:

$$SID_A = (Na^+ + K^+ + Ca^{2+} + Mg^{2+}) - (Cl^- + Lac^-)$$

Effective SID essentially includes the UC and UA in the formula but practically is calculated as the sum of the non-volatile and volatile weak acid buffer:

$$SID_E = HCO_3^- + Alb^- + Glob^- + HPO_4^- + PO_4^{2-}$$
$$= (Na^+ + K^+ + Ca^{2+} + Mg^{2+} + UC) - (Cl^- + Lac^- + UA)$$

The presence of UA or UC will cause a strong ion gap (SIG):

$$SIG = SID_A - SID_E = UC - UA.$$

UA contributing to the gap may include D-lactate, formate, ketoacids, salicylates, and sulfates. Unlike AG, a normal SIG should be 0 no matter what the albumin and phosphate levels are and is not confounded by respiratory

influences on HCO$_3^-$. Also, unlike AG, assuming a normal SIG = 0 and no confounding UC, the SIG value will equal the amount of UA present in mEq/L.

$$SID_A = (Na^+ + K^+ + Ca^{2+} + Mg^{2+}) - (Cl^- + Lac^-) \quad (8.9)$$

$$SID_E = HCO_3^- + ((Alb[g/dL] \times 10) \times ((0.123 \times pH) - 0.631))$$
$$+ ((PO_4[mg/dL] \times 0.323) \times ((0.309 \times pH) - 0.469))$$
$$(8.10)$$

The behavior of A$^-$, and more specifically albumin, differs between species and changes in pH have small effects until they become extreme. The following formula has been proposed for horses based on the behavior of horse plasma with a pH between 7.20 and 7.60:

$$SID_E = HCO_3^- + (2.25 \times Alb[g/dL]) + (1.40 \times Glob[g/dL])$$
$$+ (0.59 \times PO_4[mg/dL])$$
$$(8.11) \ (Constable, 1997)$$

It is important to realize that neither SID$_A$ nor SID$_E$ are exact determinations as there will always be some unmeasured ions. Despite this limitation, in normal individuals the SIG is nearly zero. In sepsis and other critical illnesses, such as liver failure, the SIG is often increased as high as 15 mEq/L or more, reflecting an increase in UA. This SIG acidosis is the primary origin of the otherwise unexplained acidosis often encountered in critical cases. The chemical nature of UA is largely unknown but likely the UA are from multiple sources that vary from one case to another. D-Lactate, unlike L-lactate, is not routinely measured and may be a significant contributor in some cases. Low molecular weight anions associated with intermediary metabolism may comprise up to one-half of the UA; these include ketones or sulfates induced by inflammation or other pathology, or that accumulate in the face of renal and liver dysfunction. Exogenously administered unmeasured anions (notably gelatins or acetate, citrate, and gluconate) also may contribute as UA, especially in the face of liver dysfunction. During sepsis, acute-phase proteins released from the liver, other inflammatory proteins, cytokines, and chemokines may also be significant contributors; hepatic or renal dysfunction may decrease their clearance. This may explain the connection between SIG acidosis and a poor prognosis, as the presence of these substances reflects both the magnitude of the inflammatory response and the presence of organ dysfunction. Not all metabolic acidoses have equal significance (Kellum, 2007a). The prognostic significance of a SIG acidosis in lactic acidosis is far worse than the same degree of acidosis originating from other causes such as hyperchloremia.

One flaw in the SIG is the inability to detect and account for UC. Most clinicians assume the contribution of UC is too small to consider. This may not always be true. Organic cations are numerous, but in normal horses they are not present in high amounts. Endogenous organic cations comprise many substances including amines such as epinephrine and dopamine and some amino acids. Exogenous cations are also common. Forty percent of commonly used drugs are cations. Many xenobiotics including toxins and other environmental substances are also cationic. At times critically ill neonatal foals have a negative SIG indicating a predominance of UC.

The SID and SIG can be calculated without a blood gas analysis, allowing an appreciation of the metabolic acid–base state in any case with information obtained solely from a chemistry panel. However, in order to fully evaluate the importance of the metabolic changes, the blood pH and $Paco_2$ need to be considered. Arterial samples should be used whenever possible in order to determine whether the metabolic changes are primary or appropriate compensation for respiratory abnormalities; similarly, they are used to detect if respiratory compensation is appropriate or if respiratory abnormalities are primary or coexisting. This perspective is necessary before therapeutic intervention is considered.

Modified base excess method

Various attempts have been made to combine the traditional approach with the Stewart approach to improve the understanding of the origin of the metabolic acid–base disturbance. SBE does not help to differentiate concurrent acid–base disorders leaving it less than ideal in complex situations. Gilfix and colleagues (1993) attempted to address this shortfall by combining the BE analysis and Stewart's approach into a more encompassing quantitative analysis. This analysis recognizes four conditions that can create metabolic acid–base disturbances: (i) a free water deficit or excess; (ii) changes in chloride concentration; (iii) changes in A^-; and (iv) the presence of organic UA. The following formulas describe the derivation of these four components of SBE:

$$BE_{measured} = BE_{fw} + BE_{Cl} + BE_{alb} + BE_{UA}$$

(8.12) (Gilfix et al., 1993)

where $BE_{measured}$ is the BE derived from the blood gas analysis; BE_{fw} is the free water component; BE_{Cl} is the contribution by Cl; BE_{alb} is the contribution by albumin; and BE_{UA} is the contribution by UA. These terms are calculated as follows:

$$BE_{fw}[mEq/L]) = 0.3 \times (Na_{measured} - Na_{ref})$$

$$BE_{Cl}[mEq/L] = Cl_{ref} - Cl_{Corr}$$

$$BE_{alb}(mEq/L) = 3.4 \times (Alb_{ref} - Alb_{measured})$$

So:

$$BE_{UA} = BE_{measured} - (BE_{fw} + BE_{Cl} + BE_{alb})$$

This approach allows a better understanding of the contribution of these influences on acid–base abnormalities so that each can be addressed separately in the therapeutic plan. But the reliance on normal values for Na, Cl, and albumin confounds the results. While individuals may maintain levels of these substances within a narrow range, there is no satisfactory method of choosing a normal value for the individual patient from the population normal range. Using different normal values within the expected range can greatly affect the result limiting the clinical usefulness of this type of analysis.

Metabolic acidosis

Metabolic acidosis is by far the most common and important acid–base abnormality in all equine patients whether they are adults, juveniles, or neonates (Table 8.3). Lactate is the most important metabolic acid and beyond its effect on the acid–base balance, its accumulation has important prognostic significance.

Lactic acidosis

L-Lactate is an important metabolite in normal physiologic conditions. Approximately 1500 mmol of L-lactate are produced daily, primarily from skeletal muscle, skin, brain, intestine, and red blood cells (Rachoin et al., 2010; Vernon & LeTourneau, 2010). Levels remain low as clearance keeps pace with production.

Hyperlactatemia – accumulation of excess lactate in the blood – is the most common cause of acidosis in the horse. In severe illness, L-lactate production occurs with hypoxia secondary to hypoxemia, hypoperfusion, or deficient oxygen-carrying capacity (anemia). In a low oxygen tension state, pyruvate does not enter the mitochondria for oxidative phosphorylation. Hypoxia is known to inhibit the pyruvate dehydrogenase (PDH) complex involved in aerobic breakdown of pyruvate to acetyl coenzyme A (Vernon & LeTourneau, 2010). Lactic

acidosis caused by cell hypoxia has been referred to as type A lactic acidosis. Hyperlactatemia without tissue hypoxia has been referred to as type B lactic acidosis. There are a number of causes of type B lactic acidosis, which commonly occur in sepsis. Any tissue undergoing a significant inflammatory response will be a source of lactate. Leukocytes produce large amounts of lactate during phagocytosis or when activated in sepsis in the presence of normal oxygen levels (Vernon & LeTourneau, 2010). Other causes of type B lactic acidosis include thiamine deficiency, hypermetabolism/catabolism of sepsis, β_2-adrenergic stimulation of the Na/K pump, and increased muscle activity as occurs in neonatal foals with seizures. Also, in sepsis the enzyme regulating lactate metabolism, pyruvate dehydrogenase kinase, increases in activity. This enzyme inactivates the pyruvate dehydrogenase (PDH) complex, which metabolizes pyruvate. Pyruvate and lactate may accumulate as a result, independent of any effect of diminished tissue perfusion (Rachoin et al., 2010). Catecholamine-induced and sepsis-induced alterations in glycolysis and mitochondrial function, and increased pyruvate production, combined with increased glucose entry into cells, can also lead to hyperlactatemia (Rachoin et al., 2010).

Decreased lactate clearance can be mediated by inflammatory mediators, hypoperfusion of the liver and kidneys, and liver or kidney dysfunction, and may contribute to hyperlactatemia (Vernon & LeTourneau, 2010). Lactate clearance occurs principally in the liver (60%) with important contributions from the kidney (30%) and to a lesser extent other organs (heart and skeletal muscle) (Vernon & LeTourneau, 2010). Renal lactate clearance is primarily through metabolism and not excretion (Rachoin et al., 2010). Due to reabsorption in the proximal convoluted tubule, urinary excretion of lactate is normally under 2% but can rise to 10% with markedly increased lactate concentrations once the renal threshold is exceeded (approximately 5 mmol/L) (Boyd & Walley, 2008; Vernon & LeTourneau, 2010).

Available data indicate that lactate itself is not necessarily harmful and is shuttled to tissues during stress states as a carbon backbone energy fuel. When lactate levels are increased in the blood, it may be more of an indicator of an underlying stress state and secondary metabolic disruption than the direct cause of pathogenesis (Rachoin et al., 2010; Vernon & LeTourneau, 2010). Although lactic acid accumulation is a marker of severe illness, it also potentially plays a protective role

Table 8.3 Causes of metabolic acid–base disturbances.

Abnormality	Acidosis	Alkalosis
Abnormal SID		
UA (e.g., D-lactate, keto acids)	↓SID ↑[UA⁻]	–
UC (e.g., organic cations)	–	↑SID ↑[UC⁺]
Free water excess or deficit	Water excess = dilutional	Water deficit = contraction
	↓SID + ↓[Na⁺]	↑SID ↑[Na⁺]
Chloride	↓SID ↑[Cl⁻]	↑SID + ↓[Cl⁻]
Abnormal A$_{TOT}$		
Albumin [Alb]	↑[Alb] (rare)	↓[Alb]
Phosphate [Pi]	↑[Pi]	↓[Pi]

A$_{TOT}$, total amount of weak acid species in both dissociated and non-dissociated forms; SID, strong ion difference; UA, unidentified anions; UC, unidentified cations.

especially in providing energy for the heart in the face of severe hypoglycemia (Rachoin et al., 2010). During periods of stress other organs, notably the brain, also use lactate preferentially as an energy substrate, reflecting its beneficial effects (Rachoin et al., 2010). The usefulness of increased lactate production routinely seen in sepsis may thus represent multiple adaptive processes aimed at improving the delivery of energy substrates to vital tissues (Rachoin et al., 2010).

The influence of L-lactate on the acid–base balance can best be judged by examining the SID_A. The normal SID_A is approximately 40 mEq/L. The degree to which the SID_A decreases below 40 when lactate (mmol/L) is included in the formula reflects the acidifying effect of lactate. Leaving the lactate value out of the SID_A formula will indicate what the acid–base balance will be after clearance of the lactate. Often in foals this exercise will uncover a concurrent underlying SID alkalosis. If the lactate value has not been measured, it may be a major contributor to the SIG. In cases of hyperlactatemia, the SIG gap is a good estimate of the unmeasured acid. It should also be noted that lactate (mmol/L) will have a direct effect on SBE. Again, as with SID_A, lactate will contribute to the SBE value millimole for millimole. So subtracting the lactate value from the SBE will both indicate the influence of the lactatemia on the acid–base balance and may help uncover concurrent problems. Patients with a hyperlactatemia will also have low HCO_3 levels and increased AG but since the relationship is not direct less can be learned by examining these values.

It should also be noted that the presence of hyperlactatemia does not necessarily mean an acidosis is present. It is not unusual for a foal with mixed acid–base abnormalities to have an overall metabolic alkalosis despite having a moderate hyperlactatemia.

Therapy for lactic acidosis

Interventions to correct lactic acidosis should be focused on correcting the underlying etiology. Insuring adequate perfusion and oxygen delivery and combating sepsis are the most important and indeed the most effective therapies. Sodium bicarbonate therapy is not recommended. Administration of sodium bicarbonate may significantly raise the pH and serum bicarbonate as well as the partial pressure of carbon dioxide, but this effect is transient. This therapy does not translate into improved hemodynamics or augmented sensitivity to catecholamines (Boyd & Walley, 2008). Indeed, sodium

bicarbonate administration in lactic acidosis has been shown to be detrimental in other species. Studies evaluating sodium bicarbonate in lactic acid fail to show convincing benefit and raise serious questions about its detrimental effects (Rachoin et al., 2010).

Unidentified anions (UA)

Traditionally L-lactate has been the main unidentified anion. In fact the AG analysis was developed to identify the presence of lactate. Today, with routine availability of lactate assays, L-lactate is accounted for except in cases with laboratory failures. In herbivores, D-lactate continues to be a major UA. Other major endogenous UA include ketoacids, volatile fatty acids (VFAs), and sulfates. Other sources of organic UA are ingested organic acids such as salicylates, methanol, and ethylene glycol.

The presence of UA/UC is discovered through the realization that the numbers don't "add up" and there is a "gap" (AG or SIG). Unaccounted changes in other major players, especially hypoalbuminemia, hypoglobulinemia, or the occurrence of UC, can mask the presence of UA by making it appear that the numbers do add up as they exert an opposite effect. This is the reason to use AG_{corr} or SIG and part of the reason a significant proportion of acid–base disturbances defy a full explanation. Many patients with severe disease will have at least some UA as reflected by the presence of a SIG of 4–8. The source of the UA in these cases may be D-lactate or metabolites accumulating during sepsis such as ketones, sulfates, acute-phase proteins, other inflammatory proteins, cytokines, chemokines, and other mediators. Exogenously administered unmeasured anions (notably gelatins or acetate, citrate, and gluconate, especially in the face of abnormal liver metabolism) and toxins also may contribute to UA.

Therapy for UA acidosis

Like lactic acidosis, the underlying cause for the accumulation of UA should be addressed rather than trying to correct the acidosis with the use of sodium bicarbonate (Figures 8.6 and 8.7). Improving clearance of the UA by improving liver and renal perfusion can also be important in addressing a SIG acidosis.

Hyperchloremic acidosis

A hyperchloremic metabolic acidosis can occur in two ways. First, Cl can be added to the circulation, either by way of an exogenous source (e.g., saline) or internal

Intrauterine distress birth asphyxia		mEq/L
pH	6.791	
Pco$_2$	59.6	
SID$_A$	62.9	
SID$_E$	32.9	
SIG	30	
Na	142 mmol/L	142
K	4.13 mmol/L	4.13
Cl	88 mmol/L	88
Ca^{++}	5.49 mg/dL	2.74
Mg^{++}	2.49 mg/dL	2.04
Lac	?? mmol/L	??
PO$_4$	27.8 mg/dL	16.4
Alb	2.97 g/dL	6.7
Glob	1.73 g/dL	2.4
HCO$_3$	9.2 mmol/L	9.2
SBE	−22.5 mEq/L	−22.5

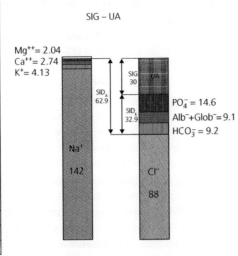

Figure 8.6 Gamblegram showing strong ion gap (SIG) and quantification of UA (unidentified anion). Blood values taken from a foal with intrauterine distress and birth asphyxia. In this case the lactate level was above the measuring limit of the analysis technique. It is likely most of the UA was lactate. SBE, standard base excess; SID$_A$, apparent strong ion difference; SID$_E$, effective strong ion difference.

Neonatal encephalopathy		mEq/L
pH	7.088	
Pco$_2$	45.9	
SID$_A$	43	
SID$_E$	34.3	
SIG	8.7	
Na	135 mmol/L	135
K	4.23 mmol/L	4.23
Cl	81 mmol/L	81
Ca^{++}	4.23 mg/dL	2.12
Mg^{++}	1.23 mg/dL	1.06
Lac	18.6 mmol/L	18.6
PO$_4$	20.53 mg/dL	12.1
Alb	2.89 g/dL	6.5
Glob	1.71 g/dL	2.4
HCO$_3$	14 mmol/L	14
SBE	−15.2 mEq/L	−15.2

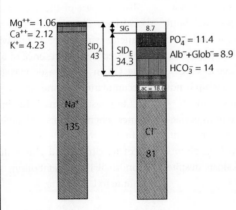

Figure 8.7 Gamblegram showing strong ion gap (SIG) and quantification of UA (unidentified anion). Blood values taken from a foal with neonatal encephalopathy. SBE, standard base excess; SID$_A$, apparent strong ion difference; SID$_E$, effective strong ion difference.

shifts (e.g., from the red cell). Second, Cl can be retained or reabsorbed while water and other ions (e.g., Na) are excreted, so that the relative concentration of Cl as compared to (Na + K) increases. Hyperchloremia is a cause of SID$_A$ acidosis and its magnitude and importance are best judged by examining the SID$_A$ (Kellum, 2005). The smaller the SID$_A$ (<40) the more important the contribution of hyperchloremia to the acidosis. The hyperchloremia will also be reflected in an equal molar decrease in SBE. Hyperchloremia is usually caused by gastrointestinal or renal disease. There is a small population of patients who have hyperchloremia that cannot be explained by renal or gastrointestinal mechanisms.

Gastrointestinal causes of hyperchloremia

Any process where Na is lost without Cl, such as severe diarrhea, will reduce the SID leading to a hyperchloremic acidosis. For example, in diarrhea, bicarbonate loss is greater than chloride loss because of failure of the

Cl/bicarbonate exchange. This will favor development of hyperchloremia. Accompanying this is extracellular volume contraction, which stimulates renal retention of sodium with chloride, because the need to conserve water by absorbing all available Na overrides the need to lose Cl in these circumstances. This will also lead to the development of hyperchloremic metabolic acidosis. In diarrhea, absorption of NH_4^+ generated by gut bacteria may also contribute to the acidosis as Cl is reabsorbed as the accompanying anion (Effros & Swenson, 2010).

The scavenging of all available Cl in cases where diarrhea results in hypovolemia as noted above can lead to a clinical picture that closely mimics renal causes of hyperchloremia, such as tubular acidosis. These clinical entities can be confused until the patient becomes volume replete with appropriate fluid therapy. Final judgment of which problem is leading to the hyperchloremia cannot be made until the kidneys no longer need to maximally conserve fluid.

Renal causes of hyperchloremia

Although the kidneys excrete many fixed acids, control of Cl reabsorption/excretion is the major renal acid–base-balancing mechanism. As a compensatory response to alkalosis, Cl is preferentially retained by the kidney. Change in Cl concentration relative to Na leading to change in SID_A is the major renal acid–base compensatory mechanism. As the normal diet usually consists of a balance of Na and Cl, the kidneys can retain or excrete the surplus Cl depending on acid–base needs. With disease, the tubular cells responsible for the regulation of Cl excretion may fail and under some circumstance may be responsible for hyperchloremic acidosis. This tubular dysfunction may be seen in the chronic stages of renal failure or in a complex of diseases causing tubular cell dysfunction in the absence of renal pathology, which is referred to as renal tubular acidosis.

Renal tubular acidosis (RTA)

Hyperchloremic acidosis is the cardinal sign of RTA, which is a sporadic disease found in horses (Ring et al., 2005; Rocher & Tannen, 1986). RTA is a collection of genetic and acquired renal tubular disorders involving proton and bicarbonate transporters as well as chloride and sodium transporters (Bagga & Sinha, 2007; Ring et al., 2005). Three types of RTA have been described in humans: proximal RTA (type 2), distal RTA (type 1), and hyperkalemic distal RTA (type 4) (Hemstreet, 2004).

Only proximal (type 2) and distal (type 1) RTA have been described in horses (Arroyo & Stampfli, 2007).

Proximal RTA (type 2) is characterized by impaired proximal recovery of bicarbonate, thought to be a Cl transporter defect. This may be combined with other proximal tubular defects referred to as Fanconi syndrome (defective reabsorption of glucose, amino acids, electrolytes, and organic acids) (Bagga & Sinha, 2007; Hemstreet, 2004; Ring et al., 2005; Rocher & Tannen, 1986). Proximal RTA is characterized by bicarbonaturia, with a fractional bicarbonate excretion greater than 15% while on bicarbonate replacement therapy (Bagga & Sinha, 2007; Ring et al., 2005). In untreated cases, the urine is usually acidic as plasma bicarbonate drops low enough for reabsorption to keep pace with the low filter load. Treatment may be difficult because administered base is often excreted at such a high rate that the desired normalization is not achieved. The acidosis in proximal RTA can be viewed in the conventional manner as loss of bicarbonate, or from the physicochemical approach to acid–base balance as the retention of chloride resulting in a hyperchloremic acidosis (decreased SID_A) (Ring et al., 2005).

Distal RTA (type 1) is characterized by impaired ability to acidify the urine in the distal tubules (Rocher & Tannen, 1986). With distal RTA ammonium (NH_4^+) ions are not excreted in amounts adequate to keep pace with a normal rate of acid production (Bagga & Sinha, 2007; Ring et al., 2005). Again the problem may be traced to a Cl transporter abnormality. Distal RTA is recognized by the inability to decrease urine pH below 5.5 in spite of metabolic acidosis; it is also characterized by a low urine Pco_2 after bicarbonate loading indicating a lack of distal hydrogen ion secretion (Bagga & Sinha, 2007; Ring et al., 2005). In humans, nephrocalcinosis and nephrolithiasis frequently occur secondary to this condition because of hypercalciuria.

Renal tubular acidosis can occur as a primary (persistent or transient) or secondary problem. In humans, secondary RTA occurs as a result of a great number of other diseases, exposure to certain drugs and toxins, a variety of genetic defects of carrier systems in the renal tubular cells, or structural disruptions of renal tubules caused by trauma or other primary renal diseases (Ring et al., 2005). Several drugs commonly used in horses have been reported to cause RTA in humans including aminoglycosides, trimethoprim potentiated sulfa drugs, carbonic anhydrase inhibitors, non-steroidal anti-inflammatory drugs, and tetracyclines (when outdated or degraded) (Arroyo & Stampfli, 2007; Firmin et al., 2007; Hemstreet, 2004). The time frame for development and recovery from drug-induced RTA is variable between individuals but may begin within a week of exposure to the drug and can resolve as quickly as 3–4 days after discontinuing the drug (Hemstreet, 2004).

Foals with RTA usually are presented with lethargy, failure to thrive, growth retardation, generalized weakness, ataxia, anorexia, colic, constipation, tachycardia, tachypnea, polyuria, and polydipsia (Arroyo & Stampfli, 2007; Bagga & Sinha, 2007). The signs may be quite vague. Any foal found to have a hyperchloremic acidosis (decreased strong ion difference, normal anion gap) with otherwise normal renal function and without possible GI or other origin hyperchloremia (such as treatment with large volumes of saline), should be suspected of having RTA.

Acidosis of progressive renal failure

Hyperchloremia without hyperkalemia is characteristic of many renal diseases associated with loss of renal tissue and a decrease in the glomerular filtration rate. Retention of acid in these patients is attributable to a decrease in the ability of the kidneys to excrete $NH_4^+Cl^-$. In these cases the decline in serum bicarbonate is relatively modest, but the chronic acidosis is associated with bone reabsorption, insulin resistance, and protein catabolism (Effros & Swenson, 2010).

Identifying the kidneys as the source of the hyperchloremia

If the origin of the hyperchloremic acidosis is extrarenal and renal function is normal, large amounts of chloride would be expected to be excreted in the urine with NH_4^+ to excrete the acid load. The urine strong ion difference (urine Na + urine K − urine Cl), which normally is positive (normal near 80) will be low (usually negative). Failure to excrete chloride in the urine in the face of acidosis confirms renal disease.

Saline infusion

Large volumes of normal saline infusion will produce a hyperchloremic acidosis. Take, for example, a normal patient (Na 140, K 5, Cl 100, SID_A 45) receiving a bolus of saline (Na 154, K 0, Cl 154, SID 0) equal to 20% of its ECF. The new values in theory would be: Na 142, K 4.17, Cl 109, and SID_A 37. It is the volume and the SID of the fluid that result in the change. To illustrate this, giving 0.5 L of 1.8% NaCl (Na 308, K 0, Cl 308, SID 0) will result in Na 163, K 3.8, Cl 125, and SID 42. So hypertonic saline will result in less acidosis than normal saline if less volume is given but the administered Na and Cl remain constant. This type of theoretical example does not take into account the alkalizing effect of diluting the buffer base (albumin, globulin, phosphorus, which are acids) with the fluid administration (Guidet et al., 2010).

Other causes of hyperchloremia

A hyperchloremic acidosis can also be induced by increased chloride salt administration in the form of saline (SID = 0), lactated Ringer's solutions (SID = 54.6 before catabolism of lactate but 26.5 after), or total parenteral nutrition (TPN) infusions. In sepsis there are occasional patients with hyperchloremic acidosis that cannot be explained by traditional sources. It has been hypothesized that this Cl originates from intracellular and interstitial compartments as a result of the partial loss of the Donnan equilibrium that is caused by albumin exiting the intravascular space. This speculation is unproven (Gunnerson et al., 2006; Kellum, 2005; Kellum et al., 2004).

Therapy for hyperchloremia

Primary hyperchloremia is best approached therapeutically by administration of $NaHCO_3$. In the traditional view this is bicarbonate replacement therapy. In the view of modifying the strong ion difference, this therapy results in the administration of Na without Cl, producing a gradual increase in the strong ion difference. When the cause of the hyperchloremia is distal RTA, correction is often accomplished using as little as 2–4 mEq/kg/day of sodium bicarbonate. When proximal RTA is the cause much larger amounts of sodium bicarbonate are needed (e.g., up to 20 mEq/kg/day) as this condition is much more refractory. When the cause of the hyperchloremia is extrarenal, correction may be accomplished with appropriate balanced crystalloid therapy without special consideration of the hyperchloremia. If sodium bicarbonate is used it should be titrated to effect.

Dilutional acidosis

Changes in free water content will change SID. As free water dilutes the strong ion concentrations, the SID will decrease resulting in a metabolic acidosis. Changes in free water are reflected by changes in sodium concentration. Any process that leads to dilution of the total number of ions will cause an acidosis, including infusion of mannitol (before the diuresis), hyperglycemia, or the increase of any osmotically active particle that may increase the volume of extracellular water without changing the net charge.

Because of this free water effect, it may be difficult to tell how much the abnormal SID is due to changes in free water and how much is due to changes in the relative concentrations of Na and Cl. To address this problem a Cl value corrected for free water can be used:

$$Cl_{Corr} = (Na_{ref} / Na_{measured}) \times Cl^-_{measured}$$

The same correction can be used on all the strong ions used. The difference between SID calculated with all measured values and the SID calculated with all corrected values (and the reference Na) will indicate how much of the acidosis is from free water. A disadvantage of this technique is that the calculations will vary depending on what value is selected as the normal Na value. It should be noted that the effect is from free water excess or deficit and will not be seen with fluid overload of strong ion balanced fluid. Fluid overload will also have a dilutional effect on the buffer base (albumin, globulin, and phosphate) – these are acids having a modulating effect on the strong ion acidosis and changes in the SIG. Unlike the dilutional effect on the SID_A, the effect on the buffer base will occur no matter what the composition of the diluting fluid (Guidet et al., 2010).

Therapy

As the magnitude of the acidosis caused by dilution is usually quite small, therapy beyond avoiding unnecessary fluid loading, especially in the face of renal compromise, is not usually necessary. However dilution rarely occurs in isolation.

Buffer base concentrations

The buffer base, also referred as A_{TOT}, is the total amount of weak acid species in both the dissociated and the non-dissociated form. The major contributors to the buffer base in plasma are albumin, globulin, and phosphate. Increase in weak acid concentration, such as occurs with hyperphosphatemia of renal failure and hyperproteinemia of hemoconcentration, will contribute to a metabolic acidosis. Each g/dL of albumin contributes

2.25 mEq/L of anion, each g/dL of globulin 1.4 mEq/L of anion, and each mg/dL inorganic phosphate 0.59 mEq/L of anion; taken together, especially in the face of unusually increased amounts, they will have a significant influence on the acid–base status of the patient.

Therapy

Treatment is focused on the underlying cause of the hyperproteinemia or hyperphosphatemia rather than directly at modifying their blood levels.

Metabolic alkalosis

Primary metabolic alkalosis is less common in horses than metabolic acidosis. It is more commonly involved in compensatory responses. But critically ill horses with complex underlying abnormalities leading to acid–base abnormalities often have alkalizing influences as well as acidifying influences. (see Table 8.3).

Hypochloremia

Although the kidneys excrete many fixed acids, control of Cl reabsorption/excretion is the major renal acid–base balancing mechanism. As a compensatory response to acidosis, Cl is preferentially excreted by the kidney. Change in Cl concentration relative to Na, leading to change in SID, is the major renal compensatory mechanism. As the normal diet usually consists of a balance of Na and Cl the kidneys can retain or excrete the surplus Cl depending on acid–base needs.

Any process that removes chloride without sodium, such as gastric reflux with pyloric obstruction or a chloriuresis, as with furosemide therapy, can lead to a hypochloremic alkalosis. Anything leading to a net loss of free water over sodium and chloride such as with a diuresis induced by hyperglycemia or use of diuretics may cause a contraction alkalosis. In this case, even though the absolute concentration of chloride will be high, the Cl concentration will not increase as rapidly as the Na concentration leading to a relative hypochloremia and an alkalosis.

Therapy

If the hypochloremia is compensatory, it should not be corrected. If it appears primary and there is evidence of volume depletion, the fluid/chloride deficit should be corrected with normal saline. If the hypochloremic metabolic alkalosis is associated with hypokalemia and total body potassium deficits, correcting the deficit with potassium chloride (KCl) will also aid in reversing the alkalosis. As the potassium deficit will be predominantly intracellular, all but a small fraction of retained potassium ends up within the cells during correction. The net effect of KCl administration is that the retained strong anion (Cl⁻) stays extracellular, whereas most of the retained strong cation disappears into the intracellular space. This will reduce plasma SID.

Unidentified cations (UC)

The presence of UC is much less common than UA. They include endogenous organic cations such as amines and exogenous organic cations such as ingested toxins and toxic levels of drugs (almost half of the organic drugs we use are cations). It is very rare for UC to be found in concentrations high enough to confound acid–base analysis; however, in equine neonatology endogenous UC can occur at significant levels. For the most part they remain unidentified, but can contribute to an alkalosis in critically ill neonates.

The presence of UC is discovered by the realization that the numbers don't "add up" and there is a "gap" (SIG). Unaccounted changes in other major players, especially hyperproteinemia or hyperphosphatemia, can mask the presence of UC; their presence makes it appear that the numbers do add up as they exert an opposite effect. As the levels of UC are usually much lower than those of UA, it is likely that in many cases the presence of UC is underappreciated. The counterbalancing effect of the presence of UC and UA cannot be detected using the analytical methods developed so far. This is part of the reason why a proportion of acid–base disturbances in our patients defy our efforts to fully explain them (Figure 8.8).

Contraction alkalosis

Changes in free water content will change SID. A free water deficit causes a metabolic alkalosis by increasing the SID through a relative increase in concentration of all strong ions. Changes in free water are particularly reflected by changes in sodium concentration. Because of this free water effect, it may be difficult to tell how much the abnormal SID is due to changes in free water and how much due to changes in the relative concentrations of Na and Cl. To address this problem a Cl value corrected for free water can be used:

$$Cl_{Corr} = \left(Na_{ref} / Na_{measured} \right) \times Cl^{-}_{measured}$$

The same correction can be used on all the strong ions used. The difference between SID calculated with all measured values and the SID calculated with all corrected values (and the reference Na) will indicate how much of the alkalosis is from a free water deficit.

FIRS, sepsis		mEq/L
pH	7.361	
Pco₂	68.3	
SID_A	39.6	
SID_E	50.6	
SIG	–11	
Na	137 mmol/L	137
K	3.73 mmol/L	3.73
Cl	102 mmol/L	102
Ca⁺⁺	4.62 mg/dL	2.31
Mg⁺⁺	1.03 mg/dL	0.84
Lac	1.3 mmol/L	1.3
PO₄	6.75 mg/dL	3.98
Alb	1.82 g/dL	4.1
Glob	2.48 g/dL	3.5
HCO₃	39.1 mmol/L	39.1
SBE	13.1	

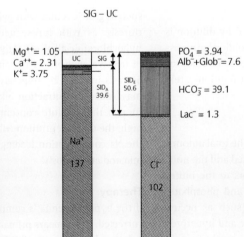

Figure 8.8 Gamblegram showing strong ion gap (SIG) and quantification of UC (unidentified cation). Blood values taken from a foal with FIRS (fetal inflammatory response syndrome) and sepsis. SBE, standard base excess; SID_A, apparent strong ion difference; SID_E, effective strong ion difference.

Albumin/phosphate concentrations

A_{TOT} is defined as the total amount of weak acid species in both the dissociated and the non-dissociated form. The major contributors to A_{TOT} in plasma are albumin and phosphate. Decreases in weak acid concentration, such as hypoproteinemia (especially hypoalbuminemia), are often present in critical patients contributing to a metabolic alkalosis. Neonates are born with low albumin concentrations but concurrently high PO_4 concentrations relative to adult horses. The two balance each other well until foals become catabolic because of neonatal illness. Albumin is an efficient buffer largely because of the multiple buffering sites on each molecule. Thus its effectiveness as a buffer is maintained at quite low concentrations. Only at the most extreme levels of hypoalbuminemia will its buffering abilities be lost. Preservation of acid buffering is not a strong indication for plasma replacement therapy in cases of hypoalbuminemia.

Respiratory acidosis

Respiratory acidosis is marked by hypercapnia, usually due to inadequate pulmonary excretion of CO_2. Hypercatabolism induced by sepsis, leading to increased CO_2 production, may also contribute. If not supplemented with oxygen therapy, hypoxemia will occur simultaneously. Increases in the HCO_3^- concentration (approximately 0.1 mEq/L for each mmHg increase in PCO_2) occurs within 5 to 10 minutes secondary to the equilibrium of CO_2 with HCO_3 influenced by the law of mass action in the presence of carbonic anhydrase. Plasma $[H^+]$ increases by approximately 0.75 nEq/L for every mmHg increase in PCO_2. The increase in HCO_3^- should not be viewed as an increase in buffer but rather the reflection of the transformation of a volatile acid (PCO_2) into a non-volatile acid (H^+). Plasma potassium concentration increases by approximately 0.1 mEq/L for every 0.1 decrease in pH as a result of intracellular acid buffering. Plasma phosphate concentration also increases slightly and plasma chloride and lactate concentrations decrease slightly. The decrease in lactate is thought to be secondary to the increased intracellular acidosis inhibiting 6-phosphofructokinase interfering with glycolysis.

After 3 to 5 days, renal conservation and generation of HCO_3^- increase (approximately 0.3–0.4 mEq/L for each mmHg increase in PCO_2) accompanied by increased renal excretion of Cl, resulting in a compensatory hypochloremic alkalosis. With compensation, plasma $[H^+]$ only increases by approximately 0.3 nEq/L for every mmHg increase in PCO_2. Compensatory changes will not completely restore the acid–base balance. When the hypercapnia resolves, a post-hypercapnic metabolic alkalosis (hypochloremic alkalosis) may persist for a few days.

Rapidly developing hypercapnic acidosis is more disruptive to the patient's physiology and more likely to be life-threatening than slowly developing, chronic disease. Hypoxemia associated with hypoventilation is the major cause of morbidity in patients with acute respiratory acidosis.

There are numerous causes of hypoventilation leading to hypercapnic respiratory acidosis. Lack of central receptor sensitivity is a common cause in foals with neonatal encephalopathy. Central depression can also result from sedatives, head trauma, cerebral edema, or encephalitis. Neuromuscular disorders leading to hypoventilation include botulism, spinal cord injury, and tetanus. Respiratory fatigue can cause hypoventilation in weak neonates with low lung compliance. Restricted ventilation can result from fractured ribs, flail chest, pneumothorax, hemothorax, or diaphragmatic hernia. Upper airway obstruction leading to hypoventilation may result from nasal obstruction, pharyngeal disease (collapse, cysts), laryngeal disease (paresis, chondroids), laryngospasm, angioedema, tracheal collapse, or aspiration as well as other abnormalities. Lower airway obstruction can result from bronchospasm, bronchiolitis, pulmonary alveolar dysfunction, pneumonia, acute respiratory distress syndrome, or pulmonary edema. Hypercapnia can also result from a pulmonary perfusion defect such as may result from cardiac defects, cardiac arrhythmias, cardiac insufficiency, hypoperfusion, or shock.

Signs of mild to moderate hypercapnia include increased cardiac output, increased blood pressure, bounding pulse, and warm skin. These signs are the manifestations of a centrally mediated adrenergic surge as a response to hypercapnia. Clinical observations suggest that this response peaks with a P_aCO_2 of approximately 80 to 100 mmHg. Even in cases that are hypotensive, such as foals suffering from septic shock, there may be a transient improvement in perfusion as a result of this adrenergic stimulation. As the P_aCO_2 continues to rise the hypercapnia will result in direct organ depression (primarily cardiac and CNS) resulting in decreased cardiac output (bradycardia and decreased myocardial contractility) and hypotension. Also systemic and cerebral vasodilation and pulmonary and renal vasoconstriction will occur. Other cardiac arrhythmias may also occur. Hypercapnic encephalopathy is primarily manifested by a transient increased central irritability followed by severe central depression, progressing to a non-responsive state and respiratory depression leading to respiratory arrest.

Therapy

When considering treatment of hypercapnia only the arterial pH should be considered. Hypercapnia should not be corrected if the arterial pH is alkalotic, normal, or mildly acidotic. With significant metabolic alkalosis, hypercapnia is appropriate. Current evidence suggests that mild hypercapnic acidosis (pH >7.2) may be beneficial in sepsis because of its anti-inflammatory effects (Curley et al., 2010; Ijland et al., 2010)). It is unclear if this mild respiratory acidosis should be corrected.

The primary method of treating respiratory acidosis is increasing alveolar ventilation. Caffeine and doxapram have been used to increase ventilation when the cause of hypercapnic acidosis is depression of central receptors in foals. A small study of anesthetic-induced respiratory acidosis suggested that doxapram could be useful (Giguère et al., 2007). A retrospective study of the use of caffeine or doxapram in equine neonatal encephalopathy cases showed that doxapram therapy did not correct the acidosis despite decreasing the P_aco_2. With caffeine therapy, the P_aco_2 did not change yet the pH tended to normalize, but there was a concurrent confounding progressive metabolic alkalosis in the caffeine cases (Giguère et al., 2008). The mild respiratory acidosis these pharmacologic agents have been used to treat may be better left uncorrected. Definitive treatment for severe respiratory acidosis is mechanical ventilation, which has been described in foals (Palmer, 2005).

When hypoventilation is caused by upper airway obstruction, stenting the airway with an endotracheal tube to prevent collapse or placing a tracheostomy may resolve the problem. When hypoventilation is caused by lower airway obstruction, use of bronchodilators may resolve the problem.

Since hypercapnia will lead to hypoxemia when breathing room air, oxygen therapy is indicated. Careful monitoring of Cl and K concentrations, and supplementation as indicated, is important to support renal compensation for the respiratory acidosis. Sodium bicarbonate therapy is contraindicated in the face of respiratory acidosis as it will add to the CO_2 load, thereby contributing to the acidosis.

Respiratory alkalosis

Respiratory alkalosis is marked by hypocapnia due to increased pulmonary excretion of CO_2. Decreases in the HCO_3^- concentration (approximately 0.2 mEq/L for each mmHg decrease in Pco_2) occurs within 5 to 10 minutes secondary to the equilibrium of HCO_3 with CO_2 influenced by the law of mass action in the presence of carbonic anhydrase. Plasma [H^+] decreases by approximately 0.75 nEq/L for every mmHg decrease in Pco_2. The decrease in HCO_3^- should not be viewed as a decrease in buffer but rather the reflection of the transformation of a non-volatile acid (H^+) into a volatile acid (Pco_2). Plasma potassium concentration decreases by approximately 0.2 mEq/L for every 0.1 increase in pH as a result of intracellular K/H exchange. Hypophosphatemia may develop and plasma chloride concentrations may increase.

There are several causes of hyperventilation. Hypoxemia stimulates hyperventilation when the P_ao_2 decreases below 60 mmHg. Central hyperventilation may occur in neonatal encephalopathy as a primary problem or secondary to hyperthermia. Hyperventilation can also be secondary to stimulation of pulmonary neuroreceptors in pneumonia, pneumothorax, hemothorax, acute respiratory distress syndrome, or interstitial lung disease. Hyperventilation may also occur secondary to pain, anxiety, fever, high adrenergic tone, meningoencephalitis, hepatic encephalopathy, or cerebral trauma. Hyperventilation may be seen in pregnancy, sepsis, liver failure, or heat exhaustion. Acute respiratory alkalosis can result in decreased cerebral blood flow because of local vasoconstriction, which may result in cerebral hypoxemia and neurologic abnormalities. This is self-limiting as the local increase in lactic acid secondary to tissue hypoxia results in vasodilation (Adrogué & Madias, 2011; Madias & Adrogué, 2009; Mehta & Emmett, 2009).

Therapy

Therapy is generally aimed at the underlying cause. In severe cases of central hyperventilation sedation with phenobarbital to depress the central receptors may be useful.

Mixed acid–base disorders

The term "mixed acid–base disorder" refers to a clinical condition in which two or more primary acid–base disorders coexist. They generally present with one obvious disturbance with what appears to be an inappropriate (excessive or inadequate) compensation. The "inappropriateness" of the compensatory process is the result of a separate primary disorder rather than the compensatory response itself. The expected degrees of compensation for primary acid–base disorders have been determined in humans by analysis of data from a large number of patients, and are expressed in the form of equations. When disorders influence the blood pH in opposite directions, the blood pH will be determined by the dominant disorder(s). If disorders cancel out each other's effects, blood pH can be normal. When there is compensation for acid–base disorders, both P_aCO_2 and HCO_3^- are expected to change in the same direction (i.e., both are high or both are low). If P_aCO_2 and HCO_3^- have changed in opposite directions, the presence of a mixed acid–base disorder is expected. Compensation may be excessive, insufficient, or appropriate. One can also have an idea about the appropriateness of compensation from the degree of pH deviation.

Mixed acid–base disorders are common in critically ill patients and can lead to dangerous extremes of pH. Four or more independent abnormalities may be contributing to the final pH. Untangling these independent abnormalities can reveal the underlying pathophysiology that is placing the patient in jeopardy. When examining the information from a patient with a complex mixed acid–base disorder it is helpful to examine the four major influences on acid–base balance:

1 SID_A excluding lactate.
2 lactate plus other organic anions (UA);
3 abnormalities in the buffer base;
4 respiratory component.

Abnormalities of the SID_A (excluding lactate), whether brought about as appropriate renal compensation or produced as a primary abnormality, take time to develop and time to resolve, suggesting chronicity. As is apparent, abnormalities in the SID_A in these cases are a result primarily of the abnormality of Na + K and Cl concentrations and are caused by renal (or placental) and/or gastrointestinal adjustments of these ions. Lactic acidosis and other organic anion acidoses are processes of abnormal intermediary metabolism, which can develop rapidly and resolve rapidly. These abnormalities imply other underlying pathophysiologic forces at work. Abnormalities of the buffer base, which can have a large influence on the acid–base balance, with extreme levels of plasma proteins and phosphate are unusual; when present they reflect still different underlying pathophysiologies. And finally changes in respiratory acid excretion may reflect attempts at normal respiratory compensation or underlying neurorespiratory abnormalities. Examining each of these parts of the puzzle in turn will help the clinician to have a better understanding of why the pH value is normal or abnormal. It also points toward a better understanding of the underlying pathophysiology that is placing the patient at peril (DuBose, 2012).

In the complex disturbances of critically ill patients, alkalinizing and acidifying disturbances may both be present concurrently and may escape detection because of their offsetting effects. There are significant differences between the mechanisms causing acid–base imbalances. There are likewise significant differences in outcomes for patients developing acidosis from dilution, poisoning, hyperchloremia, excessive use of normal saline infusions, dysoxia, and other causes of increased lactate production. The acid–base abnormalities themselves may be of less clinical significance than previously thought.

Summary

This has been a short review of the underlying causes of metabolic acid–base disturbances and the strengths and weakness of the analytic tools designed to help understand the origin of the disturbance in clinical cases. Acute metabolic acidosis can be a complex problem and may be caused by an alteration in the SID or the buffer base. An altered SID reflects a change in the relative ratio of strong anions to strong cations. This change can be caused by anion gains as occur with lactic acidosis, renal acidosis, ketoacidosis, or hyperchloremia. Alternatively, cations may be lost, as occurs with severe diarrhea or renal tubular acidosis. Acute acidosis also may reflect increased free water relative to strong ions (dilutional acidosis), which may accompany excessive hypotonic fluid intake or the presence of excessive osmoles such as with hyperglycemia or alcohol poisoning (ethanol, methanol, isopropyl alcohol, ethylene glycol). The plasma concentration of albumin and phosphate also can have an influence over acid–base balance by resulting in abnormal amounts of the buffer base, which in turn is reflected by the amount of the non-volatile weak acid present. The respiratory contribution to the acid–base balance is less complex but none the less important to consider. The techniques described in this chapter have been found useful for exploring acid–base disturbances in horses secondary to colic, diarrhea, and exercise (Navarro et al., 2005; Nappert & Johnson, 2001; Viu et al., 2010). They are equally useful in understanding acid–base abnormalities in neonatal foals as demonstrated by the examples in this chapter.

References

Adrogué HJ, Madias NE. (2011) Respiratory acidosis, respiratory alkalosis, and mixed disorders. In: Floege J, Johnson RJ, Feehally J (eds) *Comprehensive Clinical Nephrology*, 4th edn. London: Mosby, pp. 176–92.

Arroyo LG, Stampfli HR. (2007) Equine renal tubular disorders. *Vet Clin Equine* **23**:631–9.

Astrup P, Jorgensen K, Siggaard-Andersen O. (1960) Acid-base metabolism: New approach. *Lancet* **i**:1035–9.

Bagga A, Sinha A. (2007) Evaluation of renal tubular acidosis. *Indian J Pediatr* **74**:679–86.

Boyd JH, Walley KR. (2008) Is there a role for sodium bicarbonate in treating lactic acidosis from shock? *Curr Opin Crit Care* **14**:379–83.

Collings JL. (2010) Acid-base disorders. In: Marx JA, Hockberger RS, Walls RM, Adams JG, et. al. (eds) *Marx–Rosen's Emergency Medicine*, 7th edn. Philadelphia: Saunders Elsevier, pp. 1605–14.

Constable PD. (1997) A simplified strong ion model for acid-base equilibria: Application to horse plasma. *J Appl Physiol* **83**:297–311.

Corey HE. (2003) Stewart and beyond: New models of acid-base balance. *Kidney Int* **64**:777–87.

Curley G, Contreras M, Nichol AD, Higgins BD, Laffey JG. (2010) Hypercapnia and acidosis in sepsis a double-edged sword? *Anesthesiology* **112**:462–72.

DuBose TD. (2012) Disorders of acid-base balance. In: Taal MW, Chertow GM, Marsden PA, Skorecki K, Yu ASL, Brenner BM (eds) *Brenner & Rector's The Kidney*, 9th edn. Philadelphia: Elsevier, pp. 595–631.

Effros MR, Swenson ER. (2010) Acid-base balance. In: Mason CJ, Broaddus VC, Martin TR, et al. (eds) *Murray and Nadel's Textbook of Respiratory Medicine*, 5th edn. Philadelphia: Saunders Elsevier, pp. 134–58.

Emmett M, Narins RG. (1977) Clinical use of the anion gap. *Medicine* **56**:38–54.

Fencl V, Leith DE. (1993) Stewart's quantitative acid-base chemistry: Applications in biology and medicine. *Resp Physiol* **91**:1–16.

Figge J, Mydosh T, Fencl V. (1992) Serum proteins and acid-base equilibria: a follow-up. *J Lab Clin Med* **120**:713–19.

Firmin CJ, Kruger TF, Davids R. (2007) Proximal renal tubular acidosis in pregnancy. *Gynecol Obstet Invest* **63**:39–44.

Giguère S, Sanchez LC, Shih A, Szabo NJ, Womble AY, Robertson SA. (2007) Comparison of the effects of caffeine and doxapram on respiratory and cardiovascular function in foals with induced respiratory acidosis. *Am J Vet Res* **68**: 1407–16.

Giguère S, Slade JK, Sanchez LC. (2008) Retrospective comparison of caffeine and doxapram for the treatment of hypercapnia in foals with hypoxic-ischemic encephalopathy. *J Vet Intern Med* **22**:401–5.

Gilfix BM, Bique M, Magder S. (1993) A physical chemical approach to the analysis of acid-base balance in the clinical setting. *J Crit Care* **8**:187–97.

Guidet B, Soni N, Della Rocca G, et al. (2010) A balanced view of balanced solutions. *Critical Care* **14**:325–37.

Gunnerson KJ, Saul M, He S, Kellum JA. (2006) Lactate versus non-lactate metabolic acidosis: a retrospective outcome evaluation of critically ill patients. *Crit Care* **10**:R22.

Greenbaum LA. (2011) Electrolyte and acid-base disorders. In: Kliegman RM, Stanton BF, Geme III JW, Schor NF, Behman RE (eds) *Nelson Textbook of Pediatrics*, 19th edn. Philadelphia: Saunders Elsevier, pp. 212–42.

Hasselbalch KA. (1916) The calculation of blood pH via the partition of carbon dioxide in plasma and oxygen binding of the blood as a function of plasma pH. *Biochem Z* **78**:112–44.

Hemstreet BA (2004) Antimicrobial-associated renal tubular acidosis. *Ann Pharmacother* **38**:1031–8.

Henderson LJ. (1907) The theory of neutrality regulation in the animal organism. *Am J Physiol* **18**:427–48.

Ijland MM, Heunks LM, van der Hoeven JG. (2010) Bench-to-bedside review: Hypercapnic acidosis in lung injury – from 'permissive' to 'therapeutic.' *Crit Care* **14**:237–47.

Jorgensen K, Astrup P. (1957) Standard bicarbonate, its clinical significance, and a new method for its determination. *Scand J Clin Lab Invest* **9**:122–32.

Kellum JA. (2005) Determinants of plasma acid-base balance. *Crit Care Clin* **21**:329–46.

Kellum JA. (2007a) Acid-base disorders and strong ion gap. *Contrib Nephrol* **156**:158–66.

Kellum JA. (2007b) Disorders of acid-base balance. *Crit Care Med* **35**:2630–6.

Kellum JA, Song M, Li J. (2004) Lactic and hydrochloric acids induce different patterns of inflammatory response in LPS-stimulated RAW 264.7 cells. *Am J Physiol Regul Integr Comp Physiol* **286**:R686–R692.

Kurtz I, Kraut J, Ornekian V, Nguyen MK. (2008) Acid-base analysis: a critique of the Stewart and bicarbonate-centered approaches. *Am J Physiol Renal Physiol* **294**:F1009–F1031.

Latta TA. (1832) Relative to the treatment of cholera by the copious injection of aqueous and saline fluids into the veins. *Lancet* **ii**:274–7.

Madias NE, Adrogué HJ. (2009) Respiratory acidosis and alkalosis. In: Greenberg A (ed.) *Primer on Kidney Diseases*, 5th edn. Philadelphia: Saunders, pp. 91–7.

Mehta AN, Emmett M. (2009) Approach to acid-base disorders. In: Greenberg A (ed.) *Primer on Kidney Diseases*, 5th edn. Philadelphia: Saunders, pp. 98–107.

Morgan TJ, Cowley DM, Weier SL, Venkatesh B. (2007) Stability of the strong ion gap versus the anion gap over extremes of PCO_2 and pH. *Anaesth Intensive Care* **35**:370–3.

Nappert G, Johnson PJ. (2001) Determination of the acid-base status in 50 horses admitted with colic between December 1998 and May 1999. *Can Vet J* **42**:703–7.

Navarro M, Monreal L, Segura D, Armengou L, Añor S. (2005) A comparison of traditional and quantitative analysis of acid-base and electrolyte imbalances in horses with gastrointestinal disorders. *J Vet Intern Med* **19**:871–7.

O'Shaughnessy WB. (1831) Proposal of a new method of treating the blue epidemic cholera by the injection of highly-oxygenised salts into the venous system. *Lancet* **i**:366–71.

Palmer JE. (2005) Ventilatory support of the critically ill foal. *Vet Clin North Am: Equine Pract* **21**:457–86.

Rachoin JS, Weisberg LS, McFadden CB. (2010) Treatment of lactic acidosis: appropriate confusion. *J Hosp Med* **5**:E1–E7; doi: 10.1002/jhm.600.

Rastegar A. (2009) Clinical utility of Stewart's method in diagnosis and management of acid-base disorders. *Clin J Am Soc Nephrol* **4**:1267–74.

Ring T, Frische S, Nielsen S. (2005) Clinical review: Renal tubular acidosis – a physicochemical approach. *Crit Care* **9**: 573–80.

Rocher LL, Tannen RL. (1986) The clinical spectrum of renal tubular acidosis. *Ann Rev Med* **37**:319–31.

Shannon M. (2007) Acid-base, fluid, and electrolyte balance. In: Shannon M (ed.) *Haddad and Winchester's Clinical Management of Poisoning and Drug Overdose*, 4th edn. Philadelphia: Saunders Elsevier, pp. 105–18.

Siggaard-Andersen O. (1963) Blood acid-base alignment nomogram. Scales for pH, PCO_2, base excess of whole blood of different hemoglobin concentrations. Plasma bicarbonate and plasma total CO_2. *Scand J Clin Lab Invest* **15**:211–17.

Siggaard-Andersen O. (1977) The Van Slyke equation. *Scand J Clin Lab Invest* **37**(Suppl. 146):15–20.

Singer RB, Hastings AB. (1948) Improved clinical method for estimation of disturbances of acid-base balance of human blood. *Medicine (Baltimore)* **27**:223–42.

Stewart PA. (1981) How to Understand Acid Base Balance. *A Quantitative Acid–Base Primer for Biology and Medicine*. New York: Elsevier.

Van Slyke DD. (1921) Studies of acidosis: XVII. *The normal and abnormal variations in the acid base balance of the blood. J Biol Chem* **48**:153–76.

Van Slyke DD. (1928) Sendroy: Studies of gas and electrolyte equilibria in blood: XV. Line charts for graphic calculations by Henderson–Hasselbalch equation, and for calculating plasma carbon dioxide content from whole blood content. *J Biol Chem* **79**:781–98.

Vernon C, LeTourneau JL. (2010) Lactic acidosis: recognition, kinetics, and associated prognosis. *Crit Care Clin* **26**:255–83.

Viu J, Jose-Cunilleras E, Armengou L, et al. (2010) Acid-base imbalances during a 120 km endurance race compared by traditional and simplified strong ion difference methods. *Equine Vet J* **42**(Suppl. 38):76–82.

Wang Y, Xu T. (2011) Acidosis, acid-sensing ion channels, and neuronal cell death. *Mol Neurobiol* **44**:350–8.

Wooten EW. (2003) Calculation of physiological acid-base parameters in multicompartment systems with application to human blood. *J Appl Physiol* **95**:2333–44.

SECTION 2
Fluid therapy

CHAPTER 9

Preparation, supplies, and catheterization

Jamie Higgins

Idaho Equine Hospital, Nampa, ID, USA

Introduction

The primary reason for intravenous catheter placement is the continuous administration of intravenous medications, especially intravenous fluids or other continuous rate infusions (CRI). However, intravenous catheters are also placed when intermittent intravenous access is required in order to avoid the discomfort and potential complications of repeated needle insertions into the vein. This often occurs in patients hospitalized in an intensive care unit, which require frequent blood sample collection or medication administration. Patients requiring long-term intravenous medications (even if only once or twice a day) may be easier to manage with an intravenous catheter, but the risks and benefits need to be evaluated.

Intravenous catheter selection

When selecting the type of catheter to be used, there are many factors to consider including the required duration of venous access, the veins available for catheter placement, the behavior of the patient, risks of thrombophlebitis, and the cost of different catheter types. The purpose of the catheter (i.e., large-volume fluid resuscitation vs long-term medication administration) will also be a factor in selection of catheter type. Intrinsic patient characteristics such as underlying disease conditions, severity of illness, and age of the patient should be considered as well.

Catheter size

The flow rate of a fluid is defined by the Hagen–Poiseuille equation:

$$Q = \Delta P \left(\frac{\pi r^4}{8 \mu L} \right) \tag{9.1}$$

where Q = flow rate of the fluid, ΔP represents the change in pressure, r is the radius of the tube, L is the length of the tube, and μ is the viscosity of the fluid.

This equation indicates that flow rate is proportional to the catheter lumen radius (r) to the fourth power and inversely proportional to length (L) of the catheter. Therefore, the fluid administration rate will be greatest when using short, large-bore catheters. *In vitro* clinical trials indicate that fluid administration rates using large-bore catheters and tubing can reach rates of approximately 50 L/h (Nolen-Walston, 2012). When the same model was applied *in vivo*, rates were reduced by approximately 20% (Nolen-Walston, 2012). The insertion of larger-bore catheters may increase vessel wall trauma, which can predispose to catheter site complications.

If a patient has signs of hypovolemic shock and requires rapid, large-volume fluid replacement then bilateral placement of large-bore jugular venous catheters can be used. Shorter-length catheters, while delivering fluids more rapidly, have increased risk of extravasation of fluids and medications as they may be more likely to become displaced from the vein. Excessive movement of a short catheter within the vein compared to a longer length catheter can potentially induce vessel wall inflammation (Spurlock et al., 1990).

Equine Fluid Therapy, First Edition. Edited by C. Langdon Fielding and K. Gary Magdesian.
© 2015 John Wiley & Sons, Inc. Published 2015 by John Wiley & Sons, Inc.

The catheter size typically used in adult horses for long-term use is a 14-gauge catheter. When rapid fluid resuscitation is needed, a 10- or 12-gauge catheter is recommended. This size of catheter is best removed as soon as possible due to the irritation that it may cause to the vessel, predisposing the vein to complications such as thrombophlebitis. For foals or miniature horses, a 16-gauge catheter can be placed for long-term use. However, 14-gauge catheters appear safe and effective for emergency fluid resuscitation even in these smaller animals.

Smaller gauge catheters (18-gauge or less) may be easier to place in dehydrated patients or when the vein is difficult to visualize. In emergency situations, a smaller catheter can be placed for immediate venous access. When needed, a guide wire can be passed through this smaller catheter and a larger catheter can be "swapped" for the smaller one. It may be necessary to dilate the opening in the skin and/or vein to accommodate the larger catheter.

Lumen number

Single lumen

Single lumen catheters have only one port connected to a single catheter tube. They can be slightly easier to place compared to multiple lumen catheters, particularly for a less experienced clinician. However, if multiple medications are being given at the same time, especially as continuous infusions or ones that are incompatible, single lumen catheters may be less ideal. There may be interactions between the drugs including formation of a precipitate, a change in drug potency, total inactivation of a medication, or the formation of toxic or harmful products if medications can mix in a single lumen (Davie, 1977; Klein, 1984). In addition, parenteral nutrition (PN) optimally is administered through a dedicated port.

Multiple lumen

Multiple lumen catheters contain between two and four individual ports each connected to individual tubing running the length of the catheter and contained within one catheter. The lumen exits are placed along the distal catheter body and are rotated 90° around the catheter circumference to minimize mixture of infusates (Figure 9.1). The multiple ports allow for administration of medications, blood sampling, fluid replacement, and monitoring simultaneously all through one catheter.

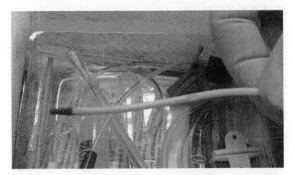

Figure 9.1 Multiple ports rotated around the circumference of the catheter to minimize mixture of infusates.

The individual lumen diameters may be of reduced size when multiple lumens are present and this will limit the fluid flow rate that can be achieved.

Catheter material

The catheter material will affect the structural integrity, rigidity, and biostability. Each of these characteristics will influence the likelihood of vascular wall irritation leading to thrombus formation and thrombophlebitis (Tan et al., 2003). Materials currently used for catheters include Teflon (fluorinated ethylene propylene polymer), polyurethane, and silicone (Dallap & Orsini, 2008). Teflon or polyurethane catheters have been associated with fewer septic complications than polyvinyl chloride or polyethylene catheters in humans, and are the types most commonly used in horses (Maki & Ringer 1987, 1991).

Teflon

Teflon catheters are prone to cracking and kinking at the insertion site due to the rigid characteristics of the material (Figure 9.2). This rigidity also causes increased vessel wall irritation, increasing the risk of thrombophlebitis (Spurlock & Spurlock, 1990; Spurlock et al., 1990; Tan et al., 2003). Teflon catheters usually lie along the vessel wall when indwelling (Spurlock et al., 1990). Teflon catheters are only recommended for a maximum use of 3 days due to the potential complications associated with the material (Dallap & Orsini, 2008; Hay, 1992; Tan et al., 2003). Teflon catheters usually are placed in a simple, over-the-needle configuration with a single lumen. With this style of catheter, the metal stylet is withdrawn as the catheter is advanced into the vein.

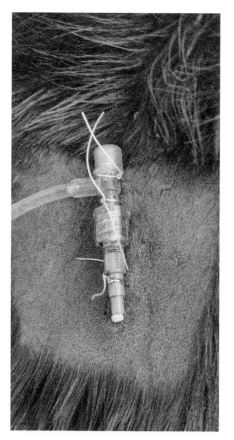

Figure 9.2 Kinking of a Teflon catheter at the insertion site.

Polyurethane and silicone

Polyurethane and silicone catheters are much less rigid, which improves the structural integrity and biostability – properties that reduce the likelihood of catheter kinking. These characteristics allow for polyurethane or silicone catheters to remain in use for up to 3–4 weeks. The softer material of polyurethane and silicone catheters is less traumatic to the vessel wall (Dallap & Orsini, 2008; Tan et al., 2003). These softer catheters usually lie within the lumen of the vessel, rather than up against the vessel wall (Spurlock et al., 1990). Soft catheters, such as polyurethane or silicone, typically require a guide-wire for catheter placement. This additional step can increase the opportunity for contamination of aseptic technique (Marino, 2007; Tan et al., 2003). Softer catheters also have an increased tendency to back out of the vein (Spurlock et al., 1990). For guide-wire catheters, an over-the-needle introduction catheter is initially placed. Once the metal stylet is removed from the

introduction catheter, a metal guide-wire is passed through the introduction catheter and the introduction catheter is removed from the vein. Next, a dilator is often passed over the wire and removed before a softer long-term catheter is passed over the guide-wire into the vein. Often, the skin at the proposed catheter entry site should be opened with a 14-gauge hypodermic needle or with a stab incision using a no. 15 scalpel blade.

Location for catheter placement

Jugular vein

The most common site for intravenous catheter placement in horses is the left or right jugular vein. The jugular vein allows for large gauge vascular access for high-volume fluid administration. The jugular vein is located in the jugular furrow, ventral to the sternomandibularis and dorsal to the brachiocephalicus muscles. The vein is lateral to the trachea, carotid artery, and vagosympathetic trunk (Hay, 1992). The best area for jugular vein placement is at the point of junction between the cranial one-third and caudal two-thirds of the cervical region. The jugular vein is most superficial at this point. Additionally, the carotid artery comes closer to the jugular vein as it courses distally down the neck decreasing the separation of the jugular vein from the carotid artery by the omohyoid muscle. The carotid artery is more likely to be entered during catheter venepuncture in the lower part of the neck (Tan et al., 2003). Inadvertent puncture of the carotid artery can lead to large hematoma formation or, more dangerously, administration of medications into the arterial circulation leading to seizures or death.

Arterial catheterization may be suspected if high-pressure, pulsatile flow is obtained from the catheter. If venous catheterization cannot be confirmed, a blood-gas analysis can be performed to more definitively determine the location of the catheter (artery vs vein). The partial pressure of oxygen in the sample is likely to be the most useful in determining the presence of the catheter in the artery; however, severe respiratory disease can complicate interpretation. If there is any concern that the catheter is located in the artery, it should not be used for administration of medications. Ultrasonographic evaluation can also assist in differentiating venous versus arterial placement.

The left jugular vein is in close proximity to the left recurrent laryngeal nerve. There are anecdotal reports of

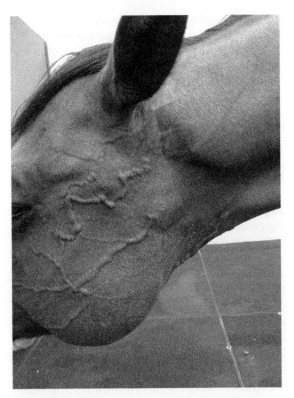

Figure 9.3 Venous distention secondary to left jugular vein thrombosis.

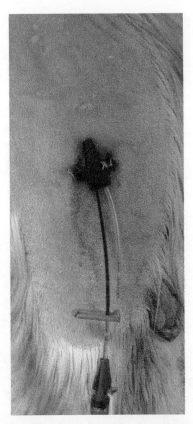

Figure 9.4 Cephalic catheter should be oriented so that the distal end of the catheter delivers fluids and medications along the direction of blood flow returning to the heart.

left laryngeal hemiplegia in association with perivascular irritation from left jugular vein catheterization or perivascular leakage of medications. The left jugular vein is also in close proximity to the esophagus. Therefore, some clinicians advocate the use of the right jugular vein in performance horses.

Prior to placement of an intravenous catheter in the jugular vein, the patency of both jugular veins should be verified. If one of the jugular veins is compromised (either significant inflammation or complete thrombosis), the other jugular vein should not be used for catheterization. With thrombosis of both jugular veins, the decreased venous drainage can lead to dramatic edema formation in the head and subsequent respiratory distress from nasal and laryngeal edema. Even with thrombosis of one jugular vein, venous distention is apparent (Figure 9.3).

Alternative catheter site locations

Alternative locations for venous catheterization include the proximal cephalic vein or the lateral thoracic vein. Over-the-wire catheters made of polyurethane or silicone are recommended for these locations. Catheters placed in these veins may require more frequent flushing (every 4 hours). The duration of patency for these catheters may also be more limited as compared to jugular vein catheters. All venous catheters should be placed in an orientation so that the distal end of the catheter delivers the fluids and medications along the direction of blood flow returning to the heart (Figure 9.4).

Cephalic vein

For cephalic vein catheterization, good restraint of the animal is important as the person placing the catheter is positioned in a potentially dangerous area. The site for insertion of the cephalic catheter is the flat region of the medial proximal antebrachium. Flexible polyurethane catheters should be used to avoid kinking as the catheter is passed proximally up the limb through the axillary region. Avoiding placement of the tip of the catheter at the elbow joint will prevent reduction in blood and fluid flow and maintain catheter patency (Tan et al., 2003). Bandaging of the catheter in this location is recommended to prevent removal by the patient. Additionally, a bandage that provides increased pressures over the insertion site may help to reduce hematoma formation particularly at the time of placement.

Lateral thoracic vein

For catheterization of the lateral thoracic vein, the vein can be identified at the level of the point of the elbow at the point of the junction between the cranial one-third and caudal two-thirds of the lateral aspect of the thorax and abdomen. A slight depression can often be palpated in the thoracoabdominal wall where the lateral thoracic vein runs in a horizontal course. If the lateral thoracic vein cannot be palpated, the vein can be found with superficial ultrasound of the region. A flexible catheter made of polyurethane should be used for this site as well, as the vein curves along the surface of the animal's trunk. Bandaging of this catheter site also is recommended to minimize risks of the catheter becoming dislodged.

Saphenous vein

The lateral branch of the saphenous vein can be catheterized in the neonatal foal. Patient compliance and mobility of the vein make this a poor choice in adult horses. Even in foals, insertion and maintenance of a catheter in this location can be challenging.

Patient characteristics affecting catheter selection

Many of the patients selected for indwelling venous catheterization have underlying inflammatory disease and may be more prone to catheter-associated complications. Colic patients, for example, have had reported rates of thrombophlebitis of 18% to 50% following colic surgery (Lankveld et al., 2001). In addition to horses with surgical colic, patients with enteritis, colitis, or pneumonia, critically ill neonates, and other groups of patients with inflammatory diseases are likely to have altered vascular flow and coagulation status, which may affect the rate of catheter-related complications. Most of these patients experience dehydration and/or hypovolemia. As such, they may be susceptible to increased risk of vascular trauma during placement of the catheter

due to poor jugular fill with consequent poor vessel visualization. In addition, they are often hypercoagulable early in the course of disease, particularly when endotoxemic (Epstein et al., 2011; Lankveld et al., 2001; Traub-Dargatz & Dargatz, 1994).

In addition to underlying medical considerations, patient behavior may affect catheter selection. For example, some horses are very reactive to pressure placed near the jugular vein (this may be from previous episodes of needle insertion) and may have better compliance for cephalic catheter placement and maintenance. Horses that are very active in the stall may be less likely to kink or displace a polyurethane catheter than a Teflon catheter.

Catheter placement

Considerations for catheter site preparation

Use of an antiseptic solution that kills or inhibits the growth of microorganisms is the basis of catheter site preparation. Removal of hair and gross skin contamination, sterilization of skin, maintenance of sterile equipment and gloves during catheter placement, and securing of the catheter to the skin are all important steps in decreasing catheter-associated complications. By reducing the patient's skin flora, the risks for developing an infection from the catheter insertion are decreased (Marino, 2007). Antiseptic solutions can be effective in the presence of hair (Hague et al., 1997). Traumatic clipping of the hair leading to abrasion of the skin can promote wound infection, so use of sharp blades to minimize skin trauma is important (Southwood & Baxter, 1996; Tan et al., 2003). Clipping of hair can remove gross environmental contamination such as mud and dirt. Hair removal can also lead to better visualization of the vein, allowing for less traumatic catheter placement, especially in miniature equids and horses with hirsutism or hypertrichosis.

Steps to prepare for catheter placement

Preparation for catheter placement involves a number of steps.

1 Confirm that all supplies necessary for catheter placement are readily available, including spare catheter supplies in the event that they become damaged or contaminated during placement of the catheter.

2 Select appropriate site for catheter placement.

3 Remove hair from skin with electric clippers (or safety razor if clippers are not available).

4 Remove gross skin contamination with gentle soap (a surgical prep sponge with povidone iodine or chlorhexidine scrub is often used).

5 Perform sterile preparation of the skin with either alternating povidone iodine solution and isopropyl alcohol or alternating chlorhexidine scrub and solution. Alternating preparation solutions with repeated applications three to seven times is recommended for sterile preparation of the skin prior to catheterization. Chlorhexidine is recommended by the Centers for Disease Control due to its residual antimicrobial activity of up to 6 hours after application (Marino, 2007). Chlorhexidine also elicits less of an inflammatory skin reaction than povidone iodine (Southwood & Baxter, 1996). This may be especially important in foals. Chlorhexidine also has better activity in the presence of organic material than povidone iodine (Southwood & Baxter, 1996). Contact time for preparation should be a minimum of 5 minutes, especially for povidone iodine to allow time for maximal antimicrobial effect (Zubrod et al., 2004). Isopropyl alcohol potentiates the antimicrobial activity of povidone iodine by increasing the release of free iodine, so should be used for the final application. Saline is recommended as the final rinse with chlorhexidine rather than alcohol to avoid decreasing the residual antimicrobial activity (Southwood & Baxter, 1996).

6 The subcutaneous tissue over the intended catheter insertion site should be desensitized with 2% lidocaine infiltration prior to a final sterile preparation of the skin. Other local anesthetics can also be used. Removing skin sensation to the area of insertion will encourage patient compliance and promote atraumatic catheter placement. Some clinicians do not desensitize the skin with a local anesthetic particularly in emergency situations when rapid catheter placement is essential.

7 Sterile surgical gloves are required for over-the-wire catheters. Individuals with less catheter placement experience should wear sterile gloves when placing all catheters to prevent contamination of the catheter material.

8 Full-thickness skin incisions using a no. 15 scalpel blade can facilitate catheter placement by decreasing tissue drag. This is frequently used for catheters in foals and for cephalic and lateral thoracic vein

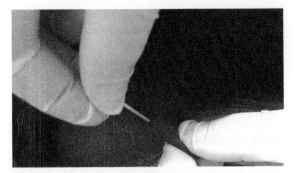

Figure 9.5 A 14-gauge needle used to puncture the skin before catheter insertion.

catheters in adult horses. Conversely, a large gauge needle (14-gauge) can be used to puncture the skin at the site of catheter insertion (Figure 9.5).

Catheter placement

There are many different strategies for successful placement of intravenous catheters (Table 9.1). The first step in catheter placement is to insert the tip of the stylet-catheter combination into a distended vein. Vein distention can be increased by lifting the head (for the jugular vein), increasing the pressure occluding the vein, or increasing the time that the vein is being held off. The tip of the stylet-catheter combination must be advanced far enough into the vein that the catheter can be successfully slid off the stylet.

The most common pitfalls resulting in failure of correct catheter placement include:

- Inadequate distention of the vein.
- Inadequate advancement of the tip of the catheter into the vein before sliding the catheter off the stylet.

Catheter insertion should not be attempted until the vein can be visualized and has been filled to maximal distention. Blind insertion into a poorly filled vein is unlikely to result in success. The location of the catheter-stylet combination within the vein can be confirmed by aspiration of blood using a syringe attached to the top of the stylet. This may be particularly useful in dehydrated patients with poor jugular fill.

Catheter maintenance

Securing the catheter

Catheter-associated complications can be related to excessive movement of the catheter at the insertion site and/or movement within the vein. Stabilization of the

Table 9.1 Tips for catheter selection and placement in specific situations.

Specific situations	Suggestions
Miniature horses	• Using over-the-wire catheters may make catheter placement easier • Polyurethane or silicon catheters are particularly helpful to prevent catheter kinking in small breeds of horse • Wrapping catheters is particularly helpful in these breeds
Severely dehydrated horses	• Lifting the head to allow venous filling will make visualization of the vein easier • Encouraging relaxation of the head and neck will also allow for easier catheter placement • If a standard over-the-stylet catheter cannot be placed, use of an over-the-wire catheter may be helpful
Foals	• Using over-the-wire catheters made of polyurethane or silicone may be easier to place and maintain • Wrapping catheters is important in these patients
Cephalic catheters	• An assistant with sterile gauze can apply pressure whenever possible during the placement of over-the-wire catheters as this will minimize hematoma formation • Wrapping catheters is important for these catheters
Lateral thoracic catheters	• Ultrasound guidance can be helpful if the vein cannot be clearly visualized
Over-the-wire placement in full-size adult horses	• Placement of a 14-gauge needle within the vein, passage of a guidewire, removal of the needle, and passage of an over-the-wire catheter can eliminate the use of a dilator, saving time and cost • Catheter wraps are often not required for these catheters

catheter with skin sutures will minimize movement. Quickset adherent glues are sometimes used for catheter stabilization, but are not recommended to be used alone for a catheter that will be in place for longer than 24–48 hours. Normal exfoliation of skin over this time period can loosen the glue's adherence of the catheter to the skin (Spurlock & Spurlock, 1990). Securing the infusion set to the halter or braided mane during fluid administration can also minimize movement and tension on the catheter, and will help to prevent kinking of the catheter (Hay, 1992).

Flushing the catheter

In order to prevent clotting of blood within the catheter and formation of a thrombus at the catheter tip, frequent flushing of the catheter is recommended. For jugular catheters flushing every 6–8 hours is usually sufficient (Hay, 1992). However, catheters placed in hypercoagulable patients may require more frequent flushing. In cephalic and lateral thoracic catheters, flushing every 4 hours may be necessary. Blood is more likely to pool in these catheters due to their directionality (against the pull of gravity), making them more prone to clotting. Saline (0.9%) should be heparinized to a concentration of 10 IU heparin/mL saline to be used as the flush solution (Hay, 1992). Preservative-free saline should be used in neonatal foals, as the preservative benzyl alcohol has been associated with morbidity and mortality in human neonatal infants in the 1980s

(Hay, 1992). Illness in infants occurred between several days and a few week of age, and was characterized by metabolic acidosis, neurologic signs (seizures), hypotension, and progression to respiratory distress. This has been referred to as "gasping syndrome" and was found to be due to the fact that the detoxification process in affected neonates is too immature to detoxify and eliminate benzyl alcohol and its metabolites. Heparinized saline appropriate for use in neonatal foals can be made by adding 5000 IU of heparin to a 500-mL bag of preservative-free 0.9% saline. In humans, flush solutions without heparin have been used for venous catheters, and these may be appropriate for horses as well (Alexander, 2010). A number of studies showed that normal saline is just as effective as or more efficacious than heparin for venous catheters (Alexander, 2010). Research evaluating non-heparinized flush solutions in horses is not available.

Catheter complications

Foals, horses with systemic inflammatory response syndrome (SIRS), and immunocompromised horses are predisposed to catheter-related complications (Ettlinger et al., 1992; Spurlock & Spurlock, 1990; Tan et al., 2003). For example, thrombophlebitis is significantly more likely to occur in patients with fevers, diarrhea, or leukopenia (Geraghty et al., 2009; Traub-Dargatz &

Dargatz, 1994). Critically ill patients, especially those with gastrointestinal disease, may have loss of endogenous anticoagulants (i.e., antithrombin) into the bowel. Systemic activation of procoagulants, predisposing to thrombus formation, may also be present because of upregulation of tissue factor and loss of endogenous anticoagulants (Divers, 2003). Patients with difficult behavior or those with intractable pain are also at increased risk of catheter problems due to potentially traumatic or non-sterile catheter placement (Divers, 2003; Tan et al., 2003). Critically ill patients also frequently stand with their heads lowered, promoting increased vascular turbulence and stasis of blood flow in the jugular veins. Administration of non-steroidal anti-inflammatory drugs (NSAIDs) while the catheter is in place has been shown to reduce the risk of catheter complications (Geraghty et al., 2009).

To minimize the potential for catheter-associated complications, it is important to examine both the catheter insertion site and the distal vein at the location of the catheter tip at least twice daily. These are the most common sites for initiation of thrombus formation. These sites should be examined for signs of perivascular swelling, heat, pain on palpation, exudate, firmness, "ropiness", or lack of vascular fill of the distal catheterized vein (Divers, 2003; Gardner & Donawick, 1992; Gardner et al., 1991; Traub-Dargatz & Dargatz, 1994). If any of these clinical signs occur, or if the patient develops fevers of unknown origin, nucleated cell count changes (complete blood count), or hyperfibrinogenemia of unknown origin, it is prudent to remove the catheter immediately (Gardner & Donawick, 1992; Gardner et al., 1991). Culture and sensitivity submission of the catheter tip or of purulent discharge from the insertion site should be performed to determine the appropriate antimicrobial regime. If intravenous access is still clinically indicated for the patient, an alternative vein should be selected for placement of the replacement catheter (Dallap & Orsini, 2008; Divers, 2003; Ettlinger et al., 1992; Tan et al., 2003). No further venepuncture should be performed at any level of the affected vessel.

Clinical evidence of thrombophlebitis might not become apparent until 24 to 48 hours after removal of the catheter, so continued examination of the catheter insertion site and vein is indicated even after removal of the catheter (Lankveld et al., 2001). Development of thrombophlebitis has been associated with increased time of indwelling catheterization (Lankveld et al.,

2001; Traug-Dargatz & Dargatz, 1994). Catheters in place for less than 10 days have been shown to be most likely colonized with bacterial organisms along the external surface of the catheter (Cicalini et al., 2004). Conversely, longer-dwelling catheters (>10 days) are more likely infected via endoluminal spread of bacteria from the hub (Cicalini et al., 2004). Newer inventions of antimicrobial-impregnated catheters might be beneficial in preventing this endoluminal bacterial colonization in longer-dwelling catheters (Cicalini et al., 2004).

Thrombophlebitis

Thrombophlebitis may develop secondary to formation of a fibrin sleeve surrounding the catheter, or where the catheter contacts and irritates the intima of the vein or a venous valve (Marino, 2007). Non-septic thrombophlebitis can occur from irritation of the vascular endothelium due to infusion of hypertonic medications or from infusion of fluids under pressure (Hay, 1992; Marino, 2007). Septic thrombophlebitis can occur from bacterial contamination of the catheter during insertion, migration of skin flora along the catheter, bacterial contamination of injected medications or fluids, or hematogenous spread from a focus of infection elsewhere in the body (Gardner et al., 1991). Use of non-sterile intravenous fluids also predisposes an animal to development of thrombophlebitis (Traub-Dargatz & Dargatz, 1994).

Clinical signs

Significant thrombophlebitis of the jugular vein will lead to venous distention of the superficial vasculature of the head on the affected side. Facial edema and oral and nasal edema secondary to decreased venous drainage from the head can lead to respiratory distress and dysphagia with the potential need for a tracheostomy (Gardner & Donawick, 1992; Hay, 1992; Tan et al., 2003). Other clinical signs include fever, perivenous edema, and neck pain leading to stiffness and a reluctance to flex the neck; in some cases purulent or serous discharge from the insertion site may be present. Jugular vein thrombosis can extend to involve the external maxillary vein and the linguofacial vein cranially, or extend down to the thoracic inlet caudally (Gardner et al., 1991). Partial or mild thrombophlebitis can remain subclinical and only detectable with ultrasonographic evaluation.

Additional complications that have been reported secondarily to jugular vein thrombophlebitis include endocarditis, pulmonary thromboembolism, and infarctive pleuropneumonia (Gardner & Donawick, 1992; Tan et al., 2003). Limb edema and cellulitis can be seen with thrombophlebitis of the cephalic vein. Thrombosed veins can potentially recanalize allowing patent blood flow again. Alternatively, they may remain either partially or completely occluded as the thrombus is replaced with fibrosis. In these cases, collateral circulation will be needed to compensate for decreased venous drainage from the affected area (Gardner & Donawick, 1992; Tan et al., 2003).

Diagnosis

Diagnosis of thrombophlebitis can be subjectively made through clinical assessment of the affected vein. Fever and perivenous edema are often present. Sequential ultrasound is a useful diagnostic tool in evaluation of veins with thrombophlebitis or local cellulitis (Figure 9.6). Ultrasound examination can aid in both initial evaluation (diagnosis and prognosis) and for monitoring progression of the thrombus (Gardner & Donawick, 1992). The degree of blood flow can also be assessed. Ultrasound of the jugular vein is performed with a high-frequency ultrasound transducer, such as a 7.5 MHz or 10 MHz transducer, using a shallow depth and focal point for evaluation of the superficial vasculature. Holding off the jugular vein at the thoracic inlet will distend the vein cranially, allowing better visualization and evaluation of the jugular vein lumen. The vein should be evaluated in both short- and long-axis planes (Gardner et al., 1991).

Aseptic thrombi are identified with ultrasound as a mass with an often homogenous echogenic appearance within the vessel lumen. Septic thrombi are often more heterogenous in appearance. There may be areas of decreased echogenicity consistent with fluid pockets and necrosis. Hyperechogenicity can also be observed if gas accumulation is present within the thrombus (Gardner & Donawick, 1992; Gardner et al., 1991; Geraghty et al., 2009). Clinical signs of pain on palpation, heat, and swelling have been significantly associated with identification by ultrasound of cavitating lesions within the thrombus suggestive of septic foci (Gardner et al., 1991).

Venous ultrasound can be used for guided aspiration of fluid-filled pockets within the thrombus for bacterial culture and susceptibility testing (Gardner & Donawick, 1992; Gardner et al., 1991). Purulent or serosanguineous

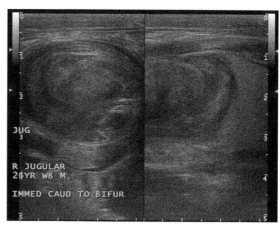

Figure 9.6 Ultrasound image of a thrombosed jugular vein. Picture courtesy of Dr Mary Beth Whitcomb.

fluid collected from cavitating lesions within these thrombi reportedly yields 55% aerobic and 8% anaerobic microorganisms (Gardner et al., 1991).

Horses at high risk of developing catheter complications can have repeated venous ultrasound evaluations to identify signs of subclinical complications such as vessel wall thickening or early thrombus formation. This technique may allow for early removal of the catheter and treatment of the vein (Geraghty et al., 2009). Ultrasound can be used for evaluation of blood flow versus blood stasis.

In order to identify and properly treat the causative bacterial organisms, bacterial culture of the catheter and/or any purulent drainage from the insertion site is indicated. To collect the catheter for culture, the skin surrounding the insertion site should be prepped aseptically with either povidone iodine or chlorhexidine, followed with alcohol, to remove potential skin contaminants. The catheter should then be removed using sterile technique and the tip of the catheter cut with sterile scissors and dropped into a sterile blood tube without anticoagulant (i.e., red top tube) or alternatively into bacterial transport medium (Ettlinger et al., 1992). This sample should be submitted for both aerobic and anaerobic bacterial culture and sensitivity. Using this technique, bacterial organisms reportedly have been isolated from catheters in up to 57% of clinical cases, with neonatal foals having the highest frequency of culture-positive catheters (Ettlinger et al., 1992). It was also found that adult horses with more severe disease, including colic and diarrhea, had increased rates of culture-positive catheters, either due to depressed immune function or due to more intensive and prolonged intravenous medical and fluid therapy (Ettlinger et al., 1992).

Bacterial microorganisms that have been associated with septic thrombophlebitis and cultured from infected catheters include aerobic skin flora such as *Staphylococcus aureus*, *Enterobacter* spp., *Streptococcus equi* ssp. *zooepidemicus*, α-hemolytic *Streptococcus* spp., *Actinobacillus*, *Klebsiella*, *Escherichia coli*, *Pseudomonas*, and *Corynebacterium* spp. (Ettlinger et al., 1992; Gardner et al., 1991; Geraghty et al., 2009; Lankveld et al., 2001; Spurlock et al., 1990; Tan et al., 2003). Anaerobic bacteria that have reportedly been cultured from septic thrombi include *Peptostreptococcus* spp. and *Fusobacterium necrophorum* (Gardner et al., 1991). Many bacteria isolated from septic thrombi and infected catheters are highly resistant or multi-drug resistant (Gardner et al., 1991). Bacterial colonization of catheters is common, but septicemia or positive blood cultures are rare (Tan et al., 2003).

Septic thrombi may not yield a positive bacterial culture due to concurrent antimicrobial administration for the underlying disease or a delay in processing collected samples. Lack of a positive culture should not rule out bacterial infection of the thrombus and the need for ongoing antimicrobial therapy (Gardner et al., 1991).

Treatment

Treatment for local cellulitis and phlebitis should include local therapy consisting of warm compress application, topical dimethyl sulfoxide, topical antimicrobial dressing, and topical diclofenac cream. Systemic antimicrobial administration is indicated if thrombophlebitis is severe or there are clinical or ultrasonographic indications of a septic thrombus or abscess. The presence of associated fevers or signs of a systemic inflammatory response may also indicate a need for antimicrobial therapy. Antimicrobial selection should be based on culture and susceptibility testing. While awaiting bacterial culture results, initial antimicrobial therapy should be broad spectrum and also include activity against staphylococcal species, as these are among the most common bacteria isolated from infections at the venepuncture site. Initial antibiotic choices include cephalosporins, penicillin/aminoglycoside combinations, chloramphenicol, and trimethoprim sulfamethoxazole (Divers, 2003). Human health hazards associated with chloramphenicol should be discussed and preventative measures, including not crushing tablets and wearing gloves when handling the pills, should be taken. Enrofloxacin can also be used; however, *in vitro* susceptibility does not necessarily correlate well with *in vivo* efficacy in the case of staphylococci, and one of the disadvantages of fluoroquinolones is that acquired resistance through genetic mutations may develop during therapy. Therefore, fluoroquinolones should not be used as monotherapy for serious staphylococcal infections.

For septic thrombi that do not respond to medical management or that are causing septicemia or other significant secondary complications, surgical resection of the affected vein may be indicated (Gardner & Donawick, 1992). Reconstruction of the jugular vein using a saphenous vein autograft has been reported (Rijkenhuizen & van Swieten, 1998).

Aspirin or systemic heparin administration can be used to prevent worsening of the thrombus by decreasing platelet aggregation and further activation of the coagulation cascade (Divers, 2003; Geraghty et al., 2009). Aspirin has been shown to prevent platelet aggregation in horses (Cambridge et al., 1991). However, the efficacy of aspirin to prevent thromboembolism in horses is controversial. Use of subcutaneous low molecular weight heparin (LMWH) is preferable to unfractionated heparin, as it is safer and more dependable in its effects (Feige et al., 2003). Heparin has both preventative and curative effects on vascular thrombosis as well as anti-inflammatory properties. Enoxaparin at a dose of 40 IU/kg or dalteparin at a dose of 50 IU/kg subcutaneously once a day is recommended (de la Rebiere de Pouyade et al., 2009; Schwarzwald et al., 2002). A study comparing unfractionated heparin with dalteparin in horses with colic found that there were significantly more jugular vein changes in horses treated with unfractionated heparin, including partial thrombosis of the jugular vein or thickening of the jugular vein wall found on ultrasound (Feige et al., 2003). These effects were significant in the surgical group only, in which dalteparin was started within 16 h postoperatively. Thrombophlebitis and thrombosis with complete occlusion of the vein did not occur in any of the horses. In addition, the packed cell volume (PCV) decreased significantly in the unfractionated heparin group, whereas it did not in the dalteparin group. Clotting times were prolonged in the unfractionated group, but not in the horses treated with LMWH (Feige et al., 2003). NSAID use may also be beneficial by reducing platelet production of thromboxane A2 (Geraghty et al., 2009).

Catheter breakage

In order to minimize the chance of catheter breakage and potential catheter embolization, frequent monitoring of the catheter for kinking at the insertion site or patient-induced trauma to the catheter is critical. When placing an over-the-stylet catheter, avoid reintroduction of the stylet into the catheter while it is in the vein. The end of the stylet can cut the catheter leading to fragmentation.

If a catheter breaks off in the vein or is inadvertently cut during removal, pressure should be applied to the distal vein to prevent migration of the catheter into the thoracic cavity. If the catheter is lost into the vascular system, thoracic radiographs, ultrasound, or fluoroscopy have been described for locating the broken catheter piece (Dallap & Orsini, 2008). In adult horses, the catheter fragment usually passes through the heart and lodges in the pulmonary vasculature, usually not causing a clinically significant problem. In neonatal foals and miniature horses or ponies, the catheter often is too large to pass through the heart and lodges in the right side of the heart. This can cause cardiac arrhythmias, sepsis, pulmonary embolism, endocarditis, or cardiac wall perforation (Ames et al., 1991; Divers, 2008; Hoskinson et al., 1991). Therefore in foals or miniature horses and ponies, or adult horses where a J wire lodges in the heart, removal of the catheter fragment or wire should be attempted (Divers, 2008).

In both horses and humans, there appears to be lower morbidity and mortality if the fragment lodges in the great veins and virtually no clinically significant complications associated with catheter fragments lodging in the peripheral lung (Ames et al., 1991). There are reports of both surgical and non-surgical removal of catheter fragments in foals and horses. If the fragment lodges in the heart, non-surgical removal can be attempted via a percutaneous, transvenous retrieval technique using a basket retrieval catheter or a retrieval snare and a small jugular phlebotomy to remove the catheter fragment (Ames et al., 1991; Hoskinson et al., 1991). Fluoroscopic guidance is recommended for this procedure, but can potentially be accomplished with ultrasound guidance if the fragment is located in the

heart (Ames et al., 1991; Hoskinson et al., 1991). A report described removal of a retained metal guidewire from the jugular vein that was lost during placement of an indwelling catheter (Nannarone et al., 2012). The retained wire was removed under standing sedation (romifidine) by percutaneous fluoroscopically assisted endovascular retrieval, using a four-pronged retrieval catheter. Another report describes removal of catheter fragments within the jugular vein and subcutaneous tissues in a 4-month-old filly after an IV catheter broke at the hub (Culp et al., 2008). Under anesthesia, an 11-F vascular access sheath was placed in the jugular vein and an 8-F guiding catheter was introduced into the sheath, followed by an endovascular snare through the catheter. Fluoroscopy was used, and the catheter pieces were removed using the loop of the snare (Culp et al., 2008). Complications in horses and humans reportedly associated with this procedure have included induction of cardiac arrhythmias, which are usually transient, and further fragmentation and embolization of the catheter fragments (Ames et al., 1991; Hoskinson et al., 1991).

Perivascular leakage

With cracking or kinking of the catheter at the insertion site, subcutaneous or perivascular leakage of the administered fluids or medications can occur. With isotonic fluids, this is usually not a significant problem and the fluids will be resorbed from the subcutaneous space. If the medication is an irritating solution or the fluids contain any irritating additives, clinical signs of pain, swelling, cellulitis, and vessel or subcutaneous necrosis may occur. Horner syndrome may be present if the perivascular leakage affects the nerves of the eye and face. The most irritating substances are those with either a high or low pH. Treatment recommendations for perivascular leakage of irritating substances include stopping the infusion and removing the damaged catheter. In addition, warm compress application, subcutaneous infiltration of the area with physiological saline, and ventral drainage and flushing may be indicated (Divers, 2008).

Venous air embolism

Air can be aspirated into the vein during catheter placement or if the infusion set or cap becomes detached from the catheter while indwelling. Air can travel down an open jugular catheter due to negative pressure created in the chest during inspiration when the head is above the level of the heart (Bradbury et al., 2005). Small air emboli are usually well tolerated clinically. Large air emboli can cause respiratory distress and non-cardiogenic pulmonary edema. Additionally, central nervous system signs such as ataxia, vestibular signs, intense pruritus, extreme agitation, and central blindness due to cerebral air embolism can be present (Bradbury et al., 2005; Holbrook et al., 2007; Tan et al., 2003).

Pulmonary edema develops as a result of acute inflammation and increased vascular permeability secondary to air in the pulmonary microvasculature. Impeded blood flow into the right atrium and pulmonary artery leading to secondary hypoxemia and systemic hypotension may also contribute to pulmonary edema (Bradbury et al., 2005; Holbrook et al., 2007).

Once the pulmonary vasculature is saturated with air, an air embolus can cross the pulmonary circulation into the systemic circulation and potentially lead to a cerebral air embolism (Bradbury et al., 2005). Recommended treatments include capping or removal of the catheter and providing nasal oxygen insufflation. Increasing the oxygen tension in the blood (P_aO_2) provides an oxygen diffusion gradient forcing oxygen into and nitrogen out of the bubbles of air of the air embolus, reducing the size of the bubbles. The administration of flunixin meglumine, furosemide, bronchodilators, dimethyl sulfoxide (DMSO), thiamine, corticosteroids, and treatment in a hyperbaric oxygen chamber may be beneficial (Bradbury et al., 2005; Holbrook et al., 2007). With time and treatment, the adverse symptoms associated with an air embolism can improve and the horse can become clinically normal (Holbrook et al., 2007).

Exsanguination

Exsanguination from a disconnected infusion port is a very rare occurrence and more likely when an underlying hemostatic disorder is present (Tan et al., 2003). Small patients, especially neonatal foals, may be at greater risk for substantial blood loss should disconnection occur. If a catheter becomes dislodged and the horse is bleeding from the insertion site, pressure should be applied to the site until bleeding stops. If large volumes of blood have been lost, intravenous fluid administration with isotonic crystalloids may be warranted. In severe cases, administration of whole blood may be required.

References

Alexander H. (2010) Heparin versus normal saline as a flush solution. *Int J Adv Sci Arts* **1**:63–75.

Ames TR, Hunter DW, Caywood DD. (1991) Percutaneous transvenous removal of a broken jugular catheter from the right ventricle of a foal. *Equine Vet J* **23**:392–3.

Bradbury LA, Archer DC, Dugdale AH, et al. (2005) Suspected venous air embolism in a horse. *Vet Rec* **156**:109–11.

Cambridge H, Lees P, Hooke RE, et al. (1991) Antithrombotic actions of aspirin in the horse. *Eq Vet J* **23**:123–7.

Cicalini S, Palmieri F, Petrosillo N. (2004) Clinical review: new technologies for prevention of intravascular catheter-related infections. *Crit Care* **8**:157–62.

Culp WTN, Weisse C, Berent AC, et al. (2008) Percutaneous endovascular retrieval of an intravascular foreign body in five dogs, a goat, and a horse. *J Am Vet Med Assoc* **232**: 1850–6.

Dallap Schaer B, Orsini JA. (2008) Intravenous catheter placement. In: Orsini JA, Divers TJ (eds) *Equine Emergencies: Treatment and Procedures.* St Louis: Saunders Elsevier, pp. 11–13.

Davie IT. (1977) Specific drug interactions in anaesthesia. *Anaesthesia* **32**:1000–8.

de la Rebiere de Pouyade G, Grulke S, Detilleus J, et al. (2009) Evaluation of low-molecular-weight heparin for the prevention of equine laminitis after colic surgery. *J Vet Emerg Crit Care* **19**:113–19.

Divers TJ. (2003) Prevention and treatment of thrombosis, phlebitis, and laminitis in horses with gastrointestinal diseases. *Vet Clin North Am Equine Pract* **19**:779–90.

Divers TJ. (2008) Adverse drug reactions. In: Orsini JA, Divers TJ (eds) *Equine Emergencies: Treatment and Procedures.* St Louis: Saunders Elsevier, pp. 781–5.

Epstein KL, Brainard BM, Gomez-Ibanez SE, et al. (2011) Thrombelastography in horses with acute gastrointestinal disease. *J Vet Intern Med* **25**:307–14.

Ettlinger JJ, Palmer JE, Benson C. (1992) Bacteria found on intravenous catheters removed from horses. *Vet Rec* **130**: 248–9.

Feige K, Schwarzwald CC, Bobeli, TH. (2003) Comparison of unfractioned and low molecular weight heparin for prophylaxis of coagulopathies in 52 horses with colic: a randomised double-blind clinical trial. *Eq Vet J* **35**:506–13.

Gardner SV, Donawick WJ. (1992) Jugular vein thrombophlebitis. In: Robinson NE (ed.) *Current Therapy in Equine Medicine* 3. Philadelphia: Saunders, pp. 406–8.

Gardner SY, Reef VB, Spencer PA. (1991) Ultrasonographic evaluation of horses with thrombophlebitis of the jugular vein: 46 cases (1985–1988). *J Am Vet Med Assoc* **199**:370–3.

Geraghty TE, Love S, Taylor DJ, et al. (2009) Assessment of subclinical venous catheter-related diseases in horses and associated risk factors. *Vet Rec* **164**:227–31.

Gulick BA, Meagher DM. (1981) Evaluation of an intravenous catheter for use in the horse. *J Am Vet Med Assoc* **178**:272–3.

Hague BA, Honnas CM, Simpson RB, et al. (1997) Evaluation of skin bacterial flora before and after aseptic preparation of clipped and nonclipped arthrocentesis sites in horses. *Vet Surg* **26**:121–5.

Hay CW. (1992) Equine intravenous catheterization. *Equine Vet Edu* **4**:319–23.

Holbrook TC, Dechant JE, Crowson CL. (2007) Suspected air embolism associated with post-anesthetic pulmonary edema and neurologic sequelae in a horse. *Vet Anaesth Analg* **34**:217–22.

Hoskinson JJ, Wooten P, Evans R. (1991) Nonsurgical removal of a catheter embolus from the heart of a foal. *J Am Vet Med Assoc* **199**:233–5.

Klein DG. (1984) The multilumen central venous catheter. *J Burn Care Rehabil* **5**:236–8.

Lankveld DP, Ensink JM, van Dinjk P, et al. (2001) Factors influencing the occurrence of thrombophlebitis after post-surgical long-term intravenous catheterization of colic horses: a study of 38 cases. *J Vet Med A Physiol Pathol Clin Med* **48**:545–52.

Maki DG, Ringer M. (1987) Evaluation of dressing regimens for prevention of infection with peripheral intravenous catheters: gauze, a transparent polyurethane dressing, and an iodophor-transparent dressing. *J Am Med Assoc* **258**:2396–403.

Maki DG, Ringer M. (1991) Risk factors for infusion-related phlebitis with small peripheral venous catheters: a randomized controlled trial. *Ann Intern Med* **114**:845–54.

Marino PL. (2007) Vascular access. In: Marino PL (ed.) *The ICU Book*. Philadelphia: Lippincott, Williams, & Wilkins, pp. 107–48.

Nannarone S, Falchero V, Gialletti R, et al. (2012) Successful removal of a guidewire from the jugular vein of a mature horse. *Eq Vet Educ* **25**:173–6.

Nolen-Waltson RD. (2012) Flow rates of large animal fluid delivery systems used for high-volume crystalloid resuscitation. *J Vet Emerg Crit Care* **22**:661–5.

Rijkenhuizen AB, van Swieten HA. (1998) Reconstruction of the jugular vein in horses with post thrombophlebitis stenosis using saphenous vein graft. *Equine Vet J* **30**:236–9.

Schwarzwald CC, Feige K, Wunderli-Allenspach H, et al. (2002) Comparison of pharmacokinetic variables for two low-molecular-weight heparins after subcutaneous administration of a single dose to horses. *Am J Vet Res* **63**:868–73.

Spurlock SL, Spurlock GH. (1990) Risk factors of catheter-related complications. *Comp Cont Educ Prac Vet* **12**:241–8.

Spurlock SL, Spurlock GH, Parker G, et al. (1990) Long-term jugular vein catheterization in horses. *J Am Vet Med Assoc* **196**:425–30.

Southwood LL, Baxter GM. (1996) Instrument sterilization, skin preparation, and wound management. *Vet Clin North Am Equine Pract* **12**:173–94.

Stefano JL, Norman ME, Morales MC, et al. (1993) Decreased erythrocyte Na+,K(+)-ATPase activity associated with cellular potassium loss in extremely low birth weight infants with nonoliguric hyperkalemia. *J Pediatr* **122**:276–84.

Tan RH, Dart AJ, Dowling BA. (2003) Catheters: a review of the selection, utilisation and complications of catheters for peripheral venous access. *Aust Vet J* **81**:136–9.

Traub-Dargatz JL, Dargatz DA. (1994) A retrospective study of vein thrombosis in horses treated with intravenous fluids in a veterinary teaching hospital. *J Vet Intern Med* **8**:264–6.

Zubrod CJ, Farnsworth KD, Oaks JL. (2004) Evaluation of arthrocentesis site bacterial flora before and after 4 methods of preparation in horses with and without evidence of skin contamination. *Vet Surg* **33**:525–30.

CHAPTER 10

Monitoring fluid therapy

Brett Tennent-Brown

Senior Lecture in Equine Medicine, Faculty of Veterinary Science, University of Melbourne, Australia

Fluids are most often administered to horses in an effort to restore tissue perfusion and oxygen delivery and often in emergency situations. However, fluids might also be administered to provide diuresis, correct electrolyte abnormalities, or to meet the maintenance requirements of horses that are either unable or unwilling to drink. Plasma-based products and synthetic colloids are not uncommonly administered to increase or maintain oncotic pressure in horses with protein loss. Fluid therapy plans in equine medicine are, by their nature, only an estimation of a patient's requirements, and fluid administration should be considered a dynamic process. Once a plan has been devised, the patient should be repeatedly monitored to ensure that the appropriate therapeutic goals are achieved. Overhydration is a real concern in equine neonates, particularly those with low oncotic pressure or increased vascular permeability. Under-resuscitation is generally of more concern than over-resuscitation in adult horses. However, excessive fluid administration is, at the very least, an unnecessary expense for owners and potentially detrimental to adult patients.

Fluid therapy should be guided by parameters that reflect the initial aims of the fluid plan. In most cases, these will be indices that reflect the adequacy of tissue and organ perfusion. However, they might also be specific electrolyte concentrations or a measure of oncotic pressure. Monitoring begins with careful clinical assessment; results from laboratory tests and monitoring equipment provide additional information that enable quantification of clinical findings. Not all monitoring techniques will be appropriate for all patients; the selection of a particular technique should be based on reliability, expense, practicality, and the value of information gained from its use. Measurements should be performed at frequent intervals as trends are generally more informative than values obtained at a single time point or infrequent measurements. The frequency with which a particular parameter is measured will depend on the stability of the patient, ease of the monitoring technique to perform, expected rate of change of a monitored variable, and the cost of each measurement. It is important to recognize that most of the monitoring techniques available to veterinarians (and human physicians) only assess global circulation and might provide only limited information on the microperfusion of individual tissue beds.

Physical examination findings

The clinical signs traditionally used to assess a patient's fluid deficit evaluate aspects of both hypovolemia and dehydration (Table 10.1) but provide only a crude estimate of fluid status (Nolen-Walston et al., 2010; Pritchard et al., 2006, 2008). However, assessment of mucous membrane character, capillary refill time, eye position, jugular fill, skin-tent duration, pulse character, extremity temperature, and heart rate furnish a practical starting point in developing a fluid plan (Table 10.1). Although one must take into account the influence of the underlying disease, serial measurement of these clinical signs can be very useful in evaluating the effectiveness of resuscitation efforts.

Equine Fluid Therapy, First Edition. Edited by C. Langdon Fielding and K. Gary Magdesian.

Table 10.1 Summary of clinical signs associated with hypovolemia and dehydration in adult horses. Note that not all signs are consistently present in all horses.

Degree	Dehydration (%)	Mucous membranes	Capillary refill time (s)	Heart rate (/min)	Other clinical signs
Mild	5–8	Normal to slightly tacky	Normal (<2)	Normal	Decreased urine production
Moderate	8–10	Tacky	Variable (often 2–3)	40–60	Decreased arterial blood pressure
Severe	10–12	Dry	Variable (often prolonged >4)	>60	Jugular fill slow; peripheral pulses weak; sunken eyes

Body weight

Unfortunately the normal or baseline body weight is rarely known with any accuracy in horses presented in an emergent situation. In addition, changes in gut fill can have a substantial effect on body weight. Despite these limitations, once or twice daily measurement of body weight can provide a useful estimate of fluid balance (and nutritional status) in hospitalized horses, particularly neonates, especially when performed serially. Sudden increases in body weight might indicate fluid retention – 1 L of fluid weighs approximately 1 kg (2.2 lb).

Laboratory results

Packed cell volume and total solids concentration

The measurement of packed cell volume (PCV) and total solids (TS) concentration is simple, quick, and inexpensive. In addition, a number of studies have shown that PCV has utility as a prognostic indicator, with higher values associated with a poorer prognosis (Proudman et al., 2005a,2005b). The microhematocrit method is the most accurate technique for measuring PCV, and good-quality refractometers provide a reliable measure of TS concentration. However, these variables are not always as useful in directing fluid therapy in horses as they are in other species (Nolen-Walston et al., 2010). In adult horses there is great individual variation in PCV, and PCV is often increased in distressed or excited animals as a result of splenic contraction. The presence of anemia will obscure the increase in PCV expected with hypovolemia (Pritchard et al., 2008). Similarly, interpretation of TS concentration can be misleading as many horses that require fluid resuscitation also experience protein loss. Nevertheless, an increase in both PCV and TS (or total protein or albumin) concentration is consistent with a loss of plasma volume. Serial measurement of PCV and TS concentration is the most informative and a decrease in these variables toward normal is expected with appropriate resuscitation.

Blood lactate concentration

A decrease in tissue perfusion and oxygen delivery (Do_2) with subsequent anaerobic metabolism is the most important cause of hyperlactatemia in large animals (Tennent-Brown et al., 2009). However, hyperlactatemia will occasionally occur in the face of apparently adequate Do_2 usually in association with intense systemic inflammation (Gore et al., 1996). Additionally, horses with advanced liver failure might have an increase in blood lactate concentration as a result of impaired metabolism (Chrusch et al., 2000). It is important to recognize that venous lactate concentrations measured in peripheral veins reflect the adequacy of global perfusion (i.e., it represents a global "average"); measured venous lactate concentrations can be normal despite significant perfusion deficits of individual tissue beds.

For clinicians with ready access to veterinary diagnostic laboratories, measurement of lactate concentrations is often performed routinely. Unless samples are collected into tubes containing sodium fluoride, erythrocyte lactate production will continue and can affect measured concentrations in samples stored for longer than 30–60 minutes. For veterinarians without immediate access to a diagnostic laboratory, lactate can be accurately measured using hand-held meters. A number of these machines have been validated for use in horses. It should be noted that some of these meters perform better with plasma than with whole blood samples, which might limit their field utility (Tennent-Brown et al., 2007). The site of blood collection (arterial vs venous, and choice of vein) has some effect on the measured lactate concentration, but these differences are typically irrelevant clinically. A slight increase in lactate concentration can occur with struggling or prolonged occlusion of the vein during sample collection. If blood samples are collected from an intravenous catheter, it is important to ensure than an adequate "waste" volume is removed before sample collection as lactate-containing fluid solutions (e.g., lactated Ringer's solution) may increase the measured lactate concentration. Conversely, fluids that do not contain lactate as a buffer will tend to decrease the measured lactate concentration in inappropriately collected samples. Historically, the anion gap (AG) has been used as an estimate of lactate concentration. However, the anion gap should be interpreted with caution as it can be increased by anions other than lactate (e.g., with azotemia) and is decreased with hypoalbuminemia (Moe & Fuster, 2003). An increase in the anion gap might also be seen with an increase in D-(bacterial) lactate concentration (Ewaschuk et al., 2003).

An increase in blood lactate concentration is strongly suggestive of hypovolemia, and serial lactate measurement is a useful guide for volume resuscitation in equine patients (Hashimoto-Hill et al., 2011; Tennent-Brown et al., 2009). The upper limit of normal for blood lactate concentration in adult horses is often considered to be 1.5 mmol/L but concentrations in euhydrated horses are usually less than 1.0 mmol/L. This is important because the increase in blood lactate concentration in hypovolemic animals can be relatively subtle until hypovolemia becomes severe (Magdesian et al., 2006). Care must be taken when evaluating neonates as the blood lactate concentration in normal newborn foals exceeds that in adults for the first 1–3 days of life (Kitchen & Rossdale, 1975; Magdesian, 2003). However, lactate concentrations above the normal age-interpreted ranges for foals, persistent hyperlactatemia, or a very slow decrease in lactate concentration in a neonatal foal should prompt concerns of a fluid deficit (Corley et al., 2005; Henderson et al., 2008; Wotman et al., 2009).

Increased blood lactate concentrations due to hypovolemia and hypoperfusion are expected to decrease to normal over 6–12 hours with effective restoration of vascular volume and tissue perfusion (Tennent-Brown et al., 2009). Additional monitoring techniques to ensure that volume replacement and D_{O_2} are adequate should be employed if hyperlactatemia persists in the face of apparently appropriate fluid resuscitation. If volume replacement and D_{O_2} are deemed appropriate, one might consider a severe inflammatory process or liver failure as other possible sources of hyperlactatemia, among several other differentials for high lactate concentrations.

Mixed or central venous hemoglobin saturation and oxygen extraction ratios

Venous oxyhemoglobin saturation ($S_{v}O_{2}$) is dependent on arterial oxyhemoglobin saturation ($S_{a}O_{2}$), cardiac output, and tissue oxygen demand. A decrease in cardiac output or an increase in tissue oxygen demand will decrease $S_{v}O_{2}$ as more oxygen is stripped from hemoglobin by the tissues. Venous oxyhemoglobin saturation is decreased in anemic patients (decreased carrying capacity with a subsequent decrease in arterial oxygen content ($C_{a}O_{2}$)) and in patients with significant pulmonary disease (impaired pulmonary gas exchange with a subsequent decrease in $S_{a}O_{2}$). Theoretically, $S_{v}O_{2}$ can be increased (or normal) in patients with mitochondrial dysfunction (i.e., the tissues are unable to utilize oxygen) or with significant shunting (i.e., the oxygen-consuming tissues are bypassed). To accurately assess global perfusion, Svo2 is ideally measured in samples collected from the pulmonary artery (PA). However, the use of information derived from mixed venous (i.e., PA) sampling has not consistently produced significant survival benefits in human studies and there are concerns related to complications associated with PA catheterization (Harvey et al., 2005). As a consequence, this procedure is now less commonly performed.

Measurement of $S_{v}O_{2}$ from a central venous catheter (i.e., placed in either the cranial or caudal vena cava) provides a good approximation of mixed venous values, is easier to perform, and is considered safer (Reinhart et al., 1989). The tip of a standard 20-cm intravenous catheter placed in the jugular vein of equine neonates often lies within the cranial vena cava and so central venous $S_{v}O_{2}$ monitoring could be easily applied to these patients. Central venous $S_{v}O_{2}$ values can also be monitored in horses that have had catheters placed for central venous pressure (CVP) measurement. In the author's experience, $S_{v}O_{2}$ measured in jugular samples (i.e., collected from standard-length catheters in adult horses) does not reliably reflect central venous $S_{v}O_{2}$.

Studies in critically ill human patients have shown that central venous S_vO_2 can be a valuable resuscitation end-point (Rivers et al., 2001). Because primary cardiac disease is relatively rare in equine patients and hypovolemia is the most common cause of decreased cardiac output, monitoring S_vO_2 could be a useful guide to fluid resuscitation. The normal or target central venous S_vO_2 used in the management of critically ill human patients is 70–75% (Rivers et al., 2001). Similar values are probably suitable for equine patients although this has not been assessed. In horses with normal pulmonary function and hemoglobin concentrations, values for S_vO_2 below 70% are suggestive of hypovolemia.

The oxygen extraction ratio (O_2ER) measures the percentage of oxygen removed from the blood as it moves through the tissues. The O_2ER therefore provides similar information to S_vO_2 but requires both mixed-venous (i.e., PA) and arterial samples. Oxygen extraction ratios can be estimated from the arterial and venous oxyhemoglobin saturations or calculated more precisely using the blood oxygen content.

$$\text{Oxygen extraction ratio}\,(\%) = (S_aO_2 - S_vO_2)/S_aO_2 \qquad (10.1)$$

$$\text{Oxygen extraction ratio}\,(\%) = (C_aO_2 - C_vO_2)/C_aO_2 \qquad (10.2)$$

$$\begin{aligned}&\text{Arterial } O_2 \text{ content [mLO}_2\text{/dL]} =\\ &\quad (1.34 \times S_aO_2 \times [\text{Hb}]) + (0.003 \times P_aO_2)\end{aligned} \qquad (10.3)$$

$$\begin{aligned}&\text{Venous } O_2 \text{ content [mLO}_2\text{/dL]} =\\ &\quad (1.34 \times S_vO_2 \times [\text{Hb}]) + (0.003 \times P_vO_2)\end{aligned} \qquad (10.4)$$

where:
[Hb] = hemoglobin concentration (g/dL);
P_aO_2 = arterial partial pressure of O_2 (mmHg);
C_aO_2 = arterial O_2 content (mL O_2/dL);
C_vO_2 = venous O_2 content (mL O_2/dL);
S_aO_2 = arterial O_2 saturation (%);
S_vO_2 = venous O_2 saturation (%).

Measurement of arterial hemoglobin saturation or oxygen content allows estimation of the contribution of pulmonary disease to a decreased S_vO_2. Normal values for O_2ER are 25–30%; a decrease in cardiac output or an increase in tissue oxygen demand increases the O_2ER. The O_2ER will also be increased in anemic patients. In the case of hypovolemia, the O_2ER is expected to be greater than 25–30% and decrease toward normal as volume is restored and cardiac output improved.

Urine output and urine specific gravity

Urine output is a marker of end-organ (i.e., renal) blood flow and, therefore, can be used as an indicator of the adequacy of fluid administration. Qualitative assessment of urine production (i.e., reduced, adequate, or excessive) based on micturition frequency and the subjective volume of urine in the stall is sufficient in many adult horse cases. In recumbent foals, urine production can be semi-quantitatively measured by weighing urine-soaked absorbent pads. Placement of an indwelling urinary catheter is required to accurately measure urine production but should be considered in hemodynamically unstable patients or those predisposed to decreased renal perfusion. Placement and securing of indwelling urinary catheters is relatively straightforward in foals and mares (Magdesian, 2004). Long-term catheterization of geldings and stallions is more difficult; harnesses and external collection devices can be used although their use can be fraught with difficulties. Urine from catheterized animals should be collected into sterile collecting systems and care must be taken to minimize the risk of infection. Urine samples from catheterized patients should be evaluated periodically to check for bacterial infections.

Urine production by adult horses is highly variable and depends on diet, water intake, and ambient conditions. The reported range for urine production by adult horses is 15 to 30 mL/kg/day (or approximately 0.6 to 1.25 mL/kg/h) (Kohn & Strasser, 1986; Rumbaugh et al., 1982) and this is probably a reasonable target for evaluating fluid administration in adult horses. Because healthy nursing foals consume large volumes of milk (approximately 8–10 mL/kg/h), they produce large volumes (approximately 4–8 mL/kg/h) of dilute urine (Brewer et al., 1991). This value for urine production by healthy foals should not be applied to critically ill neonates. Urine production in foals receiving combinations of intravenous fluids, parenteral nutrition, and other medications will be highly variable but should be approximately two-thirds of total fluid inputs if they are meeting requirements. This is a more appropriate guide for directing therapy in sick neonates receiving fluids; urine output less than one-half to two-thirds of total inputs should prompt an investigation into the cause of decreased production. Potential causes of decreased urine production might include hypovolemia or hypotension, anuric or oliguric renal disease, and obstruction of the urinary tract or uroperitoneum in foals.

Reassessment of the fluid rate should be considered if urine production exceeds two-thirds of the volume administered.

Urine specific gravity has been used by some clinicians to assess the adequacy of fluid therapy. In the absence of renal disease, hypovolemia and dehydration should result in concentrated urine (urine specific gravity >1.035). Urine specific gravity should become approximately isosthenuric (1.008 to 1.012) with adequate resuscitation with balanced polyionic fluids. However, disease in critically ill patients (e.g., endotoxemia, cantharidin toxicity) can interfere with antidiuretic hormone (ADH) function and other aspects of renal function confounding interpretation of urine specific gravity measurements (Grinevich et al., 2004; Versteilen et al., 2008). These patients can produce large volumes of dilute urine (specific gravity <1.008) in the face of hypovolemia.

Hemodynamic parameters

Central venous pressure

Central venous pressure (CVP) is the pressure within the intrathoracic portion of the vena cava and reflects the balance between the pumping ability of the heart and venous return. Central venous pressure is determined by: cardiac function; central venous blood volume; and venomotor tone. Measurement of CVP can be used to assess right side cardiac function but in large animal patients, CVP measurements are most often used to assess intravascular volume.

Measurement of CVP in horses requires placement of the tip of a fluid-filled catheter in the cranial vena cava or right atrium. In neonatal foals, the tips of standard 20-cm intravenous catheters often lie within the cranial vena cava. Special catheters (up to 90 cm in length) are commercially available (Mila International, Versailles, KY) for CVP measurement in adult horses but the use of sterile polyethylene or polypropylene tubing passed through a 10- or 14-gauge venous catheter has also been described (Fielding et al., 2004). The CVP catheter is then connected to a water manometer (Mila International, Versailles, KY) for intermittent pressure measurements or to a pressure transducer and suitable monitor for continuous monitoring. Small oscillations in the fluid meniscus (or the pressure reading) synchronized with respiration confirm the intrathoracic location of the catheter tip. Using a

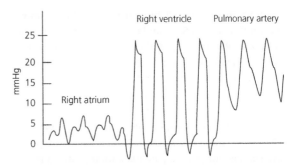

Figure 10.1 The figure shows the expected pressure waveforms and approximate pressure values as the tip of a catheter connected to a pressure transducer and monitor moves from the right atrium (or vena cava) into the right ventricle and then the pulmonary artery. The shape of the waveform and pressure values can be used to determine the location of the catheter tip.

pressure transducer and monitor, the location of the catheter tip can be confirmed by observing the appropriate waveform (Figure 10.1). The location of the catheter tip can also be confirmed using echocardiography (Wilsterman et al., 2009). Confirmation of catheters in neonatal foals can be achieved with portable thoracic radiographs. When using a water manometer, the author passes the catheter into the ventricle (recognized by the systolic pressures of approximately 20–34 cmH$_2$O) and then withdraws the catheter so that the tip lies within the right atrium or cranial vena cava as assessed by the decrease in measured pressures. When a pressure transducer is used, venous pressure tracings demonstrate a-, c-, and v-waves and x- and y-descents (Figure 10.2 and Table 10.2). Simultaneous recording of an electrocardiogram allows for accurate interpretation of the CVP pressure tracing (Figure 10.2).

Measurements of CVP in standing horses are referenced to the right atrium, so the zero mark on a water manometer or the electronic pressure transducer should be placed at the point of the shoulder; it is critical that this positioning is identical between measurements. The water manometer can be taped or fixed to a portable IV pole for consistency among measurements. The horse's head should be held in a neutral position that is constant between measurements and all intravenous infusions should be stopped during CVP measurement. In recumbent horses, CVP measurements should be zeroed to the sternal manubrium.

During spontaneous respiration, CVP is greatest during expiration (positive intrathoracic pressure) and

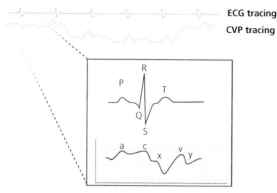

ECG tracing
CVP tracing

Figure 10.2 Central venous pressure (CVP) tracing recorded using a pressure transducer demonstrating a-, c-, and v-waves and x- and y-descents (inset). Simultaneous recording of an electrocardiogram (ECG) allows for accurate interpretation of the CVP tracing. The decrease in CVP shown in the trace is a result of the negative intrathoracic pressure generated during inspiration. The most precise measure of CVP is the mean of the a-wave at end-expiration. Note that water manometers tend to dampen the pressure changes considerably so these small deflections are typically not observed and measurements are consequently less precise.

Table 10.2 The origin of the a-, c-, and v-waves, and x- and y-descents in recordings of right atrial pressures (see Figure 10.1).

Component	Cause
a-wave	Atrial contraction
c-wave	Bulge of tricuspid valve into the atria during ventricular contraction (systole). The c-wave is increased in size with tricuspid insufficiency
x-descent	Reduction in atrial pressure during ventricular contraction and ejection
v-wave	Early atrial filling, while tricuspid valve is closed
y-descent	Rapid flow of blood into ventricle from the atria after tricuspid valve opens

lowest with inspiration (negative intrathoracic pressure). With mechanical ventilation, this relationship is reversed. In either case, CVP should be measured at end-expiration. The most precise measure of CVP is the mean of the a-wave at end-expiration when using an electronic pressure transducer and monitor. Water manometers tend to dampen the pressure changes considerably so that measurements are less precise and they can overestimate CVP by up to 5 cmH$_2$O under some circumstances. Central venous pressures in normal

neonatal foals range from 3 to 12 cmH$_2$O during the first two weeks of life (Thomas et al., 1987). Central venous pressure in healthy standing adult horses measured with a water manometer ranges between 5 and 15 cmH$_2$O (Klein & Sherman, 1977; Magdesian et al., 2006; Wilsterman et al., 2009). Pressures measured in mmHg may be converted to cmH$_2$O by multiplying by 1.36.

Although single measurements have value, trends in CVP over time are usually more informative. Low or negative CVP values are consistent with hypovolemia (or vasodilation); however, a normal CVP does not necessarily indicate euvolemia. Response to a 5–10-L bolus of crystalloid fluids over 10 to 15 minutes can also be useful in assessing vascular volume. No or a minimal increase in CVP with a rapid (<5 min) return to baseline following bolus administration is consistent with hypovolemia. A return of CVP toward baseline more slowly over 15 minutes suggests that blood volume is close to normal. A large initial increase in CVP (>4 cmH$_2$O) and a prolonged (>30 min) return to baseline implies increased venous blood volume (or reduced cardiac compliance or both). An increase in CVP suggests intravascular volume overload but can also occur with right ventricular failure, pericardial or pleural effusion, vasoconstriction, and intra-abdominal hypertension. In addition, CVP can be artifactually increased by catheter occlusion, inadvertent ventricular catheterization, and air bubbles within the manometer or fluid lines.

Blood pressure monitoring

Blood flow rather than pressure is the main determinant of tissue perfusion. However, it is rarely possible to measure flow directly and blood pressure is usually closely correlated to flow except when vessel compliance and resistance are altered (as occurs in many critical care patients). Arterial blood pressure is, therefore, commonly used as an indicator of tissue perfusion in combination with other clinical parameters. Both systolic and diastolic pressures change considerably as the pulse pressure wave moves away from the left ventricle making peripheral measurement of these variables unreliable (Dorman et al., 1998). Mean arterial pressure (MAP) also changes as the pulse pressure wave travels peripherally but the changes are not as dramatic, and peripheral measures of MAP (e.g., using a tail cuff monitor) can provide a reasonable estimate of aortic MAP (Shah & Bedford, 2001). Furthermore, MAP is the more important determinant of organ perfusion and therefore a more relevant measure than either systolic or diastolic blood pressure (Hollenberg et al., 2004).

Direct (invasive) arterial blood pressure measurement with the use of an arterial catheter can provide continuous data with the appropriate monitoring equipment and is more accurate than indirect (non-invasive) blood pressure measurement, particularly in hypovolemic or vasoconstricted patients. However, arterial catheters can be difficult to maintain in large animal patients and arterial thrombosis is a potential concern. Consequently, in large animals blood pressure is most commonly measured indirectly using an inflatable cuff to occlude an artery and some means to detect blood flow (Doppler-based techniques) or vessel wall vibration (oscillometric monitors). Indirect pressure measurements from the middle coccygeal or dorsal metatarsal arteries provide reasonably reliable measures of blood pressure in foals and adult horses (Giguere et al., 2005; Latshaw et al., 1979; Nout et al., 2002; Parry et al., 1984). The width of the internal bladder in the cuff can be important; the ideal width varies with the technique used and whether diastolic, systolic, or mean arterial pressure is measured (Parry et al., 1984). When using oscillometric techniques to measure MAP in adult horses, bladder width should be 20–25% of the circumference of the tail (Latshaw et al., 1979). The ideal bladder width for use in foals is unknown; one study in anesthetized foals found that cuff width had little effect on MAP measurement (Giguere et al., 2005). To improve accuracy, indirect measurements should be repeated until at least three consistent values are obtained. Most automated pressure monitors also measure pulse rate; if the reported rate differs from the actual heart rate, pressure measurements should be interpreted with caution. When performing indirect coccygeal blood pressure measurements in standing horses, pressure readings are typically 15–20 mmHg lower than true systolic blood pressure (referenced to the point of the shoulder). While some clinicians prefer to correct the value for the distance above the right atria, this is optional; the key is to obtain and record readings in a consistent fashion.

The blood pressure at which intervention should occur in hypotensive equine patients is unknown (Table 10.3). There is evidence from human medicine that a MAP of 65 mmHg is sufficient for adequate tissue perfusion and this is probably a reasonable target for adult horses (Bourgoin et al., 2005; LeDoux et al., 2000). A target MAP of 69 mmHg has been suggested for critically ill

Table 10.3 Systolic, diastolic, and mean arterial blood pressure values for normal foals and adult horses.

Method	Systolic (mmHg)	Diastolic (mmHg)	Mean (mmHg)
Direct			
Foals[a]			
12 hours old (mean ± SE)			88 ± 2
14 days old (mean ± SE)			100 ± 3
Adult horses			
Ponies (mean ± SE)[b]	131 ± 5	86 ± 2	110 ± 2
Horses (mean ± SE)[c]	168 ± 6	116 ± 4	133 ± 4
Indirect[d]			
Mean (± SD)	112 ± 17	77 ± 14	89 ± 14
(normal range[e])	(80–144)	(49–105)	

[a] Arterial blood pressure measured directly from the ascending aorta and referenced to the level of the mid-thorax in foals restrained in lateral recumbency (Thomas et al., 1987).
[b] Direct arterial blood pressures measured from the descending aorta and referenced to the point of the shoulder in 12 standing ponies (147 ± 13 kg) (Orr et al., 1975).
[c] Direct arterial blood pressures measured from the right carotid artery and referenced to the point of the shoulder in seven standing adult horses (Steffey et al., 1987).
[d] Indirect arterial blood pressures measured from the coccygeal artery and referenced to the point of the shoulder in 296 conscious adult horses (Parry et al., 1984). Note that presented values are not corrected for bladder width or adjusted for the height of the tail above the heart.
[e] Defined as within the 2.5th and 97.5th percentiles for all horses.

equine neonates (Corley, 2002). Unfortunately, normotension does not ensure normovolemia, and shock (defined as a life-threatening, generalized maldistribution of blood flow resulting in failure to deliver and/or utilize adequate amounts of oxygen) can occur in the absence of hypotension. In addition, some foals appear to perfuse adequately with lower pressures.

Gastric tonometry

Most available monitoring techniques assess global perfusion and may provide very little information about the perfusion of individual tissue beds. Regional perfusion can be inferred from measures of organ injury or function including: cardiac troponin I (cTnI) activity; blood urea nitrogen and creatinine concentrations and urine production; and serum liver enzyme activities. However, most traditional laboratory markers used to monitor end-organ function are relatively insensitive and/or non-specific. Methods to directly gauge individual tissue bed perfusion have concentrated on the splanchnic tissues because the hepatosplanchnic circulation often becomes compromised early in circulatory failure and the stomach is relatively accessible (at least in human patients and foals) (Cerny & Cvachovec, 2000).

Gastric tonometry (and the related technique of sublingual capnography) is based on the principle that tissue partial pressure of CO_2 (Pco_2) rises in conditions associated with poor tissue perfusion (Cerny & Cvachovec, 2000). The gastrointestinal tract is thought to have higher Do_2 requirements than other organs. Gastric mucosa is, therefore, one of the first tissues to demonstrate an increase in Pco_2 (and decrease in pH) when perfusion becomes compromised. Under anaerobic conditions, tissue Pco_2 is increased as a result of hydrogen ion buffering by bicarbonate and is exacerbated by stagnant blood flow and impaired CO_2 washout (Cerny & Cvachovec, 2000). Tissue Pco_2 is, therefore, primarily determined by tissue CO_2 production and regional blood flow but arterial CO_2 content (C_aco_2) also has an effect. Because tissue Pco_2 is influenced by arterial CO_2 content, calculation of ΔPco_2 or the difference between gastric mucosal Pco_2 and arterial Pco_2 might be more accurate (Cerny & Cvachovec, 2000).

Gastric tonometry is a reasonable predictor of outcome in severely ill human patients (Hameed & Cohn, 2003). The ability of ΔPco_2 to guide resuscitation is less clear; however, gastric tonometry has been useful in titrating vasopressor therapy to improve gastric perfusion in some human hospital populations (Lebuffe et al., 2001). The experimental use of gastric tonometry has been reported in foals. The ΔPco_2 value obtained for normal foals after fasting was 0–54 mmHg and is much wider than values obtained from humans (Valverde et al., 2006). Gastric tonometry (and ΔPco_2) has also been used to monitor the effect of vasopressors on gastric blood flow in anesthetized foals but the clinical utility of this technique remains to be determined (Valverde et al., 2006).

Other parameters to monitor during fluid therapy

Laboratory parameters

Electrolyte concentrations should be carefully monitored during fluid therapy of more than a few days duration. Many horses receiving balanced polyionic intravenous fluids that are not supplemented with additional potassium become hypokalemic with prolonged treatment, particularly if they are not eating. Some horses, particularly ill neonates, are unable to tolerate the sodium and chloride loads even when maintenance-type fluids are administered. Both hypernatremia and hyponatremia are possible complications depending on the fluid type used, especially in neonatal foals. Calcium (particularly ionized), phosphorus, and magnesium concentrations should also be monitored in inappetent animals. Hypophosphatemia is a recognized complication of insulin therapy and may occur in animals receiving dextrose infusions for prolonged periods. Blood glucose concentrations should be measured frequently in all animals receiving dextrose infusions or parenteral nutrition. Blood glucose concentrations greater than 160–180 mg/dL are likely to exceed the renal threshold for reabsorption and the subsequent osmotic diuresis could exacerbate fluid and electrolyte imbalances. The measurement of blood glucose concentrations might also have some prognostic value, with prolonged hyperglycemia suggesting a poorer prognosis (Hassel et al., 2009; Hollis et al., 2007, 2008).

Colloid osmotic pressure

Measurement of colloid osmotic pressure (COP) should be considered in hypoproteinemic animals and horses receiving synthetic colloids. Refractometery of total solids concentrations will underestimate increases in COP caused by synthetic colloids. A colloid osmometer determines COP by measuring the pressure created by water movement across a semi-permeable membrane as a result of an oncotic pressure gradient between the reference solution (saline) and a test sample. Estimates of COP can be calculated from serum total protein or albumin and globulin concentrations. While these are reasonably accurate in healthy animals they are less reliable in hospitalized (clinically ill) horses. Reported oncotic pressures for healthy equine neonates and adults range between 21 and 25 mmHg, although healthy neonatal foals have had lower values in some studies (as low as 15 mmHg; mean ± SD of 18.8 ± 1.9 mmHg) (Runk et al., 2000).

Summary

Fluid plans in equine medicine should be regarded as an estimate of a patient's fluid requirements. Optimization of a fluid plan requires selection of appropriate targets

Table 10.4 Summary of recommended resuscitation targets for adult horses.

Parameter	Target	Comment
Lactate (mmol/L)[a]	<1.0–1.5	Expect to see lactate decrease to normal concentrations over 12 to 24 hours
Venous hemoglobin-O_2 saturation (%)	70–75	Requires a venous sample collected from the vena cava (central venous) or pulmonary artery (mixed-venous) for accurate interpretation
O_2 extraction ratio (%)	25–30	Requires simultaneously collected arterial and venous samples. Venous samples should be collected from the vena cava or pulmonary artery
Urine output (mL/kg/h)[b]	0.6–1.25	
Central venous pressure (cmH$_2$O)	5–15	Serial measurements must be performed in an identical manner for accurate interpretation
Mean arterial pressure (mmHg)	65–70	

[a]Healthy newborn foals have higher blood lactate concentrations than adults. A decrease in lactate concentration toward adult values over 24 to 72 hours is expected in euvolemic foals.
[b]Urine production in healthy nursing foals can be as high as 4–8 mL/kg/h. This value should not be used as a resuscitation target in critically ill foals. Urinary output in this group should be approximately two-thirds of all fluid inputs.

followed by careful and frequent monitoring to ensure that those targets are met. Good monitoring begins with a careful clinical examination and the use of various monitoring techniques to quantify examination findings (Table 10.4). The choice of monitoring techniques and frequency with which they are performed will depend on the patient and the technique used; not all monitoring techniques will be appropriate for all patients. Finally, it is important to recognize that most monitoring techniques assess global perfusion, which might not reveal perfusion deficits of individual tissue beds.

References

Bourgoin A, Leone M, Delmas A, Garnier F, Albanese J, Martin C. (2005) Increasing mean arterial pressure in patients with septic shock: effects on oxygen variables and renal function. *Crit Care Med* **33**:780–6.

Brewer BD, Clement SF, Lotz WS, Gronwall R. (1991) Renal clearance, urinary excretion of endogenous substances, and urinary diagnostic indices in healthy neonatal foals. *J Vet Int Med* **5**:28–33.

Cerny V, Cvachovec K. (2000) Gastric tonometry and intramucosal pH – theoretical principles and clinical application. *Physiol Res* **49**:289–97.

Chrusch C, Bands C, Bose D, et al. (2000) Impaired hepatic extraction and increased splanchnic production contribute to lactic acidosis in canine sepsis. *Am J Resp Crit Care Med* **161**:517–26.

Corley KTT. (2002) Monitoring and treating hemodynamic disturbances in critically ill neonatal foals. Part 1: Haemodynamic monitoring. *Equine Vet Educ* **14**:270–9.

Corley KT, Donaldson LL, Furr MO. (2005) Arterial lactate concentration, hospital survival, sepsis and SIRS in critically ill neonatal foals. *Equine Vet J* **37**:53–9.

Dorman T, Breslow MJ, Lipsett PA, et al. (1998) Radial artery pressure monitoring underestimates central arterial pressure during vasopressor therapy in critically ill surgical patients. *Crit Care Med* **26**:1646–9.

Ewaschuk JB, Naylor JM, Zello GA. (2003) Anion gap correlates with serum D- and DL-lactate concentration in diarrheic neonatal calves. *J Vet Int Med* **17**:940–2.

Fielding CL, Balaam JL, Sprayberry KA. (2004) *How to measure central venous pressure in standing adult horses.* In: Proceedings of the American Association of Equine Practitioners Conference, Denver, CO. AAEP, pp. 415–17.

Giguere S, Knowles HA Jr, Valverde A, Bucki E, Young L. (2005) Accuracy of indirect measurement of blood pressure in neonatal foals. *J Vet Int Med* **19**:571–6.

Gore DC, Jahoor F, Hibbert JM, DeMaria EJ. (1996) Lactic acidosis during sepsis is related to increased pyruvate production, not deficits in tissue oxygen availability. *Ann Surg* **224**:97–102.

Grinevich V, Knepper MA, Verbalis J, Reyes I, Aguilera G. (2004) Acute endotoxemia in rats induces down-regulation of V2 vasopressin receptors and aquaporin-2 content in the kidney medulla. *Kidney Int* **65**:54–62.

Hameed SM, Cohn SM. (2003) Gastric tonometry: the role of mucosal pH measurement in the management of trauma. *Chest* **123**(5 Suppl.):475S–481S.

Harvey S, Harrison DA, Singer M, et al. (2005) Assessment of the clinical effectiveness of pulmonary artery catheters in management of patients in intensive care (PAC-Man): a randomised controlled trial. *Lancet* **366**:472–7.

Hashimoto-Hill S, Magdesian KG, Kass PH. (2011) Serial measurement of lactate concentration in horses with acute colitis. *J Vet Int Med* **25**:1414–19.

Hassel DM, Hill AE, Rorabeck RA. (2009) Association between hyperglycemia and survival in 228 horses with acute gastrointestinal disease. *J Vet Int Med* **23**:1261–5.

Henderson IS, Franklin RP, Wilkins PA, Boston RC. (2008) Association of hyperlactatemia with age, diagnosis, and survival in equine neonates. *J Vet Emerg Crit Care* **18**:496–502.

Hollenberg SM, Ahrens TS, Annane D, et al. (2004) Practice parameters for hemodynamic support of sepsis in adult patients: 2004 update. *Crit Care Med* **32**:1928–48.

Hollis AR, Boston RC, Corley KT. (2007) Blood glucose in horses with acute abdominal disease. *J Vet Int Med* **21**:1099–103.

Hollis AR, Furr MO, Magdesian KG, et al. (2008) Blood glucose concentrations in critically ill neonatal foals. *J Vet Int Med* **22**:1223–7.

Kitchen H, Rossdale PD. (1975) Metabolic profiles of newborn foals. *J Reprod Fert Suppl* **23**:705–7.

Klein L, Sherman J. (1977) Effects of preanesthetic medication, anesthesia, and position of recumbency on central venous pressure in horses. *J Am Vet Med Assoc* **170**:216–19.

Kohn CW, Strasser SL. (1986) 24-hour renal clearance and excretion of endogenous substances in the mare. *Am J Vet Res* **47**:1332–7.

Latshaw H, Fessler JF, Whistler SJ, Geddes LA. (1979) Indirect measurement of mean blood pressure in the normotensive and hypotensive horse. *Equine Vet J* **11**:191–4.

Lebuffe G, Robin E, Vallet B. (2001) Gastric tonometry. *Intens Care Med* **27**:317–19.

LeDoux D, Astiz ME, Carpati CM, Rackow EC. (2000) Effects of perfusion pressure on tissue perfusion in septic shock. *Crit Care Med* **28**:2729–32.

Magdesian KG. (2003) Blood lactate levels in neonatal foals: Normal values and temporal effects in the post-partum period. *J Vet Emerg Crit Care* **13**:174.

Magdesian KG. (2004) Monitoring the critically ill equine patient. *Vet Clin N Am-Equine* **20**:11–39.

Magdesian KG, Fielding CL, Rhodes DM, Ruby RE. (2006) Changes in central venous pressure and blood lactate concentration in response to acute blood loss in horses. *J Am Vet Med Assoc* **229**:1458–62.

Moe OW, Fuster D. (2003) Clinical acid-base pathophysiology: disorders of plasma anion gap. *Best Pract Res Clin Endocrinol Metab* **17**:559–74.

Nolen-Walston RD, Norton JL, Navas de Solis C, et al. (2010) The effects of hypohydration on central venous pressure and splenic volume in adult horses. *J Vet Int Med* **25**:570–4.

Nout YS, Corley KTT, Donaldson LL, Furr MO. (2002) Indirect oscillometric and direct blood pressure measurements in anesthetized and conscious neonatal foals. *J Vet Emerg Crit Care* **12**:75–80.

Orr JA, Bisgard GE, Forster HV, Rawlings CA, Buss DD, Will JA. (1975) Cardiopulmonary measurements in nonanesthetized, resting normal ponies. *Am J Vet Res* **36**:1667–70.

Parry BW, McCarthy MA, Anderson GA. (1984) Survey of resting blood pressure values in clinically normal horses. *Equine Vet J* **16**:53–8.

Pritchard JC, Barr AR, Whay HR. (2006) Validity of a behavioural measure of heat stress and a skin tent test for dehydration in working horses and donkeys. *Equine Vet J* **38**:433–8.

Pritchard JC, Burn CC, Barr AR, Whay HR. (2008) Validity of indicators of dehydration in working horses: a longitudinal study of changes in skin tent duration, mucous membrane dryness and drinking behaviour. *Equine Vet J* **40**:558–64.

Proudman CJ, Edwards GB, Barnes J, French NP. (2005a) Modelling long-term survival of horses following surgery for large intestinal disease. *Equine Vet J* **37**:366–70.

Proudman CJ, Edwards GB, Barnes J, French NR. (2005b) Factors affecting long-term survival of horses recovering from surgery of the small intestine. *Equine Vet J* **37**:360–5.

Reinhart K, Rudolph T, Bredle DL, Hannemann L, Cain SM. (1989) Comparison of central-venous to mixed-venous oxygen saturation during changes in oxygen supply/demand. *Chest* **95**:1216–21.

Rivers E, Nguyen B, Havstad S, et al. (2001) Early goal-directed therapy in the treatment of severe sepsis and septic shock. *N Engl J Med* **345**:1368–77.

Rumbaugh GE, Carlson GP, Harrold D. (1982) Urinary production in the healthy horse and in horses deprived of feed and water. *Am J Vet Res* **43**:735–7.

Runk DT, Madigan JE, Rahal CJ, et al. (2000) Measurement of plasma colloid osmotic pressure in normal Thoroughbred neonatal foals. *J Vet Intern Med* **14**:475–8.

Shah N, Bedford RF. (2001) Invasive and noninvasive blood pressure monitoring. In: Lake CL, Hines RL, Blitt CD (eds) *Clinical Monitoring: Practical Applications for Anesthesia and Critical Care*. Philadelphia: W.B. Saunders, pp. 181–203.

Steffey EP, Dunlop CI, Farver TB, Woliner MJ, Schultz LJ. (1987) Cardiovascular and respiratory measurements in awake and isoflurane-anesthetized horses. *Am J Vet Res* **48**:7–12.

Tennent-Brown BS, Wilkins PA, Lindborg S, Russell G, Boston RC. (2007) Assessment of a point-of-care lactate monitor in emergency admissions of adult horses to a referral hospital. *J Vet Int Med* **21**:1090–8.

Tennent-Brown BS, Wilkins PA, Lindborg S, Russell G, Boston RC. (2009) Sequential plasma lactate concentrations as prognostic indicators in adult equine emergencies. *J Vet Int Med* **24**:198–205.

Thomas WP, Madigan JE, Backus KQ, Powell WE. (1987) Systemic and pulmonary haemodynamics in normal neonatal foals. *J Reprod Fertil Suppl* **35**:623–8.

Valverde A, Giguere S, Sanchez LC, Shih A, Ryan C. (2006) Effects of dobutamine, norepinephrine, and vasopressin on cardiovascular function in anesthetized neonatal foals with induced hypotension. *Am J Vet Res* **67**:1730–7.

Versteilen AM, Heemskerk AE, Groeneveld AB, van Wijhe M, van Lambalgen AA, Tangelder GJ. (2008) Mechanisms of the urinary concentration defect and effect of desmopressin during endotoxemia in rats. *Shock* **29**:217–22.

Wilsterman S, Hackett ES, Rao S, Hackett TB. (2009) A technique for central venous pressure measurement in normal horses. *J Vet Emerg Crit Care* **19**:241–6.

Wotman K, Wilkins PA, Palmer JE, Boston RC. (2009) Association of blood lactate concentration and outcome in foals. *J Vet Int Med* **23**:598–605.

CHAPTER 11

Fluid overload

C. Langdon Fielding

Loomis Basin Equine Medical Center Penryn, CA, USA

Introduction

Fluid overload occurs when total body water is increased above the normal volume for a given patient. Fluid overload becomes clinically apparent when the extracellular fluid volume reaches a critical value (likely different for each patient). Many of the clinical signs of fluid overload are related to overexpansion of the vascular space with subsequent fluid accumulation within the interstitium.

Fluid overload is always a relative state because hypervolemia can be an appropriate response under certain circumstances. In cases where there is inadequate preload to maintain cardiac output, as with heart failure, total body fluid overload may allow the heart to maintain cardiac output even at the risk of subsequent volume overload. In this case total body water (specifically extracellular fluid volume) has exceeded a normal volume, but it is an appropriate expansion in order to maintain normal cardiovascular function.

The presence of fluid overload requires either excessive fluid administration or inadequate renal excretion. Particularly in adult horses, healthy kidneys are able to clear excessive fluid administration given adequate time. Therefore, nearly all cases of fluid overload occur because renal physiology does not recognize the fluid overload or is unable to excrete it.

In renal failure, the kidneys may be unable to remove the required amount of fluid from the extracellular fluid volume (ECFV) to maintain normal water balance (Figure 11.1). Most commonly this occurs due to a decreased glomerular filtration rate (GFR) as occurs in

many types of renal failure. As discussed below, when GFR is inadequate, fluid will accumulate and total body water will increase. Unless GFR can be increased, there may be limited treatment options for the excess fluid. Less commonly, GFR may be normal, but the kidneys eliminate an inappropriately low amount of water. This can be due to inappropriate release of vasopressin or an inappropriate response to a given concentration of vasopressin.

Perhaps more importantly, there are a number of conditions where renal function is adequate, but the kidneys are "tricked" into allowing fluid overload. Common examples of this scenario include increased capillary permeability, hypoproteinemia, changes in interstitial compliance, and heart failure. While each of these causes is different, in all cases the excess fluid is not recognized by the kidneys and is therefore not removed.

An example of the "tricked" kidney is an increase in capillary permeability. This permeability allows increased fluid to accumulate within the interstitium. Both ECFV and total body water (TBW) will gradually exceed normal volumes. However, the intravascular volume may be decreased (or even normal) and therefore the kidneys do not perceive a fluid overload (i.e., none of the mechanisms that recognize intravascular volume overload will be engaged). The kidneys may even perceive the need to retain additional fluid as the intravascular volume may be inadequate.

While more complex, heart failure can represent a similar problem. The kidneys perceive that additional intravascular volume is needed in order to maintain

Equine Fluid Therapy, First Edition. Edited by C. Langdon Fielding and K. Gary Magdesian.
© 2015 John Wiley & Sons, Inc. Published 2015 by John Wiley & Sons, Inc.

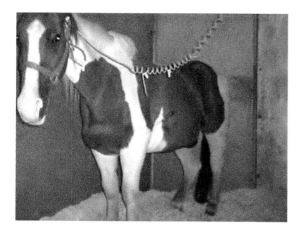

Figure 11.1 Horse with anuric renal failure and fluid overload with severe ventral edema.

cardiovascular function. This volume is maintained despite the excessive total body water and extracellular fluid volumes. A more thorough discussion of the pathophysiology of fluid overload in heart failure is found in Chapter 17.

In summary, fluid overload usually results when the kidneys either do not recognize the excess water or are unable to excrete it. Given that fluid overload can have severe consequences, such as pulmonary edema, prompt recognition of risk factors is important. Not all cases of fluid overload require immediate treatment, but increasing renal excretion of fluid is often the most practical means to resolve the excess fluid accumulation.

Risk factors for fluid overload

Identifying patients that are at increased risk for fluid overload is an essential part of fluid therapy planning. Edema formation is likely due to a combination of factors that contribute to the risk of fluid overload. In studies evaluating the risk factors for fluid overload, hypoproteinemia, heart failure, renal failure, and blood product administration have all been implicated (Malhotra & Axisa, 2009; Murphy et al., 2013). However, it is not clear whether these risk factors are actual causative agents or merely associated with sick patients that are more likely to have volume overload. Nonetheless, the presence of these risk factors can be used to identify patients with increased susceptibility to overload. Potential risk factors for fluid overload in horses are listed in Box 11.1.

Failure to recognize risk factors was implicated in fluid overload-associated morbidity in human patients (Walsh & Walsh, 2005). In this study, approximately 7% of patients were identified with fluid overload, and the authors concluded that some cases occurred due to failure to recognize the major factors contributing to excess fluid balance (Walsh & Walsh, 2005). It is likely that the risk factors in horses are similar to those in other species, and they should be carefully considered before fluid therapy is initiated.

Heart failure

The topic of heart failure and fluid balance is covered extensively in Chapter 17. A combination of physiologic compensatory mechanisms associated with heart failure can result in severe and life-threatening fluid overload.

Hypoproteinemia

Edema is a common development in many cases of hypoproteinemia in horses (Galvin et al., 2004; Nyack et al., 1984; van den Wollenberg et al., 2011). However, the importance of low plasma protein concentration in the formation of edema remains equivocal. It is particularly complicated because many conditions that result in hypoproteinemia are also associated with systemic inflammation (e.g., colitis). It is often difficult to delineate the contribution of hypoproteinemia, increased vascular permeability, and interstitial matrix compliance changes. All of these factors can lead to edema, but they are often present together.

In experimental and clinical studies, significant hypoproteinemia can be present without edema formation (Joles et al., 1989; Lecomte & Juchmes, 1978; Steyl & Van Zyl-Smit et al., 2009). The nephrotic syndrome represents a classic example of the controversies surrounding the role of hypoproteinemia in edema formation (Rondon-Berrios, 2011). A number of clinical and experimental observations have questioned the causative role of hypoproteinemia in edema formation in this syndrome (Rondon-Berrios, 2011). While no studies are available in horses, clinical observation suggests a high degree of variability in terms of edema formation in horses with hypoproteinemia. Interestingly, some horses with chronic protein loss may have marked hypoproteinemia, yet insignificant edema formation.

When considering total protein or albumin concentration, there is unlikely to be a universal cut-off value for the formation of edema. While albumin concentrations less than 1–1.5 g/dL or total protein concentrations less than 4.0 g/dL have been anecdotally implicated as a threshold for edema formation in horses, there is no research to support these conclusions. In humans, colloid osmotic pressure (associated with serum total protein concentrations) below 10–12 mmHg was identified as an edema threshold; however, this has been shown to be unreliable (Duncan & Young, 1982). In another study of postoperative patients, human patients with albumin concentrations below 2.7 g/dL prior to surgery were at higher risk for edema formation postoperatively (Malhotra & Axisa, 2009). Hypoproteinemia was associated with an increased risk of mortality in horses in one study; however, the specific presence of edema was not evaluated (Metcalfe et al., 2012).

In summary, hypoproteinemia should always be considered as a risk factor for edema formation. In cases where intravenous fluid administration will be initiated, the risk of edema formation may be even higher. In cases where edema is present, however, the identification of hypoproteinemia should not exclude the search for other causes contributing to a state of fluid overload.

Renal failure

Patients with compromised renal function will be at increased risk for fluid overload if they are unable to excrete the quantity of fluid that is being administered. In specific groups of humans with renal failure, fluid overload is an independent risk factor for mortality (Bouchard et al., 2009; Schrier, 2010). In another study chronic renal failure was identified as a risk factor for developing fluid overload (Murphy et al., 2013).

It is not always possible to evaluate renal function prior to initiating fluid therapy. If kidney values or urinalysis are available, this information should be used to assess the risk of fluid overload with intravenous fluid administration. However, acute kidney injury is recognized with as little as a 0.3 mg/dL increase in serum creatinine concentration (Khwaja, 2012). Single measurements of creatinine values at the middle or upper end of a laboratory normal range may still be associated with renal insufficiency. This may be difficult to determine if the patient's previous normal value is not available. Fractional excretion of sodium may be another means for identifying more subtle changes in renal function and patients at higher risk for fluid overload (Schrier, 2011).

Systemic inflammation

A systemic inflammatory response to a variety of diseases induces a large number of physiologic changes in critically ill patients that can affect multiple organs. There are many potential means by which the systemic inflammatory response could lead to fluid overload (Wiig et al., 2003). Specifically, changes in renal function, cardiac function, capillary permeability, interstitial compliance, and plasma protein concentrations are just a few of the possible mechanisms.

An increase in capillary permeability has consistently been thought to play a role in the pathophysiology of edema formation. The basis for this is discussed in more detail in Chapter 1 as it relates to the Starling equation. There is clinical evidence that capillary permeability increases during systemic inflammation (Basu et al., 2010; Wiig et al., 2003). The exact contribution of this increased permeability in creating fluid overload is somewhat controversial (Levick & Michel, 2010).

Interstitial compliance has also been implicated as a major contributor to edema formation (Reed & Rubin, 2010). Figure 11.2 shows an example of normal interstitial compliance; interstitial compliance is the change in interstitial volume resulting from a change in interstitial pressure. By creating greater negative pressure, it is possible for the interstitium to help increase net movement of fluid out of the vascular space. A variety of inflammatory triggers have been shown to induce changes in this pressure and result in fluid accumulation within the interstitium (Reed & Rubin, 2010).

Blood product administration

In a variety of clinical settings, transfusion of blood products has been associated with increased risk of circulatory overload (Kumar et al., 2013; Li et al., 2011; Murphy et al., 2013). The volume of transfused

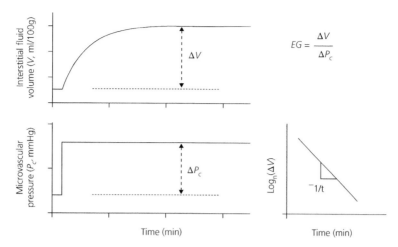

Figure 11.2 Illustration of change in interstitial fluid volume (ΔV) in response to a step increase in microvascular pressure (ΔP_c). The edemagenic gain (EG) determines the final change in interstitial fluid volume between two steady states and thus the steady-state behavior of the system. The edemagenic time constant (τ) determines the rate at which interstitial fluid volume changes and thus the transient behavior of the system. From Dongaonkar RM, Laine GA, Stewart RH, et al. Evaluation of gravimetric techniques to estimate the microvascular filtration coefficient. Am J Physiol Regul Integr Comp Physiol 2011 Jun;300(6):R1426–36. Reproduced with permission.

products and the rate of transfusion were shown to be independent risk factors for fluid overload (Li et al., 2011). Blood and/or plasma transfusions are used in equine practice but fluid overload does not appear to be commonly identified. In one study evaluating adverse reactions to plasma transfusions, edema was not noted in any of the cases (Hardefeldt et al., 2010). However, this study did not specifically look at changes in body weight or other evaluations of fluid balance.

Aggressive fluid resuscitation

Excessive fluid administration will always be a relative concept because different patients can tolerate different volumes of fluid at different rates. In healthy horses, rates of 80 mL/kg/h seem to be well tolerated over a 30-minute period (Fielding et al., 2007). When fluids are administered by gravity flow through a single IV catheter, it may not be possible to administer fluids fast enough to cause significant fluid overload in an average size horse without other risk factors (hypoproteinemia, renal failure, etc.). However, when fluid pumps, multiple catheters, or large bore catheters are used, much higher rates are possible (Nolen-Walston, 2012).

Rate of fluid administration was noted as a risk factor for fluid overload in studies in humans (Li et al., 2011). However, this study focused on the administration of colloids and did not address crystalloids. While not well

documented in horses, it seems likely that high rates of crystalloid fluid administration (>20–40 mL/kg/h for a prolonged period) could result in fluid overload particularly in patients with other risk factors.

Recognizing fluid overload

Given the significant clinical consequences of fluid overload, early detection is ideal. Techniques for identifying patients with fluid overload are listed in Table 11.1. Using a combination of clinical exam findings, laboratory testing, andr more advanced monitoring techniques is usually indicated.

Peripheral edema formation

Clinical examination is one of the best means of detecting peripheral edema formation. The ventral abdomen is a common location where small amounts of edema can be detected (see Figure 11.1). Swelling of the leg, sheath, and head are other locations that are important to evaluate. In general, dependent regions are more likely to develop edema. In critically ill neonatal foals, a "jelly" appearance of the tissues can often be visualized or palpated with edema formation. As these sick foals are often recumbent, it is less likely to accumulate in the lower legs or ventral abdomen.

Table 11.1 Clinical tools used to identify fluid overload.

Clinical exam	Edema: ventral abdomen, legs, head
	Adventitial lung sounds
	Serial body weight increases (after rehydration)
Hemodynamic monitoring	Central venous pressure
	Pulse pressure variation
Pulmonary function impairment	Partial pressure arterial oxygen
	Pulse oximetry
Other monitoring techniques	Bioelectrical impedance analysis

Changes in body weight

Perhaps one of the easiest ways of evaluating fluid overload is to monitor changes in body weight. Evaluating daily trends is more useful than a single measurement. Body weight on presentation can be particularly challenging to interpret as patients may be severely dehydrated and a gain in body weight after fluid administration may be entirely appropriate.

Body weight changes also do not address the location of the excess fluid. For example, a horse with colitis may accumulate significant fluid in the intestinal tract but still be hypovolemic. In general, a patient who is at risk for fluid overload and consistently gains weight each day may be accumulating excess fluid. Ideally, other examination and laboratory factors should be considered in conjunction with body weight.

Central venous pressure monitoring

Central venous pressure (CVP) represents the pressure within the intrathoracic vena cava. A more complete discussion of this topic is available in Chapter 10; however, CVP monitoring is a method to detect volume overload. Specifically, elevated CVP (>15 cmH$_2$O) may indicate the potential for fluid overload. Likewise, a rise in CVP (>4 cmH$_2$O) in response to a fluid challenge could also indicate a risk for edema formation unless hypovolemia is present and baseline CVP is low.

The use of CVP monitoring to detect fluid overload is controversial (Marik et al., 2008). Experimental studies indicate that it could have some benefit as a marker of fluid overload (Taguchi et al., 2011). CVP monitoring has been described in horses for detection of dehydration and hypovolemia, but its ability to detect volume overload in horses is unclear (Magdesian et al., 2006).

Pulmonary function deterioration

Deterioration in pulmonary function during fluid therapy may be another way to detect fluid overload. However, it is important to recognize that horses with systemic inflammation may be at risk for pulmonary disease (acute respiratory distress syndrome: ARDS) as well as fluid overload. The excess fluid may not be a direct cause of the pulmonary dysfunction; rather the systemic inflammatory response may be the primary cause of excessive pulmonary fluid. Pulse oximetry and arterial blood gas monitoring are practical means of monitoring oxygenation and pulmonary function. Any deterioration in these variables could indicate fluid overload and should be investigated.

Advanced monitoring techniques

The ideal monitoring technique for fluid overload would be able to quantitate the amount of water accumulating in different fluid compartments. Bioimpedance analysis (BIA) is designed to make these determinations and quantify the size of the ECFV, intracellular fluid volume (ICFV), and TBW. The use of BIA in horses is described and appears to detect acute volume changes in healthy horses (Fielding et al., 2007; Latman et al., 2011). The technology is also used in humans undergoing hemodialysis in order to maintain appropriate fluid volumes in these patients (Celik et al., 2011).

There is unfortunately little research evaluating BIA in sick horses in the clinical setting. There is evidence that BIA may be influenced by electrolyte imbalances, which are common in critically ill patients, representing a disadvantage of this technology. While BIA is relatively non-invasive, it requires patients to remain still for short periods and avoid contact with metal, neither of which is necessarily practical for hospitalized horses. Continued research may better define the role of BIA in equine critical care.

Evaluation of the respiratory changes in arterial pressure has been a recent focus of research for evaluating fluid responsiveness and preventing fluid overload. Pulse pressure variation (PPV) can be used to evaluate the need for fluid volume in patients undergoing mechanical ventilation. This calculated value is based on the difference between systolic and diastolic arterial pressure during the inspiratory and expiratory phases of

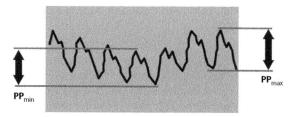

Figure 11.3 Graphical example of the arterial waveform during mechanical ventilation and the location for measurement of pulse pressure variation (PPV).

positive pressure ventilation (Figure 11.3); PPV has been described in horses (Fielding & Stolba, 2012).

In humans, PPV values of approximately 12–13% have been used to discriminate between patients who will benefit from additional intravenous fluids and those in whom additional fluids could be detrimental (Marik et al., 2009). A PPV value greater than 13% would indicate the need for additional intravenous fluids. In horses, most mechanically ventilated patients are under general anesthesia, but these animals pose some unique risks for fluid overload. The PPV can be calculated using Equation 11.1 (Fielding & Stolba, 2012):

$$Pulse\ pressure\ variation =$$
$$\left\{ \left(Sys_{Ins} - Dias_{Ins} \right) - \left(Sys_{Exp} - Dias_{Exp} \right) \right\} / \quad (11.1)$$
$$\left\{ \left[\left(Sys_{Ins} - Dias_{Ins} \right) + \left(Sys_{Exp} - Dias_{Exp} \right) \right] / 2 \right\}$$

where:
Sys_{Ins} = maximum systolic pressure during the inspiratory phase of PPV;
$Dias_{Ins}$ = maximum diastolic pressure during the inspiratory phase of PPV;
Sys_{Exp} = minimum systolic pressure during the expiratory phase of PPV;
$Dias_{Exp}$ = minimum diastolic pressure during the expiratory phase of PPV.

Treatment of fluid overload

Once fluid overload is recognized, the clinician must decide whether treatment is warranted. Treatment is indicated for the following reasons:

1 Fluid overload is contributing to impairment of normal pulmonary function and oxygenation is inadequate.

2 Fluid overload is contributing to impairment of normal cardiovascular function and perfusion is inadequate.

3 Renal function is impaired and the fluid overload is unlikely to improve with time.

If none of these criteria are present, normal kidney function should gradually resolve the excess fluid and return the patient to a normal volume status, provided large volumes of additional fluids are not administered. In these cases, careful monitoring of hydration and perfusion parameters is warranted, but no additional treatment may be needed. If treatment is warranted to improve fluid overload, the main components of treatment include: (i) modify/eliminate fluids being administered; (ii) increase renal excretion of fluids if possible; and (iii) remove fluid accumulations (pleural, peritoneal, etc.) if possible.

Modification of the fluid therapy plan

Modifying the fluid therapy plan should always be considered when fluid overload is recognized. All sources of fluid administration (intravenous, oral, etc.) need to be evaluated. In some cases, simply decreasing the rate of fluid administration may be all that is required. However, for critically ill patients with poor perfusion, a high rate of fluids may be required to maintain cardiac output. In these cases, if the rate cannot be safely decreased, it may be possible to change fluid type. For example, colloids may be more likely to result in intravascular volume overload (Murphy et al., 2013). Therefore, switching to an isotonic crystalloid fluid at the same rate may help to mitigate the volume overload.

Increased renal excretion of fluid

Increasing the renal excretion of fluids is the most common way to treat severe fluid overload. Common drugs used to induce diuresis in horses include furosemide and mannitol. However, in cases of impaired renal function, particularly oliguria or anuria, mannitol could result in further volume overload because it cannot be eliminated. Furosemide infusions have been described in horses and are administered at a continuous rate of 0.12 mg/kg/h preceded by a loading dose of 0.12 mg/kg IV (Johansson et al., 2003). When a continuous rate infusion (CRI) is not possible, intermittent bolus administration can be used.

Furosemide infusions are used in humans to address volume overload, particularly in cases of impaired renal function (Mirhosseini et al., 2013; Thomsen et al., 2012). Furosemide is generally effective in achieving a negative fluid balance (Thomsen et al., 2012). However, furosemide has the potential to cause deterioration in renal function and to worsen electrolyte imbalances (Thomsen et al., 2012). In a study of heart transplant patients with fluid overload, furosemide was considered inferior to renal replacement therapy in humans (Mirhosseini et al., 2013). However, furosemide is more readily available in equine intensive care units.

In cases of renal failure, there continues to be controversy over the benefits of furosemide. Furosemide may decrease oxygen consumption in the loop of Henle and therefore be protective by decreasing potential ischemic injury. If furosemide is able to increase urinary flow, this could also improve intratubular obstruction. Results of clinical trials are conflicting with some studies implicating furosemide in association with a worsening of renal function as compared to other treatments (Kelly et al., 2008; Mirhosseini et al., 2013).

In horses, furosemide likely represents the most practical and safe option to induce fluid diuresis and resolve volume overload. However, it is possible that renal function and electrolyte balance may be negatively affected by furosemide; therefore, monitoring of kidney values and electrolytes is important. In some cases, continued fluid administration (even hypertonic fluid) in combination with furosemide administration may be needed to maintain an appropriate fluid balance.

Removal of fluid accumulations

In some cases of fluid overload, there may be fluid effusions within third spaces such as the peritoneal or pleural spaces. If these effusions are small volume, they are unlikely to have significant detriment. However, in cases of large-volume fluid accumulation, removal may improve respiratory function (particularly in cases of pleural effusion) and help to restore fluid balance. These fluid accumulations are typically removed using a chest tube or teat cannula. However, if fluid removal is too rapid, severe hypotension can result. Removing large volumes of fluid slowly (over hours) may be safer and allow for a more gradual restoration of fluid balance.

Prognosis in fluid overload

The prognosis for survival following fluid overload depends on the inciting cause and the severity of overload. If the inciting cause can be resolved and renal function is adequate, fluid balance is likely to return to normal. For example, in cases of iatrogenic volume overload due to overly aggressive fluid therapy, renal excretion of fluid will gradually remove the excess fluid. However, if fluid accumulation is severe and due to renal failure following severe sepsis, the fluid accumulation may be difficult to resolve and the prognosis may be guarded/poor. In general, renal function is one of the more significant determinants of prognosis in cases of volume overload. In addition, the prognosis of the underlying disease also dictates the outcome despite resolution of fluid overload.

In cases of severe overload, pulmonary function may be severely compromised. Even if the underlying cause of the overload is treatable, respiratory failure may result before the excess fluid can be removed. In these cases, treatment with furosemide should be initiated as quickly as possible.

Prevention of fluid overload

Prevention of fluid overload is not always possible. Aggressive fluid resuscitation may be warranted and necessary for treatment of the underlying primary disease and some degree of fluid overload may be unavoidable. However, clinicians should recognize the risk factors for fluid overload and be cognizant of treatments that may precipitate it. In addition to recognizing at-risk patients, the following strategies can be used to prevent fluid overload.

Selection of fluid type

Colloid administration has been implicated in fluid overload, but it depends on the rate and volume administered (Murphy et al., 2013). Its use should be considered carefully particularly in cases where crystalloids have equal efficacy. If colloids are required (i.e., blood transfusion), the rate of fluid administration should be considered and moderated if possible.

Selection of fluid rate

The rate of fluid administration should be modified in patients where fluid overload is deemed likely. Often, 50% of the "maintenance rate" may be used in these high-risk patients. Renal function needs to be monitored carefully, however. Fluid boluses should be used only when absolutely necessary as they may cause a more rapid, albeit temporary, increase in central venous pressures than continuous rate administration.

Diuretic treatment

In some cases, rapid fluid resuscitation may be needed in a patient that already has significant fluid overload. For example, a horse with chronic hyponatremia may have significant edema and fluid accumulation. However, acute worsening of the underlying disease may necessitate rapid fluid administration in order to stabilize the patient. This patient is likely to have worsening fluid accumulation; administration of a diuretic (i.e., furosemide) in conjunction or shortly following fluid resuscitation may help to mitigate the fluid overload. As discussed above, furosemide is likely the most practical, effective, and safe diuretic to use for these purposes.

Neonatal foals

Similar to adult human patients, there is clinical evidence that fluid overload is associated with increased mortality in specific groups of ill infants (Askenazi et al., 2013). Risk factors for fluid overload in neonates also include kidney failure, heart failure, hypoproteinemia, and inflammatory conditions (Nguyen et al., 2006). However, many critical neonatal foals (e.g., those delivered from severe dystocia) appear to be prone to fluid overload particularly with treatment of intravenous fluids. This may be due to differences in capillary permeability or the compliance of their interstitium (Palmer, 2004). It is extremely important to manage the fluid balance of such patients carefully given the detrimental effects of fluid overload.

In the treatment of neonatal foals with fluid overload, similar therapeutic options exist as described for adult horses. Modifying fluid administration is one consideration, but increasing fluid urinary excretion may be required with significant volume overload. Furosemide infusions are used in neonatal foals as well. In humans, furosemide has a much longer half-life in infants as compared to adults but is still used to treat fluid overload (Nguyen et al., 2006; Pacifici, 2012). While neonatal foals respond differently to furosemide than adult horses, the pharmacokinetics have not been well described (Broughton et al., 1984). Furosemide infusions are often very effective at removing excess fluid from foals, but fluid and electrolyte balance must be monitored.

References

Askenazi DJ, Koralkar R, Hundley HE, et al. (2013) Fluid overload and mortality are associated with acute kidney injury in sick near-term/term neonate. *Pediatr Nephrol* 28:661–6.

Basu S, Bhattacharya M, Chatterjee TK, et al. (2010) Microalbuminuria: A novel biomarker of sepsis. *Indian J Crit Care Med* 14:22–8.

Bouchard J, Soroko SB, Chertow GM, et al. (2009) Program to Improve Care in Acute Renal Disease (PICARD) Study Group. Fluid accumulation, survival and recovery of kidney function in critically ill patients with acute kidney injury. *Kidney Int* 76:422–7.

Broughton Pipkin F, Ousey JC, Wallace CP, et al. (1984) Studies on equine prematurity 4: Effect of salt and water loss on the renin–angiotensin–aldosterone system in the newborn foal. *Equine Vet J* 16:292–7.

Celik G, Kara I, Yilmaz M, et al. (2011) The relationship between bioimpedance analysis, haemodynamic parameters of haemodialysis, biochemical parameters and dry weight. *J Int Med Res* 39:2421–8.

Dongaonkar RM, Laine GA, Stewart RH, et al. (2011) Evaluation of gravimetric techniques to estimate the microvascular filtration coefficient. *Am J Physiol Regul Integr Comp Physiol* 300:R1426–36.

Duncan A, Young DS. (1982) Measurements of serum colloid osmotic pressure are of limited usefulness. *Clin Chem* 28:141–5.

Fielding CL, Magdesian KG, Carlson GP, et al. (2007) Estimation of acute fluid shifts using bioelectrical impedance analysis in horses. *J Vet Intern Med* 21:176–83.

Fielding CL, Stolba DN. (2012) Pulse pressure variation and systolic pressure variation in horses undergoing general anesthesia. *J Vet Emerg Crit Care* 22:372–5.

Galvin N, Dillon H, McGovern F. (2004) Right dorsal colitis in the horse: minireview and reports on three cases in Ireland. *Ir Vet J* 57:467–73.

Hardefeldt LY, Keuler N, Peek SF. (2010) Incidence of transfusion reactions to commercial equine plasma. *J Vet Emerg Crit Care (San Antonio)* 20:421–5.

Johansson AM, Gardner SY, Levine JF, et al. (2003) Furosemide continuous rate infusion in the horse: evaluation of enhanced efficacy and reduced side effects. *J Vet Intern Med* 17:887–95.

Joles JA, Willekes-Koolschijn N, Braam B, et al. (1989) Colloid osmotic pressure in young analbuminemic rats. *Am J Physiol* 257:F23–28.

Kelly AM, Dwamena B, Cronin P, et al. (2008) Meta-analysis: effectiveness of drugs for preventing contrast-induced nephropathy. *Ann Intern Med* 148:284–94.

Khwaja A. (2012) KDIGO Clinical Practice Guidelines for Acute Kidney Injury. *Nephron Clin Pract* 120:179–84.

Kumar R, Kumar S, Lata S. (2013) Albumin infusion may deleteriously promote extracellular fluid overload without improving circulating hypovolemia in patients of advanced cirrhosis with diabetes mellitus and sepsis. *Med Hypotheses* 80:452–5.

Latman NS, Keith N, Nicholson A, et al. (2011) Bioelectrical impedance analysis determination of water content and distribution in the horse. *Res Vet Sci* 90:516–20.

Lecomte J, Juchmes J. (1978) So-called absence of edema in analbuminemia. *Rev Med Liege* 33:766–70.

Levick JR, Michel CC. (2010) Microvascular fluid exchange and the revised Starling principle. *Cardiovasc Res* 87:198–210.

Li G, Rachmale S, Kojicic M, et al. (2011) Incidence and transfusion risk factors for transfusion-associated circulatory overload among medical intensive care unit patients. *Transfusion* 51:338–43.

Magdesian KG, Fielding CL, Rhodes DM, et al. (2006) Changes in central venous pressure and blood lactate concentration in response to acute blood loss in horses. *J Am Vet Med Assoc* 229:1458–62.

Malhotra K, Axisa B. (2009) Low plasma albumin linked to fluid overload in postoperative epidural patients. *Ann R Coll Surg Engl* 91:703–7.

Marik PE, Baram M, Vahid B. (2008) Does central venous pressure predict fluid responsiveness? A systematic review of the literature and the tale of seven mares. *Chest* 134:172–8.

Marik PE, Cavallazzi R, Vasu T, et al. (2009) Dynamic changes in arterial waveform derived variables and fluid responsiveness in mechanically ventilated patients: A systematic review of the literature. *Crit Care Med* 37:2642–7.

Metcalfe LV, More SJ, Duggan V, Katz LM. (2012) A retrospective study of horses investigated for weight loss despite a good appetite (2002–2011). *Equine Vet J* 45:340–5.

Mirhosseini SM, Fakhri M, Asadollahi S, et al. (2013) Continuous renal replacement therapy versus furosemide for management of kidney impairment in heart transplant recipients with volume overload. *Interact Cardiovasc Thorac Surg* 16:314–20.

Murphy EL, Kwaan N, Looney MR, et al. Risk factors and outcomes in transfusion-associated circulatory overload. *Am J Med* 126:357.e29–357.e38.

Nguyen TH, Nguyen TL, Lei HY, et al. (2006) Volume replacement in infants with dengue hemorrhagic fever/dengue shock syndrome. *Am J Trop Med Hyg* 74:684–91.

Nolen-Walston RD. (2012) Flow rates of large animal fluid delivery systems used for high-volume crystalloid resuscitation. *J Vet Emerg Crit Care (San Antonio)* 22:661–5.

Nolen-Walston RD, Norton JL, Navas de Solis C, et al. (2011) The effects of hypohydration on central venous pressure and splenic volume in adult horses. *J Vet Intern Med* 25:570–4.

Nyack B, Padmore CL, Dunn D, et al. (1984) Splenic lymphosarcoma in a horse. *Mod Vet Pract* 65:269–70, 272.

Pacifici GM. (2012) Clinical pharmacology of the loop diuretics furosemide and bumetanide in neonates and infants. *Paediatr Drugs* 14:233–46.

Palmer JE. (2004) Fluid therapy in the neonate: not your mother's fluid space. *Vet Clin Equine* 20:63–75.

Reed RK, Rubin K. (2010) Transcapillary exchange: role and importance of the interstitial fluid pressure and the extracellular matrix. *Cardiovasc Res* 87:211–17.

Rondon-Berrios H. (2011) New insights into the pathophysiology of oedema in nephrotic syndrome. *Nefrologia* 31: 148–54.

Schrier RW. (2010) Fluid administration in critically ill patients with acute kidney injury. *Clin J Am Soc Nephrol* 5:733–9.

Schrier RW. (2011) Diagnostic value of urinary sodium, chloride, urea, and flow. *J Am Soc Nephrol* 22:1610–13.

Steyl C, Van Zyl-Smit R. (2009) Mechanisms of oedema formation: the minor role of hypoalbuminaemia. *S Afr Med J* 99:57–9.

Taguchi H, Ichinose K, Tanimoto H, et al. (2011) Stroke volume variation obtained with Vigileo/FloTrac™ system during bleeding and fluid overload in dogs. *J Anesth* 25:563–8.

Thomsen G, Bezdjian L, Rodriguez L, et al. (2012) Clinical outcomes of a furosemide infusion protocol in edematous patients in the intensive care unit. *Crit Care Nurse* 32: 25–34.

van den Wollenberg L, Butler CM, Houwers DJ, et al. (2011) Lawsonia intracellularis-associated proliferative enteritis in weanling foals in the Netherlands. *Tijdschr Diergeneeskd* 136: 565–70.

Walsh SR, Walsh CJ. (2005) Intravenous fluid-associated morbidity in postoperative patients. *Ann R Coll Surg Engl* 87:126–30.

Wiig H, Rubin K, Reed RK. (2003) New and active role of the interstitium in control of interstitial fluid pressure: potential therapeutic consequences. *Acta Anaesthesiol Scand* 47:111–21.

CHAPTER 12

Replacement fluids therapy in horses

K. Gary Magdesian

Professor in Critical Care and Emergency Medicine, School of Veterinary Medicine, University of California, Davis, CA, USA

Introduction

Replacement of blood volume and interstitial deficits is the cornerstone of replacement fluid therapy. Hypoperfusion, associated with hypovolemia, hypotension, and/or reduced cardiac output, is the priority during triage of critically ill horses; left unchecked, it is associated with multiple organ dysfunction and mortality. After addressing hypovolemia, interstitial and then intracellular fluid losses must also be treated, although they are prioritized after circulating volume. Acute abdominal crises (e.g., colic), colitis, acute hemorrhage, endotoxemia, and sepsis are among the most common equine medical disorders associated with shock and requiring rapid fluid replacement.

Just what is the optimal fluid type and rate for replacement in horses lacks scientific consensus, making fluid therapy subject to clinician preference. As a consequence there are many different protocols for fluid therapy. Added to that, the detection of dehydration in horses is highly insensitive, with the earliest clinical detection occurring at 3–5% of body weight loss in fluid. Even more challenging is estimation of the percent loss from each of the fluid subcompartments, including those of the extracellular fluid (ECF) compartment (plasma volume, interstitium, and transcellular space) and intracellular fluid (ICF). Extravascular losses (interstitial), without concurrent intravascular deficits, are particularly difficult to detect. Little peer-reviewed data are available to guide the equine clinician's choice of fluids, including different isotonic crystalloids, hypertonic crystalloids,

and/or colloids. The reader is referred to Chapter 22 for replacement fluid therapy of foals.

Background

The need for replacement fluids stems from the importance of fluid volume as it relates to stroke volume and cardiac output. Blood pressure is dependent upon cardiac output and peripheral vascular resistance. Cardiac output, along with hemoglobin and oxygenation status, is a primary determinant of oxygen delivery. Cardiac output is determined by stroke volume and heart rate. Stroke volume is where the beneficial effects of fluids are most evident. Stroke volume is determined by contractility, preload, and afterload. Preload is influenced by venous return, and hence blood volume. By increasing stroke volume, fluid therapy results in an increase in cardiac output with resultant increase in arterial blood pressure and perfusion. End-organ perfusion requires a minimum mean arterial pressure of 60 mmHg, and this is the minimum blood pressure goal for fluid therapy (Kirchheim et al., 1987).

There are four major decisions in formulating replacement fluid therapy (the "TROL" plan adapted from the human medical literature) (Vincent & Weil, 2006):

1 Type
2 Rate
3 Objectives
4 Limits

Equine Fluid Therapy, First Edition. Edited by C. Langdon Fielding and K. Gary Magdesian.
© 2015 John Wiley & Sons, Inc. Published 2015 by John Wiley & Sons, Inc.

The TROL approach

Type of fluid

A physiologic approach to selection of fluid type is adopted. Fluids types available for replacement include: (i) isotonic crystalloids, (ii) hypertonic crystalloids, and (iii) colloids. Hypotonic fluids are "maintenance" as opposed to "replacement" fluids and include 0.45% NaCl/2.5% dextrose (hypotonic *in vivo*), Plasma-Lyte 56 (Baxter Healthcare Corporation, Deerfield, IL), Normosol™-M (Abbott Laboratories, North Chicago, IL), and 5% dextrose in water (D5W). These are not replacement fluids because they distribute among all fluid compartments, including the ICF, based on osmolarity. These hypotonic fluids should never be administered as a rapid bolus because of their propensity to expand the ICF and potential for intracellular edema.

There is considerable debate and no consensus in the veterinary or human medical communities regarding the optimal fluid type for resuscitation of hypovolemia. Numerous meta-analyses and systematic reviews have shown no clear benefit for either crystalloids or colloids for use in human patients (Ribeiro et al., 2009). The conclusions in most of these reports are that crystalloids are preferred over colloids under most circumstances due to cost differences because there are no clear benefits of using colloids (Roberts, 2011). Despite a lack of benefit, there is also evidence for increased risk of side effects of colloids, including anaphylaxis, coagulopathies, and acute renal dysfunction. A recent meta-analysis of over 10,000 human patients in 38 clinical trials questioned the safety of hetastarch (Zarychanski et al., 2013). When seven trials (590 patients) were excluded due to retraction of the original studies because of scientific misconduct on the part of the lead author, hydroxyethyl starch was found to be associated with increased mortality and increased renal failure (Zarychanski et al., 2013). There are no reports of renal failure secondary to hydroxyethyl starch (HES) administration in horses, and no studies have evaluated mortality in horses receiving colloids, but the results of this meta-analysis raise concern.

There is no similar debate over the use of isotonic crystalloids versus hypertonic saline, because hypertonic saline is regarded as a supplement to, rather than a replacement for, isotonic fluids. Isotonic fluids are electrolyte-containing fluids that have a composition similar to that of the ECF compartment, and have the same or similar osmolarity as equine plasma; the osmolarity ranges from 270 to 308 mOsm/L in these commercial fluids as compared to equine plasma, which has an osmolarity of 270–300 mOsm/L (Carlson & Rumbaugh, 1983; Carlson et al., 1979; Pritchard et al., 2006). They may also contain dextrose or acid–base components (namely, sodium lactate, acetate, or gluconate). These isotonic replacement crystalloids are commonly used to expand the intravascular and interstitial spaces, and do not significantly affect the osmolarity of the ECF in patients with a normal plasma osmolarity. Therefore, there is no osmotic drive for the fluids to distribute intracellularly; as a consequence these fluids are considered replacement products by virtue of the fact that they are primarily ECF expanders.

Isotonic crystalloids distribute among the entire ECF, with approximately 20–25% of the administered volume remaining within the plasma volume, and 75–80% distributing extravascularly to the interstitium under normal circumstances. Hypovolemia results in reduced filtration fraction at the level of the capillary, a higher plasma oncotic pressure, and increased lymphatic return; therefore, a higher percentage of the administered volume may remain within the plasma. Due to this distribution pattern, the maximum hemodynamic effects of crystalloids occur immediately after infusion, because distribution is thought to occur within 30–60 minutes. Conventionally three to four times the estimated intravascular deficit in isotonic crystalloid has been recommended because of this extravascular distribution for cases of controlled, acute hemorrhage or acute hypovolemia (Dutton, 2007). However, due to concerns over interstitial and tissue edema with this approach, some authors have questioned the need for this large volume of fluids (Bauer et al., 2009).

Colloids distribute virtually entirely within the vascular compartment in normal animals; however, animals with systemic inflammatory response syndrome (SIRS) or severe trauma may have altered capillary permeability resulting in increased extravasation of colloid particles into the interstitium. If this occurs, the extravasated colloids would potentiate edema formation by raising interstitial oncotic pressure and increasing interstitial water content.

The administration of both crystalloids and colloids simultaneously or serially has advantages in some circumstances, particularly when concurrent hypovolemia and hypoproteinemia are present as might be present in

Table 12.1 Composition of replacement crystalloids (all values in mEq/L).

Crystalloid	Sodium	Potassium	Chloride	Calcium	Magnesium	Osmolarity	Organic anion
LRS	130	4	109	3	0	272	28 lactate
Saline (0.9%)	154	0	154	0	0	308	0
Plasma-Lyte 148	140	5	98	0	3	295	27 acetate/23 gluconate
Plasma-Lyte A	140	5	98	0	3	295	27 acetate/23 gluconate
Normosol-R	140	5	98	0	3	295	27 acetate/23 gluconate

LRS, lactated Ringer's solution.

horses with acute colitis or foals with *Lawsonia intracellularis* enteropathy. Isotonic and hypertonic crystalloids can be administered in conjunction as a rapid volume-expanding combination in adult horses with such conditions. Plasma can be administered concurrently; however, it should be administered slowly initially to monitor for transfusion reactions. The concerns raised about hetastarch (see earlier) should warrant close monitoring of creatinine concentration in horses administered it.

Isotonic crystalloids (Table 12.1)

Isotonic crystalloids are conveniently available in 5-L bags for use in adult horses. These include 0.9% saline, lactated Ringer's solution (LRS), Plasma-Lyte® A or 148 (Baxter Healthcare Corporation, Deerfield, IL) and Normosol™ R (Abbott Laboratories, North Chicago, IL).

Saline

Isotonic saline solution (0.9%; also termed "normal saline" and "physiological saline") contains only sodium and chloride ions. Because it lacks additional electrolytes or constituents, it is not considered a balanced electrolyte solution like the others. Physiological saline (0.9%) is the author's least preferred isotonic crystalloid for use in horses, except for those with marked hyperkalemia or hypochloremic metabolic alkalosis. The reason for its limited applicability is its tendency to produce hyperchloremic metabolic acidosis (HCMA), which has been noted to occur in both humans and horses (Roche & James, 2009; Stewart, 1983). Normal saline has a higher concentration of sodium and chloride (154 mEq/L of each) than does equine ECF (including plasma). The chloride content is relatively greater than the normal equine ECF or plasma chloride concentration, as compared to the increase in sodium. The normal chloride concentration of horse plasma is approximately 90–102 mEq/L, whereas normal sodium concentration is approximately 130–140 mEq/L. Therefore, saline provides a relatively greater amount of chloride than sodium and the net effect of these differences is that 0.9% saline produces a mild hyperchloremia, which is a form of strong ion acidosis. Another way of looking at this is that the sodium-chloride and strong ion difference of saline is 0, yielding an inorganic acidosis because the normal strong ion difference in horses is approximately 40. Hyperchloremic acidosis has a number of potential adverse effects, including renal afferent arterial vasoconstriction, renal dysfunction, coagulopathies, inflammatory cytokine release, and possibly additional organ dysfunction observed in humans and other species (Chowdhury et al., 2012; Kellum et al., 2004). A retrospective study of human patients who had undergone emergency abdominal surgery showed that patients given saline suffered a higher mortality rate and increased complications including acidosis, infection, renal failure requiring dialysis, blood transfusion, and electrolyte disturbances compared to those administered Plasma-Lyte 148 (Shaw et al., 2012).

One advantage of 0.9% saline in some circumstances is that it is free of potassium and is the only commercially available crystalloid as such. Because it is potassium free, it is a potential volume expander during hyperkalemic crises in horses such as hyperkalemic period paralysis or uroperitoneum. However, administration of large volumes of saline to normokalemic horses could result in dilutional hypokalemia. Saline is also indicated in cases with primary metabolic alkalosis due to hypochloremia, such as competing endurance horses; again, this is because of the effects of saline on raising ECF (and plasma) chloride concentrations. It is also compatible with many drugs, blood products, and sodium bicarbonate. Ideally saline should be avoided in cases of rhabdomyolysis unless severe hyperkalemia is present. The reason for this is that aciduria potentiates myoglobin-induced nephrosis, whereas alkaline urine appears to be protective, at least in humans (Cho et al., 2007).

Lactated Ringer's solution (LRS)

Lactated Ringer's solution is commonly administered to horses; it is a balanced electrolyte solution meaning it is closer to plasma in composition, and contains less chloride and sodium, than saline. Even so, LRS is still mildly hyperchloremic (109 mEq/L) relative to equine plasma (90–102 mEq/L), and it is therefore possible to increase plasma chloride concentration with large-volume or chronic administration of LRS, especially if renal dysfunction is present. The sodium concentration is at the lower limit of normal for horses (130 mEq/L). Therefore, the sodium–chloride difference of LRS is 21 mEq/L, which is smaller than that in the ECF and plasma of horses (~40). The in vivo strong ion difference of LRS (after metabolism of lactate) is 28. This may be a slight disadvantage when treating animals with hyperchloremic or hyponatremic acidoses (e.g., renal tubular acidosis; some forms of gastrointestinal disease), compared to using fluids with a lower chloride and higher sodium concentration, such as Plasma-Lyte 148/A or Normosol-R (Cl=98 mEq/L; Na=140 mEq/L); this also makes LRS slightly acidifying when considering it solely from an electrolyte standpoint independent of the effects of sodium lactate.

Lactated Ringer's solution contains sodium lactate (28 mEq/L as the L-lactate form) as an alkalinizing salt, which is ultimately metabolized to glucose (through gluconeogenesis) or carbon dioxide and water (through oxidation), and in both cases yielding a minor contribution of base. These processes are believed to take approximately 30 minutes. In humans, L-lactate did not accumulate at doses up to 100 mmol/h unless there was severe liver dysfunction (Shin et al., 2011). Racemic LRS should be avoided, as D-lactate is not metabolized by mammalian tissues and is proinflammatory. In the past some commercial formulations of LRS were racemic, but now the majority contain only L-lactate. LRS is not the optimal fluid choice for horses with severe liver disease or failure, because they may have reduced ability to metabolize lactate in the liver (the primary site of lactate metabolism). This inadequate metabolism in the face of large-volume administration could theoretically cause a mild increase in plasma lactate concentration; even so, this will not contribute directly to an acidosis because the lactate in LRS is present as the sodium salt rather than the acid. In addition, dogs with lymphosarcoma do not metabolize lactate normally, but whether this holds true in horses with lymphoma has not been studied (Touret et al., 2010). Lactic acidosis as occurs with hypoperfusion or endotoxemia is not a contraindication to using LRS, as infusion of LRS does not result in an increase in blood lactate (unless the plasma lactate concentration is >9 mmol/L or the horse has significant hepatic dysfunction). In fact, lactate concentrations usually decrease with the associated increase in perfusion after administration of LRS to hypovolemic horses, unless the hepatic dysfunction is severe.

Lactated Ringer's solution should not be administered through the same infusion lines as blood or plasma products because it contains calcium, which will bind citrate or other calcium antagonists present in the anticoagulant. In addition, sodium bicarbonate should not be directly added to LRS because of a potential for precipitation of calcium carbonate. LRS is an excellent replacement fluid choice for cardiopulmonary cerebral resuscitation (CPCR) and situations where rapid volume expansion is required, as with hypovolemic shock. The potassium concentration of LRS is 4 mEq/L and must be considered when treating critically ill horses that are potentially hyperkalemic, such as horses with hyperkalemic periodic paralysis or acute renal failure.

For horses with botulism LRS is an excellent fluid choice because it lacks magnesium and contains calcium. Magnesium can potentiate neuromuscular blockage (Kim et al., 2012). However, if alternatives are available (such as Plasma-Lyte A) LRS should be avoided in cases where calcium is contraindicated or potentially harmful, such as those with myocardial damage from glycoside toxicity (e.g., oleander poisoning or digoxin overdose), and those with brain injury where calcium may play a role in pathogenesis.

Plasma-Lyte 148, Plasma-Lyte A, and Normosol-R

Normosol-R and Plasma-Lyte A or 148 are commercial fluids with the composition most similar to equine plasma in terms of electrolytes. This may make them the most physiologic commercial fluid available for horses, and they are the author's preferred fluid types under most circumstances, except as noted below (Table 12.2).

These fluids (Plasma-Lyte 148, Plasma-Lyte A, and Normosol-R) have an identical composition. The only difference among them is their pH as supplied in the

Table 12.2 Comparison of fluid composition of commercial crystalloids with that of plasma in horses.

	Lactated Ringer's solution	Normal saline	Plasma-Lyte A	Plasma-Lyte 148	Normosol-R	Equine plasma
Sodium (mEq/L)	130	154	140	140	140	130–140
Potassium (mEq/L)	4	0	5	5	5	3.0–4.9
Chloride (mEq/L)	109	154	98	98	98	90–100
Calcium (mEq/L)	3	0	0	0	0	5.7–7.1
Magnesium (mEq/L)	0	0	3	3	3	1.3–1.9
Base (mEq/L)	28L[a]	0	27A 23G[a]	27A 23G[a]	27A 23G[a]	23–32B[a]
Osmolality (mOsm/kg)	272	308	295	295	295	279–296
Calories (kcal/L)	9	0	21	21	21	NA
pH in bag	6.5	5.5	7.4	5.5	6.6	7.36–7.48

[a]L, lactate; A, acetate; G, gluconate; B, bicarbonate.

bag: Plasma-Lyte A has a pH of 7.4, Plasma-Lyte 148 has a pH of 5.5, and Normosol-R has a pH of 6.6, making Plasma-Lyte A the most physiologic. While the titratable acidity contained in each bag is likely negligible relative to patient acid–base physiology, it is possible that the 7.4 pH of Plasma-Lyte A may be best tolerated by the vein endothelium upon entry of the fluid, especially with long-term fluid therapy, but this remains to be studied. These fluids contain magnesium rather than calcium and therefore can be administered along with plasma or blood products and sodium bicarbonate. They contain acetate (27 mEq/L) and gluconate (23 mEq/L) rather than lactate as the alkalinizing salts, which is an advantage for horses with liver dysfunction. These provide more net alkalinizing effect than does LRS. Whereas lactate is primarily metabolized by the liver and kidney, acetate is metabolized by muscle and other tissues in addition to liver and kidney; gluconate is metabolized by a number of tissues and is also excreted unchanged in the urine. Gluconate is metabolized slowly, but there is no evidence of toxicity in clinical or experimental studies. In fact, supraphysiologic concentrations of gluconate have shown protection against post-ischemic myocardial dysfunction and oxidative injury (Murthi et al., 2003).

These "acetated" fluids (Plasma-Lyte and Normosol) have a sodium and chloride content of 140 mEq/L and 98 mEq/L, respectively, yielding a sodium–chloride difference of 42 mEq/L. The sodium:chloride ratio is greater than that of LRS (Na = 130, Cl = 109 mEq/L), yielding a larger simplified strong ion difference (SID), and is similar to that of normal horse plasma or ECF (approximately 40). The "effective" *in vivo* SID (assuming complete metabolism of acetate and gluconate upon administration) of these acetated fluids is:

$$(Na + K + Mg) - (Cl) = (140 + 5 + 3) - (98) = 50 \, mEq/L$$

A fluid with higher SID is advantageous for patients with metabolic acidosis because of the net alkalinizing effect of an increasing SID. The clinical significance of these differences between these fluids and LRS may be small; however, they allow for tailoring of fluid therapy to individual patients. For comparison purposes, the *in vivo* SID of LRS is 28.

There is concern over the vasodilatory properties of concentrated acetate solutions, which contain far more acetate than Plasma-Lyte or Normosol; the hypotension is suspected to be due to acetate-stimulated release of adenosine from the muscle (Bunger & Soboll, 1986). In addition concentrated acetate solutions have demonstrated proinflammatory, myocardial depressant, and hypoxemia-promoting properties in renal replacement fluids, leading to removal of acetate from these fluids (Bingel et al., 1987; Veech & Gitomer, 1988). This has led some clinicians to exhibit empiric caution over the use of commercial acetated replacement solutions such as Plasma-Lyte or Normosol as rapid blood volume resuscitating fluids where vasodilation or hypotension may already be present. However, there is no evidence that the commercial fluids containing acetate have any of the aforementioned effects seen with concentrated and high-dose acetate solutions. In fact, in humans acetate has advantages over L-lactate found in LRS. It is very rapidly metabolized, and up to 300 mmol/h infusion rate is tolerated without significant accumulation (Morgan, 2013). This is far lower than is provided through Plasma-Lyte or Normosol (27 mmol/L). Because acetate is metabolized in several extrahepatic tissues, especially muscle, it is less subject to accumulation than lactate in shock states or with severe liver dysfunction. A study performed by the author in standing, healthy horses did not reveal hypotension associated with rapid boluses of Plasma-Lyte A (40 mL/kg over 30 min) (Hall & Magdesian, 2009).

Because of their lack of calcium, and possibly due to their magnesium content, these fluids are good choices in horses with myocardial damage and necrosis (e.g., oleander toxicity), ventricular dysrhythmias, and brain injury. In addition, they are indicated for use in cases with liver dysfunction where lactate metabolism may be reduced.

Cases where these fluids optimally should be avoided include those where exogenous magnesium is contraindicated, such as animals with botulism or neuromuscular weakness, because magnesium potentiates neuromuscular blockade (Kim et al., 2012). These fluids contain 3 mEq/L of magnesium. In addition, they should not be administered to animals where potassium should be avoided (horses with significant hyperkalemia).

Hypertonic saline

The primary hypertonic crystalloid solution available for small-volume fluid replacement in horses is hypertonic saline (7–7.5%). Hypertonic saline results in a rapid rise in plasma osmolarity (through sodium), causing a shift of extravascular fluids into the vascular space. Initially fluid is shifted from the interstitial compartment, and later from the intracellular fluids, into the intravascular space. Hypertonic saline expands the blood volume by approximately 3.5 times the infused volume, and can expand blood volume by 12% at 30 minutes post-infusion (4 mL/kg) in dogs (Silverstein et al., 2005). In addition to its plasma volume expanding effects, hypertonic saline has a number of other benefits. It has mild inotropic, anti-inflammatory, and anti-edema effects, which may be of benefit in horses with endotoxemia (Bulger et al., 2007). These include mitigation of endothelial and erythrocyte edema (Monafo, 1970; Moylan et al., 1973. It has also demonstrated anti-inflammatory effects in lab animals, with reduced neutrophil activation and lung and bowel injury (Murao et al., 2003a,b). Anti-inflammatory effects have also been shown in humans (Junger et al., 1997). Whether the inotropic effects of hypertonic saline are direct or indirect remains to be proven, but it has been shown to increase cardiac contractility in experimentally induced hemorrhagic shock in horses (Schmall et al., 1990). Hypertonic saline can be utilized to treat increased intracranial pressure as occurs with head trauma. In limited studies with isovolume administration, hypertonic saline has demonstrated similar to greater efficacy as mannitol, though additional studies are required especially using different dosages of each drug (Vialet et al., 2003).

Administered doses of hypertonic saline should not exceed 4 mL/kg in order to prevent dangerous hypernatremia. It should be administered along with isotonic crystalloids, as the plasma expansion effects are transient and short-lived. Contraindications to administration of hypertonic saline include pre-existing hypernatremia or hyperosmolarity and uncontrolled hemorrhage, as it can cause transient increases in blood pressure, which may interfere with clot stabilization. Serum sodium should not be allowed to rise more than 12 mEq/L in a 24-hour period, in order to prevent central pontine myelinolysis (Laureno & Karp, 1997). Hypertonic saline should be used with caution in neonatal foals, as they appear less tolerant of rapid swings in plasma sodium concentrations. In animals with marked dehydration, isotonic crystalloids should be administered prior to or at the same time as hypertonic saline to provide fluid volume to be drawn back into the vascular space. Given that the sodium to chloride difference is 0, hypertonic saline is also mildly acidifying as is isotonic saline.

Colloids

Colloids have the theoretical advantage of primarily intravascular distribution; this could lead to more rapid plasma volume expansion than a similar volume of isotonic crystalloids, which distribute among the entirety of the ECF. Colloids are iso-osmotic and hence do not alter the intracellular fluid volume directly. In normal horses colloids raise plasma colloid osmotic pressure (COP) and lead to plasma expansion. However, horses with SIRS or sepsis often have altered vascular integrity, which can lead to increased permeability to colloids as well as to water. This makes the administration of colloids somewhat challenging in critically ill horses. Large volumes of crystalloids could potentiate pulmonary edema in horses with acute respiratory distress syndrome (ARDS), making colloids an attractive choice of fluids for these cases. However, without knowledge of the state of the capillary permeability to proteins, it is impossible to know whether administered colloids would also extravasate into the lungs and actually potentiate pulmonary edema. Because of this, the author cautions against the use of colloids in horses with ARDS; deterioration of clinical signs (respiratory rate, respiratory effort), oxygen saturation (S_pO_2), or arterial blood gas parameters (P_aO_2) after colloid administration warrants reconsideration of colloid use. Horses receiving colloids should be serially monitored for development or worsening of edema.

Colloids have been in the medical news recently due to the discovery that a clinical trial published by Professor Joachim Boldt (Riesmeier et al., 2009) had some fabricated components. This has cast some doubt on the authenticity of other studies by the same author and a number of his published studies have been retracted. These events have called the safety of colloids into question for use in human patients. In addition, a recent meta-analysis evaluated critically ill patients requiring acute volume resuscitation with hetastarch versus other fluids (Zarychanski et al., 2013). The results of this meta-analysis, which included 38 trials and 10,880 patients, showed that hetastarch did not decrease mortality. Moreover, when seven trials (590 patients) by Boldt were excluded due to retraction, hydroxyethyl starch was found to be associated with increased mortality among the remaining 10,290 patients (RR 1.90; 95% CI: 1.02–1.17). In addition, there was increased renal failure among patients who received HES (Zarychanski et al, 2013).

These concerns aside, it should also be noted that several studies performed over decades have failed to show a benefit of colloids over crystalloids for volume resuscitation in terms of mortality among human patients. The 2011 Cochrane review of colloids versus crystalloids concluded that there is no evidence from randomized controlled trials (whether or not the trials by Boldt et al. were removed from analyses) that fluid replacement with colloids reduces the risk of death as compared to resuscitation with crystalloids in critically ill human patients, including trauma, burn, and postoperative patients (Perel & Roberts, 2011). The review concluded that "As colloids are not associated with an improvement in survival, and as they are more expensive than crystalloids, it is hard to see how their continued use in these patients can be justified outside the context of RCTs" (Perel & Roberts, 2011).

Plasma and hetastarch are the main colloids available for use in horses. The most commonly utilized synthetic colloids in veterinary practice include dextran-70 and hydroxyethyl starch (hetastarch). Dextran-70 is a 6% solution with particles ranging from 15,000 to 3,400,000 daltons. The number average molecular weight (M_n) is 41,000, average molecular weight (M_w) is 70,000 daltons, and its colloid osmotic pressure (COP) is 60 mmHg. Dextrans are associated with an increased risk of side effects (coagulopathies, allergic reactions, and renal failure) as compared to hetastarch and have similar cost, therefore they offer no advantage over hetastarch.

Hetastarch is also available as a 6% solution, with a molecular weight range of 10,000 to 1,000,000 daltons, and an average molecular weight (M_w) of 450,000 daltons. The number average molecular (M_n) weight is 69,000 daltons, with a COP of 30–34 mmHg. The substitution ratio of number of hydroxyethyl groups per 10 molecules of glucose is also used to define hetastarch. Hydroxyethyl starch is available as suspended in either isotonic saline (Hespan®) or in a lactated electrolyte solution similar to LRS (Hextend®). These are defined as 450/0.7, meaning they have an average molecular weight of 450,000 daltons and a substitution ratio of 0.7.

Hetastarch has dose-dependent effects on coagulation. These include interference with platelet function and induction of a von Willebrand-like state with reduction in plasma factor VIII concentrations and activity of von Willebrand factor (vWf) antigen (Jones et al., 1997). Studies in horses have demonstrated dose-dependent prolongation in partial thromboplastin time (PTT) with hetastarch at doses of 15 mL/kg but not after 10 mL/kg (Reickhoff et al., 2002). Because of these effects on coagulation and platelets, colloids should not be used in hemorrhaging patients and those with significant thrombocytopenia or prolonged clotting times. In human sepsis, hetastarch rarely has been reported with induction of hyperoncotic renal injury (Zarychanski et al., 2013). Although there are no reports of this in horses, hetastarch should be used with caution in horses with renal dysfunction until more specific information is available. In a study evaluating the administration of hetastarch in hypoproteinemic horses with GI diseases, COP exhibited an increase above baseline for 6 h after administration of 8–10 mL/kg/d, whereas in another study in normal ponies, hetastarch (10–20 mL/kg/d) increased COP above baseline for up to 5 days (Jones et al., 1997, 2001). Beyond the 6-hour increase in horses with GI diseases, oncotic pressure was maintained for up to 24 hours in the face of decreasing total protein and albumin concentrations.

Pentastarch is a more homogenous, in terms of molecular weight variability, derivative of hetastarch. Its average molecular weight is lower than hetastarch, being 264,000–280,000 daltons. However, the number average MW is higher than hetastarch (120,000 daltons), making pentastarch more homogenous than hetastarch. The COP of pentastarch is 40 mmHg, as compared to 30 mmHg for hetastarch, providing more profound increases in COP and efficient volume expansion as compared to hetastarch. Pentastarch has additional advantages, in that it is associated with fewer adverse effects on coagulation in humans. It also has fewer low molecular weight particles that could escape extravascularly through compromised vasculature. Pentastarch is not currently available in the USA. Tetrastarches (e.g. Vetstarch) are currently available in the U.S. They may be associated with fewer side effects than hetastarch, however further studies are required.

Plasma is not well suited for use as a replacement fluid; it must be thawed slowly to prevent denaturation of proteins, and rapid bolus administration should be avoided due to the potential for anaphylaxis, anaphylactoid, and other adverse reactions (Wilson et al., 2009). Plasma has the benefits of providing albumin, antithrombin, and specific antibodies. Potential disadvantages other than the adverse inflammatory reactions include the provision of additional clotting factors to horses that may already be prothrombotic, such as those with "DIC" at the end of this sentence that currently ends with 'already be prothrombotic.' i.e., the sentence should read: 'already be prothrombotic', such as those with DIC. Human albumin solution and plasma protein fraction are used as colloids in human patients; however,a recent Cochrane review (Bunn et al., 2011) comparing different types of colloids (both natural and synthetic) found no evidence that one colloid solution is more effective or safer than any other. However, many comparisons had wide confidence intervals and therefore warrant larger randomized clinical trials. The reader is referred to the chapters on Colloids (Chapter 24) and Blood transfusions (Chapter 23) for more information on colloid use in horses.

Rate of administration

Predicting the volume and rate of fluid required to resolve hypovolemia and dehydration in horses is difficult. Signs of dehydration (reduced skin turgor, tacky membranes) can be insensitive, and deciphering the distribution of fluid deficits (plasma, interstitium, intracellular) based on clinical signs is even less accurate.

Clinical signs of hypovolemia, such as tachycardia and decreased extremity temperature, are also somewhat insensitive. Indicators of extravascular losses (i.e., dehydration), such as mucous membrane dryness and skin test, were not valid or repeatable measures of dehydration in one study of working horses (Pritchard et al., 2006). Both fluid overload and persistent hypovolemia are detrimental and can result in organ dysfunction, reflecting the importance of careful fluid resuscitation.

The traditional approach to estimating fluid deficits and planning replacement strategies has been to assign a percentage dehydration to a patient based on clinical signs. A horse with moderate dehydration would have 5–6% dehydration, marked dehydration would be indicative of 8–10% dehydration, and severe dehydration would be as much as 10–15% dehydrated. Because of the inaccuracy of estimating fluid deficits based on physical examination indicators, and the near impossibility of correctly predicting the amount of deficit from the varying fluid compartments, there is considerable error with this approach.

A simpler and potentially safer approach to replacement fluid therapy than trying to calculate absolute fluid deficits and one that is likely subject to fewer complications is that of the "fluid challenge"; this is a method for guiding fluid repletion in human critical care (Vincent & Weil, 2006). This technique allows for prompt correction of fluid deficits in hypovolemic patients, while minimizing the risks of fluid overload and edema through an incremental approach and frequent reassessment.

With the fluid challenge method, defined volumes of fluid are administered rapidly over predetermined intervals until either: (i) clinical signs and laboratory indicators of hypoperfusion abate or plateau, or (ii) central venous pressures increase to a maximum safe level (12 and 15 cmH$_2$O in foals and horses, respectively). It should be noted that central venous pressure (CVP) does not always accurately predict intravascular preload and volume, because it is also dependent on other physiologic influences such as ventricular compliance and afterload. However, CVP can serve as an accurate "cap" or upper limit to fluid loading in horses. Clinical parameters that are markers of improvement in volume status include heart rate (less reliable in neonatal foals), extremity temperature, capillary refill time, pulse quality, jugular refill, mentation, blood lactate, packed cell volume, total protein concentration, and arterial blood pressure (Box 12.1). While any one of these perfusion

---

> **Box 12.1 Clinical perfusion parameters in horses.**
>
> - Mentation
> - Heart rate
> - Extremity temperature (ears, limbs)
> - Mucous membrane color
> - Capillary refill time
> - Pulse quality
> - Jugular refill
> - Urine output (if present indicates renal perfusion)

parameters or tools may not be definitive, the combination of several is useful to assess response to fluid loading. Urine output in particular is an important marker of adequacy of end-organ perfusion as represented by the kidney, and is a very practical guide to replacement fluid therapy; the production of moderately dilute urine is one end-point to fluid bolus administration in horses.

Guidelines for fluid administration rates with the fluid challenge method include giving 6–20 mL/kg of isotonic crystalloid over 20–30 minutes, followed by reassessment of the clinical and laboratory perfusion parameters (Ribeiro et al., 2009; Vincent & Weil, 2006). Which end of the range (6 vs 20 mL/kg) is used depends on the degree of hypovolemia and signs of shock. These incremental infusions are repeated over 30–60 minutes until either perfusion parameters improve (e.g., urine production begins), they plateau (i.e., no further improvement in the clinical indicators of perfusion), or limits to fluid loading are reached (especially CVP ceilings, other markers such as edema are insensitive) (Corley, 2002). Most hypovolemic horses require two to three boluses of 10–20 mL/kg (e.g., 10–20 L total for a 500-kg horse) before the rate can be decreased from bolus administration to a maintenance or twice maintenance rate. The number of these fluid challenges is determined by serial reassessment of clinical, laboratory, and monitoring indicators of perfusion. The importance of reassessment is reflected in avoidance of excessive administration of isotonic crystalloids, because of risks of tissue edema, worsened tissue oxygenation, and possibly even compartment syndrome in organs (Ribeiro et al., 2009).

If colloids are selected as part or all of the initial replacement fluid, a smaller volume should be administered due to relative greater retention within the vascular space (unless capillary permeability is abnormally increased). Doses of 3–10 mL/kg can be used for

hetastarch, although a total daily dose of 10 mL/kg should not be exceeded due to the risk of coagulopathies at higher doses. The primary indication for colloid use in horses is the presence of concurrent hypovolemia and hypoproteinemia. Colloids should be administered along with or shortly following administration of isotonic fluids because they do not rehydrate the interstitial space. The volume of colloid administered should replace three to four times that in isotonic crystalloid, because only approximately one-quarter of isotonic crystalloid would remain within the vascular space. For example, 1 L of hetastarch should replace approximately 3 L of LRS in the initial fluid plan. If hypertonic saline (7–7.5%) is used for initial fluid resuscitation it should be coadministered with isotonic fluids because its effects are transient and the hypernatremia and hyperchloremia it induces must be corrected.

Objectives of replacement fluid therapy

The primary goal of fluid administration during the replacement phase is to re-establish tissue perfusion. The immediate priority is restoration of circulating volume in order to increase blood pressure. Hypovolemia may be absolute or relative; absolute hypovolemia occurs with either external or internal losses of circulating plasma volume. Examples of external losses of plasma volume include acute hemorrhage and diarrhea, whereas internal losses may include increased capillary permeability with expansion of the interstitial space and third spacing of fluids (effusions). Hypovolemia may also be relative; this occurs when venous capacitance increases with venodilation, due to release of inflammatory mediators as might occur during sepsis or SIRS, or with administration of anesthetic agents or vasodilatory pharmaceuticals.

Replenishment of interstitial losses is next in priority after plasma volume replacement. The interstitium serves as a reserve for plasma volume, as they are both components of the ECF. Finally, intracellular losses can be replaced more slowly, often over several hours as third in priority for the fluid replacement phase. Additional immediate goals in fluid therapy include addressing acid–base and electrolyte abnormalities. The primary metabolic acid–base derangement with hypovolemia is lactic acidosis, although sodium and chloride abnormalities can also contribute to overall acid–base balance.

Specific goals during replacement fluid therapy include normalization of clinical perfusion parameters: mentation, heart rate, extremity temperature, pulse quality, mucous membrane color, capillary refill time, and urine

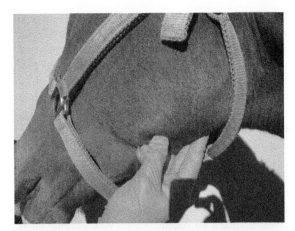

Figure 12.1 Palpation of the facial artery for pulse quality.

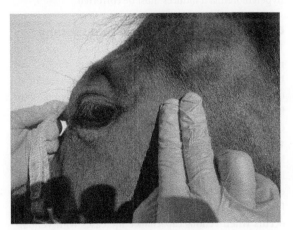

Figure 12.2 Palpation of the transverse facial artery for pulse quality.

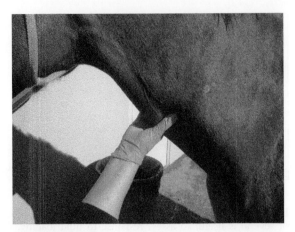

Figure 12.3 Jugular fill as a physical exam marker of blood volume status in horses.

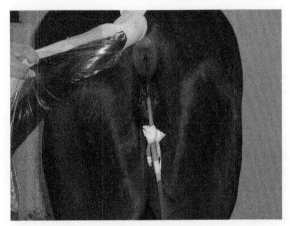

Figure 12.4 Urinary catheter placed in a mare.

production. Pulse quality can be palpated along the facial or transverse facial artery (Figures 12.1 and 12.2). Jugular fill can be used as another indirect marker of blood volume, except in horses with heart failure or intrathoracic disease, because of the ease of visualization and palpation of the jugular vein in this species (Figure 12.3). Urine production is a key indicator of the adequacy of fluid bolus loading. Urine can be measured through catheterization, which is particularly easy to perform in mares (Figure 12.4). Once urine flow begins, the replacement phase of fluid therapy can generally be slowed and maintenance fluid therapy or multiples thereof if necessary (including ongoing losses or diuresis if desired) can begin. Laboratory perfusion parameters include lactate concentration, venous oxygen saturation and oxygen extraction ratio, urine specific gravity, serial packed cell volume, and serial total protein concentrations. Ultimately, improvement in arterial blood pressure is sought as a marker of the potential for adequate tissue perfusion. An increase in mean arterial blood pressure to or over 60 mmHg is a reasonable minimal goal, with normalization of pressure optimal. Arterial blood pressure can be measured using an indirect blood pressure monitor and tail cuff over the coccygeal artery (Figure 12.5). Optimizing filling pressures, most practically in the form of central venous pressure (CVP), is a controversial goal of fluid replacement. There is considerable debate over the value of CVP as an indicator of volume status. While this is controversial, CVP is a reasonable indicator of a limit to fluid loading as discussed above.

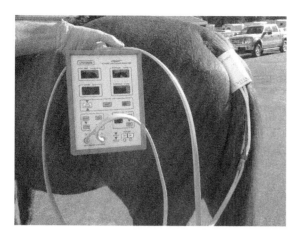

Figure 12.5 Indirect arterial pressure measurement.

Limits to fluid therapy

The primary clinical limit to fluid administration is edema. Edema can be immediately life threatening in the form of pulmonary edema, particularly in adult horses with SIRS that have increased capillary permeability and reduced oncotic pressure, or those with ARDS. Slower onset edema can have consequences on tissue oxygenation and organ dysfunction through "secondary" compartment syndromes (Roche & James, 2009). "Secondary compartment syndrome" is a form of abdominal compartment syndrome in the absence of abdominal injury, and is thought to be a consequence of early and overzealous crystalloid administration. In addition, oxygen diffusion distance is increased when tissue edema is present. The risks of edema and compartment syndrome in response to fluid therapy are receiving renewed interest and they are associated with worse outcomes in human patients (Roche & James, 2009; Sakr et al., 2005; Van Biesen et al 2005). Another potential drawback of excessive fluid administration is induction of inflammatory cytokine release; this has been demonstrated to occur with administration of some types of fluids, such as physiological saline or racemic LRS.

Despite these cautions against overhydration, under-resuscitation of hypovolemia has its own risks of organ injury through inadequate oxygen delivery and hypoperfusion; these potential adverse effects warrant close and repetitive monitoring of patients undergoing replacement fluid therapy.

Colloids have been regarded as having a reduced predilection for interstitial edema; however, recently

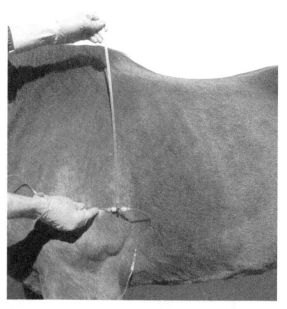

Figure 12.6 Central venous pressure measurement with a water manometer.

this has been questioned. During volume loading, if the volume of colloid administered is greater than the actual blood volume deficit, then the colloids may distribute extravascularly. Up to 60% of the infused volume can distribute into the interstitial space (Jacob et al., 2009; Rehm et al., 2001). Therefore, colloid administration should be monitored as closely and frequently as is recommended for crystalloid administration.

Identification of under- or overloading of fluid therapy in the clinical setting is difficult. Filling pressures, usually measured as CVP, can be misleading as indicators of volume repletion. However, they are likely reasonable indicators of ceilings or limits to fluid loading. That is, once a high normal CVP is reached – 12–15 cmH$_2$O (8.8–11.0 mmHg) in adult horses – fluid bolus administration should cease (Figure 12.6). CVP can be measured with a water manometer or a pressure transducer for continuous recordings. If a water manometer is used, it can be taped to a fluid pole to allow for the same reference point for every reading, for consistent readings (Figure 12.7). At that point fluid therapy should be changed over to maintenance fluid requirements in addition to ongoing losses or slightly higher rates for fluid diuresis.

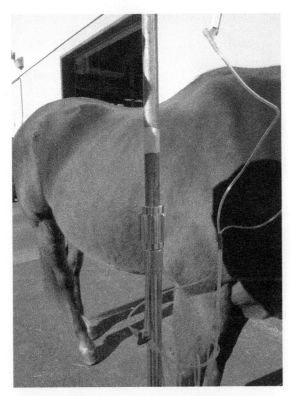

Figure 12.7 Water manometer is taped to the fluid pole for consistent readings.

Exceeding these CVP values could result in edema formation. Unfortunately CVP measurement in the adult horse requires specialized catheterization and is therefore not performed on a routine basis. Hence, the clinician must rely on other clinical parameters as indicators of fluid overload. Measurement of CVP is certainly warranted in disease states where blood volume status is of critical importance and hypervolemia could lead to significant adverse effects; these include oliguric or anuric renal failure, heart failure, and ARDS.

When CVP is not measured, other less sensitive markers of limits to fluid administration must be relied upon. These include a decrease in arterial oxygen saturation during fluid loading. A drop in the S_aO_2 or P_aO_2 during fluid therapy, without another obvious cause, warrants reassessment of fluid volume. An increase in respiratory rate or character is another possible indicator of development of pulmonary edema and fluid overload, but is not very sensitive.

Because there are no practical, highly sensitive, and reliable indicators of fluid overload available for the clinical setting, indicators of circulating volume adequacy can be used as end-points to bolus administration in order to avoid fluid overload. Urine production is a very useful and important indicator of end-organ perfusion. Therefore, once urine flow begins the bolus rates can usually be slowed. The presence of dilute urine production is an indirect marker of renal perfusion and therefore circulating volume adequacy. Though serial body weight measurement is a useful means of monitoring maintenance fluid therapy, it is not useful during replacement fluid therapy because weight gain is expected.

Conclusion

Fluid resuscitation of hypovolemic horses is challenging and dynamic. Fluid delivery is highly individual and varies from patient to patient. The "fluid challenge" method of fluid replacement with serial reassessment used in human critical care is a safe means of providing volume replacement rapidly and can be applied to horses. The decades-long debate over whether crystalloids or colloids are more effective for fluid resuscitation has not yielded definitive support for either. Because of recent meta-analyses demonstrating increased mortality and morbidity with the use of hetastarch, as well as increased costs, isotonic crystalloids should remain the mainstay of replacement fluid therapy in horses; colloid use should be regarded as a supplement when concurrent hypovolemia and hypoproteinemia are present. There has been a movement away from 0.9% saline as the crystalloid of choice for treatment of hypovolemia in human patients, due to its propensity to cause hyperchloremic metabolic acidosis and the associated deleterious effects. Saline has been shown to cause HCMA in horses as well and therefore balanced electrolyte solutions may be more physiologic for horses than 0.9% saline. The commercial acetated fluids (Plasma-Lyte, Normosol) may be more ideal for use in horses, as their electrolyte composition is close to that of equine plasma. Hypertonic saline has several hemodynamic and physiologic benefits and is useful as an adjunct to isotonic fluids in volume resuscitation of horses.

References

Bauer M, Korgten A, Hartog C, et al. (2009) Isotonic and hypertonic crystalloid solutions in the critically ill. *Best Pract Res Clin Anaesth* **23**:173–81.

Bingel M, Lonnemann G, Koch KM, et al. (1987) Enhancement of in-vitro human interleukin-1 production by sodium acetate. *Lancet* **i**:14–16.

Bulger EM, Cuschieri J, Warner K, et al. (2007) Hypertonic resuscitation modulates the inflammatory response in patients with traumatic hemorrhagic shock. *Ann Surg* **245**:635–41.

Bunger R, Soboll S. (1986) Cytosolic adenylates and adenosine release in perfused working hearts. *Eur J Biochem* **159**:203–13.

Bunn F, Trivedi D, Ashraf S. (2011) Colloid solutions for fluid resuscitation. Cochrane Database Syst Rev (Art. no. CD001319). doi: 10.1002/14651858.CD001319.pub3.

Carlson GP, Rumbaugh GE, Harrold D. (1979) Physiologic alterations in the horse produced by food and water deprivation during periods of high environmental temperatures. *Am J Vet Res* **40**:982–5.

Carlson GP, Rumbaugh GE. (1983) Response to saline solution of normally fed horses and horses dehydrated by fasting. *Am J Vet Res* **44**:964–8.

Cho YS, Lim H, Kim SH. (2007) Comparison of lactated Ringer's solution and 0.9% saline in the treatment of rhabdomyolysis induced by doxylamine intoxication. *Emerg Med J* **24**:276.

Chowdhury AH, Cox EF, Francis ST, et al. (2012) A randomized, controlled, double-blind crossover study on the effects of 2-L infusions of 0.9% saline and Plasma-Lyte(R) 148 on renal blood flow velocity and renal cortical tissue perfusion in healthy volunteers. *Ann Surg* **256**:18–24.

Corley KTT. (2002) Monitoring and treating hemodynamic disturbances in critically ill neonatal foals. Part II: assessment and treatment. *Eq Vet Educ* **14**:328–36.

Dutton RP. (2007) Current concepts in hemorrhagic shock. *Anesth Clin* **25**:23–34.

Hall TL, Magdesian KG. (2009) Acid-base and blood pressure effects of physiologic saline compared to PlasmaLyte A in horses. *J Vet Emerg Crit Care* **19**(S1):A11–A12.

Jacob M, Chappell D, Rehm M. (2009) The 'third space' – fact or fiction? *Best Pract Res Clin Anaesth* **23**:145–57.

Jones PA, Tomasic M, Gentry PA. (1997) Oncotic hemodilutional, and hemostatic effects of isotonic saline and hydroxyethyl starch solutions in clinically normal ponies. *Am J Vet Res* **58**:541–8.

Jones PA, Bain FT, Byars TD, et al. (2001) Effect of hydroxyethyl starch infusion on colloid oncotic pressure in hypoproteinemic horses. *J Am Vet Med Assoc* **218**;1130–5.

Junger WG, Coimbra R, Liu FC, et al. (1997) Hypertonic saline resuscitation: a tool to modulate immune function in trauma patients? *Shock* **8**:235–41.

Kaplan LJ, Kellum JA. (2010) Fluids, pH, ions and electrolytes. *Curr Opin Crit Care* **16**:323–31.

Kellum JA, Song M, Venkataraman R. (2004) Effects of hyperchloremic acidosis on arterial pressure and circulating inflammatory molecules in experimental sepsis. *Chest* **125**:243–8.

Kim MH, Oh AY, Jeon YT, et al. (2012) A randomized controlled trial comparing rocuronium priming, magnesium pretreatment and a combination of the two methods. *Anaesthesia* **67**:748–54.

Kirchheim HR, Ehmke H, Hackenthal E, Lowe W, Persson P. (1987) Autoregulation of renal blood flow, glomerular filtration rate and renin release in conscious dogs. *Pflugers Arch* **410**:441–9.

Laureno R, Karp BI. (1997) Myelinolysis after correction of hyponatremia. *Ann Intern Med* **126**:57–62.

Monafo WW. (1970) The treatment of burn shock by the intravenous and oral administration of hypertonic lactated saline solution. *J Trauma* **10**:575–86.

Morgan TJ. (2013) The ideal crystalloid – what is "balanced"? *Curr Opin Crit Care* **19**:299–307.

Moylan JA, Reckler JM, Mason AD Jr. (1973) Resuscitation with hypertonic lactate saline in thermal injury. *Am J Surg* **125**:580–4.

Murao Y, Loomis W, Wolf P, et al. (2003a) Effect of dose of hypertonic saline on its potential to prevent lung tissue damage in a mouse model of hemorrhagic shock. *Shock* **20**:29–34.

Murao Y, Hata M, Ohnishi K, et al. (2003b) Hypertonic saline resuscitation reduces apoptosis and tissue damage of the small intestine in a mouse model of hemorrhagic shock. *Shock* **20**:23–8.

Murthi SB, Wise RM, Weglicki WB, et al. (2003) Mg-gluconate provides superior protection against postischemic dysfunction and oxidative injury compared to Mg-sulfate. *Mol Cell Biochem* **245**:141–8.

Patanwala AE, Amini A, Erstad BL. (2010) Use of hypertonic saline injection in trauma. *Am J Health Syst Pharm* **67**:1920–8.

Perel P, Roberts I. (2011) Colloid versus crystalloids for fluid resuscitation in critically ill patients (review). *Cochrane Database Syst Rev* **3**. doi: 10.1002/14651858.CD000567.pub4.

Pritchard JC, Barr AR, Whay HR. (2006) Validity of a behavioural measure of heat stress and a skin tent test for dehydration in working horses and donkeys. *Equine Vet J* **38**:433–8.

Rehm M, Haller M, Orth V, et al. (2001) Changes in blood volume and hematocrit during acute preoperative volume loading with 5% albumin or 6% hetastarch solutions in patients before radical hysterectomy. *Anesthesiology* **95**:849–56.

Reickhoff K, Forster H, Weidhase R, et al. (2002) Administration of 10% hydroxyethyl starch 200/0.5 solution in normovolaemic horses. In: *Scientific Proceedings, 7th International Equine Colic Research Symposium*. Manchester, UK: British Equine Veterinary Association, p. 23.

Riesmeier A, Schellhaass A, Boldt J, Suttner S. (2009) Crystalloid/colloid versus crystalloid intravascular volume administration before spinal anesthesia in elderly patients: the influence on cardiac output and stroke volume. *Anesth Analg* **108**:650–4 [now retracted].

Roberts PP . (2011) Colloids versus crystalloids for fluid resuscitation in critically ill patients (Review). *Cochrane Database Syst Rev Issue* **3**: CD000567.

Roche AM, James MFM. (2009a) Colloids and crystalloids: does it matter to the kidney? *Curr Opin Crit Care* **15**:520–4.

Roche AM, James MFM. (2009b) Colloids and crystalloids: does it matter to the kidney? *Curr Opin Crit Care* **15**:520–4

Ribeiro Jr MA, Epstein MG, Alves LD. (2009) Volume replacement in trauma. *Turk J Trauma Emerg Surg* **15**:311–16.

Sakr Y, Vincent JL, Reinhart K, et al. (2005) High tidal volume and positive fluid balance are associated with worse outcome in acute lung injury. *Chest* **128**:3098–108.

Schertel ER, Schneider DA, Zissimos AG. (1996) Evaluation of a hypertonic sodium chloride dextran solution for treatment of traumatic shock in dogs, *J Am Vet Med Assoc* **208**:366.

Schmall LM, Muir WW, Robertson JT. (1990) Haemodynamic effects of small volume hypertonic saline in experimentally induced haemorrhagic shock. *Equine Vet J* **22**:273–7.

Shaw AD, Bagshaw SM, Goldstein SL, et al. (2012) Major complications, mortality, and resource utilization after open abdominal surgery: 0.9% saline compared to Plasma-Lyte. *Ann Surg* **255**:821–9.

Shin WJ, Kim YK, Bang JY, et al. (2011) Lactate and liver function tests after living donor right hepatectomy: a comparison of solutions with and without lactate. *Acta Anaesthesiol Scand* **55**:558–64.

Silverstein DC, Aldrich J, Haskins SC, et al. (2005) Assessment of changes in blood volume in response to resuscitative fluid administration in dogs. *J Vet Emerg Crit Care* **15**:185.

Stewart PA. (1983) Modern quantitative acid-base chemistry. *Can J Physiol Pharmacol* **61**:1444–61.

Touret M, Boysen RS, Madeau ME. (2010) Prospective evaluation of clinically relevant hyperlactatemia in dogs with cancer. *J Vet Int Med* **24**:1458–61.

Vail DM, Ogilvie Gk, Fettman MJ. (1990) Exacerbation of hyperlactatemia by infusion of lactated ringer's solution in dogs with lymphoma. *J Vet Int Med* **4**; 228–32.

Van Biesen W, Yegenaga I, Vanholder R, et al. (2005) Relationship between fluid status and its management on acute renal failure (ARF) in intensive care unit (ICU) patients with sepsis: a prospective analysis. *J Nephrol* **18**:54–60.

Veech RL, Gitomer WL. (1988) The medical and metabolic consequences of administration of sodium acetate. *Adv Enzyme Regul* **27**:313–43.

Vialet R, Albanese J, Thomachot L, et al. (2003) Isovolume hypertonic solutes (sodium chloride or mannitol) in the treatment of refractory posttraumatic intracranial hypertension: 2 mL/kg 7.5% saline is more effective than 2 mL/kg 20% mannitol. *Crit Care Med* **31**:1683–7.

Vincent JL, Weil MH. (2006) Fluid challenge revisited. *Crit Care Med* **34**:1333–7.

Wilson EM, Holcombe SJ, Lamar A, et al. (2009) Incidence of transfusion reactions and retention of procoagulant and anticoagulant factor activities in equine plasma. *J Vet Int Med* **23**:323–8.

Zarychanski R, Abou-Setta AH, Turgeon AF, et al. (2013) Association of hydroxyethyl starch administration with mortality and acute kidney injury in critically ill patients requiring volume resuscitation: a systematic review and meta-analysis. *JAMA* **309**:678–88.

CHAPTER 13

Maintenance fluid therapy in horses

K. Gary Magdesian

Professor in Critical Care and Emergency Medicine, School of Veterinary Medicine, University of California, Davis, CA, USA

Introduction

Maintenance fluid therapy is the provision of fluid and electrolytes necessary to maintain homeostasis of body water and electrolyte content on a daily basis. Maintenance fluids are generally considered to be hypotonic, unless free water needs are met through drinking; maintenance fluids often contain a higher concentration of potassium than do replacement fluids intended for the extracellular fluid (ECF) as potassium is the primary intracellular cation. Potassium may become deficient in horses off feed and receiving IV fluids without potassium supplementation. Provision of free water through hypotonic fluids allows for hydration of the intracellular space as well as the ECF in horses not allowed access to oral water. Because maintenance fluids distribute into all body fluid compartments, including the intracellular fluid space, they should not be administered as a bolus; rapid administration could predispose to development of tissue edema, with concerns over cerebral or pulmonary edema. In addition to electrolytes, maintenance fluids may also contain dextrose; these dextrose-containing maintenance fluids may be isotonic *in vitro*, but effectively hypotonic as soon as dextrose is metabolized *in vivo*.

Fluid physiology of horses

The key to understanding maintenance fluid and electrolyte requirements in horses is to recognize that they originate with basal metabolic needs. Metabolic rate is relatively high in the neonatal foal, and decreases to become much lower in adult horses. Because of this decline in metabolic rate, adult horses generate less heat and waste solutes from metabolism per unit body weight than do foals; this decreases the fluid and electrolyte requirements per unit of body weight as both heat dissipation (through insensible evaporative skin losses and exhalation of water vapor) and elimination of waste products (through urine) require water. Because of the distinct requirements of foals, fluid therapy for the foal is discussed in a separate chapter (Chapter 22).

Water is the major component of body mass in horses, comprising approximately 61–71% of adult body mass (0.61–0.71 L/kg) (Andrews et al., 1997; Fielding et al., 2004; Forro et al., 2000; Julian et al., 1956; Spurlock et al., 1985). The extracellular fluid (ECF) volume consists of plasma, interstitial, lymph, and transcellular fluids, and ranges from 21 to 31% (0.21–0.31 L/kg) of body mass (Carlson et al., 1979a,b; Crandall & Anderson, 1934; Epstein, 1984; Evans, 1971; Fielding et al., 2004; Kohn et al., 1978; Muir et al., 1978). Extracellular water is therefore approximately 33 to 40% of total body water (TBW).

Plasma is estimated to be 5–6% of body weight. Interstitial and lymphatic fluids are approximately 8–10%, and transcellular fluid is 6–8% of body weight (Schott, 2011). The transcellular fluid consists primarily of gastrointestinal fluid (feces comprise 71–81% water), although body cavity, cerebrospinal fluid (CSF), joint, and aqueous fluids are additional transcellular components. Intracellular fluid is 40–46% of body weight (0.46±0.06 L/kg), and represents about two-thirds of TBW in horses (Fielding et al., 2004).

Movement of water between the subcompartments of the ECF, namely the plasma and interstitial spaces, is governed by Starling's forces. These include the gradient between capillary and interstitial hydrostatic pressure (favors filtration), the gradient between capillary and interstitial oncotic pressure (counters filtration), and permeability characteristics of the endothelium. The interaction of these physiological variables is illustrated in the Starling equation:

$$J_v = K_f \left[\left(P_c - P_i \right) - \sigma \left(\pi_c - \pi_i \right) \right] \qquad (13.1)$$

where :

J_v = net fluid movement;
P_c = capillary hydrostatic pressure;
P_i = interstitial hydrostatic pressure;
π_c = capillary oncotic pressure;
π_i = interstitial oncotic pressure;
K_f = filtration coefficient;
σ = reflection coefficient.

The movement of water between the ECF and intracellular fluid (ICF) is governed by osmotic forces, as these are maintained in osmotic equilibrium. The ECF (and therefore plasma) osmolality is maintained in a narrow range of 280–300 mOsm/kg in horses (Lumsden et al., 1980).

Water balance, which is at the core of determining fluid maintenance needs, is the difference between fluid input and output. Fluid intake is through water and feed, whereas losses occur through urine, feces, and insensible evaporative losses through sweat and respiratory secretions (Table 13.1).

Because fecal losses account for 30–55% of daily water loss, horses off feed and defecating minimally require less fluid intake than those that are eating and defecating regularly; rates as low as 0.75–1.0 mL/kg/h have been suggested as being adequate based on resultant urine specific gravity of 1.010–1.020, but this requires further study (Schott, 2011). Horses eating alfalfa-timothy hay in one study produced a urine volume of 5.5 L per horse per day, yielding 12.5 mL/kg/day, or 0.52 mL/kg/h (range: 0.38–0.75 mL/kg/h) (Tasker, 1967a). The Groenendyk study found urine output was 9.9 L per horse per day, equating to 23 mL/

kg/day, or 1 mL/kg/h (range: 0.7–1.3 mL/kg/day) (Groenendyk et al., 1988). Finally, a study by Rumbaugh et al. showed urine output to be 1.24±0.38 mL/kg/h (range: 0.62–2.01) in 11 healthy horses fed alfalfa hay with free access to salt, during periods of high environmental temperatures (53–92 °F; 11–33 °C) (Rumbaugh et al., 1982). During feed and water deprivation (72 h), the urine output was 0.55±0.19, 0.29±0.09, and 0.28±0.009 mL/kg/h during 0–24, 24–48, and 48–72 h of feed and water deprivation (Rumbaugh et al., 1982). The conclusion from these studies is that urine production varies with the ambient temperature, feed intake, type of feeds fed, and access to salt. In general, horses on feed and water should be making 0.4–2 mL/kg/h urine, while those off feed and water will produce far less (0.13–0.5, up to 1 mL/kg/h depending on duration) (Groenendyk et al., 1988; Rumbaugh et al., 1982).

Fecal water approximated as a mean of 14–14.8 L/day (means 1.3–1.4 mL/kg/h; range 1–1.7 mL/kg/h) (Tasker, 1967a) and 7.2 L/horse/day (mean 0.7; range 0.5–1 mL/kg/h) (Groenendyk et al., 1988) in these two studies. This is similar to the range for urine output.

An increase in insensible losses, as might occur with hyperhidrosis or increased minute ventilation due to high ambient temperatures or illness, results in increased fluid requirements. Insensible losses were estimated to represent 0.55–0.8 mL/kg/h in horses at rest on a hay diet in the Tasker study (Tasker, 1967a). In the study by Groenendyk, insensible water (evaporative) was determined to be 1 mL/kg/h (range 0.7–1.4 mL/kg/h) (Groenendyk et al., 1988). Metabolic water is water arising from metabolism by the organism; Tasker extrapolated metabolic production of water from humans to horses, and came up with 0.26 mL/kg/h. This was confirmed with metabolic stalls by Groenendyk, who determined metabolic water to be 0.28 mL/kg/h in horses (Groendendyk et al., 1988).

Maintenance water requirements of adult horses

Studies have estimated the daily maintenance water requirement of horses to be 55–65 mL/kg/day (Groenendyk et al., 1988; Tasker, 1967a). Most of this is through water intake (45–55 mL/kg/day), with the balance coming from feed. This equates to 2–3 mL/kg/h, which can be considered the average daily fluid

Table 13.1 Water input and output in normal horses.

Water/fluid requirements	2–3 mL/kg/h
Urine output	0.4–2 mL/kg/h
Fecal water losses	0.5–1.7 mL/kg/h
Insensible losses	0.7–1.4 mL/kg/h
Metabolic water	0.26–0.28 mL/kg/h

requirement for adult horses (non-breeding, non-working). In the study by Tasker the mean water intake of four healthy horses (mean weight of 440 kg) at 40–70 °F (4.4–21 °C) was 2.2–2.3 mL/kg/h (range 1.6–3.5 mL/kg/h) and hay provided an additional 0.1 mL/kg/h of water. These values are supported by another study that found that horses (mean weight 501.5 kg) lost 28.5 kg of body weight after 24 hours of water deprivation, which would extrapolate to 2.4 mL/kg/h (Carlson, 1979b). Another study evaluated the daily water intake of five horses at 60–77 °F (15.6–25 °C) (Groenendyk et al., 1988). In this study, the water intake (through drinking) was 2.3±0.4 (range 1.9–3.0) mL/kg/h. Total water input, including free water, water from feed, and water from metabolism, was 2.7±0.5 (range 2.3–3.5) mL/kg/h. It should be noted that hotter environmental temperatures, exercise, and diet can greatly increase daily water requirements above those listed here.

Another study evaluating pregnant mares offered intermittent or continuous access to water; these mares had a mean water intake, described on an hourly basis, of 1.75–2.3 mL/kg/h (range 1.24–3.1 mL/kg/day among 42 mares) (Freeman et al., 1999). This study also supports the wide inter-individual variation in water intake, even among gravid mares. Another study of six pregnant mares found *ad libitum* water intake to be 2.9 mL/kg/h of water under the conditions of that study, including an *ad libitum* diet of non-legume hay and box stall confinement (Houpt et al., 2000). With water restriction to 40 mL/kg/day (1.67 mL/kg/h), both daily hay intake and body weight decreased indicating this was in adequate for the mares of that study.

Based on the totality of these studies, water or fluid requirements for adult horses can be extrapolated as **2.7 mL/kg/h**, with a range of **2–3 mL/kg/h** for horses on feed. Those off feed may require less, about **1 mL/kg/h**, although this varies widely. The wide range represents the inter-individual variation in water requirements in horses, and emphasizes the need for frequent reassessment and close monitoring of horses on IV fluids.

Electrolytes

The reader is referred to the specific chapters dealing with electrolyte balance (Chapters 2–8). In addition, clinical applications of electrolyte additives for IV fluid therapy are discussed later in this chapter.

Electrolyte requirements of horses are met through intake of feed under natural circumstances. In a study by Tasker, the electrolyte content of drinking water to horses was found to be negligible (Tasker, 1967a). The only significant source of electrolytes for the horses in that study was hay. Hay provided 3930 mEq of potassium and only 329 mEq of sodium per day (0.75 mEq/kg/day sodium and 9 mEq/kg/day of potassium). Urinary and fecal excretion of sodium was quite low as well, being 7 and 116 mEq of sodium per day respectively (123 mEq/day combined or 0.01 mEq/kg/h for both fecal and urinary losses), reflecting the low intake. Respiratory losses of sodium are negligible because water is lost as water vapor. Insensible evaporative loss from the skin is similar; however, sweat is different and is high in sodium, chloride, and other electrolytes.

Urinary and fecal elimination of potassium is substantially greater than that of sodium, found to be 2196 and 993 mEq/day for urine and feces, respectively (0.3 mEq/kg/h combined) (Tasker, 1967a). It should be emphasized that these horses were at rest– sweat losses would markedly alter these amounts in exercising horses. Of note from these studies also is the relatively low sodium and high potassium intake of horses through consumption of hay, and the importance of renal sodium conservation and elimination of potassium. In the study by Groenendyk et al. the mean output of sodium in urine and feces combined was 79% of intake, and was 95, 84, 74, and 75% for potassium, chloride, calcium, and magnesium, respectively.

Electrolyte losses can be substantive with disease and far exceed those under normal circumstances. In general, gastrointestinal and transudative losses are sodium rich, whereas radiant losses are sodium-free (Roberts, 2001).

Candidates for maintenance fluid therapy

Horses that are unable to maintain adequate hydration through oral means are candidates for intravenous maintenance fluid therapy. The reader is referred to the chapter on "Enteral fluid therapy" (Chapter 21) for information about oral fluids. Clearly, horses with gastric or gastroduodenal reflux are candidates for IV fluids. Horses with severe dysphagia such as those with botulism or neurologic diseases may require IV fluids if long-term nasogastric intubation is not feasible. Horses with losses greater than their ability or willingness for water and electrolyte intake are also candidates for IV fluids, especially if nasogastric (NG) intubation is not possible or poorly tolerated due to ileus. The prime example of horses with severe fluid losses that are unable to replace those through voluntary oral intake is acute colitis. Diarrhea is often so severe that losses must be replaced with IV fluids. Many of these horses have dysmotility or malabsorption and do not tolerate enteral intubation with water and electrolytes. Some horses are behaviorally intolerant of long-term NG intubation, and others develop pharyngeal or esophageal trauma (Hardy et al., 1992).

In deciding whether a horse is ready for maintenance fluid therapy, it should meet two additional requirements. First the horse should not be suffering from shock, which would necessitate replacement fluid therapy. Second, it should not be dehydrated. If either is present, then the horse still requires some form of replacement fluid therapy; a maintenance fluid plan can be commenced once replacement has occurred and if the horse is unwilling or unable to maintain its own hydration status through drinking.

Assessment of needs

As described in the earlier section on fluid requirements, healthy, resting adult horses on feed have a daily water intake of approximately 2.7 (range 2.0–3.9) mL/kg/day, although this can vary considerably depending on horse and environmental circumstances; some horses drink as little as 1–1.25 mL/kg/h, especially if off feed. For practicality and ease, the author suggests using a rate of 2.5 mL/kg/day as a starting point for maintenance fluid therapy.

These rates are an initiation point for maintenance fluid plans in clinically ill horses. They should not be stringently adhered to without re-evaluation. Each horse has unique fluid requirements, defined by its specific illness, activity level, feed intake, and the ambient temperature. Therefore, horses should be serially and frequently monitored for adequacy of IV fluid therapy, and to ensure avoidance of fluid overload. Frequent reassessment and monitoring may dictate modification of this initial rate.

Horses with medical problems often have fluid and electrolyte requirements in excess of these standard maintenance rates. These are associated with abnormal

or "ongoing" losses. Horses with increased gastrointestinal, renal, cutaneous, or respiratory losses require higher fluid rates to maintain fluid balance. Fever requires additional fluid to dissipate the increased body heat. Horses with endocrine disorders (e.g., diabetes mellitus, diabetes insipidus) may also experience excessive losses. Specific examples of excessive ongoing losses include gastric reflux, diarrhea, polyuric renal failure, hyperhidrosis, and hyperventilation. Catabolic horses with increased metabolism often require more water in order to eliminate increased waste solutes through urine. Third space losses, as occur with peritonitis, also contribute to ongoing losses.

In one study, horses with experimentally induced diarrhea defecated 19.5 ± 3.7 liters of fecal water per day (Tasker, 1967b), and horses with naturally acquired colitis likely have greater fluid losses than this. With "ongoing losses", the component of the fluid rate required to account for the diarrhea, above that required for maintenance needs, should be provided with administration of replacement fluids rather than hypotonic fluids. The additional fluid losses occurring with diarrhea or reflux are from the ECF and are generally electrolyte rich, thereby necessitating isotonic fluid for replacement. For example, if the target fluid rate for this horse is 5 mL/kg/h, only half of the rate should be supplied with a maintenance fluid (if hypotonic, see below) and the other half as a replacement fluid. This is because hypotonic fluids should not be used to replace losses from the ECF.

The reader is referred to specific chapters for fluid therapy of specific organ dysfunctions.

Monitoring techniques during maintenance fluid therapy

Physical examination

A component of monitoring the adequacy of maintenance fluid therapy is evaluation for clinical signs of dehydration. However, physical examination signs of dehydration are fairly insensitive and may not manifest until late. For example, in one study evaluating the response to feed and water withholding for 8 days, there was no change in skin turgor until day 3 of water withholding (Tasker, 1967a). After 5 days there was a "tucked-up" appearance of the abdomen. Interestingly, no change in mucous membrane moisture could be recognized at any point in the study, despite horses

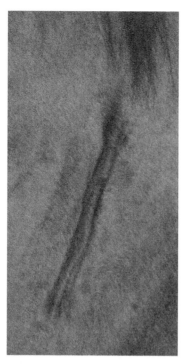

Figure 13.1 Skin turgor is a marker of hydration status (extravascular water); however, studies have raised questions about its accuracy.

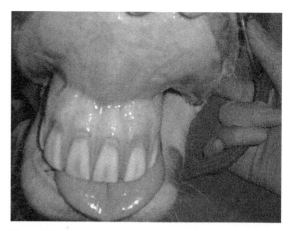

Figure 13.2 Mucous membrane color reflects perfusion, while texture can reflect hydration status.

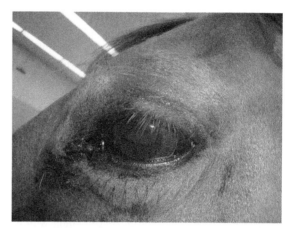

Figure 13.3 Corneal texture and tear film quality also reflect extravascular hydration status.

losing approximately 10% of body weight. In another study of food and water deprivation during hot ambient temperatures, horses lost 10.7% of body weight over 3 days (Carlson, 1979b). At that point, the horses exhibited only signs of "moderate" dehydration in terms of skin turgor and degree of eyeball retraction, despite having severe dehydration (Figure 13.1). Interestingly, but consistent with a lack of sensitivity of the skin tenting test, a study of working horses under hot ambient temperatures (30–44 °C) showed that skin tent duration had no significant association with plasma osmolarity or water intake (Pritchard et al., 2008). Rather, skin tenting was affected by side of animal, anatomical location, and degree of coat moisture, as well as age of animal. Older horses, neck site location, and left side of horse had a longer skin tent duration than younger horses, the point of the shoulder location, and the right side, respectively. Coats with wet sweat had the longest tent duration, followed by damp sweat, and dry coat, while dried sweat produced the shortest (Pritchard et al., 2008). Similarly, there was no significant relationship between degree of mucous membrane dryness

(Figure 13.2) and water intake, plasma osmolarity, or environmental temperature (Pritchard et al., 2008). Heart rate was a more reliable indicator of dehydration; animals with higher heart rates drank more water. (Pritchard et al., 2008). Corneal texture is also an indicator of hydration status; however, dry corneas are also a late sign and likely not very sensitive (Figure 13.3).

These findings are consistent among a number of studies, indicating that physical examination parameters may not be sensitive indicators of dehydration. In a study in which horses lost $4 \pm 1\%$ of body weight 8 hours after furosemide administration, pulse pressure, skin turgor, capillary refill time, and jugular distensibility remained unchanged throughout the study period despite the degree of body water loss (Freestone et al., 1988). In a more recent model of dehydration in horses, water deprivation for 24 hours led to 7% loss of body weight, yet there were minimal to no physical examination findings (Lester et al., 2013).

Laboratory indicators: packed cell volume (PCV), total protein (TP), electrolytes

Laboratory means of monitoring hydration include serial packed cell volume (PCV) and total protein (TP) concentrations. As with clinical signs, PCV may not be a very sensitive indicator of hydration status (Lester et al., 2013). In four horses deprived of water for 8 days, PCV did not significantly change throughout the duration of the study (Tasker, 1967a). However, total protein concentration increased from 6.8 (range 5.4–7.6) to 7.7 (range 6.5–8.5) g/dL. The study by Carlson et al., in which water was withheld for 3 days in hot ambient temperatures, had similar findings (Carlson et al., 1979b). In that study, the PCV increased slightly over the 72-hour period; however, this was not statistically significant. The TP concentration increased significantly by 24 hours and continued to do so throughout the study (from baseline of 7.0 ± 0.9 to 8.0 ± 0.9 g/dL).

In the study with an 8-day food and water withholding period at cooler temperatures, plasma sodium concentrations did not change, whereas potassium concentrations decreased (by 0.3–0.9 mEq/L) (Tasker, 1967a). Plasma pH decreased, as did bicarbonate concentration with a concomitant increase in P_{CO_2} (Tasker, 1967a). The study in a hotter climate revealed that both sodium and chloride concentrations increased (from 137.2 ± 1.9 to 143.6 ± 3.1, and from 99.3 ± 2.4 to 105.8 ± 2.8 mEq/L, respectively), likely representing increased insensible free water losses with the hotter ambient temperatures (Carlson et al., 1979b). Not surprisingly, plasma osmolarity increased concomitant with the increase in sodium concentration (Carlson et al., 1979b). Interestingly, in that study potassium did not decrease (Carlson et al., 1979b). In addition, the horses in the Tasker study developed diarrhea, which may have netted increased fecal sodium losses and contributed to the lack of increase in sodium concentration in that study (Tasker, 1967a). A model of dehydration through water deprivation for 24 hours caused a significant increase in plasma total protein

and sodium concentrations, and an increase in plasma osmolarity, but no change in PCV (Lester et al., 2013).

In summary, total protein concentration is a reliable indicator of plasma volume decrease, provided pathologic protein loss or gain is not present (e.g., protein-losing enteropathy or gammopathy, respectively). Packed cell volume may not be as sensitive or consistent an indicator of dehydration. Hypernatremia or hyperosmolarity, when present, should signal free water loss. For maintenance fluid therapy purposes, a downward plateau of PCV and TP concentration is desired, without rapid or significant changes in magnitude.

Osmolarity

Osmolarity, particularly when measured serially, is a good indicator of dehydration associated with water restriction. After water restriction to 30 mL/kg/day in pregnant mares (*ad libitum* water intake was 69 mL/kg/day), plasma osmolarity increased from 282 ± 0.7 to 292.2 ± 1.76 mOsm/L (Houpt et al., 2000). In another study, a 19-hour duration of water deprivation led to a 10 mOsm/L increase in osmolarity, while those with 36 h deprivation had an increase of 17 mOsm/L (Mueller & Houpt, 1991). A third study with 72 h duration of water deprivation in horses showed an increase of 25 mOsm/L in plasma osmolarity (Sneddon et al., 1991, 1993). Finally, a study of dehydration in working horses found plasma osmolarity to be a predictor of water intake after work, and horses with a higher osmolarity drank significantly more water and engaged in longer and more frequent drinking bouts (Pritchard et al., 2008). Plasma osmolarity dropped from 283 ± 1.2 to 274 ± 0.8 mOsm/L within 30 minutes of access to water. Changes in plasma sodium and chloride concentrations paralleled those of plasma osmolarity (Pritchard et al., 2008). Plasma osmolarity increased in yet another model of dehydration in healthy horses, whereas PCV did not change (Lester et al., 2013). In summary, these studies indicate that osmolarity is a reasonably good indicator of hydration status; because baseline osmolarity may not be known for a particular individual horse, serial measurements are most useful. For example, a serial drop in osmolarity after drinking water is consistent with rehydration, with plateau indicating that water repletion may be complete. Serum osmolality in adult horses ranges from 271 ± 8 to 281 ± 9 mOsm/kg H_2O (Carlson & Rumbaugh, 1983; Carlson et al., 1979b; Pritchard et al., 2006).

Body weight

Serial body weight measurements, whenever possible, are very useful for monitoring maintenance fluid therapy over time. Once the patient is rehydrated (see Chapter 12), body weight should not fluctuate in response to IV fluid therapy. A rapid increase in body weight overnight, for example, should warrant re-evaluation of fluid therapy rates, as well as renal and GI function. A study evaluating dehydrated working horses in hot ambient temperatures showed that body weight increased following access to water; the increase in body weight after working was significantly associated with water intake (Pritchard et al., 2008). A study evaluating the effects of furosemide (1 mg/kg IM) showed an increase in urine volume and decrease in body weight by 19.2 ± 5.2 kg or $4 \pm 1\%$ of body weight over an 8-hour period (Freestone et al., 1988).

Urine output

Measurement or estimation of urine output and degree of renal concentration are important means of monitoring the adequacy of maintenance fluid therapy. Normal horses produce 0.4–2 mL/kg/h of urine, with an average of approximately 1 mL/kg/h (Groenendyk et al., 1988; Rumbaugh et al., 1982). Therefore, horses undergoing maintenance fluid therapy should be producing at least 0.7–1 mL/kg/h as an indicator of maintaining adequate hydration status. Healthy adult feral mares urinate every 3–4.5 hours, while stallions may urinate more frequently (up to every 2 h) (Kownacki et al., 1978; Tyler, 1969). These can be used as guidelines for monitoring horses on fluids, indicating that a horse on an adequate maintenance fluid rate should be urinating at least every 3–4 hours. It should be noted that this applies to horses in which the goal is maintenance of hydration and not ones in which diuresis or superhydration of GI contents is the goal, where higher fluid rates are required. A horse that is urinating several times an hour may be receiving an excess volume of fluids, unless diuresis is the goal.

Urine specific gravity is helpful in monitoring fluid therapy as well. In adult horses, highly concentrated urine such as that with a specific gravity exceeding 1.030 suggests that the provided fluids may be inadequate. Similarly, urine from an adult horse with a specific gravity of less than 1.010 may indicate that fluid rates can be decreased, as long as renal dysfunction is not at the root of the isosthenuria. These values do not apply to foals, where dilute urine is normal.

Central venous pressure (CVP)

While central venous pressure (CVP) may not accurately reflect adequacy of blood or plasma volume, it is a reasonable upper limit to fluid administration (Boecxstaens et al., 2009). Said differently, a normal CVP does not necessarily signify an adequate blood volume, but a high normal CVP should be regarded as a limit to further fluid volume expansion for safety reasons, namely to prevent edema. The reader is referred to the chapters on "Replacement fluids" (Chapter 12)" and "Monitoring fluid therapy" (Chapter 9) for more on central venous pressure. During the maintenance phase of fluid therapy, maintenance of a normal CVP should be a goal. In adult horses, CVP is not routinely measured except in cases where fluid overload is a real possibility, such as horses with heart failure, and with oliguric or anuric renal failure. Normal CVP in adult horses has been reported to range from 7.5 ± 0.9 to 12 ± 6 cmH$_2$O (Hall, 1975; Klein et al., 1977).

Lactate

Blood or plasma lactate concentration optimally should not change abruptly during maintenance fluid therapy. While useful as one possible indicator of perfusion status during the fluid resuscitation phase, it should remain fairly stable, or continue to slowly decrease, during the maintenance phase. A sudden increase in lactate concentration during maintenance fluid therapy should warrant investigation as to possible causes.

Complications of maintenance fluid therapy

Adverse effects of maintenance fluid therapy include fluid overload, catheter-related problems, and electrolyte disturbances. Fluid overload can be sudden or gradual in onset, depending on the administered rate and the propensity for edema formation. Horses with hypoproteinemia or increased vascular permeability are at increased risk of tissue edema. See elsewhere in this book for further discussion of catheter-related complications (Chapter 9), fluid overload (Chapter 11), and electrolyte disturbances (Chapters 2–8).

Clinical applications of maintenance fluid therapy

Administration of maintenance fluids

Maintenance fluids are generally provided continuously at an even rate (Figure 13.4). In hospitalized horses where staff members are available for monitoring fluid administration, this is optimal. When continuous infusion is not possible, intermittent administration of fluids is an option, especially when isotonic fluids are utilized. If intermittent infusions are utilized, isotonic crystalloids should be used. Rapid boluses of

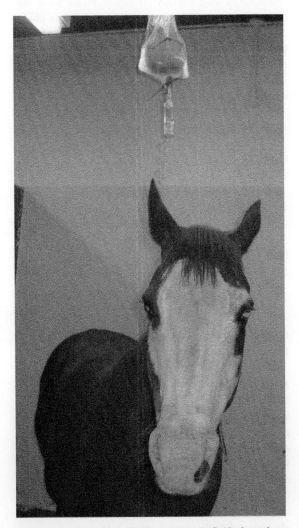

Figure 13.4 Adult horse receiving continuous fluids through a coiled IV administration set.

hypotonic fluids should be avoided in order to avoid rapidly decreasing plasma sodium concentration and osmolarity.

In addition to the rate of administration (e.g., maintenance rate of 2.5 mL/kg/h in adult horses and determination of whether higher or lower rates are required), additional considerations of fluid therapy include the **type** of fluid. In selecting the specific type of fluid, one of the most significant decisions is between hypotonic and isotonic crystalloids.

Hypotonic fluids are indicated in horses that are not drinking or are held off water for a period of time, because those horses need an alternate source of free water over the long term. In the short term (2–3 days, depending on underlying disease process and renal function), and when animals can drink water, isotonic fluids can be used for maintenance purposes. Isotonic replacement crystalloids are commonly used for maintenance fluid therapy in veterinary practice, because most horses are able to excrete electrolytes that are administered in excess of needs. This practice is convenient and reduces the risk of hyponatremia, which is a possible response to administration of large volumes of hypotonic fluids. In addition, many clinically ill horses experience ongoing abnormal electrolyte losses, as with diarrhea or gastric reflux, and poor to no feed intake; these animals benefit from administration of replacement fluids to account for these electrolyte losses or lack of intake.

Dangerous hyponatremia associated with the administration of "true" hypotonic maintenance fluids has not been reported in the equine veterinary literature. However, in the human medical literature there have been some concerns over development of hyponatremia in response to administration of hypotonic maintenance fluids, especially in the pediatric sector. Therefore, if hypotonic fluids are used, sodium should be monitored serially to ensure lack of free water excess and hyponatremia.

On the other hand, prolonged use of replacement fluids may lead to hypernatremia, hyperosmolarity, and subsequent contraction of the ICF especially in neonatal foals, which may be less tolerant of the administration of large amounts of sodium over time. Adult horses that are not allowed to drink water and those with renal disease are also at risk for developing hypernatremia over time. As when hypotonic fluids are used, plasma sodium concentrations should be serially monitored.

Types of maintenance fluids (Table 13.2)

Plasma-Lyte 56 or Normosol™-M

Plasma-Lyte 56 (Baxter Healthcare Corporation, Deerfield, IL) and Normosol™-M (Abbott Laboratories, North Chicago, IL) are hypo-osmolar relative to the ECF (111 mOsm/L as compared to 270–300 mOsm/L). The sodium concentration is lower (40 vs 140 mEq/L), and potassium concentration is higher (13 vs 5 mEq/L) than in replacement fluids such as Plasma-Lyte 148 or Plasma-Lyte A. Like their "replacement" counterparts, the maintenance versions of Plasma-Lyte or Normosol contain magnesium (3 mEq/L) rather than calcium. Acetate (16 mEq/L) is the only alkalinizing salt. Another difference from the analogous replacement fluids (Plasma-Lyte 148 or Normosol-R) is that the sodium to chloride ratio is 1:1 in these maintenance fluids, a slight disadvantage for acidotic patients with hyperchloremia. Unfortunately, these fluids are currently commercially unavailable.

0.45% Sodium chloride/2.5% dextrose

A commercially available maintenance fluid is termed "half strength" saline and dextrose (0.45% sodium chloride and 2.5% dextrose in water). Despite its isotonicity in the bag (280 mOsm/L), it is a maintenance fluid and provides a source of free water once the dextrose is metabolized *in vivo*. The sodium:chloride ratio in this solution is also 1:1 (77 mEq/L each of sodium and chloride), and it lacks potassium or other electrolytes, as well as alkalinizing agents. An advantage of this solution is that it is ready to use without having to add dextrose. It is ideal for maintenance of hydration in patients with hyperkalemia and in those that require an energy source. Potassium should be added for normo- and hypokalemic patients.

5% Dextrose in water

Dextrose 5% in water (D5W) is neither a replacement nor a maintenance fluid as it contains no electrolytes. Rather, it is simply a source of free water and dextrose. The solution is near isotonic (252 mOsm/L) as commercially prepared. However, due to metabolism of the dextrose after administration, it becomes a hypotonic fluid *in vivo*. It can be utilized as a means of carefully delivering free water to animals with free water deficits (hypernatremia) or losses as occurs with diabetes insipidus. Serum sodium concentration should not be decreased at a rate faster than 0.5 mEq/h in horses with significant hypernatremia in order to avoid CNS edema. For these same reasons dextrose 5% in water should never be bolused as a rapid infusion because it can cause acute reductions in osmolarity and risks causing cerebral edema. In addition to free water, D5W also provides 170 kcal/L of digestible energy.

"Home-made maintenance fluids": making hypotonic maintenance fluids from replacement fluids

When commercial maintenance fluids are not available, and hypotonic fluids are desired, such maintenance fluids can be developed from concomitant administration of replacement fluids and free water. This can be accomplished through the administration of half the desired fluid rate as 5% dextrose in water (D5W) and half the desired rate as a replacement fluid such as lactated Ringer's solution (LRS) or Plasma-Lyte A. This will result in an *"in vivo"* (i.e., after metabolism of dextrose) osmolarity of approximately 136 are used. If glucose is not desired, sterile water can be used

Table 13.2 Composition of maintenance fluids.

Crystalloid	Sodium	Chloride	Potassium	Calcium	Magnesium	Organic anion	Osmolarity
Normosol-M	40	40	13	0	3	16 Acetate	112
Plasma-Lyte 56	40	40	13	0	3	16 Acetate	112
0.45%NaCl/2.5% dextrose	77	77	0	0	0	0	280 (140 *in vivo*)
5% dextrose	0	0	0	0	0	0	252 (0 *in vivo*)
Plasma-Lyte A mixed with sterile water (1:1 ratio)	70	49	2.5	0	1.5	13.5 Acetate 11.5 Gluconate	148

instead of D5W as the free water source. If bagged sterile water is used, then it is critical that the water be mixed with the isotonic fluid prior to reaching the vein. Sterile water alone can lead to osmotic hemolysis.

Discontinuation of fluid therapy

Maintenance fluids optimally should be discontinued gradually, in order to avoid transient dehydration until horses develop an osmolar or volume drive to drink. This is particularly true in horses with colic or renal disease, where dehydration could have negative consequences. In a study utilizing a model of dehydration, horses were water deprived for 24 hours in order to mimic a clinical scenario possibly associated with impaction colic (Lester et al., 2013). This led to 7% loss of body weight, and a significant increase in plasma osmolality, sodium, and total plasma protein concentration. After abrupt discontinuation of IV fluid therapy at 75 mL/kg/day (3.1 mL/kg/h) horses were allowed free access to water. These horses continued to produce large volumes of urine even after completion of IV fluid administration, yet had minimal water intake. The effect was an apparent state of rebound dehydration, because body weight was similar 24 h after discontinuation of fluids as it was immediately after the initial 24-hour period of water deprivation (Lester et al., 2013). This would be particularly relevant to horses with intestinal impactions. In contrast, intragastrically administered water did not lead to a similar period of decreased water intake, and body weights in these horses 24 h after discontinuation of enteral fluids were similar to those prior to water restriction (Lester et al., 2013). In that study, enteral water resulted in greater hydration of intestinal contents than did IV fluids at 25, 50, or 75 mL/kg/day (Lester et al., 2013).

Based on these observations, fluid rates should be decreased gradually over 24 hours or longer in order to minimize this transition period of transient lack of drinking after IV fluid therapy. For example, fluid rates can be decreased by 50% for 12–24 h, and then to 25% of the rate for another 12–24 h prior to discontinuation. With a slow rate of discontinuation, the goal is to gradually provide a drive to drink (either through osmolarity or blood volume/pressure stimulus) without allowing significant dehydration.

Additives for maintenance fluid therapy

The reader is referred to the chapters on potassium (Chapter 3), magnesium (Chapter 6), phosphorus (Chapter 7), and calcium disorders (Chapter 5) as well as parenteral nutrition (Chapter 25) for more detail. The intent here is to provide concise clinical suggestions for fluid additives along with brief justification.

Potassium

Potassium supplementation is important in horses with partial to complete anorexia. Horses off feed rapidly can become depleted of body stores of potassium, because grasses and hays are relatively high in potassium content. Because potassium is primarily intracellular, means of determining total body status are not conducive to the hourly or even daily management of fluid status. Tissue concentrations of potassium would likely be the most accurate representation of total body stores of potassium. However, this is not practical for the clinical setting. Measurement of urinary fractional excretion (FE) of potassium can add to an understanding of potassium dynamics in a particular patient; however, the wide reference range may limit its clinical usefulness. Urinary fractional excretions require concurrent measurement of plasma and urine concentrations of electrolytes and creatinine and are calculated as:

$$FE_x = \frac{x(urine)}{x(plasma)} \times \frac{Cr(plasma)}{Cr(urine)} \qquad (13.2)$$

where X = electrolyte under investigation, and Cr = creatinine. This value can then be multiplied by 100 to express it as a percentage.

The reported range of the FE of potassium is 15–80% and is highly diet dependent, with most horses having values somewhere between 20 and 50% (Beech et al., 1993; King, 1994; Kohn & Strasser, 1986; Harris & Colles, 1988). One study showed a low of 10.8% for the FE of potassium in horses (Traver et al., 1977). A low FE (<11–15%) implies total body depletion of potassium; however, the sensitivity of this measurement has not been evaluated. Horses with renal dysfunction or magnesium deficiency may have altered or inaccurate FE of potassium. The FE of potassium in neonatal foals is lower than in adult horses, with a reported range of

9–18% (Brewer et al., 1991). Anorexia predisposes to hypokalemia, as do fluid diuresis and renal tubular acidosis. Administration of replacement crystalloids often results in diuresis in order to eliminate the administered excess sodium, which causes a concomitant loss of urinary potassium. Experimentally induced endotoxemia has been shown to decrease plasma potassium concentrations as well, while simultaneously increasing insulin concentrations (Toribio et al., 2005).

Despite a lack of practical means of measuring total body potassium, measurement of plasma concentrations remains important because ECF potassium is clinically more relevant than ICF stores in terms of neuromuscular transmission. Supplementation of potassium in response to ECF (or plasma) concentrations in horses often is based on experience and clinician preference rather than specific consensus guidelines. The maximum safe rate of potassium administration is 0.5 mEq/kg/h, except under very special circumstances (such as when insulin is co-administered). Horses with renal dysfunction or other causes of hyperkalemia should receive rates below this upper maximum limit, and potassium should be monitored especially frequently in those horses.

Most commonly, 20–40 mEq/L of potassium chloride (KCl) is added to crystalloid fluids during maintenance fluid therapy (2–3 mL/kg/h of fluids). While recommendations for specific cut-off values for supplementation of potassium vary from clinician to clinician, the author utilizes the following approximate guidelines: a plasma potassium below 3.5 mEq/L warrants supplementation of fluids with a rate of 10–20 mEq/L, whereas a potassium level below 3.2 mEq/L should be supplemented with 20 mEq/L. A potassium concentration below 3 mEq/L may indicate supplementation with 30–40 mEq/L. It should be noted that LRS contains 4 mEq/L of potassium, and commercial acetated polyionic fluids, such as Plasma-Lyte A or Normosol-R, have 5 mEq/L, so that the supplemented potassium should be added to these concentrations for determination of final concentration. Commercial "maintenance" fluids, such as Plasma-Lyte 56 or Normosol-M, contain a higher potassium concentration (13 mEq/L) since these fluids are intended for both the ECF and ICF spaces. In addition, horses with hyperchloremia can be supplemented with potassium phosphate as opposed to KCl, as long as hyperphosphatemia is not present.

It should be noted that horses with hypokalemia that is refractory to potassium supplementation may have concurrent magnesium depletion. Hypomagnesemia is often associated with hypokalemia and kaliuresis (Whang et al., 1984, 1992). Magnesium is a cofactor for Na/K-ATPases, and hypomagnesemia therefore leads to decreased intracellular potassium and increased intracellular sodium concentrations, respectively, leading to lowered resting membrane potential. Therefore, hypomagnesemia leads to loss of intracellular potassium stores, and to reduced reabsorption of potassium in the kidney (kaliuresis). This can result in increased potential for spontaneous cardiac depolarization, as well as increased Purkinje cell excitability and increased likelihood of dysrhythmia generation.

Calcium

Mild hypocalcemia is common in horses that are partially to completely anorexic. In addition, surgical colic or colitis, prolonged exercise with heavy sweating, endotoxemia, or small intestinal disease (especially of the duodenum, where most calcium absorption occurs) often causes hypocalcemia in horses (Schryver et al., 1970). Ionized calcium should be measured whenever possible, because it is the active form in plasma. Experimentally induced ionized hypocalcemia (<0.83 mmol/L, or 3.52 mg/dL) has been associated with dysrhythmias (4/7 ponies) and was fatal in 2/7 ponies (Glazier et al., 1979). Horses on maintenance fluid should therefore have ionized calcium measured daily, particularly if they are off feed. Calcium administration should be thoughtful and careful where calcium may be participating in pathology of disease, as with severe white muscle disease, calciphylaxis, myocardial necrosis, or brain injury (Lazarewicz 1996). During endotoxemia calcium may decrease, as has been shown in experimental models in horses; this was associated with a concurrent increase in parathyroid hormone (Toribio et al., 2005). In addition, horses undergoing exploratory laparotomy for acute abdominal disease (colic) commonly have ionized hypocalcemia (Dart et al., 1992; Delesalle et al., 2005; Garcia-Lopez et al., 2001).

While mild hypocalcemia is common among clinically ill horses, studies in rats with sepsis have shown an increase in mortality with administration of calcium (Malcolm et al., 1989; Zaloga et al., 1992). Because of that, overzealous use of calcium should be avoided during sepsis or endotoxemia in horses. There is no consensus on the level of ionized calcium that should be treated in horses. Supplementation should certainly occur at values at or below 1.0 mmol/L (4.0 mg/dL) because of the associated potential for dysrhythmias when values below 0.9 are reached (Borer & Corley, 2006). However, some horses may benefit from supplementation at higher concentrations depending on clinical status. Anecdotally, many clinicians supplement calcium when ionized calcium is below 1.2–1.3 mmol/L (4.8–5.2 mg/dL). Horses with refractory hypocalcemia should have their plasma ionized magnesium concentrations evaluated. Magnesium is needed for parathyroid hormone (PTH) synthesis and secretion, as well as tissue responsiveness to PTH.

A 550-kg horse (non-working, non-breeding adult) requires 22 g of calcium per day (which equates to 40 mg/kg/day) through dietary intake (NRC, 2007). Because oral calcium has an absorption rate of 50 to 67%, the intravenous calcium requirement would be 20–27 mg/kg/day (Shryver et al., 1970). The conversion of milligrams to milliequivalents is 0.05 mEq per mg. Therefore, adult horses at rest would require 1–1.35 mEq/kg/day. Calcium gluconate (23%) contains 1.069 mEq/mL of calcium. Therefore, adult horses would meet their resting calcium requirement with 0.94–1.26 mL/kg/day of 23% calcium gluconate, or 517–695 mL per day (i.e., 1 to $1^2/_5$ of a 500-mL bottle of 23% calcium gluconate for a 550 kg horse). Calcium should be diluted in crystalloids (e.g., 25–50 mL 23% calcium gluconate per liter of crystalloid fluid) add administered over 2–3 h in order to avoid bradycardia or other cardiac dysrhythmias. This rate of administration is also reasonable for horses on maintenance fluids that are anorexic.

Phosphorus

The clinical implications of hypophosphatemia in horses are poorly understood. Like potassium, the majority of phosphorus is intracellular. Generally phosphorus is not added to fluids unless significant hypophosphatemia is present. In humans, ruminants, and small animals it can be associated with hemolysis, rhabdomyolysis, ventricular dysrhythmias, and cardiac or skeletal muscle dysfunction (Bugg & Jones, 1998; Maloney et al., 2002). Hypophosphatemia has been described in horses with endotoxemia, ileus, and colic, as well as renal disease (Elfers et al., 1986; Tennant et al., 1982; Toribio et al., 2005). Mild hypophosphatemia is also common with anorexia. Other potential causes of decreased plasma phosphorus include alkalosis, excessive magnesium administration, and large colon resection. The latter is

true because the sites of phosphorus absorption are the large and small colon (Schryver et al., 1972). The absorption efficiency of phosphorus by the equine gut appears to be approximately 40% (Schryver et al., 1972).

The daily phosphorus requirement in the adult, non-working, non-breeding 550-kg horse is 15 g, which works out to 27 mg/kg/day. Given that the absorption is approximately 40%, the requirement provided IV would be 10.8 mg/kg/day, or 0.35 mmol/kg/day since phosphorus is often represented as mmol/L. However, in humans recommendations for supplementation have included a maximum rate of 0.24 mmol/kg/day unless marked hypophosphatemia was present, due to potential adverse effects of excessive phosphorus supplementation (including hyperphosphatemia-associated ventricular dysrhythmias and precipitation with calcium). This is the maximum phosphorus administration rate that the author currently recommends for horses, unless severe hypophosphatemia is present. This works out to 0.01 mmol/kg/h.

Inorganic phosphate exists as monobasic and dibasic anions, with the proportion of valences dependent on pH. Therefore, ordering by milliequivalent amounts is unreliable and risks large dosing errors. In addition, IV phosphate supplements are available in the sodium and potassium salt (sodium phosphate and potassium phosphate); therefore, the content of sodium or potassium must be considered when supplementing phosphate. For these reasons, the most reliable method of supplementing IV phosphate is by millimoles (mmol), then specifying the potassium or sodium salt form.

It should be kept in mind that potassium phosphate contains 3 mmol/mL and 4.4 mEq/mL of phosphorus and potassium, respectively. Sodium phosphate contains 3 mmol/mL of phosphorus and 4 mEq/mL of sodium. At 0.01 mmol/kg/h of phosphorus supplementation, a 550-kg horse would receive 5.5 mmol/h of phosphorus and either 8.1 mEq/h of potassium or 7.3 mEq/h of sodium. As with calcium, phosphorus should be diluted in fluids and administered slowly.

Magnesium

Ionized magnesium concentrations may be low in horses with anorexia and those with gastrointestinal diseases, especially those with strangulating lesions, endotoxemia, and ileus (Garcia-Lopez et al., 2001; Toribio et al., 2005). Increased losses may also be present in horses with clinically significant gastroduodenal reflux, some forms of diarrhea, renal disease particularly with diuresis, hyperhidrosis, and even renal tubular acidosis (Johansson et al., 2003).

Hypomagnesemia has been associated with ileus in horses, although a causal effect remains to be determined. Other clinical signs of chronic hypomagnesemia in horses include ventricular dysrhythmias, muscle tremors, hyperhidrosis, seizures, and ataxia followed by collapse (Harrington, 1974). These were signs observed in foals fed a purified diet containing low levels of magnesium, and the hypomagnesemia eventually led to death after a few weeks (Harrington, 1974).

Hypomagnesemia is associated with increased inflammatory mediator production and with increased risk of death in human intensive care units (Malpuech-Brugere et al., 1999; Weglicki et al., 1992). Similarly, equine endotoxemia is associated with a decrease in both total and ionized magnesium (de Rouffignac et al., 1993). In hospitalized horses hypomagnesemia is associated with GI dysfunction, infectious respiratory diseases, and multiorgan disease although a relationship with mortality has not been established in horses (Johansson et al., 2003). Hypomagnesemia may increase intracellular calcium concentrations, potentially making the myocardium and other tissues more susceptible to cardiotoxicity from glycosides and other cardiotoxins, as well as to consequences of ischemia (Tossiello, 1996).

Most dietary magnesium is absorbed by the small intestine. The daily dietary requirement for non-working horses is 13–15 mg/kg (Hintz & Schryver, 1972). With an estimated oral absorption of 40–50% this would equate to an IV dose of 5.2–7.5 mg/kg/day IV (Hintz & Schryver, 1972). In converting to mEq/kg/day, this would equate to 0.43–0.62 mEq/kg/day (1 mEq = 12.156 mg). For a 550-kg horse, this means 237–341 mEq/day. A 550-kg horse receiving 1 L/h of Plasma-Lyte A, Plasma-Lyte 148, or Normosol-R would receive 3 mEq/h, or 21–30% of their daily magnesium requirement. Magnesium supplementation is indicated for refractory hypokalemia or hypocalcemia because magnesium is required for renal reabsorption of potassium and PTH release, respectively.

Dextrose

Dextrose supplementation may be administered concurrent to maintenance fluids, either in the crystalloid bag (as a percentage, e.g., 2% dextrose) or separately as a "piggyback" into the fluid line connected to the crystalloid bag. Dextrose as 50% optimally should not

contact the endothelium and erythrocytes directly without dilution due to hyperosmolarity (2530 mOsm/L). A solution of 5% dextrose in water has an osmolarity of approximately 252 mOsm/L and its osmolarity will be additive to those of the fluids it is diluted in. It has a caloric content of 170 kcal/L at 5% and would therefore add 170 kcal/L to fluids in which it was diluted (e.g., LRS, Plasma-Lyte). At a rate of 1 L/h for a 500-kg horse (2 mL/kg/h), this 5% solution would provide approximately 4080 kcal/day, which is 35.5% of the resting digestible energy requirement. This supplies approximately 1.7 mg/kg/min of dextrose to a 500-kg horse. Blood glucose concentrations should be monitored.

References

Andrews FM, Nadeau JA, Saabye L, Saxton AM. (1997) Measurement of total body water content in horses, using deuterium oxide dilution. *Am J Vet Res* **58**:1060–4.

Beech J, Lindborg S, Braund KG. (1993) Potassium concentrations in muscle, plasma and erythrocytes and urinary fractional excretion in normal horses and those with chronic intermittent exercise-associated rhabdomyolysis. *Res Vet Sci* **55**:43–51.

Boecxstaens V, Deleyn AM, Stas M, Wever ID. (2009) Prevention of postoperative pulmonary edema on the ward by application of a central venous pressure rule. *The Open Surgery Journal* **3**:1–8.

Borer KE, Corley KTT. (2006) Electrolyte disorders in horses with colic. Part 2: calcium, sodium, chloride, and phosphate. *Equine Vet Educ* **18**:320–5.

Brewer BD, Clement SF, Lotz WS, Gronwall R. (1991) Renal clearance, urinary excretion of endogenous substances, and urinary diagnostic indices in healthy neonatal foals. *J Vet Int Med* **5**:28–33.

Bugg NC, Jones JA. (1998) Hypophosphataemia: Pathophysiology, effects and management on the intensive care unit. *Anaesthesia* **53**:895–902.

Carlson GP, Rumbaugh GE. (1983) Response to saline solution of normally fed horses and horses dehydrated by fasting. *Am J Vet Res* **44**:964–8.

Carlson GP, Harold D, Rumbaugh GE. (1979a) Volume dilution of sodium thiocyanate as a measure of extracellular fluid volumes in horses. *Am J Vet Res* **40**:587–9.

Carlson GP, Rumbaugh GE, Harrold DR. (1979b) Physiologic alterations produced by food and water deprivation during periods of high environmental temperatures. *Am J Vet Res* **40**:982–5.

Crandall LA, Anderson MX. (1934) Estimation of the state of hydration of the body by the amount of water available for the solution of sodium thiocyanate. *Am J Dig Dis Nutr* **1**:126–31.

Dart AJ, Snyder JR, Spier SJ, Sullivan KE. (1992) Ionized calcium concentrations in horses with surgically managed gastrointestinal disease: 147 cases (1988–1990). *J Am Vet Med Ass* **201**:1244–8.

Delesalle C, Dewulf J, Lefebvre RA, Schuurkes JA, Van Vlierbergen B, Deprez P. (2005) Use of plasma ionized calcium levels and Ca2+ substitution response patterns as prognostic parameters for ileus and survival in colic horses. *Vet Q* **27**:157–72.

de Rouffignac C, Mandon B, Wittner M, di Stefano A. (1993) Hormonal control of renal magnesium handling. *Miner Electrolyte Metab* **19**:226–31.

Elfers RS, Bayly WM, Brobst DF, et al. (1986) Alterations in calcium, phosphorus and C-terminal parathyroid hormone levels in equine acute renal disease. *Cornell Vet* **76**:317–29.

Epstein V. (1984) Relationship between potassium administration, hyperkalemia, and the electrocardiogram: an experimental study. *Equine Vet J* **16**:453–6.

Evans JW. (1971) Effect of fasting, gestation, lactation and exercise on glucose turnover in horses. *J Anim Sci* **33**:1001–4.

Fielding CL, Magdesian KG, Elliott DA, Cowgill LD, Carlson GP. (2004) Use of multifrequency bioelectrical impedance analysis for estimation of total body water and extracellular and intracellular fluid volumes. *Am J Vet Res* **65**:320–6.

Forro M, Cieslar S, Ecker GL, et al. (2000) Total body water and ECFV measured using bioelectrical impedance analysis and indicator dilution in horses. *J Appl Physiol* **89**:663–71.

Freeman DA, Cymbaluk NF, Schott HC 2nd, Hinchcliff K, McDonnell SM, Kyle B. (1999) Clinical, biochemical, and hygiene assessment of stabled horses provided continuous or intermittent access to drinking water. *Am J Vet Res* **60**:1445–50.

Freestone JF, Carlson GP, Harrold DR, Church G. (1988) Influence of furosemide treatment on fluid and electrolyte balance in horses. *Am J Vet Res* **49**:1899–902.

Garcia-Lopez JM, Provost PJ, Rush JE, Zicker SC, Burmaster H, Freeman LM. (2001) Prevalence and prognostic importance of hypomagnesemia and hypocalcemia in horses that have colic surgery. *Am J Vet Res* **62**:7–12.

Glazier DB, Littledike ET, Evans RD. (1979) Electrocardiographic changes in induced hypocalcemia and hypercalcemia in horses. J Equine Med Surg 489–94.

Groenendyk S, English PB, Abetz I. (1988) External balance of water and electrolytes in the horse. *Equine Vet J* **20**:189–93.

Hall LW. (1975) Measurement of central venous pressure in horses. *Vet Rec* **97**:66–9.

Hardy J, Stewart RH, Beard WL, Yvorchuk-St-Jean K. (1992) Complications of nasogastric intubation in horses: nine cases (1987–1989). *J Am Vet Med Assoc* **201**:483–6.

Harrington DD. (1974) Pathological features of magnesium deficiency in young horses fed purified rations. *Am J Vet Res* **35**:503–13.

Harris P, Colles C. (1988) The use of creatinine clearance ratios in the prevention of equine rhabdomyoslysis: a report of four cases. *Equine Vet J* **20**:459–63.

Hintz HF, Schryver HF. (1972) Magnesium metabolism in the horse. *J Anim Sci* **35**:755–9.

Houpt KA, Eggleson A, Kunkle K, Houpt TR. (2000) Effect of water restriction on equine behavior and physiology. *Equine Vet J* **32**:341–4.

Jeffcott L. (1972) Observations on parturition in crossbred pony mares. *Equine Vet J* **4**:209–13.

Johansson AM, Gardner SY, Jones SL, Fuquay LR, Reagan VH, Levine JF. (2003) Hypomagnesemia in hospitalized horses. *J Vet Intern Med* **17**:860–7.

Julian LM, Lawrence JH, Berlin NI, et al. (1956) Blood volume, body water and body fat of the horse. *J Appl Physiol* **8**:651–3.

King C. (1994) Practical use of urinary fractional excretion. *J Equine Vet Sci* **14**:464–8.

Klein L, Sherman J. (1977) Effects of preanesthetic medication, anesthesia, and position of recumbency on central venous pressure in horses. *J Am Vet Med Assoc* **170**:216–19.

Kohn CW, Muir WW, Sams R. (1978) Plasma volume and extracellular fluid volume in horses at rest and following exercise. *Am J Vet Res* **59**:871–4.

Kohn CW, Strasser SL. (1986) 24-hour renal clearance and excretion of endogenous substances in the mare. *Am J Vet Res* **47**:1332–7.

Kownacki M, Sasimowski E, Budzynski M, et al. (1978) Observations of the twenty-four hour rhythm of natural behavior of Polish primitive horse bred for conservation of genetic resources in a forest reserve. *Genet Pol* **19**:61–77.

Lazarewicz JW. (1996) Calcium transients in brain ischemia: role in neuronal injury. *Acta Neurobiol Exp* **56**:299–311.

Lester GD, Merritt AM, Kuck HV, Burrow JA. (2013) Systemic, renal, and colonic effects of intravenous and enteral rehydration in horses. *J Vet Int Med* Epub Apr 3.

Lumsden JH, Rowe R, Mullen K. (1980) Haematology and biochemistry reference values for the light horse. *Can J Comp Med* **44**:32–42.

Magdesian KG. (2011) *The physiology of IV fluids.* In: Proceedings, International Veterinary Emergency and Critical Care Society (IVECCS), Nashville, TN, g5.

Malcolm DS, Zaloga GP, Holaday JW. (1989) Calcium administration increases the mortality of endotoxic shock in rats. *Crit Care Med* **17**:900–3.

Maloney DG, Appadural IR, Vaughan RS. (2002) Anions and the anaesthetist. *Anaesthesia* **57**:140–54.

Malpuech-Brugere C, Nowacki W, Rock E, Gueux E, Mazur A, Rayssiguier Y. (1999) Enhanced tumor necrosis factor-alpha production following endotoxin challenge in rats is an early event during magnesium deficiency. *Acta Biochem Biophys* **1453**:35–40.

Mueller PJ, Houpt KA. A comparison of the responses of donkey (*Equus asinus*) and ponies (*Equus caballus*) to 36 hours of water deprivation. In: Fielding D, Pearson RA (eds) *Donkeys, Mules and Horses in Tropical Agricultural Development.* Edinburgh: University of Edinburgh, pp. 86–95.

Muir WW, Kohn CW, Sam SR. (1978) Effects of furosemide on plasma volume and extracellular fluid volumes in horses. *Am J Vet Res* **39**:1688–91.

National Research Council (NRC). (2007) *Nutrient Requirements of Horses*, 6th revised edition. Washington DC: National Academy Press.

Pritchard JC, Barr AR, Whay HR. (2006) Validity of a behavioural measure of heat stress and a skin tent test for dehydration in working horses and donkeys. *Equine Vet J* **38**:433–8.

Pritchard JC, Burn CC, Barr ARS, Whay HR. (2008) Validity of indicators of dehydration in working horses: a longitudinal study of changes in skin tent duration, mucous membrane dryness, and drinking behavior. *Equine Vet J* **40**:588–64.

Roberts KB. (2001) Fluid and electrolytes: parenteral fluid therapy. *Pediatr Rev* **22**:380–7.

Rumbaugh GE, Carlson GP, Harrold D. (1982) Urinary production in the healthy horse and in horses deprived of feed and water. *Am J Vet Res* **43**:735–7.

Schott II HC. (2011) Water homeostasis and diabetes insipidus in horses. *Vet Clin Equine* **27**:175–95.

Schryver HF, Craig PH, Hintz HF, Hogue DE, Lowe JE. (1970) The site of calcium absorption in the horse. *J Nutr* **100**:1127–32.

Schryver HF, Hintz HF, Craig PH, Hogue DE, Lowe JE. (1972) Site of phosphorus absorption form the intestine of the horse. *J Nutr* **102**:143–8.

Sneddon JC, van der Walt JG, Mitchell G. (1991) Water homeostasis in desert-dwelling horses. *J Appl Physiol* **71**:112.

Sneddon JC, van der Walt JG, Mitchell G, Hammer S, Taljaard JJF. (1993) Effects of dehydration and rehydration on plasma vasopressin and aldosterone in horses. *Physiol Behav* **54**:223–8.

Spurlock GH, Landry SL, Soms R, et al. (1985) Effect of endotoxin administration on body fluid compartments in the horse. *Am J Vet Res* **46**:1117–20.

Tasker JB. (1967a) Fluid and electrolyte studies in the horse. III. Intake and output of water, sodium, and potassium in normal horses. *Cornell Vet* **57**:649–57.

Tasker JB. (1967b) Fluid and electrolyte studies in the horse V. The effects of diarrhea. *Cornell Vet* **57**:668–77.

Tennant B, Bettleheim P, Kaneko JJ. (1982) Paradoxic hypercalcemia and hypophosphatemia associated with chronic renal failure in horses. *J Am Vet Med Assoc* **180**:630–4.

Toribio RE, Kohn CW, Hardy J, Rosol TJ. (2005) Alterations in serum parathyroid hormone and electrolyte concentrations and urinary excretion of electrolytes in horses with induced endoxoemia. *J Vet Intern Med* **19**:223–31.

Tossiello L. (1996) Hypomagnesemia and diabetes mellitus. *Arch Intern Med* **156**:1143–8.

Traver DS, Salem C, Coffman JR, et al. (1977) Renal metabolism of endogenous substances in the horse: volumetric vs clearance ratio methods. *J Equine Med Surg* **1**:378–82.

Tyler SJ. (1969) *The behaviour of a population of New Forest ponies.* Dissertation, University of Cambridge, UK.

Weglicki W, Phillips T, Freedman AM, Cassidy MM, Dickens BF. (1992) Magnesium-deficiency elevated circulating levels of inflammatory cytokines and endothelin. *Mol Cell Biochem* **110**:169–73.

Whang R, Oei TO, Aikawa JK, et al. (1984) Predictors of clinical hypomagnesemia. Hypokalemia, hypophosphatemia, hyponatremia, and hypocalcemia. *Arch Intern Med* **144**:1794–6.

Whang R, Whand D, Ryan M. (1992) Refractory potassium repletion: a consequence of magnesium deficiency. *Arch Intern Med* **152**:40–5.

Zaloga GP, Sager A, Black KW, Prielipp R. (1992) Low dose calcium administration increases mortality during septic peritonitis in rats. *Circ Shock* **37**:226–9.

CHAPTER 14
Fluid therapy for renal failure

C. Langdon Fielding

Loomis Basin Equine Medical Center, Penryn, CA, USA

Fluid and electrolyte balance is particularly challenging in patients with renal dysfunction, and intensive management is often required. Significant morbidity and mortality have been associated with excess fluid administration in renal failure in humans, and this may be the case in horses as well (Mehta & Bouchard, 2011). This chapter focuses on the recognition and fluid management of renal failure in horses with a particular emphasis on the treatment of acute kidney injury (AKI).

Acute kidney injury (AKI)

Acute kidney injury refers to a sudden fall in the estimated glomerular filtration rate (GFR). The severity of AKI is often staged in terms of an increased serum creatinine concentration and a decrease in urine output. It has become increasingly clear over the last decade that even mild decreases in GFR may be associated with significant increases in mortality (Hoste et al., 2006). Early recognition of AKI requires clinical and biochemical monitoring as well as a thorough knowledge of the associated risk factors. Immediate intervention is important to minimize long-term kidney dysfunction.

Recognizing AKI

Three separate staging criteria have been proposed to recognize and categorize the level of AKI in humans (Hoste et al., 2006; Kellum & Lemeire, 2013; Ronco et al., 2007). While variations exist between the criteria, all classifications include the staging of renal dysfunction based on creatinine concentration and urine output. Table 14.1 describes the most recent guidelines put forth

by Kidney Disease Improving Global Outcomes (KDIGO), which can be easily translated for use in horses (Kellum & Lameire, 2013).

Clinicians should pay particular attention to the relatively small increase (0.3 mg/dL) in serum creatinine required to recognize AKI in many of the recent guidelines. A normal creatinine range in horses may span 0.9–1.9 mg/dL or higher depending on the analyzer. Horses with AKI may have a serum creatinine value that falls in the normal range even though it has recently increased (change >0.3 mg/dL) from its baseline value. The importance of serial creatinine measurements in patients at risk for AKI cannot be emphasized enough.

Urine output that falls below 0.5 mL/kg/h is a second aspect of AKI recognition in humans. Monitoring urine output is more challenging in adult horses but is easily accomplished in neonatal foals (Chapter 10). Urination frequency and serial body weight measurements can be used to help determine if adequate urination is being maintained in hospitalized patients.

Risk factors for AKI are shown in Box 14.1.These include hypotension (typically from hypovolemia), a variety of toxins, and sepsis. Serial creatinine measurements and urine output monitoring should be performed in all patients with known risk factors. In one study evaluating renal dysfunction in horses presenting with gastrointestinal disease, hypochloremia and the presence of gastric reflux were associated with persistent azotemia despite fluid therapy (Groover et al., 2006). Many horses are presented to equine emergency departments with varying degrees of dehydration and all of these horses should be considered at risk for AKI.

Equine Fluid Therapy, First Edition. Edited by C. Langdon Fielding and K. Gary Magdesian.
© 2015 John Wiley & Sons, Inc. Published 2015 by John Wiley & Sons, Inc.

Table 14.1 A summary of criteria for acute kidney injury (AKI) according to KDIGO (Kellum & Lameire, 2013).

Stage	Serum creatinine	Urine output
1	≥0.3 mg/dL increase OR 1.5–1.9 × baseline	<0.5 mL/kg/h for 6–12 h
2	2.0–2.9 × baseline	<0.5 mL/kg/h for ≥12 h
3	≥4.0 mg/dL OR 3.0 × baseline	<0.3 mL/kg/h for ≥24 h OR anuria for ≥12 h

---

Box 14.1 Common risk factors for the development of acute kidney injury (AKI) in horses.

- Hypotension (Divers et al., 1987)
- Toxins:
  - NSAIDs (Mozaffari et al., 2010)
  - Aminoglycosides (Brashier et al., 1998)
  - Oxytetracycline (Vivrette et al., 1993)
  - Pigments (myoglobin and hemoglobin) (Alward et al., 2006; el-Ashker, 2011)
  - Cantharadin (Helman & Edwards, 1997)
- Sepsis (Cotovio et al., 2008)

Treatment of AKI

The most important treatment for patients with evidence of AKI and/or that are at risk for AKI is intravenous fluid therapy. By restoring or maintaining perfusion to the kidney, further damage is mitigated and renal function may improve with time. In cases where the evidence of AKI is equivocal, moderate intravenous fluid administration has few contraindications and may prevent significant morbidity. In cases of anuria, intravenous fluids are still warranted, but they may carry a bigger risk if administration is excessive.

In addition to intravenous fluids, decreased perfusion can be improved with ionotropes and/or vasopressors that improve arterial blood pressure. In patients with adequate perfusion but diminished urine production, other medications such as loop diuretics, mannitol, and dopamine can be considered. These medications have shown mixed benefits in clinical trials but are often used in horses. Given the limited availability of renal replacement therapy (RRT) and the questionable benefits of medications to induce urine flow, early and aggressive treatment with intravenous fluids is extremely important in horses with AKI.

Intravenous fluids
Type of fluid

An isotonic crystalloid fluid such as lactated Ringer's fluid, a commercially available acetated fluid (Normosol™-R, Plasma-Lyte®-A or Plasma-Lyte 148), or 0.9% saline may be an appropriate initial choice for fluid resuscitation in horses with AKI. These fluids provide expansion of the extracellular fluid volume (more than a hypotonic fluid) and increased perfusion to the kidneys. Some recent studies and reviews have suggested a possible benefit to lower chloride fluids (i.e., Plasma-Lyte 148/Normosol-R) as compared to 0.9% saline (Chowdhury et al., 2012; Godin et al., 2013; Yunos et al., 2012). In fact, a "chloride restrictive" strategy was shown to have positive effects on specific renal outcome measures in one clinical trial (Yunos et al., 2012). In a clinical trial comparing Normosol-R and 0.9% saline for rehydration in horses, the 0.9% saline group showed a significant increase in plasma chloride concentrations (Fielding et al., 2012).

Hypertonic saline offers some unique advantages in equine practice as it can be administered very quickly and is relatively inexpensive (on a per dose basis) compared to other crystalloids and colloids. A dose of 4 mL/kg of 7.2% sodium chloride can be used in place of the initial 20 mL/kg isotonic crystalloid dose for a horse with AKI. Compared to 0.9% saline, hypertonic saline decreased time to first urination and produced greater falls in packed cell volume and total protein concentration in endurance horses (Fielding & Magdesian, 2011). In an experimental study comparing it to an isotonic crystalloid, hypertonic saline reduced renal injury in a model of hemorrhagic shock (Sharma et al., 2012). However, hypertonic saline can produce more significant electrolyte abnormalities (specifically hyperchloremia), which may be more difficult to correct in a horse with renal insufficiency than in one with normal function (Fielding & Magdesian, 2011; Gasthuys et al., 1992). As discussed above, the excess chloride in hypertonic saline may have detrimental effects (Chowdhury et al., 2012; Godin et al., 2013; Yunos et al., 2012). In the specific case of AKI induced by rhabdomyolysis, the potentially acidifying effects of hypertonic saline may not be optimal, as alkalinizing solutions have shown benefit in human studies with myoglobin-induced kidney injury (Scharman & Troutman, 2013).

The use of sodium bicarbonate for the treatment and/or prevention of AKI remains a controversial topic in human medicine. Numerous meta-analyses have examined the data available and have not reached a clear conclusion (Jang et al., 2012; Zacharias et al., 2013). The use of sodium bicarbonate to treat AKI associated with rhabdomyolysis in humans is frequently discussed, but the evidence remains equivocal (Zimmerman & Shen, 2013). Horses tend to have a higher urine pH than humans and therefore the benefits of sodium bicarbonate therapy may be even less clear.

Supplementation of intravenous fluids with potassium in cases of AKI should be considered carefully. If urine production is diminished, then additional potassium should be avoided. In cases of documented hypokalemia, potassium supplementation should be considered but serum potassium concentrations should be monitored carefully.

Calcium supplementation of intravenous fluids was shown in one study to diminish the nephrotoxic effects of aminoglycosides in horses (Brashier et al., 1998). However, in an experimental study of sepsis, calcium supplementation exacerbated kidney dysfunction (Collage et al., 2013). In cases of documented hypocalcemia, calcium supplementation should be considered. However, when clinical and laboratory evidence of sepsis is present, calcium supplementation should be avoided.

Main conclusion: Initiate fluid therapy for AKI using lactated Ringer's solution or Normosol-R unless specific electrolyte derangements require a different type of fluid.

Rate of administration

An initial 20 mL/kg bolus of an isotonic crystalloid (over 30–60 min) or a 4 mL/kg bolus of hypertonic saline (over 10 min) can be used for rehydration in horses with AKI. Figure 14.1 depicts a treatment algorithm for AKI in horses. Treatment typically begins with this bolus administration unless signs of fluid overload are present (Chapter 11). Following each 20 mL/kg bolus of fluids, clinical exam findings and other fluid balance variables – central venous pressure (CVP) and arterial blood pressure if available – should be reviewed. If urine output has begun or increased, the patient can be changed to a rate of 2–4 mL/kg/h with careful monitoring of continued urination. If significant urine is not being produced (>1–2 mL/kg/h) but signs of hypovolemia have resolved, additional medications to produce urine flow should be considered. If signs of fluid overload (edema, respiratory dysfunction) develop, fluid administration should be stopped until urine production develops.

Ultrasound of the urinary bladder may be a particularly useful way to monitor urine production in horses and particularly in foals. A change in bladder size is one way to assess the production of urine if urination is not observed. In foals that may not be emptying their bladder, it is essential to document change in bladder size if a urinary catheter is not in place.

The ideal rate of fluid administration for patients with AKI is unknown and likely different for each animal. Given the association between fluid overload

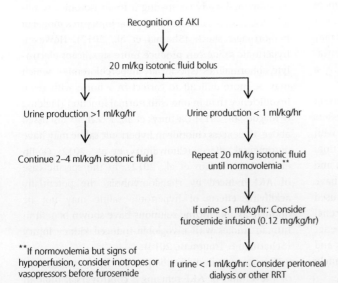

Recognition of AKI

↓

20 ml/kg isotonic fluid bolus

↓   ↓

Urine production >1 ml/kg/hr   Urine production < 1 ml/kg/hr

↓   ↓

Continue 2–4 ml/kg/h isotonic fluid   Repeat 20 ml/kg isotonic fluid
                                        until normovolemia**

↓

If urine <1 ml/kg/hr: Consider
furosemide infusion (0.12 mg/kg/hr)

↓

**If normovolemia but signs of
hypoperfusion, consider inotropes or   If urine < 1 ml/kg/hr: Consider peritoneal
vasopressors before furosemide   dialysis or other RRT

Figure 14.1 Algorithm for the treatment of acute kidney injury (AKI) in horses. RRT, renal replacement therapy.

and mortality in patients with AKI, a more conservative approach has been recently advocated (Bouchard et al., 2009; Godin et al., 2013; Heung et al., 2012). This approach targets a neutral or even slightly negative fluid balance once normovolemia has been attained. In horses, frequent and repeated body weight measurements are very important as they may be the easiest guide to ongoing fluid balance. Ideally, fluid "ins" and "outs" would be monitored and balanced for each patient as this appears to be a better method for assessing fluid balance than estimations from weight changes (Schneider et al., 2012)

Main conclusion: Utilize 20 mL/kg crystalloid fluid boluses and reassess perfusion and hydration status after each is administered. Once urine production has normalized, decrease to a rate of 2 mL/kg/h. If urine production is minimal (<1 mL/kg/h) despite adequate volume administration, consider medications to increase urine flow.

Endpoint

The endpoint to fluid administration depends on the rate of urine production, persistence of risk factors (i.e., ongoing nephrotoxic medications), and the ability/willingness of the patient to drink. In horses that are maintaining a normal fluid balance (urine production matching fluid administration/intake) and where risk factors for AKI have been discontinued, intravenous fluids can often be stopped after 24–48 hours if renal values – blood urea nitrogen (BUN), creatinine – have returned to normal. Even if renal values have not completely normalized, it may be possible to stop intravenous fluids if the patient is drinking an adequate amount to maintain renal perfusion. However, continuing fluid administration until renal values have normalized may be the safest strategy if water intake and urination cannot be closely monitored.

If azotemia persists despite therapy, intravenous fluid administration can continue until there is no longer a decrease in creatinine over a 48–72-hour period. Serum creatinine values may continue to decrease over 5–10 days or longer, and fluid administration can continue during this time. The benefit of this prolonged fluid administration strategy is unknown and some horses will continue to have improvement in creatinine levels even after intravenous fluids are stopped. Some of this improvement may occur over a period of several weeks after the insult.

Ionotropes and vasopressors

If perfusion is considered to be inadequate despite appropriate fluid therapy, then blood pressure can be improved with the use of dobutamine, norepinephrine (noradrenaline), or similar medications. These catecholamines are typically administered by constant-rate infusion and are used more commonly in foals and adult horses under anesthesia. Norepinephrine and fenoldopam have both been shown to increase urine output in healthy foals (Hollis et al., 2006, 2008) but the effects in horses with AKI are unknown.

Medications to increase urine production

The challenges in providing renal replacement therapies to horses make the continuing production of urine essential to case management. Without urine production, fluid overload and severe electrolyte derangements can develop. Medications that have been used to increase urine production in AKI include furosemide, dopamine, and mannitol. More recently, aminophylline has been described as well (Olowu & Adefehinti, 2012). While many authors agree that these medications can increase the production of urine, there is considerable doubt as to whether they alter the long-term outcome of the case in human patients. Poor fluid management may necessitate the use of these medications, but their benefit to the kidneys is questionable. Furosemide should be considered as a treatment for fluid overload and as a means to attempt to increase urine production in anuric/oliguric horses, but not necessarily as a treatment for AKI.

Loop diuretics

Loop diuretics can theoretically reduce renal tubular oxygen demand by decreasing the energy requirements of the cells in the thick ascending limb of the loop of Henle (Heyman et al., 1994). Based on this finding, one would expect the loop diuretics to decrease the severity of kidney damage in AKI. However, numerous studies have evaluated the use of furosemide in patients with AKI or at risk for developing AKI and have shown no clear benefit (Cantarovich et al., 2004; Grams et al., 2011; van der Voort et al., 2009). While furosemide produces an increase in urine flow, it does not appear significantly to alter renal outcome (Cantarovich et al., 2004). Numerous authors have concluded that there is no survival or renal outcome benefit to the use of furosemide in AKI (Bagshaw et al., 2007; Ho & Sheridan, 2006; Sampath et al., 2007).

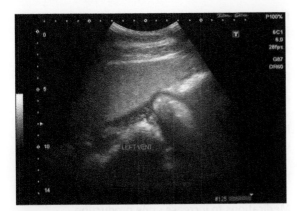

Figure 14.2 Ultrasound showing intestinal edema in a horse with fluid overload.

Furosemide is the most commonly used loop diuretic in horses and has a significant role in the management of fluid overload and electrolyte derangements. It can be given both as a bolus administration (0.1–1.0 mg/kg) and as a continuous-rate infusion (CRI) (0.12 mg/kg/h) to horses (Johansson et al., 2003). It has been shown to increase urine flow in healthy horses (Johansson et al., 2003), but there is little research available for horses with AKI.

In horses with evidence of anuria or fluid overload, furosemide is an essential part of the treatment plan (Figure 14.2). However, clinicians should realize that it is unlikely to improve renal damage. However, it may give more time for the clinician to address ongoing risk factors and electrolyte derangements, and possibly time for the kidneys to heal. In horses with AKI, furosemide should be considered as a primary treatment for fluid overload and electrolyte derangements but not as a primary treatment for AKI.

Main conclusion: In cases of anuria or fluid overload, administer intravenous furosemide (0.12 mg/kg loading dose followed by 0.12 mg/kg/h) until urine production has normalized and fluid overload is corrected.

Dopamine

Low-dose dopamine (0.5–3 μg/kg/min) has been shown to increase renal blood flow, promote natriuresis, and increase urine flow in the first 24 hours of treatment in humans (Denion et al., 1996; Friedrich et al., 2005). Similar to furosemide and mannitol, however, there is no evidence to suggest that it actually alters the outcome in AKI (Friedrich et al., 2005). If fluid therapy and

furosemide have not increased urine production in a horse with AKI and fluid overload, low-dose dopamine is a reasonable treatment to try.

Mannitol

Similar to furosemide, mannitol has been shown to increase urine flow, which can have benefits in the management of fluid overload associated with AKI (Bragadottir et al., 2012). Clinical trials have not been able to show benefit of mannitol administration to patients with AKI (Brown et al., 2004). In cases where furosemide and dopamine are not able to increase urine production, mannitol may be considered. However, monitoring of fluid balance and prevention of fluid overload need to be carefully addressed. In horses, mannitol has been used as a diuretic at a dose of 1–2 mg/kg/min after a slow intravenous bolus of 0.25–0.5 g/kg (G. Magdesian, personal communication, 2013). A total dose of 1 g/kg should not be exceeded if urine production has not been initiated by that point. If fluid overload is present, mannitol should not be bolused as it can further expand plasma volume, but the low CRI dose can be tried for a few hours as long as CVP and clinical status are monitored closely.

Aminophylline

A couple of recent studies have described the use of aminophylline to improve renal excretory function and augment urine output (Axelrod et al., 2014; Olowu & Adefehinti, 2012). These authors did not observe any negative effects of the medication, but more research is needed to evaluate the use of this medication in people and in horses. With more information, aminophylline may present an alternative to other medications used to increase urine production.

Renal replacement therapies (RRTs)

Renal replacement therapies include hemodialysis, peritoneal dialysis, hemofiltration, and kidney transplant. Of these, peritoneal dialysis has been the most commonly described in clinical cases of renal failure in horses (Chapter 27). Hemodialysis has been described for the treatment of oxytetracycline-induced acute renal failure in a neonatal foal though additional reports are lacking (Vivrette et al., 1993). More recently, continuous venovenous hemodiafiltration has been described in a group of experimental, healthy horses (Wong et al., 2013).

In clinical cases of AKI that develop anuria, renal replacement therapies may be an option for some horses. However, availability and financial considerations may limit applicability in many cases. In humans, there is some evidence that earlier initiation of RRT may improve outcome in AKI, but a clear consensus is lacking (Oh et al., 2012). Considerably more experience with RRTs is needed in horses before any recommendations about the timing of RRT can be made in this species.

Recommendations: Horses with AKI that cannot be managed with intravenous fluids and medications to increase urine production (furosemide, dopamine, etc.), should be considered candidates for RRT. At this time, peritoneal dialysis may be the most practical for equine veterinary practices.

Foals and AKI

Many of the causes of AKI are similar in adults and foals. Critically ill neonatal foals are at particular risk of developing acute kidney injury, and serial creatinine should be monitored frequently in such foals. Sick newborn foals often present to equine hospitals with gastrointestinal, neurologic, and renal dysfunction as a triad of problems possibly associated with a period of hypoxia surrounding parturition. Additionally, sepsis is a common abnormality in newborn foals that has been associated with AKI in many species.

The criteria for diagnosing AKI in humans may be more difficult to apply in newborn foals due to the presence of increased serum creatinine concentrations without acute renal failure (Chaney et al., 2010). This was termed "spurious hypercreatinemia" and refers to foals with increased serum creatinine concentrations at birth that rapidly decline over the first 24–48 hours (Chaney et al., 2010).

The treatment options are similar for foals as for adult horses. However, neonatal foals have different fluid balance physiology (see Chapter 1) and may be more prone to fluid overload as compared to adult horses (Chapter 11). Monitoring fluid balance by comparing "ins" and "outs" is extremely important in this group of patients. Early recognition of fluid retention should warrant immediate modification of the fluid therapy plan and treatment to promote fluid removal (e.g., furosemide) should be instituted. As with other age groups in humans, there is an association between AKI, fluid retention, and mortality in neonates (Askenazi et al., 2013).

Chronic kidney disease

Fluid therapy is likely to be far more important in cases of AKI than in cases of chronic kidney disease (CKD). Clinicians should be aware of cases that develop AKI on top of pre-existing CKD. Intravenous fluid administration should be carefully considered for patients with CKD and a conservative rate of administration is often indicated. Fluid overload is a common problem in humans with chronic kidney disease (Tsai et al., 2013). Horses are likely prone to similar problems with fluid overload when CKD is present. Hypercalcemia is common in horses with CKD, and additional supplementation should be avoided.

References

Alward A, Corriher CA, Barton MH, et al. (2006) Red maple (Acer rubrum) leaf toxicosis in horses: a retrospective study of 32 cases. *J Vet Intern Med* **20**:1197–201.

Askenazi DJ, Koralkar R, Hundley HE, et al. (2013) Fluid overload and mortality are associated with acute kidney injury in sick near-term/term neonate. *Pediatr Nephrol* **28**:661–6.

Axelrod DM, Anglemyer AT, Sherman-Levine SF, et al. (2014) Initial experience using aminophylline to improve renal dysfunction in the pediatric cardiovascular ICU. *Pediatr Crit Care Med* **15**:21–7.

Bagshaw SM, Delaney A, Haase M, et al. (2007) Loop diuretics in the management of acute renal failure: A systematic review and meta-analysis. *Crit Care Resusc* **9**:68.

Bouchard J, Soroko SB, Chertow GM, et al. (2009) Fluid accumulation, survival and recovery of kidney function in critically ill patients with acute kidney injury. *Kidney Int* **76**:422–7.

Bragadottir G, Redfors B, Ricksten SE. (2012) Mannitol increases renal blood flow and maintains filtration fraction and oxygenation in postoperative acute kidney injury: a prospective interventional study. *Crit Care* **16**:R159.

Brashier MK, Geor RJ, Ames TR, et al. (1998) Effect of intravenous calcium administration on gentamicin-induced nephrotoxicosis in ponies. *Am J Vet Res* **59**:1055–62.

Brown CV, Rhee P, Chan L, et al. (2004) Preventing renal failure in patients with rhabdomyolysis: do bicarbonate and mannitol make a difference? *J Trauma* **56**:1191–6.

Cantarovich F, Rangoonwala B, Lorenz H, et al. (2004) High-dose furosemide for established ARF: a prospective, randomized, double-blind, placebo-controlled, multicenter trial. *Am J Kidney Dis* **44**:402–9.

Chaney KP, Holcombe SJ, Schott HC 2nd, et al. (2010) Spurious hypercreatininemia: 28 neonatal foals (2000–2008). *J Vet Emerg Crit Care (San Antonio)* **20**:244–9.

Chowdhury AH, Cox EF, Francis ST, et al. (2012) A randomized, controlled, double-blind crossover study on the effects of 2-L infusions of 0.9% saline and Plasma-Lyte® 148 on renal blood flow velocity and renal cortical tissue perfusion in healthy volunteers. *Ann Surg* **256**:18–24.

Collage RD, Howell GM, Zhang X, et al. (2013) Calcium supplementation during sepsis exacerbates organ failure and mortality via calcium/calmodulin-dependent protein kinase kinase signaling. *Crit Care Med* **41**:e352–60.

Cotovio M, Monreal L, Navarro M, et al. (2007) Detection of fibrin deposits in horse tissues by immunohistochemistry. *J Vet Intern Med* **21**:1083–9.

Denion MD, Chertow GM, Brady HR. (1996) "Renaldose" for the treatment of acute renal failure: scientific rationale, experimental studies and clinical trials. *Kidney Int* **50**: 504–14.

Divers TJ, Whitlock RH, Byars TD, Leitch M, Crowell WA. (1987) Acute renal failure in six horses resulting from haemodynamic causes. *Equine Vet J* **19**:178–84.

el-Ashker MR. (2011) Acute kidney injury mediated by oxidative stress in Egyptian horses with exertional rhabdomyolysis. *Vet Res Commun* **35**:311–20.

Fielding CL, Magdesian KG. (2011) A comparison of hypertonic (7.2%) and isotonic (0.9%) saline for fluid resuscitation in horses: a randomized, double-blinded, clinical trial. *J Vet Intern Med* **25**:1138–43.

Fielding CL, Magdesian KG, Meier CA, et al. (2012) Clinical, hematologic, and electrolyte changes with 0.9% sodium chloride or acetated fluids in endurance horses. *J Vet Emerg Crit Care (San Antonio)* **22**:327–31.

Friedrich JO, Adhikari N, Herridge MS, et al. (2005) Meta-analysis: low-dose dopamine increases urine output but does not prevent renal dysfunction or death. *Ann Intern Med* **142**:510–24.

Gasthuys F, Messeman C, De Moor A. (1992) Influence of hypertonic saline solution 7.2% on different hematological parameters in awake and anaesthetized ponies. *Zentralbl Veterinarmed A* **39**:204–14.

Godin M, Bouchard J, Mehta RL. (2013) Fluid balance in patients with acute kidney injury: emerging concepts. *Nephron Clin Pract* **123**:238–45.

Grams ME, Estrella MM, Coresh J, et al. (2011) Fluid balance, diuretic use, and mortality in acute kidney injury. *Clin J Am Soc Nephrol* **6**:966–73.

Groover ES, Woolums AR, Cole DJ, LeRoy BE. (2006) Risk factors associated with renal insufficiency in horses with primary gastrointestinal disease: 26 cases (2000-2003). *J Am Vet Med Assoc* **228**:572–7.

Helman RG, Edwards WC. (1997) Clinical features of blister beetle poisoning in equids: 70 cases (1983–1996). *J Am Vet Med Assoc* **211**:1018–21.

Heung M, Wolfgram DF, Kommareddi M, et al. (2012) Fluid overload at initiation of renal replacement therapy is associated with lack of renal recovery in patients with acute kidney injury. *Nephrol Dial Transplant* **27**:956–61.

Heyman SN, Rosen S, Epstein FH, Spokes K, Brezis ML. (1994) Loop diuretics reduce hypoxic damage to proximal tubules of the isolated perfused rat kidney. *Kidney Int* **45**:981–5.

Ho KM, Sheridan DJ. (2006) Meta-analysis of frusemide to prevent or treat acute renal failure. *Br Med J* **333**:420.

Hollis AR, Ousey JC, Palmer L, et al. (2006) Effects of fenoldopam mesylate on systemic hemodynamics and indices of renal function in normotensive neonatal foals. *J Vet Intern Med* **20**:595–600.

Hollis AR, Ousey JC, Palmer L, et al. (2008) Effects of norepinephrine and combined norepinephrine and fenoldopam infusion on systemic hemodynamics and indices of renal function in normotensive neonatal foals. *J Vet Intern Med.* **22**:1210–15.

Hoste EA, Clermont G, Kersten A, et al. (2006) RIFLE criteria for acute kidney injury are associated with hospital mortality in critically ill patients: a cohort analysis. *Crit Care* **10**:R73.

Jang JS, Jin HY, Seo JS, et al. (2012) Sodium bicarbonate therapy for the prevention of contrast-induced acute kidney injury – a systematic review and meta-analysis. *Circ J* **76**:2255–65.

Johansson AM, Gardner SY, Levine JF, et al. (2003) Furosemide continuous rate infusion in the horse: evaluation of enhanced efficacy and reduced side effects. *J Vet Intern Med* **17**:887–95.

Kellum JA, Lameire N; for the KDIGO AKI Guideline Work Group. (2013) Diagnosis, evaluation, and management of acute kidney injury: a KDIGO summary (Part 1). *Crit Care* **17**:204.

Mehta RL, Bouchard J. (2011) Controversies in acute kidney injury: effects of fluid overload on outcome. *Contrib Nephrol* **174**:200–11.

Mozaffari AA, Derakhshanfar A, Alinejad A, et al. (2010) A comparative study on the adverse effects of flunixin, ketoprofen and phenylbutazone in miniature donkeys: haematological, biochemical and pathological findings. *N Z Vet J* **58**:224–8.

Oh HJ, Shin DH, Lee MJ, et al. (2012) Early initiation of continuous renal replacement therapy improves patient survival in severe progressive septic acute kidney injury. *J Crit Care* **27**:743.e9–18.

Olowu WA, Adefehinti O. (2012) Aminophylline improves urine flow rates but not survival in childhood oliguric/anuric acute kidney injury. *Arab J Nephrol Transplant* **5**:35–9.

Ronco C, Levin A, Warnock DG, et al. (2007) AKIN Working Group. Improving outcomes from acute kidney injury (AKI): Report on an initiative. *Int J Artif Organs* **30**:373–6.

Sampath S, Moran JL, Graham PL, et al. (2007) The efficacy of loop diuretics in acute renal failure: Assessment using Bayesian evidence synthesis techniques. *Crit Care Med* **35**:2516–24.

Scharman EJ, Troutman WG. (2013) Prevention of kidney injury following rhabdomyolysis: a systematic review. *Ann Pharmacother* **47**:90–105.

Schneider AG, Baldwin I, Freitag E, et al. (2012) Estimation of fluid status changes in critically ill patients: fluid balance chart or electronic bed weight? *J Crit Care* **27**:745.e7–e12.

Sharma P, Benford B, Karaian JE, et al. (2012) Effects of volume and composition of the resuscitative fluids in the treatment of hemorrhagic shock. *J Emerg Trauma Shock* **5**:309–15.

Tsai YC, Tsai JC, Chen SC, et al. (2013) Association of fluid overload with kidney disease progression in advanced CKD: a prospective cohort study. *Am J Kidney Dis doi:* 10.1053/j.ajkd.2013.06.011.

van der Voort PH, Boerma EC, Koopmans M, et al. (2009) Furosemide does not improve renal recovery after hemofiltration for acute renal failure in critically ill patients: a double blind randomized controlled trial. *Crit Care Med* **37**:533–8.

Vivrette S, Cowgill LD, Pascoe J, et al. (1993) Hemodialysis for treatment of oxytetracycline-induced acute renal failure in a neonatal foal. *J Am Vet Med Assoc* **203**:105–7.

Wong DM, Witty D, Alcott CJ, et al. (2013) Renal replacement therapy in healthy adult horses. *J Vet Intern Med.* **27**: 308–16.

Yunos NM, Bellomo R, Hegarty C, et al. (2012) Association between a chloride-liberal vs chloride-restrictive intravenous fluid administration strategy and kidney injury in critically ill adults. *JAMA* **308**:1566–72.

Zacharias M, Mugawar M, Herbison GP, et al. (2013) Interventions for protecting renal function in the perioperative period. Cochrane Database Syst Rev 9 (CD 003590). doi: 10.1002/14651858.CD003590.pub4.

Zimmerman JL, Shen MC. (2013) Rhabdomyolysis. *Chest* **144**:1058–65.

CHAPTER 15

Fluid therapy for hepatic failure

Thomas J. Divers

Cornell University, Ithaca, NY, USA

Introduction

There are a limited number of publications on fluid therapy for liver failure in human medicine (Masaya et al., 2001). Most research focuses on the treatment of humans with acute liver failure (ALF). These publications indicate that volume expansion with crystalloids and colloids is needed to combat hypotension and that glucose is given for hypoglycemia (O'Grady & Williams, 1986; Trotter, 2009). Hypertonic saline is frequently mentioned as a treatment for hepatoencephalopathy (HE) and the accompanying cerebral edema (Bauer et al., 2009; Singh et al., 2011). More extensive discussion on fluid therapy is provided for the treatment of cirrhosis and ascites where the advantages of normal or low-sodium-concentration fluid administration is frequently discussed (Ackermann, 2009; Ginès & Guevara, 2008).

These basic concepts of fluid therapy for humans with liver failure (LF) cannot always be directly applied to horses with LF. There appear to be some substantial differences in fluid and electrolyte abnormalities between the two species during LF. This chapter on fluid therapy for equine hepatic failure will discuss intravenous fluid administration for intravascular volume expansion; glucose and nutritional support; correction of acid–base, sodium, and potassium; and hepatic-derived protein abnormalities.

Correction of intravascular volume deficits

Correction of intravascular volume deficits should be the initial focus for fluid therapy in most horses with liver failure. Expansion of the vascular volume can improve perfusion to the diseased liver and other organs that may be secondarily involved. Horses with LF may have intravascular volume deficits for several reasons including: lack of fluid intake, decreased vascular tone and/or endothelial dysfunction, and increased urinary loss. The decrease in vascular tone may be the most important factor. In humans it has been associated with abnormally high cytokine and prostanoid release caused by the diseased liver (Trotter, 2009).

Humans with ALF often have a hyperdynamic phase of shock (vasodilation with increased cardiac output) and, although this has not been evaluated in horses with ALF, the clinical picture (reddish-brown membranes with slow capillary refill but a "pounding" heart with a mild-to-moderate tachycardia) suggests there might be similar pathophysiologic phenomena in the horse (Trotter, 2009). Increased urinary loss of fluid may in some cases (Theiler's disease and chronic fibrosis) be associated with a decrease in hepatic urea synthesis and a low serum blood urea nitrogen (BUN). This results in a decrease in urea-associated renal interstitial osmolality, which would decrease the effectiveness of vasopressin (antidiuretic hormone) on renal water resorption. Although this physiologic concept seems reasonable, it has not been proven and many horses with hepatic failure do not have low serum urea nitrogen concentrations (Durham et al., 2003).

Hypertonic saline (7.5%, 4 mL/kg) can be administered in adult horses with LF if there is clinical or measurable evidence of severe hypotension and abnormally low cardiac preload. The decision to provide resuscitation fluid therapy can be based upon the initial clinical findings. Possible disadvantages of hypertonic

Equine Fluid Therapy, First Edition. Edited by C. Langdon Fielding and K. Gary Magdesian.
© 2015 John Wiley & Sons, Inc. Published 2015 by John Wiley & Sons, Inc.

saline administration would be the large-volume urination that usually occurs following treatment causing potassium loss in the urine (kaliuresis) (see "Potassium abnormalities in horses with hepatic failure" below). A brief decrease in vascular tone may accompany the administration of hypertonic saline but this does not appear to be clinically important (Gold et al., 2008).

An alternative to the administration of hypertonic saline as a resuscitation fluid would be to administer in the first hours of therapy 50 mL/kg of a balanced crystalloid with 50 g of dextrose and 20 mEq of KCl added to each liter. This would provide a volume of fluid nearly equal to a normal intravascular plasma volume. Ideally, a crystalloid with an acetate buffer (e.g., Plasma-Lyte®) should be used rather than one with a lactate buffer (see "Abnormalities in acid–base balance and hepatic disease" below), although the volume of the fluid administered is most important (Box 15.1).

After administration of the initial resuscitation fluid, the cardiovascular status of the horse should be evaluated by checking heart rate, mucus membrane color and refill, urine production, and speed of jugular vein distention after being manually obstructed. Measuring packed cell volume (PCV) and plasma total solids (TS) is also helpful in assessing the resuscitation effort. Persistent elevations in PCV in spite of favorable findings for other parameters are not unusual in horses with either ALF, chronic liver disease that is severe, or hepatic neoplasia (Durham et al., 2003; Gold et al., 2008). The exact cause of this persistently elevated PCV is unknown but does appear to reflect a true circulating erythrocytosis. The presumption is that the erythrocytosis is a result of extramedullary erythrocytosis, although this is unproven. The increased PCV may simply be the result of decreased storage of red blood cells in the spleen and liver.

Early in the evaluation process of horses with liver failure, glucose and lactate should be measured on point-of-care instruments such that the concentration of glucose administered in the initial and maintenance fluids can be

---

Box 15.1 Resuscitation fluids for horses with liver failure

- Hypertonic saline (7.2%): 4 mL/kg
- Isotonic crystalloid with acetate buffer qs to 5% dextrose and 20 mEq KCl/L: 50 mL/kg

---

Box 15.2 Fluid therapy following resuscitation for horses with liver failure

- Acetate-buffered balanced electrolyte solution qs to 5–10% dextrose and 20–40 mEq KCl/L

---

adjusted (see discussion on glucose abnormalities below). Glucose treatment in foals with ALF or in miniature horses or ponies with hepatic lipidosis may vary from what is described above in the initial polyionic crystalloid therapy. A decline in plasma lactate would be an indication of improved perfusion and is likely a favorable prognostic finding. Since the liver is a major organ for lactate metabolism and lactated Ringer's may sometimes be given for resuscitation, it is possible that tissue perfusion has been improved but might not be reflected by a comparative decline in plasma lactate (Heinig et al., 1979). Potassium, sodium, P_{CO_2}, creatinine, and calcium should be monitored in horses with ALF and appropriate adjustments made in therapy in an attempt to correct abnormalities.

Following initial successful resuscitation, approximately twice maintenance fluid rate (120 mL/kg/day) with an acetate-buffered balanced electrolyte solution is indicated. Dextrose (generally 50–100 g/L) and KCl (generally 20–40 mEq/L) should be continued, depending upon the clinical condition of the horse, laboratory chemistry monitoring, and oral consumption of fluids (Box 15.2).

Cerebral dysfunction with liver failure

In humans with ALF, hepatic encephalopathy (HE) is strongly linked to ammonia/ammonium toxicity, often resulting in cytotoxic cerebral edema (Arya et al., 2010; Frederick, 2011). The frequent occurrence of cerebral edema in humans with LF mandates strict attention to changes in serum sodium and glucose concentrations that may exacerbate the cytotoxic edema and cause osmotic edema. Horses that have died from LF characteristically have Alzheimer type II cells in the brain but have not been documented to have cerebral edema (Bergero & Nery, 2008). Alzheimer type II cells are reactive astrocytes that are mostly a result of hyperammonemia.

Regardless of the notable absence of reports of cerebral edema in horses with HE the following should be

---

Box 15.3 Factors to avoid in horses with hepatic encephalopathy

- Overhydration
- Respiratory acidosis or alkalosis
- Serum sodium derangements
- Hypokalemia
- Serum calcium derangements
- Hypo-oncotic states
- Low head position
- Excessive sedation
- Hypovolemia/hypotension
- Hyperthermia

---

avoided in hopes of preventing the possibility of cerebral edema: "overhydration"; respiratory acidosis; marked abnormalities in plasma sodium, ionized calcium, and oncotic pressure; and abnormally low position of the head (often due to tranquilization). Excessive sedation, in an attempt to control abnormal behavior in horses with HE, should be avoided (Box 15.3). In addition to the possibility of causing an abnormal head position, the same sedatives may decrease ventilation, increase P_{CO_2}, and result in vasodilation within the brain. This vasodilation could contribute to cerebral edema.

Although ammonia/ammonium are not the only neurotoxins involved in HE, they may be the most important. All efforts should be made to decrease their production, prevent their diffusion into the central nervous system, and increase their elimination (also see "Potassium abnormalities in horses with hepatic failure" below). Maintaining adequate urine production and normal plasma K^+ concentration will enhance renal ammonia/ammonium excretion. Although numerous reports have described horses with HE and blood ammonia measured within the normal range, this does not exclude the possibility that prior hyperammonemia or intracellular accumulation of ammonium are involved in the HE (McGorum et al., 1999; West, 1996).

Colloid therapy and abnormalities in hepatic-derived proteins in liver failure

Colloids can be used as an adjunct fluid therapy to crystalloids. However, colloid therapy will substantially increase the cost of treatment without proven benefit. If colloids are used, fresh-frozen plasma (FFP) or 25% human albumin may have some therapeutic advantages. Plasma albumin treatment may increase plasma oncotic pressure, which will prolong and enhance the plasma volume restoration effect of crystalloid therapy. In addition, albumin may provide an antioxidant effect and potentially bind endogenous toxins that may be involved in the pathophysiology of HE (Ahya et al., 2006; Polli & Gattinoni, 2010).

Although the liver is the sole producer of albumin, severe hypoalbuminemia is rare in horses with either acute or chronic LF. This is different from the more marked hypoalbuminemia that may occur in other species with LF. This difference may be related to either the longer half-life of equine albumin (20 days) or the ability of the equine liver to produce albumin in spite of tremendous loss of function. Most horses with chronic LF have mild decreases in serum albumin. The decrease may be partially due to a systemic inflammatory response causing a decrease in albumin production and an increase in acute-phase proteins, which are common in most cases of equine liver failure (Parraga et al., 1995). Administration of 25% human albumin would have a more dramatic effect on plasma oncotic pressure than would fresh frozen equine plasma but it is rarely used in horses. It would be a foreign antigen and does not provide regulating coagulation/inflammatory factors as does equine FFP. Fresh-frozen plasma provides many proteins other than albumin that may be decreased with severe liver disease. These proteins include the non-endothelial derived clotting factors (II, V, VII, IX, X, XI, XIII) and other regulatory proteins such as protein C, protein S, antithrombin III, and fibronectin.

Although prothrombin time (PT) can very quickly be prolonged following LF (the half-life of factor VII is approximately 8 h), naturally occurring bleeding abnormalities are uncommon in horses with LF. Liver biopsy rarely causes notable hemorrhage in horses with LF in spite of prolonged clotting times, possibly because of normal platelet counts in most horses with LF. Nasogastric intubation should be performed with caution in horses with LF, because nasal hemorrhage following this procedure is not uncommon in affected horses. Horses with LF that require nasogastric intubation, or those in need of surgery (i.e., cholelithiasis), could be given FFP in an attempt to improve clotting function prior to the procedure. Large amounts of plasma (10–15 mL/kg) may be needed to return PT and partial thromboplastin time (PTT) to normal ranges. Smaller amounts (2–8 mL/kg) would be less expensive, decrease the chances of volume overload, and may reduce the possibility of hemorrhage even if clotting function tests remain outside of the normal values.

Ammonia concentrations in equine citrated FFP have not been reported, but plasma therapy would not be expected to contribute significantly to the patient's blood ammonium level. The need for whole blood in LF would be unusual, but may be required with uncontrolled nasal bleeding associated with nasogastric tubing, bleeding following liver biopsy, or hemorrhage during abdominal surgery to remove choleliths. If a whole blood transfusion is needed, it should be freshly collected. Even with proper collection and storage for a short time (days), high ammonia concentrations can occur in the transfused blood and this should be avoided (Mudge et al., 2004).

Hetastarch is best avoided in horses with LF as it may further prolong clotting times and its storage in hepatocytes and Kupffer cells may cause further deterioration in hepatic function (Christidis et al., 2001; Jones et al., 1997).

Sodium abnormalities in hepatic failure

Hyponatremia appears to be the most discussed and presumably the most important electrolyte abnormality in humans with LF. Hyponatremia in humans with LF is thought to decrease the effective circulating volume and may increase the risk of cerebral edema (Ackermann, 2009; Palm et al., 2011). Hyponatremia associated with LF in humans is a result of cirrhosis and accompanying ascites, which results in a relative water excess with dilution of plasma sodium. Additionally, these patients have reduced effective circulating plasma volume. This results in increases of plasma vasopressin concentrations and increased renal water absorption with further dilution of the plasma sodium. Although the plasma sodium concentration is low with dilutional hyponatremia, the total body sodium is usually high (Ackermann 2009; Ginès & Guevara, 2008).

Ascites caused by LF is rarely reported in horses. Equine hepatic lipidosis sometimes causes marked ventral edema and, although not reported in the literature, ascites may also be present (Watson et al., 1992).

The cause of ventral edema in horses with hyperlipemia and hepatic lipidosis is unknown, but might be the result of an acute increase in hydrostatic pressure in the subcutaneous abdominal veins. This increased hydrostatic pressure may be caused by the acute need for these veins to carry an increased blood volume from the abdomen to the heart; this demand for alternate venous return may be due to the resistance to portal flow caused by the rapidly enlarging liver. Affected ponies and miniature horses are also frequently hyperglycemic, which may further contribute to dilutional hyponatremia (Watson et al., 1992). It is also possible that a part of the hyponatremia observed in horses with hepatic lipidosis may be spurious. Hyperlipemia may cause a false decrease in the sodium as calculated by some chemistry machines (Lippi & Aloe, 2010). Ponies and miniature horses with hepatic lipidosis, hyperlipemia, and ventral edema may best be treated with a lower sodium fluid such as 0.45% NaCl + 2.5% dextrose + 20–40 mEq/L of KCl for maintenance purposes (assuming urination is occurring) and 0.1 U insulin/kg while monitoring both glucose and potassium concentrations.

Potassium abnormalities in horses with hepatic failure

Potassium homeostasis may be more important than sodium abnormalities in most horses with LF. Horses consume remarkable amounts of potassium in feed daily and when they become anorexic, as would be expected with LF, total body potassium and extracellular potassium may be quickly depleted. Additionally, a decrease in effective plasma volume as expected with LF would likely increase plasma aldosterone concentrations, which may further decrease plasma potassium through enhanced loss in the urine. Although total body K^+ content would almost certainly be low in most horses with LF, plasma potassium concentrations may be variable depending upon renal function, acid–base abnormalities, and plasma glucose concentrations. These factors can cause changes in potassium elimination and the intracellular–extracellular shifting of potassium.

Horses with Theiler's disease and those with endstage liver disease may occasionally develop intravascular hemolysis, which may increase plasma potassium

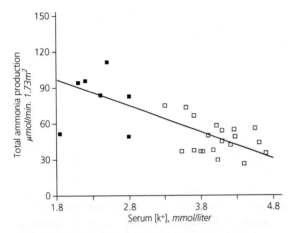

Figure 15.1 Relationship between total renal ammonia production and serum potassium. From Tizianello et al. Renal ammoniagenesis in humans with chronic potassium depletion. Kidney International. 1991; 40. Nature Publishing Group. Reproduced with permission.

concentration. Fluid therapy used to correct and maintain an adequate circulating intravascular volume will in most cases cause a net loss of potassium (even when added to the fluids) because of increased urine production and kaliuresis.

It has been proposed that potassium deficiency is a pathophysiologic factor in HE and efforts should be made to maintain plasma potassium concentration within the normal range (Baertl et al., 1963). The direct association between hypokalemia and HE is unproven but may be a result of a relationship between potassium and ammonia metabolism (Tizianello et al., 1991). Hypokalemia has been shown to alter the metabolism of ammonium by the kidney and to increase plasma ammonia and ammonium concentrations as shown in Figure 15.1 (Tizianello et al., 1991). The exact mechanisms for this increase are unknown, but may be related to enhancement of ammoniagenesis during hypokalemia (Tizianello et al., 1991; Wall, 2003).

Administration of potassium has been shown to decrease blood ammonia concentrations (Baertl et al., 1963). In horses with LF that are producing urine following rehydration, potassium should be supplemented at 20–40 mEq/L. Although many crystalloids contain a small amount of potassium, rapid intravenous administration of those crystalloids would likely reduce serum potassium concentration due to the diuresis and kaliuresis that

occurs. Increases in plasma and cerebrospinal fluid (CSF) ammonia (NH_3) concentrations will also be expected to increase ammonium (NH_4^+) in those fluid compartments since there is a pH-adjusted equilibration between ammonia and ammonium (Bosoi & Rose, 2009). Since K^+ and NH_4^+ are comparable in many aspects, abnormalities with either potassium or NH_4^+ will affect membrane potential, depolarizing both neurons and astrocytes (Bosoi & Rose, (2009).

Abnormalities in glucose homeostasis with liver failure

The liver is the primary organ responsible for glucose production. Glucose support should be considered in the fluid therapy plan for all patients with LF. This is especially important in foals with LF as they are much more likely to be hypoglycemic than are adult horses. Biochemistry findings in adult horses with LF may differ in several ways from those in many other species with LF. However, the major difference is that adult horses with LF are rarely hypoglycemic (McGorum et al., 1999).

Most adult horses with LF are normoglycemic or even hyperglycemic, although those with LF caused by neoplasia and some cases of hepatic lipidosis may be hypoglycemic. Hyperglycemia in equine LF may be at least partially the result of hyperammonemia; high NH_3 both enhances the release of glucagon and causes insulin resistance (the insulin resistance may be especially pronounced in some horses with hyperlipemia) (Roller et al., 1982). Glucose as a 5% solution should initially be added to the crystalloid fluids provided to horses with LF but may need to be adjusted after plasma glucose concentrations are known. For marked hypoglycemia, as is common in foals with LF, the initial intravenous fluid dextrose concentration should be 10%.

Insulin should be administered to equines with hyperlipemia and blood glucose concentrations above 180 mg/dL. Glucose and/or insulin administration will decrease plasma potassium concentration, and this should be monitored carefully in those patients. If the horse with LF is still eating, or in ponies or miniature horses with hepatic lipidosis fed with a feeding tube, intravenous glucose supplementation may not be necessary.

Intravenous nutritional support for hepatic failure

Glucose will be the predominant intravenously administered nutritional support for horses with LF. Although forced enteral feeding is preferred in ponies, donkeys, or miniature horses with hepatic lipidosis, partial parenteral nutrition using amino acids and glucose can be life-saving in those that cannot be fed enterally (i.e., esophageal choke) (Durham, 2006). The amino acid solution can be mixed with a balanced electrolyte solution and/or glucose. If glucose is used, its plasma concentrations should be monitored to determine an acceptable concentration of glucose in the parenteral nutrition (5–25%) and/or need for insulin therapy (Oikawa et al., 2006).

The form of protein provided in the parenteral nutrition, or for that matter in enteral support, is controversial for patients with liver disease. Products high in branched-chain amino acids are generally preferred (Charlton, 2006). Studies in humans and other non-equine species have shown improvement in HE when a high ratio of branched-chain to aromatic amino acids protein nutrition was provided (Charlton, 2006). Therefore, the use of high branched-chain formulations for parenteral nutrition would be recommended for horses with HE. The less expensive standard protein solutions of crystalline amino acids might be equally useful in ponies, donkeys, and miniature horses with hyperlipemia that cannot be fed enterally (Durham, 2006).

Most horses with LF have a negative energy balance and any protein supplements will be primarily "burned" for calories (approximately 4 cal/g). Horses with LF should not be maintained for more than 5 days on dextrose alone without provision of some protein, as this may cause hepatic lipidosis. All horses with LF should be administered multi-B vitamins to support cellular metabolism in the liver and other organs. These should be given intravenously slowly (e.g., diluted in crystalloids) each day while the horse is anorexic and receiving fluid therapy.

Abnormalities in acid–base balance and hepatic disease

The liver is important in acid–base physiology. It is involved in metabolism of organic acid anions (i.e., lactate), metabolism of ammonia, and production of albumin (Häussinger, 1997). Acid–base abnormalities in horses with LF may be different from those commonly seen in other species. In humans with LF, primary respiratory alkalosis with accompanying metabolic acidosis or alkalosis is common (Ahya et al., 2006). The respiratory alkalosis may be caused by hyperventilation resulting from HE.

In horses with LF, the predominant acid–base disturbance appears to be metabolic acidosis and acidemia. There may be a partial compensatory respiratory alkalosis in horses with HE, but these horses may be more prone to respiratory acidosis due to hypoventilation. Metabolic acidosis in horses with ALF is likely a result of hypoperfusion, increased anaerobic metabolism, and production of lactic acid. There is also a decrease in the clearance of lactate by the failing liver and as a response to hyperammonemia (Luft, 2001; Visek, 1979). The liver is responsible for at least 50% of lactate metabolism and when sufficient hepatic function is lost lactate metabolism is slowed. Hyperammonemia without liver disease in horses consistently causes both hyperglycemia and metabolic acidosis associated with increased lactate concentrations (Peek et al., 1997). The reason for the direct association between hyperammonemia and lactic acidosis is likely a result of high ammonia interference with the tricarboxylic acid cycle and aerobic metabolism (Visek, 1979).

Lactic acidosis in horses with LF should be treated as it may cause impaired myocardial contractility and decrease vascular response to catecholamines. Treatment of L-lactate acidosis in horses with LF should focus on improving cardiac output and improving perfusion of all tissues including the liver. This is best accomplished by administration of non-lactate-containing crystalloids and correction of electrolyte abnormalities (i.e., calcium and potassium abnormalities) that may be undermining normal cardiac and endothelial cell (or vascular) function. It is important to normalize glucose concentrations and inhibit inflammatory cytokines and prostanoids. Blood ammonia concentration can be reduced by decreasing the intestinal absorption of ammonia and increasing its clearance.

Sodium bicarbonate should not be used in the treatment of horses with metabolic acidosis and LF. Sodium bicarbonate may rapidly increase the plasma ammonia concentration by shifting the ammonium: ammonia equilibration toward gaseous ammonia (NH_3), which readily crosses an intact blood–brain barrier (Pandha, 1992). In addition, bicarbonate therapy may be harmful in treating HE as it may lower plasma ionized calcium and potassium concentrations, and even increase respiratory acidosis in horses with HE that are hypoventilating. Tranquilizers used to sedate horses with HE should be used cautiously to avoid possible adverse effects such as hypoventilation, abnormally low head position, and decreased cardiac output. These could all could negatively impact the treatment of LF.

References

Ackermann D. (2009) Treatment of ascites, hyponatremia and hepatorenal syndrome in liver cirrhosis. *Ther Umsch* **66**: 747–51.

Ahya SN, José Soler M, Levitsky J, Battle D. (2006) Acid–base and potassium disorders in liver disease. *Semin Nephrol* **22**: 466–70.

Arroyo V, Fernandez J. (2011) Pathophysiological basis of albumin use in cirrhosis. *Ann Hepatol* **10**:S6–S14.

Arya R, Gulati S, Deopujari S. (2010) Management of hepatic encephalopathy in children. *Postgrad Med J* **86**: 34–41.

Baertl JM, Sancetta SM, Gabuzda GJ. (1963) Relation of acute potassium depletion to renal ammonium metabolism in patients with cirrhosis. *J Clin Invest* **42**:696–706.

Bauer M, Kortgen A, Hartog C, Riedermann N, Reinhart K. (2009) Isotonic and hypertonic crystalloid solutions in the critically ill. *Best Pract Res Clin Anaesthesiol* **23**:173–81.

Bergero D, Nery J. (2008) Hepatic diseases in horses. *J Anim Physiol An N* **92**:345–55.

Bosoi CR, Rose CF. (2009) Identifying the direct effects of ammonia on the brain. *Metab Brain Dis* **24**:95–102.

Charlton M. (2006) Branched-chain amino acid enriched supplements as therapy for liver disease. *J Nutr* **136**:295S–298S.

Christidis C, Mal F, Ramos, J. Senejoux A, et al. (2001) Worsening of hepatic dysfunction as a consequence of repeated hydroxyethyl starch infusions. *J Hepatol* **35**:726–32.

Durham AE. (2006) Clinical application of parenteral nutrition in the treatment of five ponies and one donkey with hyperlipaemia. *Vet Rec* **158**:159–64.

Durham AE, Newton JR, Smith KC, et al. (2003) Retrospective analysis of historical, clinical, ultrasonographic, serum biochemical and haematological data in prognostic evaluation of equine liver disease. *Equine Vet J* **35**:542–7.

Frederick RT. (2011) Current concepts in the pathophysiology and management of hepatic encephalopathy. *Gastroenterol Hepatol* **7**:222–33.

Ginès P, Guevara M. (2008) Hyponatremia in cirrhosis: pathogenesis, clinical significance, and management. *Hepatology* **48**:1002–10.

Gold JR, Warren AL, French TW, Stokol T. (2008) What is your diagnosis? Biopsy impression smear of a hepatic mass in a yearling Thoroughbred filly. *Vet Clin Pathol* **37**:339–43.

Häussinger D. (1997) Liver regulation of acid-base balance. *Miner Electrolyte Metab* **23**:249–52.

Heinig RE, Clarke EF, Waterhouse C. (1979) Lactic acidosis and liver disease. *Arch Int Med* **139**:1229–32.

Jones PA, Tomasic M, Gentry PA. (1997) Oncotic, hemodilutional, and hemostatic effects of isotonic saline and hydroxyethyl starch solutions in clinically normal ponies. *Am J Vet Res* **58**:541–8.

Kramer GC. (2003) Hypertonic resuscitation: physiologic mechanisms and recommendations for trauma care. *J Trauma* **54**:S89–S99.

Lippi G, Aloe R. (2010) Hyponatremia and pseudohyponatremia: first, do no harm. *Am J Med* **123**:E17.

Luft FC. (2001) Lactic acidosis update for critical care clinicians. *J Am Soc Nephrol* **12**:S15–S19.

Masaya Y, Kazuaki I, Makoto Y. (2001) Fluid replacement therapy. *Fluid therapy of liver disease. Clin All-Round* **50**:3030–5.

McGorum BC, Murphy D, Love S, Milne EM. (1999) Clinicopathological features of equine primary hepatic disease: a review of 50 cases. *Vet Rec* **145**:134–9.

Mudge MC, Macdonald MH, Owens SD, Tablin F. (2004) Comparison of 4 blood storage methods in a protocol for equine pre-operative autologous donation. *Vet Surg* **33**:475–86.

O'Grady JG, Williams R. (1986) Management of acute liver failure. *Schweiz Med Wochenschr* **116**:541–4.

Oikawa S, McGuirk S, Nishibe K, et al. (2006) Changes of blood biochemical values in ponies recovering from hyperlipemia in Japan. *J Vet Med Sci* **68**:353–9.

Palm C, Wagner A, Gross P. (2011) Hypo- and hypernatremia. *Dtsche Med Wochenschr* **136**:29–33.

Pandha HS. (1992) Treating acidosis in fulminant hepatic failure: the case against use of bicarbonate solutions. *N Z Med J* **105**:271.

Parraga ME, Carlson GP, Thurmond M. (1995) Serum protein concentrations in horses with severe liver disease: a retrospective study and review of the literature. *J Vet Int Med* **9**:154–61.

Peek SF, Divers TJ, Jackson CJ. (1997) Hyperammonaemia associated with encephalopathy and abdominal pain without evidence of liver disease in four mature horses. *Equine Vet J* **29**:70–4.

Polli F, Gattinoni L. (2010) Balancing volume resuscitation and ascites management in cirrhosis. *Curr Opin Anaesthesiol* **23**:151–8.

Roller MH, Riedermann GS, Romkema GE, Swanson RN. (1982) Ovine blood chemistry values measured during ammonia toxicosis. *Am J Vet Res* **43**:1068–71.

Singh RK, Poddar B, Singhal S, Azim A. (2011) Continuous hypertonic saline for acute liver failure. *Indian J Gastroenterol* **30**:178–80.

Tizianello A, Garibotto G, Robaudo C, et al. (1991) Renal ammoniagenesis in humans with chronic potassium depletion. *Kidney Int* **40**:772–8.

Trotter JF. (2009) Practical management of acute liver failure in the intensive care unit. *Curr Opin Crit Care* **15**:163–7.

Visek WJ. (1979) Ammonia metabolism, urea cycle capacity and their biochemical assessment. *Nutr Rev* **37**:273–82.

Wall SM. (2003) Mechanisms of NH_4^+ and NH_3 transport during hypokalemia. *Acta Physiol Scand* **179**:325–30.

Watson TD, Murphy D, Love S. (1992) Equine hyperlipaemia in the United Kingdom: clinical features and blood biochemistry of 18 cases. *Vet Rec* **13**:48–51.

West HJ. (1996) Clinical and pathological studies in horses with hepatic disease. *Equine Vet J* **28**:146–56.

CHAPTER 16

Fluid therapy for gastrointestinal disease

Diana M. Hassel

Associate Professor – Equine Emergency Surgery & Critical Care, Department of Clinical Sciences, Colorado State University, USA

Fluid therapy is often the mainstay of treatment for horses with gastrointestinal disorders, including various forms of colitis (salmonellosis, clostridiosis, grain overload, etc.), functional inflammatory disorders of the small intestine (duodenitis/proximal jejunitis), and strangulating or non-strangulating obstructive disorders resulting in colic. This chapter is designed to review features of fluid therapy specifically pertaining to the adult horse with gastrointestinal disease, including intravenous catheter selection, most commonly encountered fluid and electrolyte abnormalities, secondary renal disorders, and recommended methods of fluid and fluid additive delivery. The goal of this chapter is to help provide the tools for successful development of a fluid administration and monitoring plan in the adult colic or colitis patient.

Catheter selection

Although a comprehensive review of catheter materials and types can be found in Chapter 9 of this textbook, there follows a brief review of catheter selection as it pertains to the patient with gastrointestinal disease. Teflon, over-the-needle 14-gauge 5.5-inch catheters, and 14-gauge polyurethane catheters available in both over-the-needle and over-the-wire formats, are commonly used in equine practice. Choice of catheter material and size in the colic or colitis patient is best dictated by the systemic status of the patient. A colic patient with a non-strangulating simple obstruction that will likely not require the presence of an indwelling intravenous catheter for more than 72 hours, may be effectively managed with an inexpensive 14-gauge polytetrafluoroethylene (PTFE, Teflon®), over-the-needle catheter (e.g., Abbocath®: Abbott Laboratories, Abbott Park, IL; 14-gauge 5½ in). Acute colic patients with strangulating obstructions or other surgical lesions may be best managed with a longer term, less thrombogenic material such as polyurethane. An over-the-needle polyurethane catheter (e.g., Mila International, Florence, KY; 14-gauge 5¼ in) can be more rapidly placed than over-the-wire varieties, and may be a more practical choice for the acute colic patient. Colitis patients may benefit from the longer term over-the-wire polyurethane catheter (e.g., Mila International, Florence, KY; 14-gauge 8 in) inserted using the Seldinger technique as they are at high risk for venous thrombosis and thrombophlebitis. Unique athrombogenic coated catheters have recently shown promise in human medicine in reducing catheter-related complications (Hitz et al., 2012).

Intravenous catheters of 10-gauge or 12-gauge may be optimally utilized in the acutely hypovolemic preoperative patient with a severe strangulating obstruction to facilitate administration of a more rapid fluid bolus for resuscitation and preparation for anesthesia with minimal delays. A fluid pump administration system allows for much more rapid administration of intravenous fluids than gravity (Figure 16.1).

Exceeding a rate of 200 mL/min is not recommended when using a standard 14-gauge catheter due to an increased potential for injury to the endothelium from recoil that may occur at the distal end of the catheter.

Equine Fluid Therapy, First Edition. Edited by C. Langdon Fielding and K. Gary Magdesian.

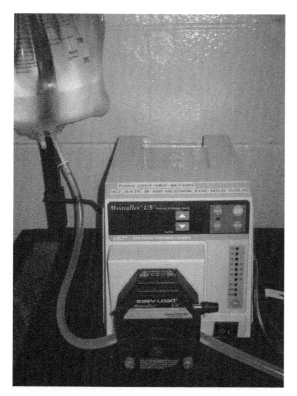

Figure 16.1 Fluid administration pump for rapid intravenous infusion in patients with acute severe hypovolemia and dehydration.

More rapid administration of fluids can be achieved through either larger gauge catheters or by placement of a second catheter. Large-bore catheters should only be used when necessary, however, as they may carry increased thrombogenic risk.

Fluid and electrolyte disorders in gastrointestinal disease

Hypovolemia and dehydration

There are two common scenarios in evaluating the body water status of horses with gastrointestinal disease. Horses with chronic colic of more than 1 day duration are likely to show clinical signs of dehydration (extracellular fluid volume depletion), largely as a consequence of reduced water intake. These clinical signs become apparent as a horse approaches a 5% level of dehydration. In a 500-kg horse, this would represent an estimated 25 L fluid deficit and would primarily be manifest

as tacky oral mucous membranes and mild delays in recovery of tented skin. As gastrointestinal tract contents serve as a substantial reserve of both water and electrolytes, a reduction in water intake often results in dehydration of colonic contents from fluid absorption in an effort to maintain adequate body water levels. A common consequence of this is colic secondary to impaction of the large colon.

The second scenario is found in cases of more acute, severe colic or colitis that have concurrent hypovolemia as a consequence of intravascular fluid losses due to changes in endothelial permeability along with intestinal mucosal malabsorptive and hypersecretory processes (Argenzio, 1992). Expected clinical findings in adult horses with intravascular fluid losses of as little as 8–10 L (or an estimated 20–25% of intravascular fluid volume) include tachycardia, cool extremities, delayed jugular vein filling, decreased urine output, and diminished pulse quality. These acute, severely hypovolemic patients often have losses as a consequence of both reduction in fluid intake and increased fluid losses into the gastrointestinal tract and interstitium. Concurrent severe protein losses are characteristic of more critical conditions and may assist with early assessment of prognosis. Low preoperative total plasma protein concentration in combination with high preoperative packed cell volume (PCV) is associated with increased risk of death in horses with surgical disease of the small intestine (Proudman et al., 2005).

When considering fluid replacement therapy in horses with gastrointestinal disease, it is essential to include ongoing losses specific to the gastrointestinal tract such as those due to mechanical obstruction of the bowel, small or large intestinal ileus, nasogastric reflux, diarrhea, and peritoneal effusion if peritonitis is present. These ongoing losses must be accounted for and added to those required for both maintenance and pre-existing dehydration and hypovolemia when formulating a fluid therapy plan (Figure 16.2).

Electrolyte and acid–base disturbances

Electrolyte and acid–base abnormalities are common in horses with obstructive disorders of the gastrointestinal tract; however, they are most severe in horses with colitis, enterocolitis, and proximal jejunitis/duodenitis. Minimum electrolyte monitoring in the colic patient on intravenous fluids should include measuring sodium, potassium, chloride, potassium, calcium, and magnesium

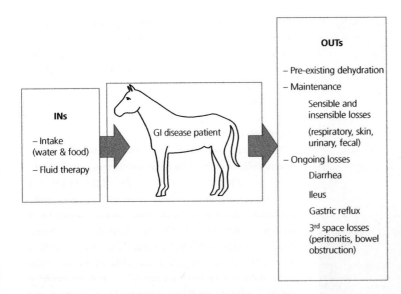

Figure 16.2 Fluid requirements to take into consideration when designing a fluid therapy plan for horses with gastrointestinal disease.

concentrations in plasma. Mild electrolyte abnormalities occur frequently among all forms of colic, with the most prevalent abnormalities including hypokalemia, hypocalcemia, and hypomagnesemia. Studies have shown that 54% of horses admitted for surgical colic have low serum ionized magnesium, and 86% have low serum ionized calcium concentrations (Dart et al., 1992; Garcia-Lopez et al., 2001). Similarly, 44–54% of colic patients after surgery are hypokalemic (Costa et al., 1999; Garcia-Lopez et al., 2001; Protopapas, 2000), speculated to be associated with reduced intake, altered absorption, excess loss from the gastrointestinal tract (Gennari, 1998; Nappert & Johnson, 2001), a dilutional effect from fluid therapy, renal losses, or secondary to treatment with drugs such as penicillin and gentamicin (Gennari, 1998). Hypokalemia that is refractory to supplementation with potassium may be a consequence of hypomagnesemia (Fiaccadori et al., 1988; Olerich & Rude, 1994). Magnesium has the potential to benefit the colic patient as there is evidence in animal models that it may exert anti-inflammatory effects during endotoxemia and may be protective during ischemia-reperfusion injury (Kim et al., 2011; Lee et al., 2011).

The prevalence of hyponatremia in postoperative surgical colic patients is 30% (Protopapas, 2000), and severe hyponatremia and hypochloremia are common in the colitis patient (Stewart et al., 1995). Fluid sequestration into the GI tract is a typical cause (Adrogue & Madias, 2000), and others may include excess secretion of antidiuretic hormone in response to pain, diarrhea,

renal failure, and iatrogenic fluid overloading from repeated nasogastric intubation with plain water (Adrogue & Madias, 2000; Lopes, 2003). Hypernatremia is less common in the equine GI patient, but may be associated with water deprivation.

As most electrolyte disorders in the GI patient fall within the mild or moderate category, routine electrolyte monitoring with concurrent supplementation of potassium, calcium, magnesium, and sodium chloride as needed is appropriate. Maintenance doses often administered are:

- 20 mEq/L of KCl added to isotonic fluids (avoid during bolus administration so as not to exceed 0.5 mEq/kg/h);
- 20–25 mL 23% calcium gluconate/L with mild to moderate hypocalcemia (total dose: 500 mL/day 23% calcium borogluconate for a 500-kg horse);
- 0.5–2 g/L of $MgSO_4$ (total dose of 25–150 mg/kg/day depending on monitoring) with mild to moderate hypomagnesemia;
- normal saline with mild to moderate hypochloremia. Treatment of hyponatremia is dependent on acid–base and concurrent chloride status, with either sodium chloride, sodium bicarbonate, or balanced electrolyte solutions with a sodium concentration at or above that of normal equine plasma (e.g., Plasma-Lyte® A, Normosol™-R).

Metabolic acidosis in the severe colic patient is often a consequence of hyperlactatemia from hypovolemia and reduced tissue perfusion or from extensive bowel ischemia (Tennent-Brown, 2012). Replenishment of intravascular volume with restoration of tissue perfusion is the essential first step to manage acidosis. Persistent metabolic acidosis may occur in some horses with continuing electrolyte loss into the gastrointestinal tract as is seen with some colitis cases, and costs and benefits of sodium bicarbonate supplementation are discussed in Chapter 8. Due to the high prevalence of strong ion imbalances and hypoproteinemia in horses with severe gastrointestinal disease, a quantitative approach to acid–base assessment is recommended to better characterize acid–base disorders, and this is discussed more thoroughly in Chapter 8 (Navarro et al., 2005).

Renal dysfunction in gastrointestinal disease

Although fluid therapy for renal disease is covered in detail in Chapter 14, renal dysfunction with particular reference to gastrointestinal tract disorders merits a mention. Hemodynamic alterations as a consequence of profound dehydration and endotoxemia that often accompany gastrointestinal tract disorders can contribute to significant renal hypoperfusion and subsequent azotemia (Divers et al., 1987; Seanor et al., 1984). In addition, many horses with colitis or colic are treated with nephrotoxic drugs such as non-steroidal anti-inflammatory drugs (NSAIDs), aminoglycoside antimicrobials, and polymyxin B sulfate. The NSAIDs in particular are often administered early in the course of the disease with repeated dosing, often prior to adequately addressing fluid deficits. As a result, clinicians in referral hospitals are frequently presented with horses with both gastrointestinal disease and azotemia associated with one or more causes (Groover et al., 2006). Initial differentiation of prerenal from renal azotemia can be difficult, but azotemia that fails to resolve after 48 to 72 hours of adequate fluid administration is generally considered an indicator of renal insufficiency in hospitalized human patients (Miller et al., 1978).

Colitis and colic patients with systemic inflammatory response syndrome (SIRS) are frequently in need of colloidal support to promote adequate intravascular volume and colloid oncotic pressure. The higher molecular weight synthetic colloids have been associated with an increased incidence of acute renal failure in critically ill septic human patients, but there are currently no reports of alteration of kidney function in horses in response to synthetic colloid therapy (Bayer et al., 2011; Brunkhorst et al., 2008). Recently hetastarch has been associated with an increased mortality rate in human patients, which has called the safety of these synthetic colloids into question (Zarychanski et al, 2013).

Critically ill horses with severe gastrointestinal disorders that entail substantial and prolonged ongoing losses due to the presence of either profuse watery diarrhea or nasogastric reflux may be at risk for medullary washout and a subsequent inability to concentrate urine when fluid rates are slowed or discontinued. This is believed to be a result of increased renal blood flow and polyuria from high-volume fluid administration presumably resulting in washout of medullary interstitial osmoles. Careful monitoring of urine specific gravity to avoid hyposthenuria (urine SG <1.010) may help avoid this complication (Southwood, 2005).

Specific gastrointestinal disorders

Colic

There are numerous causes for abdominal pain in horses, but the majority of horses with obstructive disorders will fall into one of two categories: non-strangulating mechanical obstruction or strangulating obstruction. A third, less common cause is duodenitis/proximal jejunitis leading to a functional obstruction, or motility dysfunction secondary to inflammation of the small intestine. Each has unique characteristics that influence the optimal type of fluid administered and method of administration.

Non-strangulating obstructions

Non-strangulating mechanical obstructions resulting in colic cover a wide variety of conditions including feed impactions of the large colon, colonic displacements, foreign body obstructions, sand impactions, and enteroliths, among others. Most of these horses show only mild signs of systemic dehydration or electrolyte abnormalities and rarely develop hypovolemia. The basis for fluid therapy in the majority of these cases is simple rehydration, and in the case of impaction, hydration of colonic contents to allow passage of ingesta. Large colon displacements can also sometimes be successfully managed medically with IV fluid therapy, exercise, and analgesics (McGovern et al., 2011). Traditionally, colonic hydration has been approached by administration of large volumes of intravenous fluids to promote systemic overhydration combined with administration through a nasogastric tube of a laxative, such as mineral oil or magnesium sulfate (Freeman et al., 1992; White & Dabareiner, 1997). Systemic overhydration achieved by rapid intravenous infusions of large volumes of fluids has been shown to be inferior to enteral infusions of similar volumes in promoting colonic hydration and may contribute to electrolyte derangements, hemodilution, and increased urine output (Lopes et al., 2002). However, tolerance of enteral fluid therapy may vary between individuals and may be impaired as a consequence of bowel obstruction. Severe cecal or colonic distention in itself may limit fluid absorption simply due to compression of the proximal small intestine and subsequent inability to pass fluids beyond the duodenum for fluid absorption or hydration of colonic content. Colic or the onset of development of nasogastric reflux is common with initiation of aggressive enteral fluid therapy programs in horses with impactions (Lopes et al. 2001). Balanced electrolyte solutions (Box 16.1) are the optimum media for colonic hydration via the enteral route; administration may be through intermittent bolus administration or continuous enteral infusion (Lopes et al., 2004).

A potential benefit of bolus administration (5–8 L every 1–2 h in an adult) is promotion of the gastro-colic reflex associated with gastric filling to promote motility in the colon (Freeman et al., 1992; Merritt et al., 1995; Roger & Ruckebusch, 1987; Sellers et al., 1979). However, horses with impactions are able to tolerate larger volumes of fluid (5 L/h) when administered with continuous enteral administration versus bolus administration (Lopes et al., 2001). Enteral fluid therapy has been shown to resolve large colon

impactions more rapidly and is associated with shorter hospitalization times over parenteral fluid therapy alone (Hallowell, 2008). The author's preference for fluid therapy in horses with extensive palpable impactions of the large colon, prolonged colic due to an impaction, or clinical evidence of dehydration equal to or exceeding 5%, is administration of a 5-liter bolus of balanced electrolyte solution every 2 hours through an indwelling nasogastric tube combined with concurrent IV fluid therapy with balanced isotonic crystalloids. Based on the level of dehydration, a 10–60 L/kg IV bolus is initially administered followed by 2–4 mL/kg/h until fecal passage is observed. Chapter 21 provides a more detailed review of enteral fluid therapy indications, types, and rates.

When intravenous fluids are administered in horses with simple obstructions, polyionic isotonic replacement fluids such as lactated Ringer's solution (LRS), Normosol-R, and Plasma-Lyte A are good choices. Although 0.9% saline would be adequate when no other fluid sources are available, the high sodium and chloride content (154 mEq/L) will likely lead to electrolyte imbalances when administered to horses with normal sodium and chloride concentrations, particularly hyperchloremia. Regardless of the presence or absence of electrolyte abnormalities in the non-strangulating obstructive colic patient, if an initial IV bolus of polyionic fluids is administered, electrolyte supplementation should be avoided until the fluid rate has been slowed to 2–6 mL/kg/h.

Monitoring

Although hypokalemia, hypocalcemia, and hypomagnesemia are common among horses with colic and anorexia, for simple obstructions or non-strangulating displacements whose treatments consist primarily of analgesics and balanced polyionic fluid therapy, intensive monitoring and supplementation of electrolytes are often unnecessary. Monitoring of packed cell volume (PCV) and total plasma protein concentration will provide useful information on efficacy of fluid therapy in restoring fluid deficits. If an impaction or displacement persists through initial aggressive fluid therapy and further medical treatment is indicated, a more thorough evaluation with assessment of plasma electrolyte concentrations is appropriate. Stall-side portable analyzers have become readily available in recent years allowing rapid and easy evaluation of electrolyte values.

Box 16.1 Balanced electrolyte solution for continuous or intermittent bolus enteral fluid therapy via nasogastric tube.

- Mix the following in 5 L warm water:
NaCl	28 g
$NaHCO_3$	17 g
KCl	3 g
- Simplified recipe for 5 L volume of warm water:
NaCl	30 g
KCl	15 g

Functional obstructions (duodenitis/ proximal jejunitis)

Duodenitis/proximal jejunitis (DPJ), also known as proximal enteritis or anterior enteritis, is characterized by inflammation of the proximal small intestine resulting in ileus and fluid accumulation in the stomach and small intestine, and is often accompanied by SIRS (systemic inflammatory response syndrome). Although a definitive cause is unknown, some evidence supports *Clostridium* spp. as an important pathogen in the development of DPJ (Arroyo et al., 2006; Edwards, 2000). The hallmark of DPJ is the development of ileus with large volumes of nasogastric reflux resulting in colic that is partially responsive to gastric decompression. Other features of the disease are depression, tachycardia, prerenal azotemia, dehydration, hypovolemia, fever, leukocytosis, and electrolyte abnormalities (Johnston & Morris, 1987; Seahorn et al., 1992; White et al., 1987). The severity of the disease and presence of SIRS is highly variable but in all cases fluid therapy and gastric decompression remain the mainstays of treatment. Additional common therapies include NSAIDs, lidocaine ($50 \mu g/kg/min$) or other prokinetic therapy, treatment for endotoxemia, and restriction of food and water intake. Although some advocate surgical management based on evidence for a clostridial etiology for the disease (Edwards, 2000), more recent work suggests surgical decompression provides no benefit (Underwood et al., 2008).

Unique fluid therapy considerations in DPJ

Dysfunction of the proximal small intestine and stomach prevents enteral fluid therapy as a viable option. Unlike simple obstructions of the gastrointestinal tract, moderate to severe electrolyte abnormalities are common in horses presented with DPJ; this is because excessive fluid and electrolyte secretion occurs as a result of the inflammatory process. Sodium and chloride are actively secreted into the intestinal lumen and water follows through highly permeable intercellular spaces (McConnico, 2004; Powell, 1991). The average adult horse is capable of carrying 2.66 L of fluid per meter (0.81 L of fluid per foot) of small intestine, suggesting a fluid capacity of nearly 50 L, which contains 100 mmol/L Na^+, 22 mmol/L K^+, and 66 mmol/L Cl^- (Schott, 2012). The length of the small intestine in horses with strangulating obstructions is reported to increase by 29–36%, reflecting a possible underestimation of this potential volume loss (Freeman & Kilgallon,

2001). Passive secretion of protein-rich fluid into the lumen follows, with the end result of small intestinal distention, ileus, nasogastric reflux, dehydration, hypoproteinemia, and circulatory shock (McConnico, 2004). Loss of luminal bicarbonate through repeated fluid evacuation from the stomach with nasogastric intubation, combined with lactate accumulation from tissue hypoperfusion, may lead to metabolic acidosis. Classic findings on biochemical panels in these horses include hyponatremia, hypochloremia, hypokalemia, elevated blood creatinine concentration, and elevated anion gap.

Hypoproteinemia may develop during the course of therapy with persistent DPJ as a result of continued enteric protein losses and systemic protein catabolism. Fluid therapy in these cases should be directed toward rapid correction of the fluid deficit, correction of electrolyte abnormalities, and maintenance of adequate colloid osmotic pressure (COP) when a hypo-oncotic state is present. Partial parenteral nutrition with glucose-amino acid solutions is also recommended with DPJ that persists for more than 48 hours as anorexia, cachexia, and continued protein loss are expected. Enteral nutrition and water intake are restricted until resolution of ileus has occurred. Refer to Chapter 25 for a more extensive discussion of partial or complete parenteral nutrition including formulations, rates of administration, and common complications.

Correction of the fluid deficits in the DPJ case should take into account presenting deficits (percent dehydration × body weight in kg), maintenance requirements (2–3 mL/kg/h), and ongoing losses (nasogastric reflux volume) (see Figure 16.2). Once initial deficits have been addressed and adequate tissue perfusion and renal function have been restored, excessive fluid administration should be avoided. There is a strong correlation between excessive intravascular volume and subsequent mortality, morbidity, and length of stay in human ICU patients (Shields, 2008). In the DPJ patient, excessive fluid administration combined with reduced intravascular oncotic pressure may further result in increased capillary perfusion pressure, which may accelerate flux of fluid from the vasculature into the intestinal lumen (McConnico, 2004).

Monitoring

In severe cases of DPJ with concurrent SIRS and severe derangements in fluid and electrolyte status, regular and repeated use of advanced monitoring techniques such as arterial blood pressure monitoring, central venous pressure, urine specific gravity, venous blood gas evaluation, and serial abdominal ultrasound to assess efficacy of treatment and progression of ileus may be advantageous (Feary & Hassel, 2006; Magdesian, 2004). Detection of trends in these monitored variables as well as packed cell volume, total plasma protein, serum electrolytes, creatinine, hepatic enzymes, lactate, and colloid osmotic pressure will provide more useful information to guide fluid therapy. An observed increase in packed cell volume accompanied by no change or a decrease in total plasma protein concentration can provide an early clue that further fluid and protein losses are occurring. If this is observed and an indwelling nasogastric tube is not present, a tube should be passed to allow for gastric decompression. Frequent abdominal ultrasound will also provide useful information pertaining to restoration of small intestinal function through observation of the degree of small intestinal distention. Motility patterns of the small intestine, and presence or absence of fluid or gas distention within the stomach evident as observation of the stomach wall beyond the 13th intercostal space, can also be evaluated.

Colloid osmotic pressure (COP) should be monitored in all cases of DPJ that are severely hypoproteinemic or are receiving synthetic colloid therapy. Colloid therapy is most commonly needed in the colitis patient as discussed below, and a more in-depth discussion of indications and types is provided in Chapter 24.

Strangulating obstructions

Strangulating obstructive diseases in horses span a variety of conditions leading to ischemia of a segment of small or large intestine; they include, but are not limited to, large colon volvulus, strangulating lipoma, epiploic foramen entrapment, gastrosplenic ligament entrapment, mesenteric rent, small intestinal volvulus, intussusception, inguinal hernia, and diaphragmatic hernia. Fluid therapy is an integral component of therapy as hypovolemic shock, endotoxemia, and SIRS are commonly encountered.

Unique fluid therapy considerations for strangulating obstructions

As horses with colic secondary to strangulating obstructions are surgical emergencies, fluid therapy in these patients has two phases. Phase one consists of emergency resuscitation to prepare for anesthesia, and phase two

encompasses the postoperative period. Unlike those with non-strangulating obstructions, many of these patients require rapid intravascular expansion with hypertonic solutions with or without synthetic colloids, as well as ongoing colloidal support in the postoperative period.

During the acute presentation of a horse with a strangulating obstruction, a rapid physical assessment of hydration and blood volume status should be performed to determine whether adequate stabilization can be achieved with prompt delivery of isotonic crystalloids, or if there is a need for accelerated volume expansion prior to initiation of anesthesia. A simple test to aid in this decision is a PCV. Horses with marked elevations in PCV (>50%) should be treated aggressively by rapid blood volume expansion with hypertonic saline solution (HSS) or synthetic colloids in combination with isotonic crystalloid therapy.

In the postoperative period, horses with strangulating obstructive disease often exhibit SIRS in response to exposure to bacterial antigens and endotoxin both before and after surgery. Translocation of endotoxin and other bacterial by-products continues in the postoperative period as a consequence of injury to the mucosa from either direct ischemia or secondary to distention and tissue manipulation. Hypoproteinemia, hemoconcentration, and electrolyte disturbances are common sequelae.

In horses with strangulating small intestinal disease, postoperative ileus occurs commonly and eliminates the capacity for enteral feeding. The use of partial parenteral nutrition may be indicated, similar to that described for horses with DPJ.

Types of fluid and fluid additives

Hypertonic saline solution (7.2–7.5% sodium chloride) should be administered in the acute strangulating obstructive colic patient when signs of shock with inadequate tissue perfusion are present. The volume administered is 2–6 mL/kg and it has approximately eight times the tonicity of plasma (approximately 1200 mOsm/L Na^+; 1200 mOsm/L Cl^-). HSS increases intravascular volume, improves cardiac contractility, improves cardiac output, reduces systemic vascular resistance through arteriolar vasodilation, and decreases tissue edema. It also improves microcirculation, blood viscosity, oxygen transport, and immunomodulation (Fielding & Magdesian, 2011; Kien & Kramer, 1989; Kien et al., 1991, 1996; Kreimeier et al., 1997; Oliveira et al., 2002a; Pantaleon, 2010). These beneficial hemodynamic effects last approximately 30 minutes and in large part are attributed to an increase in intravascular volume derived from both intracellular and interstitial compartments because of the hyperosmolar concentration gradient. This necessitates administration of isotonic fluids immediately following HSS administration to help restore these deficits. HSS also has been shown to promote vasopressin release, which may further enhance its ability to increase intravascular volume (Batista et al., 2009). Of particular benefit in horses with gastrointestinal disease is the proposed benefit of HSS on microvascular circulation and mitigation of intestinal edema development (Pascual et al., 2003; Radhakrishnan et al., 2009). Combination therapy with HSS (5 mL/kg) and a synthetic colloid (hetastarch: 10 mL/kg) in endotoxemic horses was superior to isotonic fluid therapy alone in protecting against endotoxemia-mediated hypocalcemia (Pantaleon et al., 2007).

Electrolyte deficiencies in horses with strangulating obstructions should be managed with the addition of potassium, magnesium, calcium, sodium, and chloride as was discussed earlier in this chapter. Ionized hypomagnesemia and hypocalcemia are particularly prevalent among surgical colic cases, reported at 54% and 84%, respectively (Garcia-Lopez et al., 2001).

Partial parenteral nutrition for postoperative small intestinal resection cases may initially consist of 2.5% dextrose added to intravenous fluids. However, the rate of fluid administration needs to be considered when calculating the amount of dextrose to be added; for example, 2.5% dextrose at a maintenance fluid rate of 2.5 mL/kg/h (1.25 L/h for a 500-kg horse) would equate to 1 mg/kg/min of dextrose. This is a reasonable starting point for adult horses that are euglycemic. Blood glucose monitoring may be relevant if dextrose supplementation is pursued as the mean blood glucose level at presentation in horses with strangulating obstructions is 212 mg/dL and persistent hyperglycemia should be avoided (Hassel et al., 2009). Further caloric supplementation with parenteral nutrition sources including 50% dextrose and amino acids may be appropriate when prolonged anorexia occurs due to persistent nasogastric reflux. Hypertriglyceridemia is present in nearly all postoperative colics (Underwood et al., 2010), and is negatively associated with survival, so the addition of lipid to parenteral nutrition solutions should be used with caution. See Chapter 25 for a detailed discussion of parenteral nutrition.

Monitoring

As was described for monitoring in severe cases of DPJ, use of advanced monitoring techniques such as arterial blood pressure monitoring, central venous pressure, urine specific gravity, and venous blood gas evaluation may be advantageous (Feary & Hassel, 2006; Magdesian 2004). More importantly, serial abdominal ultrasonography for both postoperative strangulating small intestinal lesions and large colon volvulus can provide valuable insight into progress or development of complications. Early detection of ileus and fluid losses in the postoperative small intestinal strangulating obstruction may be evident as progressive small intestinal distention, intestinal stasis, and gastric and duodenal distention detectable with abdominal ultrasonography. Detection of trends in PCV and total plasma protein concentration can provide further insight into whether ongoing losses of fluids and electrolytes are occurring in the small intestine or colon. An increase in PCV accompanied by a reduction in total plasma proteins is consistent with ongoing gastrointestinal fluid losses.

Ultrasonographic monitoring of the large colon in the postoperative large colon volvulus patient can aid in the identification of those patients at risk for developing multiple organ dysfunction syndrome (MODS) (Sheats et al., 2010). A prolonged period to postoperative involution of wall edema is associated with increased morbidity and mortality.

As in horses with DPJ, colloid osmotic pressure (COP) should be monitored in all postoperative hypoproteinemic patients receiving synthetic colloid therapy. Colloid therapy is commonly needed in the postoperative large colon volvulus and colitis patient, and a more in-depth discussion of indications and types is provided in Chapter 24.

Colitis

Acute colitis is a therapeutic challenge for clinicians, and fluid therapy remains a principal and essential component of therapy. Specific disease entities that are known to cause colitis in the adult horse include salmonellosis, clostridiosis, Potomac horse fever, proliferative enteropathy (*Lawsonia intracellularis*), and parasitic enteritis (Feary & Hassel, 2006). As a causative agent is often not identified in acute colitis patients, it is likely that other, as yet unrecognized, pathogens play an important role in the pathogenesis of this condition. Most recently, it has been proposed that colitis is a disease of intestinal dysbiosis, rather than a result of the overgrowth of an individual pathogen (Costa et al., 2012). Except in cases with a known pathogen, such as *Clostridium difficile, Cl. perfringens, Neorickettsia risticii,* and cyathostomiasis or strongylosis, treatment for acute colitis is primarily supportive in nature. Replacement of fluid and electrolyte losses, control of enteric inflammation, reduction of fluid secretion into the gastrointestinal lumen, control of endotoxemia and SIRS, and re-establishment of normal gastrointestinal flora are the principal goals of treatment.

Unique fluid therapy considerations in colitis

The first priority in acute colitis is to stabilize the patient hemodynamically with fluid and electrolyte therapy. In horses exhibiting signs of shock, rapid administration of an isotonic fluid bolus (20–40 mL/kg) in the first hour, or hypertonic saline solution followed by balanced polyionic fluids may be appropriate. However, the optimum method for fluid resuscitation should be tailored to the patient, utilizing serial monitoring of perfusion and oxygenation parameters to guide resuscitation (Driessen & Brainard, 2006), as well as electrolyte status.

Considering the inflammatory process occurring in the gastrointestinal tract in horses with colitis, use of enteral fluid therapy is generally not recommended (Ecke et al., 1998a), although voluntary ingestion of water or water with electrolytes is encouraged. In some cases, small intestinal ileus also may occur in advanced stages of SIRS/endotoxemia or with disease processes that affect the intestine diffusely, preventing the use of the enteral route for fluid therapy.

Horses with acute severe colitis often present with marked electrolyte and acid–base abnormalities as a consequence of increased secretion and diminished intake and absorption of electrolytes. Most (80%) of horses with enterocolitis have ionized hypocalcemia (Toribio et al., 2001) attributed to sequestration in the gastrointestinal tract lumen from loss or poor absorption associated with inflammation (Nakamura et al., 1998), renal losses (Zaloga et al., 1988), impaired calcium mobilization (Dandona et al., 1994), tissue sequestration, or impairment of calcium release by target tissue in response to parathyroid hormone (Zaloga et al., 1988).

Hypomagnesemia is another common finding seen often in combination with hypocalcemia in horses with colitis. Unlike calcium, which has complex regulatory mechanisms to safeguard homeostasis, regulation of magnesium concentration is dependent upon gastrointestinal tract absorption and renal absorption with little endocrine control (Kayne & Lee, 1993; Toribio et al., 2001). It is likely that hypomagnesemia in horses with colitis is a consequence of reduced intake, reduced absorption, and possibly a reduction in renal reabsorption of magnesium (Toribio et al., 2001). Magnesium has the potential to benefit horses with gastrointestinal disease as there is evidence in animal models that it may exert anti-inflammatory effects during endotoxemia and may be protective during ischemia-reperfusion injury (Kim et al., 2011; Lee et al., 2011).

Hypokalemia, hyponatremia, and hypochloremia are common electrolyte disturbances seen in the colitis patient. The ratio of intracellular to extracellular potassium may be affected by the acid–base status, with hydrogen moving into cells during acidosis to maintain electroneutrality, leading to a relative hyperkalemia (Corley & Marr, 1998). Correction of volume deficits and subsequent resolution of hyperlactatemia often results in a rapid correction of hyperkalemia, and hypokalemia may result. Close monitoring of electrolyte status during volume resuscitation is essential to avoid rapid changes in potassium status. Extracellular potassium is critical for neuromuscular transmission and is more relevant to clinical signs than whole body potassium stores (Rose & Post, 2001). Hypokalemia is speculated to be a result of reduced intake and altered absorption or excess loss from inflammation in the colon wall (Nappert & Johnson, 2001). Other potential sources of potassium loss are the kidneys (Gennari, 1998), an effect of chronic fluid therapy with isotonic fluids such as lactated Ringer's solution, which contains small quantities of potassium and may result in sodium-induced diuresis (Atkins, 1999). Drug-induced hypokalemia has been associated with beta-adrenergic agonists, glucocorticoids, insulin, diuretics, and antibiotics (Borer & Corley, 2006a; Gennari, 1998).

Sodium is a major contributor to plasma tonicity and osmolality, and abnormalities in serum sodium status are associated with disruptions in water homeostasis (Adrogue & Madias, 2000; Edelman et al., 1958). Substantial losses of sodium occur into the feces of horses with colitis, either as a consequence of sodium secretion, failure to absorb sodium in the large colon, or a combination of both (Ecke et al., 1998b). Failure to correct severe hyponatremia may result in clinical signs such as decreased mentation, seizures, weakness, lethargy, hypotension, and tachycardia (Borer & Corley, 2006b). When severe hyponatremia is present and is chronic in nature, the rate of correction should not exceed 8–12 mEq/L/day to avoid the risk of osmotic demyelination syndrome (Sterns et al., 1986). Losses of sodium without concomitant losses of chloride may also result in worsening of metabolic acidosis associated with absolute or relative hyperchloremia. However, hypochloremia is also commonly observed in the colitis patient and is readily corrected in most cases with 0.9% sodium chloride or hypertonic saline solution (HSS) if correction is warranted (i.e., metabolic alkalosis present). HSS has the potential added benefits of more rapid resolution of hypovolemia (Fielding & Magdesian, 2011) and reduction of tissue damage and organ failure from its purported anti-inflammatory effects in critically ill patients (Oliveira et al., 2002b; Pantaleon, 2010). Although HSS is reported to have an anticoagulant and antiplatelet effect (Wilder et al., 2002), this has not been recognized in the horse in a model of endotoxemia (Pantaleon et al., 2007).

Acid–base disturbances are common in acute colitis patients due to the failure of the colon to reabsorb bicarbonate, loss of bicarbonate into the gastrointestinal tract, and lactic acidosis as a consequence of hypovolemia and poor tissue perfusion related to SIRS and endotoxemia (Atherton et al., 2010). Most acute colitis patients will respond to IV fluid therapy with restoration of tissue perfusion, but chronic, persistent acidosis may occur in some cases from ongoing gastrointestinal losses. These horses may benefit from sodium bicarbonate supplementation. If considering bicarbonate therapy for treatment of metabolic acidosis in the colitis patient, normal respiratory function must be present. Bicarbonate supplementation should begin with administration of one-half of the deficit slowly followed by reassessment prior to additional therapy. Intravenous bicarbonate should not be administered with calcium-containing fluids, and oral bicarbonate is an excellent means of dealing with ongoing losses ($1 g NaHCO_3 = 12 mEq HCO_3$).

Colloid therapy is an integral component of fluid therapy in the severe colitis patient as hypoproteinemia and subsequent hypovolemia are prominent from the increased vascular permeability and low plasma oncotic pressures accompanying SIRS. In human patients, no differences have been detected in safety or efficacy of different types of colloid solutions for volume resuscitation (Bunn & Trivedi, 2012). However, a recent review and meta-analysis showed that after exclusion of seven trials performed by a researcher whose publications have been retracted because of scientific misconduct, hydroxyethyl starch was associated with a significant increased risk of mortality and acute kidney injury (Zarychanski et al., 2013). How this applies to horses is as yet unknown.

In humans with severe sepsis, there is some evidence that administration of albumin compared to saline may decrease the risk of death, and albumin administration did not negatively impact renal or other organ function (Finfer et al., 2011). Concentrated albumin solutions have been intermittently available for use in horses (Belli et al., 2008), but fresh frozen plasma and synthetic colloid solutions such as hetastarch (6% Hetastarch, Abbott Laboratories, IL), Hextend® (Abbott Laboratories, IL), and pentastarch (DuPont Critical Care, IL) are the most commonly used products in horses with colitis. Duration of oncotic support is dictated by the product itself and the severity of the systemic inflammatory process. Hetastarch (10 mL/kg) has been shown to increase colloidal oncotic pressure for as much as 24 hours in hypoproteinemic horses (Jones et al., 2001). Synthetic colloids have the advantage over natural colloids of lower cost and antigenicity, but caution should be exhibited when using higher doses of hetastarch (20 mL/kg), as it may contribute to prolongation of clotting times. The recommended dose is 8–10 mL/kg/day. Renal function should be monitored closely in horses receiving hetastarches. Concurrent use of both crystalloids and colloids may obviate the need for administration of large volumes of crystalloids, minimize the risk of interstitial edema, and more rapidly contribute to restoration of blood volume (Magdesian, 2003). See Chapter 24 for a more in-depth discussion of colloid therapy.

Monitoring

Perhaps even more so than in postoperative colics or horses with DPJ, advanced monitoring techniques play an important role in the colitis patient. Trends observed from obtaining repeated measurements tend to be much more useful than single measurement values.

The minimum database for acute colitis patients should consist of hematocrit, white blood cell count and differential, serum biochemistry analysis, and total plasma protein, fibrinogen, electrolytes, and lactate concentrations. Additional useful fluid therapy monitoring techniques include colloid osmotic pressure, urine output, urine specific gravity, urinalysis, arterial blood pressure, central venous pressure, and occasionally electrocardiography and coagulation profiles. Colloid osmotic pressure (COP) should be monitored in all hypoproteinemic colitis patients receiving synthetic colloid therapy, as indirect methods to estimate COP are no longer accurate.

Serial PCV or hematocrit and total plasma protein (TP) concentration measurements are particularly useful as a rough guideline to dictate intravenous fluid therapy rates of administration. Colitis patients typically are presented in a hypovolemic and dehydrated state and have SIRS resulting in vascular leakage of fluid and protein. Fluid therapy will result in a reduction in the PCV with a more profound reduction in TP. Initially this can be used to dictate the need for colloid therapy, but efficacy of colloid treatment should be determined by measurement of COP and clinical parameters. Often horses with colitis will have a persistently high PCV in the face of aggressive fluid therapy. Chronic, aggressive fluid therapy may result in renal medullary washout so monitoring of urine specific gravity to avoid hyposthenuria may aid in prevention of this iatrogenic complication. Serial blood lactate measurement may serve as an additional guide for efficacy of fluid therapy (Prittie, 2006; Tennent-Brown, 2012)

Monitoring changes in body weight, when practical, can provide useful insight into fluid therapy monitoring in the colitis patient, as total body water is approximately two-thirds of body weight. The water content of the equine gastrointestinal tract in its normal state is estimated to account for 6–10% of a horse's body weight (Robb et al., 1972). This method of monitoring may be particularly useful in the severely hypoproteinemic patient with diarrhea, as the effects of the gastrointestinal tract on water balance can be catastrophic when the integrity of the mucosal barrier is compromised. Alterations in fluid balance may occur as a result of venous pooling, peripheral vasodilation, mobilization of fluid from the intravascular to the interstitial compartments, and sequestration of fluid within the bowel lumen (Spier & Meagher, 1989).

References

Adrogue HJ, Madias NE. (2000) Hyponatremia. *N Engl J Med* **342**:1581–9.

Argenzio RA. (1992) Pathophysiology of diarrhea. In: NV Anderson (ed.) *Veterinary Gastroenterology*. Philadelphia: Lea & Febiger, pp. 163–72.

Arroyo LG, Stampfli HR, Weese JS. (2006) Potential role of Clostridium difficile as a cause of duodenitis-proximal jejunitis in horses. *J Med Microbiol* **55**:605–8.

Atherton R, McKenzie HC, Furr MO. (2010) Treating acute colitis in the horse. *Tieraerztliche Praxis Ausgabe Grosstiere Nutztiere* **38**:381–90.

Atkins CE. (1999) *Cardiac Manifestations of Systemic and Metabolic Disease*. Philadelphia: W.B. Saunders.

Batista MB, Bravin AC, Lopes LM, et al. (2009) Pressor response to fluid resuscitation in endotoxic shock: involvement of vasopressin. *Crit Care Med* **37**:2968–72.

Bayer O, Reinhart K, Sakr Y, et al. (2011) Renal effects of synthetic colloids and crystalloids in patients with severe sepsis: a prospective sequential comparison. *Crit Care Med* **39**:1335–42.

Belli CB, Michima LES, Latorre SM, Fernandes WR. (2008) Equine concentrated albumin solution in the fluid therapy in horses with slight to moderate dehydration. *Arq Bras Med Vet Zootec* **60**:30–5.

Borer KE, Corley KTT. (2006a) Electrolyte disorders in horses with colic. Part 1: potassium and magnesium. *Equine Vet Educ* **18**:266–71.

Borer KE, Corley KTT. (2006b) Electrolyte disorders in horses with colic. Part 2: calcium, sodium, chloride and phosphate. *Equine Vet Educ* **18**:320–5.

Brunkhorst FM, Engel C, Bloos F, et al. (2008) Intensive insulin therapy and pentastarch resuscitation in severe sepsis. *N Engl J Med* **358**:125–39.

Bunn F, Trivedi D. (2012) Colloid solutions for fluid resuscitation. Cochrane Database Syst Rev (CD001319) doi: 10.1002/14651858.CD001319.pub5.

Corley KTT, Marr CM. (1998) Pathophysiology, assessment and treatment of acid–base disturbances in the horse. *Equine Vet Educ* **10**:255–65.

Costa LR, Eades SE, Tulley RT, Richard SD, Seahorn TL, Moore RM. (1999) Plasma magnesium concentrations in horses with gastrointestinal tract disease [Abstr.]. *J Vet Intern Med* **13**:274.

Costa, MC, Arroyo LG, Allen-Vercoe E, et al. (2012) Comparison of the fecal microbiota of healthy horses and horses with colitis by high throughput sequencing of the V3-V5 region of the 16S rRNA gene. *PLoS One* **7**:e41484.

Dandona P, Nix D, Wilson MF, et al. (1994) Procalcitonin increase after endotoxin injection in normal subjects. *J Clin Endocrinol Metab* **79**:1605–8.

Dart AJ, Snyder JR, Spier SJ, Sullivan KE. (1992) Ionized calcium concentration in horses with surgically managed gastrointestinal disease: 147 cases (1988–1990). *J Am Vet Med Assoc* **201**:1244–8.

Divers TJ, Whitlock RH, Byars TD, Leitch M, Crowell WA. (1987) Acute renal failure in six horses resulting from haemodynamic causes. *Equine Vet J* **19**:178–84.

Driessen B, Brainard B. (2006) Fluid therapy for the traumatized patient. *J Vet Emerg Crit Care* **16**:276–99.

Ecke P, Hodgson DR, Rose RJ. (1998a) Induced diarrhoea in horses part 2: Response to administration of an oral rehydration solution. *Vet J* **155**:161–70.

Ecke P, Hodgson DR, Rose RJ. (1998b) Induced diarrhoea in horses. Part 1: Fluid and electrolyte balance. *Vet J* **155**:149–59.

Edelman IS, Leibman J, Omeara MP, Birkenfeld LW. (1958) Interrelations between serum sodium concentration, serum osmolarity and total exchangeable sodium, total exchangeable potassium and total body water. *J Clin Invest* **37**:1236–56.

Edwards GB. (2000) Duodenitis-proximal jejunitis (anterior enteritis) as a surgical problem. *Equine Vet Educ* **12**:318–21.

Feary DJ, Hassel DM. (2006) Enteritis and colitis in horses. *Vet Clin North Am Equine Pract* **22**:437–79, ix.

Fiaccadori E, Del Canale S, Coffrini E, et al. (1988) Muscle and serum magnesium in pulmonary intensive care unit patients. *Crit Care Med* **16**:751–60.

Fielding CL, Magdesian KG. (2011) A comparison of hypertonic (7.2%) and isotonic (0.9%) saline for fluid resuscitation in horses: a randomized, double-blinded, clinical trial. *J Vet Intern Med* **25**:1138–43.

Finfer S, McEvoy S, Bellomo R, McArthur C, Myburgh J, Norton R. (2011) Impact of albumin compared to saline on organ function and mortality of patients with severe sepsis. *Intensive Care Med* **37**:86–96.

Freeman DE, Kilgallon EG. (2001) Effect of venous strangulation obstruction on length of equine jejunum and relevance to small-intestinal resection. *Vet Surg* **30**:218–22.

Freeman DE, Ferrante PL, Palmer JE. (1992) Comparison of the effects of intragastric infusions of equal volumes of water, dioctyl sodium sulfosuccinate, and magnesium sulfate on fecal composition and output in clinically normal horses. *Am J Vet Res* **53**:1347–53.

Garcia-Lopez JM, Provost PJ, Rush JE, Zicker SC, Burmaster H, Freeman LM. (2001) Prevalence and prognostic importance of hypomagnesemia and hypocalcemia in horses that have colic surgery. *Am J Vet Res* **62**:7–12.

Gennari FJ. (1998) Hypokalemia. *N Engl J Med* **339**:451–8.

Groover ES, Woolums AR, Cole DJ, LeRoy BE. (2006) Risk factors associated with renal insufficiency in horses with primary gastrointestinal disease: 26 cases (2000–2003). *J Am Vet Med Assoc* **228**:572–7.

Hallowell GD. (2008) Retrospective study assessing efficacy of treatment of large colonic impactions. *Equine Vet J* **40**:411–13.

Hassel DM, Hill AE, Rorabeck RA. (2009) Association between hyperglycemia and survival in 228 horses with acute gastrointestinal disease. *J Vet Intern Med* **23**:1261–5.

Hitz F, Klingbiel D, Omlin A, Riniker S, Zerz A, Cerny T. (2012) Athrombogenic coating of long-term venous catheter for cancer patients: a prospective, randomised, double-blind trial. *Ann Hematol* **91**:613–20.

Johnston JK, Morris DD. (1987) Comparison of duodenitis/proximal jejunitis and small intestinal obstruction in horses: 68 cases (1977–1985). *J Am Vet Med Assoc* **191**:849–54.

Jones PA, Bain FT, Byars TD, David JB, Boston RC. (2001) Effect of hydroxyethyl starch infusion on colloid oncotic pressure in hypoproteinemic horses. *J Am Vet Med Assoc* **218**:1130–5.

Kayne LH, Lee DB. (1993) Intestinal magnesium absorption. *Miner Electrolyte Metab* **19**:210–17.

Kien ND, Kramer GC. (1989) Cardiac performance following hypertonic saline. *Braz J Med Biol Res* **22**:245–8.

Kien ND, Reitan JA, White DA, Wu CH, Eisele JH. (1991) Cardiac contractility and blood flow distribution following resuscitation with 7.5% hypertonic saline in anesthetized dogs. *Circ Shock* **35**:109–16.

Kien ND, Antognini JF, Reilly DA, Moore PG. (1996) Small-volume resuscitation using hypertonic saline improves organ perfusion in burned rats. *Anesth Analg* **83**:782–8.

Kim JE, Jeon JP, No HC, et al. (2011) The effects of magnesium pretreatment on reperfusion injury during living donor liver transplantation. *Korean J Anesthesiol* **60**:408–15.

Kreimeier U, Thiel M, Peter K, Messmer K. (1997) Small-volume hyperosmolar resuscitation. *Acta Anaesthesiol Scand Suppl* **111**:302–6.

Lee CY, Jan WC, Tsai PS, Huang CJ. (2011) Magnesium sulfate mitigates acute lung injury in endotoxemia rats. *J Trauma* **70**:1177–85.

Lopes MA, Johnson S, White NA. (2001) Enteral fluid therapy: Slow infusion versus boluses. In: Proceedings of the 11th Annual ACVS Veterinary Symposium (Abstr.), p. 13.

Lopes MA, Walker BL, White NA 2nd, Ward DL. (2002) Treatments to promote colonic hydration: enteral fluid therapy versus intravenous fluid therapy and magnesium sulphate. *Equine Vet J* **34**:505–9.

Lopes MA, White NA 2nd, Donaldson L, Crisman MV, Ward DL. (2004) Effects of enteral and intravenous fluid therapy, magnesium sulfate, and sodium sulfate on colonic contents and feces in horses. *Am J Vet Res* **65**:695–704.

Lopes MAF. (2003) Administration of enteral fluid therapy: methods, composition of fluids and complications. *Equine Vet Educ* **15**:107–12.

Magdesian KG. (2003) Colloid replacement in the ICU. *Clin Tech Equine Pract* **2**:130–7.

Magdesian KG. (2004) Monitoring the critically ill equine patient. *Vet Clin North Am Equine Pract* **20**:11–39.

McConnico RS. (2004) Duodenitis-proximal jejunitis (anterior enteritis, proximal enteritis). In: Reed SM, Bayly WM, Sellon

DC (eds) *Equine Internal Medicine*. Philadelphia, PA: W.B. Saunders, pp. 873–7.

McGovern KF, Bladon BM, Fraser BS, Boston RC. (2011) Attempted medical management of suspected ascending colon displacement in horses. *Vet Surg* **41**:391–403.

Merritt AM, Panzer RB, Lester GD, Burrow JA. (1995) Equine pelvic flexure myoelectric activity during fed and fasted states. *Am J Physiol* **269**:G262–8.

Miller TR, Anderson RJ, Linas SL, et al. (1978) Urinary diagnostic indices in acute renal failure: a prospective study. *Ann Intern Med* **89**:47–50.

Nakamura T, Mimura Y, Uno K, Yamakawa M. (1998) Parathyroid hormone activity increases during endotoxemia in conscious rats. *Horm Metab Res* **30**:88–92.

Nappert G, Johnson PJ. (2001) Determination of the acid-base status in 50 horses admitted with colic between December 1998 and May 1999. *Can Vet J* **42**:703–7.

Navarro M, Monreal L, Segura D, Armengou L, Anor S. (2005) A comparison of traditional and quantitative analysis of acid-base and electrolyte imbalances in horses with gastrointestinal disorders. *J Vet Intern Med* **19**:871–7.

Olerich, MA, Rude RK. (1994) Should we supplement magnesium in critically ill patients? *New Horiz* **2**:186–92.

Oliveira RP, Velasco I, Soriano FG, Friedman G. (2002a) Clinical review: Hypertonic saline resuscitation in sepsis. *Crit Care* **6**:418–23.

Oliveira RP, Weingartner R, Ribas EO, Moraes RS, Friedman G. (2002b) Acute haemodynamic effects of a hypertonic saline/dextran solution in stable patients with severe sepsis. *Intensive Care Med* **28**:1574–81.

Pantaleon L. (2010) Fluid therapy in equine patients: small-volume fluid resuscitation. *Compend Contin Educ Vet* **32**:E1–7.

Pantaleon LG, Furr MO, McKenzie HC, Donaldson L. (2007) Effects of small- and large-volume resuscitation on coagulation and electrolytes during experimental endotoxemia in anesthetized horses. *J Vet Int Med* **21**:1374–9.

Pascual JL, Khwaja KA, Chaudhury P, Christou NV. (2003) Hypertonic saline and the microcirculation. *J Trauma* **54**: S133–40.

Powell DW. (1991) Immunophysiology of intestinal electrolyte transport. *Handbook of Physiology: The Gastrointestinal System*. Bethesda, MD: American Physiological Society, sect. 6, vol. IV, ch. 25, pp. 591–641.

Prittie J. (2006) Optimal endpoints of resuscitation and early goal-directed therapy. *J Vet Emerg Crit Care* **16**:329–39.

Protopapas K. (2000) Studies on metabolic disturbances and other post-operative complications following equine surgery. D Vet Med thesis, Royal Veterinary College: University of London.

Proudman CJ, Edwards GB, Barnes J, French NR. (2005) Factors affecting long-term survival of horses recovering from surgery of the small intestine. *Equine Vet J* **37**:360–5.

Radhakrishnan RS, Shah SK, Lance SH, et al. (2009) Hypertonic saline alters hydraulic conductivity and up-regulates mucosal/submucosal aquaporin 4 in resuscitation-induced intestinal edema. *Crit Care Med* **37**:2946–52.

Robb J, Reid JT, Rhee MSS, et al. (1972) Chemical composition and energy value of body fatty-acid composition of adipose-tissue, and liver and kidney size in horse. *Anim Prod* **14**: 25–34.

Roger, T, Ruckebusch Y. (1987) Pharmacological modulation of postprandial colonic motor activity in the pony. *J Vet Pharmacol Ther* **10**:273–82.

Rose BD, Post TW. (2001) *Clinical Physiology of Acid-Base and Electrolyte Disorders*. New York: McGraw Hill.

Schott HC. (2012) Volume of distended small intestine and ionic compsition of gastric reflux and small intestinal fluid in horses. *J Vet Int Med* **26**:731 (Abstr.).

Seahorn TL, Cornick JL, Cohen ND. (1992) Prognostic indicators for horses with duodenitis-proximal jejunitis. 75 horses (1985–1989). *J Vet Intern Med* **6**:307–11.

Seanor JW, Byars TD, Boutcher JK. (1984) Renal disease associated with colic in horses. *Mod Vet Pract* **65**:A26–29.

Sellers AF, Lowe JE, Brondum J. (1979) Motor events in equine large colon. *Am J Physiol* **237**:E457–64.

Sheats MK, Cook VL, Jones SL, Blikslager AT, Pease AP. (2010) Use of ultrasound to evaluate outcome following colic surgery for equine large colon volvulus. *Equine Vet J* **42**:47–52.

Shields CJ. (2008) Towards a new standard of perioperative fluid management. *Ther Clin Risk Manag* **4**:569–71.

Southwood LL. (2005) Critical care of the postoperative colic patient: advanced. *AAEP Focus Meeting*. Quebec, Canada. International Veterinary Information Service; available at: http://www.ivis.org/proceedings/aaepfocus/2005/Southwood2.pdf

Spier, SJ, Meagher DM. (1989) Perioperative medical care for equine abdominal surgery. *Vet Clin North Am Equine Pract* **5**:429–43.

Sterns RH, Riggs JE, Schochet SS Jr. (1986) Osmotic demyelination syndrome following correction of hyponatremia. *N Engl J Med* **314**:1535–42.

Stewart MC, Hodgson JL, Kim H, Hutchins DR, Hodgson DR. (1995) Acute febrile diarrhoea in horses: 86 cases (1986–1991). *Aust Vet J* **72**:41–4.

Tennent-Brown BS. (2012) Interpreting lactate measurement in critically ill horses: diagnosis, treatment, and prognosis. *Compend Contin Educ Vet* **34**:E1–6.

Toribio RE, Kohn CW, Chew DJ, Sams RA, Rosol TJ. (2001) Comparison of serum parathyroid hormone and ionized calcium and magnesium concentrations and fractional urinary clearance of calcium and phosphorus in healthy horses and horses with enterocolitis. *Am J Vet Res* **62**: 938–47.

Underwood C, Southwood LL, McKeown LP, Knight D. (2008) Complications and survival associated with surgical compared with medical management of horses with duodenitis-proximal jejunitis. *Equine Vet J* **40**:373–8.

Underwood C, Southwood LL, Walton RM, Johnson AL. (2010) Hepatic and metabolic changes in surgical colic patients: a pilot study. *J Vet Emerg Crit Care (San Antonio)* **20**:578–86.

White NA 2nd, Dabareiner RM. (1997) Treatment of impaction colics. *Vet Clin North Am Equine Pract* **13**:243–59.

White NA 2nd, Tyler DE, Blackwell RB, Allen D. (1987) Hemorrhagic fibrinonecrotic duodenitis-proximal jejunitis in horses: 20 cases (1977–1984). *J Am Vet Med Assoc* **190**:311–15.

Wilder DM, Reid TJ, Bakaltcheva IB. (2002) Hypertonic resuscitation and blood coagulation: in vitro comparison of several hypertonic solutions for their action on platelets and plasma coagulation. *Thromb Res* **107**:255–61.

Zaloga GP, Malcolm D, Chernow B, Holaday J. (1988) Endotoxin-induced hypocalcemia results in defective calcium mobilization in rats. *Circ Shock* **24**:143–8.

Zarychanski R, Abou-Setta AH, Turgeon AF, et al. (2013) Association of hydroxyethyl starch administration with mortality and acute kidney injury in critically ill patients requiring volume resuscitation: a systematic review and meta-analysis. *JAMA* **309**:678–88.

CHAPTER 17

Fluid therapy and heart failure

Sophy A. Jesty

Assistant Professor in Cardiology, University of Tennessee, USA

Introduction

While many disease processes improve with the supplementation of intravenous fluids, heart failure typically requires a decrease in overall body fluid volume (cardiac tamponade is an exception). This chapter will discuss the pathophysiology of heart failure and fluid balance in these patients. A review of the treatments for heart failure and cardiac tamponade is also included.

Heart failure

Pathophysiology of heart failure

Heart failure is a clinical syndrome in which cardiac dysfunction leads to the inability of the heart to pump adequate blood forward. Heart failure can be caused by three mechanisms: (i) volume overload; (ii) pressure overload; and (iii) primary myocardial disease. Volume overload is the most common cause in horses.

There are two hemodynamic consequences of heart failure: (i) increased ventricular filling pressure, which leads to venous congestion (i.e., congestive heart failure); and (ii) reduced cardiac output (i.e., output failure). Congestive heart failure is much more commonly recognized than output failure, but they probably occur simultaneously in many cases.

In horses, the most common causes of heart failure include: (i) congenital cardiac defects leading to left-to-right shunting (i.e., ventricular septal defect in younger horses leading to left-sided heart failure); (ii) chronic degenerative valve disease in older horses (leading to

left-sided, right-sided, or bilateral heart failure); and (iii) pericardial disease resulting in cardiac tamponade (leading to signs of right-sided heart failure). Less common causes include systolic dysfunction, myocarditis, and tachycardiomyopathy.

Specific clinical signs depend on which side of the heart is failing. The consequence of left-sided congestive heart failure is pulmonary edema. Clinical signs associated with left-sided congestive heart failure include cough, tachypnea, dyspnea, hemoptysis, and frothy nasal discharge (a grave prognostic indicator if due to pulmonary edema). The consequence of left-sided output failure is systemic hypoperfusion. Clinical signs associated with left-sided output failure include exercise intolerance, weakness, lethargy, cool extremities, and hypothermia.

The consequences of right-sided congestive heart failure can include subcutaneous edema, peripheral venous distention, hepatomegaly, and ascites. Clinical signs associated with right-sided congestive heart failure include ventral edema, abdominal distention, and peripheral venous distention. The consequence of right-sided output failure is pulmonary hypoperfusion (which can lead to left-sided output failure as well). Clinical signs associated with right-sided output failure include exercise intolerance, weakness, and lethargy.

In horses, as opposed to other species, left-sided congestive heart failure can lead secondarily to right-sided congestive heart failure, therefore horses can present with signs of bilateral (sometimes called biventricular) heart failure. This is postulated to be due to a propensity for pulmonary vascular remodeling and

Equine Fluid Therapy, First Edition. Edited by C. Langdon Fielding and K. Gary Magdesian.
© 2015 John Wiley & Sons, Inc. Published 2015 by John Wiley & Sons, Inc.

vasoconstriction with increased left-sided filling pressure in this species (Reef et al., 1998).

Regardless of the underlying heart disease, once heart disease results in a decline in cardiac output, neurohormonal compensatory mechanisms temporarily preserve organ perfusion. These compensatory mechanisms are helpful in restoring tissue perfusion in the early stages of heart failure , but some of the compensatory mechanisms become detrimental once heart failure develops. These neurohormonal systems include the sympathetic nervous system (which causes tachycardia, increased inotropy, and vasoconstriction), the renin-angiotensin-aldosterone system (RAAS, which causes sodium and water retention, increased thirst, and vasoconstriction), the vasopressinergic system (which causes water retention and vasoconstriction), endothelin (which causes vasoconstriction), the kallikrein-kininogen-kinin system (which causes vasodilation), and the natriuretic peptide system (which causes diuresis) (Lee & Tkacs, 2008; Mann, 1999; McMurray & Pfeffer 2002a,b). Only the kallikrein-kininogen-kinin and the natriuretic peptide systems are beneficial in heart failure, and unfortunately they become overwhelmed with chronic or severe heart failure. The other compensatory mechanisms exacerbate cardiac dysfunction by increasing preload, afterload, and myocardial oxygen demand. Heart failure treatment strategies target these detrimental compensatory mechanisms.

Fluid balance in heart failure

The paradox of fluid balance in patients with heart failure is the simultaneous arterial hypovolemia in the face of total extracellular fluid (ECF) overload (with venous hypervolemia). The decrease in effective forward arterial flow as cardiac output declines with heart failure is sensed by baroreceptors in the carotid sinus, aortic arch, and the renal afferent arteriole (Schrier 1988a,b; Szady & Hill, 2009). Sodium and water retention and vasoconstriction result from activation of the sympathetic nervous system, the RAAS, and the vasopressinergic system. The imbalance between effective forward flow and total body fluid volume makes treating chronic heart failure a medical challenge. Treating one of these may exacerbate the other. The necessity of decreasing total body fluid volume results in a further decrease in arterial blood volume and tissue perfusion.

Treatment of heart failure

The most important consequence of heart failure is congestion leading to pulmonary edema (left-sided) and subcutaneous edema and ascites (right-sided). These manifestations of heart failure are secondary to increased hydrostatic pressure in the pulmonary and systemic capillary systems, respectively. Decreasing hydrostatic pressure by decreasing blood volume is essential. Fluid administration is contraindicated in cases of congestive heart failure. Immediate treatment for acute congestive heart failure (specifically left-sided, which is a true medical emergency) should include diuretics and oxygen supplementation. Treatment of chronic heart failure should include diuretics and (ideally) angiotensin-converting enzyme (ACE) inhibitors. There are many medications available to treat heart disease and heart failure in horses, including diuretics, vasodilators, positive inotropes, and antiarrhythmic drugs. In this chapter, only treatments that directly affect fluid and electrolyte balance will be discussed.

Loop diuretics

Furosemide, a loop diuretic, has long been the diuretic of choice in humans and animals for a number of reasons:

1 For a given level of natriuresis, furosemide produces superior diuresis when compared with other diuretics.
2 Furosemide will work despite the presence of renal impairment, which is common with heart failure.
3 There is increasing response to increasing doses (i.e., it is a "high ceiling" diuretic) (Opie & Gersh, 2005).

Furosemide inhibits the luminal $Na^+/K^+/2Cl^-$ cotransporter in the thick ascending loop of Henle, thereby reducing reabsorption of these electrolytes (and therefore water) and resulting in very effective diuresis. In horses, IV administration results in a decrease in blood volume, ECF volume, left ventricular filling pressure, and pulmonary capillary pressure (Muir et al., 1976).

The initial emergency dose in horses is 1–2 mg/kg (IV bolus), depending on the severity of the clinical signs. This can be followed by additional IV boluses as early as 30–60 minutes or as late as 6–8 hours after the first dose. If the horse requires significant diuresis to clear the pulmonary edema, a continuous IV infusion should be used. Furosemide infusions (0.12 mg/kg/h) have been shown to result in a greater and more consistent decrease in plasma volume with fewer adverse effects on renal function than equivalent IV bolus dosing

(Johansson et al., 2003; Yelton et al., 1995). In cases of severe, acute heart failure in horses, furosemide infusions appear very effective in the author's experience. The infusion rate should be decreased or increased as necessary depending on improvement or worsening of clinical signs. Although there are adverse consequences of using furosemide (as discussed below), high dosages are often required. There is no standard total daily dose of furosemide for a horse in acute heart failure; the dose that should be used is the minimum amount needed to clear the pulmonary edema. A dose sufficient to clear the pulmonary edema **must** be used, or the horse's life will remain in danger. The adverse consequences can be addressed once the immediate life-threatening scenario of pulmonary edema has been resolved.

For chronic heart failure (left, right, or bilateral), furosemide is also the cornerstone of treatment. When given orally, furosemide is both poorly and variably absorbed in horses (Johansson et al., 2004), so furosemide should not be administered orally in this species. Other routes of administration (subcutaneous, intramuscular, intravenous) can be used. The suggested dose for chronic heart failure management in horses is 1–2 mg/kg two to three times daily. In other species, increasing the dose of furosemide throughout the course of heart failure management (up to at least 12 mg/kg daily) results in increased diuresis and improved clinical signs. One of the reasons that the life expectancy of horses with heart failure may be shorter than that for small animals with heart failure is that furosemide dosing is less aggressive in horses (Reef et al., 1998). Anecdotally, the author has started to increase the daily dose of furosemide in chronic heart failure horses with positive outcomes. Throughout diuretic therapy in horses, access to water at all times is recommended in order to avoid inadvertent and severe dehydration. In humans, water and salt restriction is part of the management of heart failure, but fluid balance in human medicine can be more closely monitored than in equine medicine. This is especially true once the horse leaves the hospital.

In cases of right-sided congestive heart failure in which there is significant pleural or abdominal effusion, thoraco- and abdominocentesis with drainage should be considered an important part of the treatment protocol. Medical management should increase the time between drainage procedures, but will not render this procedure unnecessary.

There are other loop diuretics (torsemide, bumetanide) that may be used in refractory cases of heart failure or may completely replace furosemide at some point in the future (Wargo & Banta, 2009). More research is needed to evaluate these medications in horses. Currently, furosemide should be considered the first-line diuretic of choice.

The adverse consequences of furosemide relate to its mechanism of action. Furosemide activates deleterious neurohormonal systems (sympathetic nervous system, RAAS, and the vasopressinergic system), induces hypovolemia and dehydration, and creates electrolyte and acid–base imbalances (hyponatremia, hypochloremia, hypokalemia, and metabolic alkalosis). Furosemide's activation of various neurohormonal systems increases sodium and water retention and causes vasoconstriction, both undesirable in the treatment of heart failure. It also has direct adverse fibrotic remodeling effects on the myocardium via angiotensin II and aldosterone, worsening cardiac function (Swedberg et al., 1990; Szady & Hill, 2009; Tan et al., 1991; Thohan et al., 2004; Weber & Brilla 1991). For this reason, furosemide should be administered with medications to blunt the RAAS, in order to avoid hastening progression of heart disease.

As furosemide decreases blood volume, decreased tissue perfusion and cellular dehydration can result. Renal function may be jeopardized by reducing renal blood flow. In one study, diuretic use was a predisposing factor for humans presenting for non-obstructive acute renal failure (Calvino et al., 1997). In another study, a third of elderly human patients with acute renal failure were being treated at the time of failure with diuretics, ACE inhibitors, and/or non-steroidal anti-inflammatories (NSAIDs) (Ng et al., 2008). Seventy-five percent of these people recovered with discontinuation of the medications. Finally, studies show that renal function worsens in 22% of people treated for acute heart failure (Valle et al., 2011), and that a smaller decline in glomerular filtration rate is seen when low-dose furosemide is used instead of high doses (Peacock et al., 2009). Although complete discontinuation of diuretics is unlikely to be feasible, a reduction in dose and discontinuation of ACE inhibitors and NSAIDs should be considered in patients developing renal failure.

Furosemide can cause hypokalemia and hyponatremia. Hypokalemia can be ameliorated by increasing potassium ingestion (potassium-rich feeds such as alfalfa or orchard grass hay can be used). Oral supplementation with potassium chloride (KCl) may be necessary if significant hypokalemia develops (**note:** salt supplementation should not include sodium). Hyponatremia is a consequence both of heart failure itself and of chronic furosemide use. In fact, hyponatremia has long been considered a marker for the activation of the sympathetic system and RAAS that occurs with heart failure (Levine et al., 1982; Lilly et al., 1984). Of particular importance for the development of hyponatremia is the release of arginine vasopressin (AVP), which acts to insert aquaporin channels into the collecting ducts. Aquaporin channels increase the permeability to free water, allowing for solute-free (hypo-osmolar) absorption, which would more readily contribute to hyponatremia than other mechanisms of water retention that rely on sodium retention. AVP release is stimulated by two mechanisms at play during heart failure: a decrease in arterial blood pressure and angiotensin II. AVP release is inhibited by a decrease in plasma osmolality, but this negative feedback mechanism is overwhelmed during heart failure, as hypotension is prioritized as a stimulus for release of AVP. Multiple studies in humans have shown that hyponatremia is one of the strongest predictors of cardiac mortality in patients with heart failure (Ghali, 2008; Lee & Packer, 1986; Lee et al., 2003; Velavan et al., 2010; Wong et al., 2002), probably because it denotes the ability of the neurohormonal systems to retain fluids despite treatment with medications aimed at reversing fluid retention.

The hyponatremia encountered with chronic heart failure and diuretic use should not be corrected with sodium supplementation. In fact, in veterinary medicine, this hyponatremia is often ignored since animals do not present with attributable clinical signs. In humans, fluid restriction is one way to reverse the hyponatremia, but compliance is poor because thirst becomes unbearable. Fluid restriction in veterinary patients is dangerous because of the relative lack of monitoring of hydration status once the animal leaves the hospital. A more recent method for managing hypervolemia (i.e., congestive heart failure) and hyponatremia in humans is the simultaneous use of a hypertonic saline infusion with high-dose furosemide infusion. Although initially counterintuitive, this combination allows for an osmotic draw of water into the vascular compartment, which is then quickly excreted through the kidneys by the action of the diuretic. In humans this strategy leads to both water loss and sodium retention, effects that account for

improvement in symptoms, decreased readmissions, and improvement in mortality (Licata et al., 2003; Paterna et al., 2000) This approach may be appropriate in severe heart failure cases (particularly with hyponatremia) refractory to initial treatment but the author has not used this combination in clinical practice. In humans, arginine vasopressin antagonists have been recently developed to combat hypo-osmolar fluid retention, but these are prohibitively expensive to consider for use in horses at this time.

Although the loop diuretics are very effective, sequential nephron blockade (or diuretic stacking) can be helpful because it furthers diuresis with fewer adverse consequences. Sequential nephron blockade mitigates diuretic resistance when compared with continually increasing the loop diuretic dose (Opie & Gersh, 2005). While loop diuretics should be considered as a first choice, other diuretics can be combined with a loop diuretic as the disease progresses and management requires more aggressive treatment. Thiazide diuretics (which the author uses in horses) and the aldosterone antagonists (not commonly used in horses) are possible choices for chronic management of equine heart failure when additional diuretics are required.

Thiazide diuretics

Hydrochlorothiazide inhibits the NaCl cotransporter in the distal convoluted tubule, reducing the reabsorption of sodium and chloride (and therefore water). Because much of the filtered sodium has already been reabsorbed by the time it reaches the distal convoluted tubule, thiazide diuretics are less effective than the loop diuretics. Hydrochlorothiazide has been used in horses to control the signs of hyperkalemic periodic paralysis (HYPP) (Beech & Lindborg, 1995). Thiazide diuretics can cause serious hyponatremia (Spital, 1999) and hypokalemia (even more so than loop diuretics) (Opie & Gersh, 2005), so if hydrochlorothiazide is combined with furosemide, it should be initiated at a low starting dose (0.5 mg/kg PO q 24 h). Electrolytes should be monitored as the dose is increased.

Aldosterone antagonists

Spironolactone works by competitively inhibiting aldosterone in the late distal convoluted tubule, thereby reducing sodium reabsorption (and therefore water) and enhancing potassium reabsorption. Again, because much of the sodium has already been absorbed by the time the filtrate reaches the distal convoluted tubule, the aldosterone antagonists are less effective diuretics than the loop diuretics. Aldosterone antagonists are commonly used as the second diuretic (to be paired with furosemide) in small animal heart failure cases, for two reasons: (i) the potassium-sparing effect can blunt the hypokalemia that can occur with furosemide use; and (ii) the aldosterone antagonists have been shown to improve morbidity and mortality for people and dogs in heart failure despite being weak diuretics (The RALES Investigators, 1996; Bernay et al., 2010; Guyonnet et al., 2010). Aldosterone has a proinflammatory and profibrotic effect within the myocardium and therefore is a direct effector of adverse cardiac remodeling (Carey, 2010). At this time, spironolactone is somewhat expensive to be used in most horses with heart failure, but it is possible that aldosterone antagonists may become more cost effective for future use in equine medicine. If they are to be used, care should be taken to monitor electrolytes because they can result in hyperkalemia in human patients.

ACE inhibitors

Ideally, in chronic heart failure cases, furosemide should be paired with ACE inhibition. As blood volume decreases following a dose of furosemide (due to increased urine output), the body's natural response will be activation of the RAAS. This RAAS activation counteracts the previous dose of furosemide by increasing blood volume until the next dose of furosemide is given. ACE inhibitors decrease production of angiotensin II and therefore aldosterone. The most commonly used ACE inhibitor used in small animal cardiology (enalapril) has proven to be fairly ineffective in horses when given at the same dose (0.5 mg/kg PO) (Gardner et al., 2004; Sleeper et al., 2008). In horses, the most effective ACE inhibitor studied to date is benazepril (0.5 mg/kg once daily), which results in a peak reduction of serum ACE activity of 87% (Afonso et al., 2013). In this study, benazepril outperformed both ramipril and quinapril, the other most studied ACE inhibitors in horses (Afonso et al., 2013).

Renal impairment is an adverse consequence of ACE inhibition, as blocking the production of angiotensin II alters intrarenal hemodynamics. While itself vasoconstrictive, angiotensin II stimulates the production of prostaglandins, which are vasodilatory and protective for renal perfusion. ACE inhibition effectively blocks the synthesis of these protective prostaglandins, which can lead to renal ischemia, a decline in glomerular filtration pressure, and acute renal failure.

Cardiac tamponade

Pathophysiology of cardiac tamponade

Cardiac tamponade is a clinical syndrome that occurs when intrapericardial pressure increases and then exceeds the normal diastolic filling pressure within the cardiac chambers. This results in equilibration of the intrapericardial and cardiac filling pressures (i.e., the intrapericardial pressure dictates the cardiac filling pressure). The transmural pressure gradient decreases, which affects right heart filling before left heart filling since the right heart normally operates at a lower transmural filling pressure. Pericardial fluid accumulates and leads to collapse of the cardiac chambers, decreased cardiac filling during diastole, and therefore decreased cardiac output during systole. Cardiac tamponade is a medical emergency.

The development of cardiac tamponade depends on three factors: the volume of the pericardial fluid, the rate at which the fluid accumulates, and properties of the pericardium itself (e.g., compliance). Clinical signs are similar to those of right-sided congestive heart failure (Freestone et al., 1987; Worth & Reef, 1998); these include tachycardia, peripheral venous congestion, jugular pulsation, subcutaneous edema, ascites, and hepatomegaly. Despite the similarity in clinical signs, the two entities are quite distinct and need to be managed differently. Other clinical signs in horses with cardiac tamponade are both nonspecific (fever, anorexia, lethargy, weight loss, colic, tachypnea) and specific (tachycardia, quiet heart sounds, pericardial friction rubs, weak arterial pulses, and pulsus paradoxus).

Pericardial effusions in horses have been associated with viral and bacterial infections (equine herpesvirus 1 (EHV-1), EHV-2, influenza virus, *Streptococcus* spp., *Actinobacillus equuli, Pseudomonas* spp., *Pasteurella multocida, Staphylococcus aureus, Acinetobacter* spp., *Escherichia coli, Enterococcus fecalis, Corynebacterium pyogenes, Mycoplasma felis, Propionibacterium acnes, Corynebacterium pseudotuberculosis, Clostridium* spp.), immune-mediated diseases such as eosinophilic pericarditis, neoplasia, trauma, or through contiguous spread of a nearby infectious or inflammatory process. Many cases of pericarditis in horses, however, are considered idiopathic.

As diastolic filling and cardiac output decline, the resulting arterial hypovolemia will activate the neurohormonal systems that are activated in heart failure (sympathetic nervous system, RAAS, vasopressinergic system, endothelin, the kallikrein-kininogen-kinin system, and the natriuretic peptide system). Unlike in heart failure, however, the water retention and vasoconstriction that these systems cause is beneficial in cardiac tamponade because preload is the only factor that can combat the intrapericardial pressure increase (in other words, increasing preload will improve cardiac filling). Increasing afterload is not detrimental because systolic function is usually normal.

Fluid balance in cardiac tamponade

As there is a paradox or an imbalance between arterial and venous fluid compartments in heart failure, there is the same imbalance in cardiac tamponade, with arterial hypovolemia in the face of systemic venous hypervolemia. Unlike with heart failure, in which preload must be decreased because cardiac dysfunction is the underlying cause for congestion, in cardiac tamponade preload must be increased to drive cardiac filling.

Treatment of cardiac tamponade

The most important aspect of managing cardiac tamponade is to relieve the intrapericardial pressure by reducing the pericardial effusion. This can only be accomplished with pericardiocentesis (Azam & Hoit, 2011), which will result immediately in a decline in the intrapericardial pressure and therefore a normalization of cardiac filling and cardiac output. In humans, pericardiocentesis is a fairly safe procedure, with a major complication rate of only 1% (Azam & Hoit, 2011). In horses, pericardiocentesis appears to be a safe procedure although adverse consequences can occur. Nonetheless, the risks of not performing pericardiocentesis far outweigh the risks of the procedure. In the short term, prior to pericardiocentesis, IV fluids (isotonic intravenous solutions) should be supplemented at twice the normal maintenance rate. Increasing preload by supplementing with IV fluids will enhance right heart filling and can lead to hemodynamic improvement in the short term. During and after pericardiocentesis, fluids should be continued at one to two times the normal maintenance rate since cardiac output and urine production surge once the cardiac tamponade has been relieved. The pericardial fluid can be drained through a 16-28 Fr trocar catheter (the largest diameter that can be safely used in the individual patient should be used). Some clinicians drain the pericardial fluid slowly out of a concern for hemodynamic shifts, but the pericardial volume is comparatively small and reaccumulation does not happen immediately.

Diuretics, while tempting to consider, are absolutely contraindicated in cases of cardiac tamponade. Not only are diuretics incapable of mobilizing large-volume third space fluids in a short time (as would be necessary in cardiac tamponade), they would serve to decrease preload through increased urine output. Decreasing preload would exacerbate the hemodynamic abnormalities associated with cardiac tamponade, worsening the situation for the horse.

As with heart failure, there are additional aspects of treating pericardial disease and cardiac tamponade in horses that are discussed in other texts and articles. The aspects of treatment that relate to fluid balance are covered in this text.

Conclusions

This chapter reviews two clinical syndromes of cardiac dysfunction (heart failure and cardiac tamponade) that are directly and intimately related to fluid balance. These syndromes are both characterized by a decrease in arterial blood volume with a concomitant increase in venous blood volume. Treatment differs for the two disease processes because of the differing underlying physiologies. Heart failure is caused by true cardiac dysfunction while cardiac tamponade is not. An understanding of the fluid balance in these two clinical syndromes is essential to the development of a useful management strategy.

References

Afonso T, Giguère S, Rapoport G, Berghaus LJ, Barton MH, Coleman AE. (2013) Pharmacodynamic evaluation of 4 angiotensin-converting enzyme inhibitors in healthy adult horses. *J Vet Int Med* **27**:1185–92.

Azam S, Hoit BD. (2011) Treatment of pericardial disease. *Cardiovasc Ther* **29**:308–14.

Beech J, Lindborg S. (1995) Prophylactic efficacy of phenytoin, acetazolamide and hydrochlorothiazide in horses with hyperkalemic periodic paralysis. *Res Vet Sci* **59**:95–101.

Bernay F, Bland JM, Haggstrom J, et al. (2010) Efficacy of spironolactone on survival in dogs with naturally occurring mitral regurgitation caused by myxomatous mitral valve disease. *J Vet Int Med* **24**:331–41.

Calvino JA, Romero R, Novoa D, Guimil D, Cordal T, Sanchez-Guisande D. (1997) Acute renal failure related to nonsteroidal antiinflammatory drugs and angiotensin-converting enzyme inhibitors. *Nefrologia* **17**:405–10.

Carey RM. (2010) Aldosterone and cardiovascular disease. *Curr Opin Endocrinol Diabetes Obes* **17**:194–8.

Freestone JF, Thomas WP, Carlson GP, Brumbaugh GW. (1987) Idiopathic effusive pericarditis with tamponade in the horse. *Equine Vet J* **19**:38–42.

Gardner SY, Atkins CE, Sams RA, Schwabenton AB, Papich MG. (2004) Characterization of the pharmacokinetic and pharmacodynamic properties of the angiotensin-converting enzyme inhibitor, enalapril, in horses. *J Vet Int Med* **18**:231–7.

Ghali JK. (2008) Mechanisms, risks, and new treatment options for hyponatremia. *Cardiology* **111**:147–57.

Guyonnet J, Elliott J, Kaltsatos V. (2010) A preclinical pharmacokinetic and pharmacodynamic approach to determine a dose of spironolactone for treatment of congestive heart failure in dog. *J Vet Pharmacol Ther* **33**:260–7.

Johansson AM, Gardner SY, Levine JF, et al. (2003) Furosemide continuous rate infusion in the horse: Evaluation of enhanced efficacy and reduced side effects. *J Vet Int Med* **17**:887–95.

Johansson AM, Gardner SY, Levine JF, et al. (2004) Pharmacokinetics and pharmacodynamics of furosemide after oral administration to horses. *J Vet Int Med* **18**:739–43.

Lee CS, Tkacs NC. (2008) Current concepts of neurohormonal activation in heart failure: Mediators and mechanisms. *AACN Adv Crit Care* **19**:364–85; quiz 386–7.

Lee DS, Austin PC, Rouleau JL, Liu PP, Naimark D, Tu JV. (2003) Predicting mortality among patients hospitalized for heart failure. *JAMA, J Am Med Assoc* **290**:2581–7.

Lee W, Packer M. (1986) Prognostic importance of serum sodium concentration and its modification by converting-enzyme inhibition in patients with severe chronic heart failure. *Circulation* **73**:257–67.

Levine TB, Franciosa JA, Vrobel T, Cohn JN. (1982) Hyponatraemia as a marker for high renin heart failure. *Brit Heart J* **47**:161–6.

Licata G, Pasquale PD, Parrinello G, et al. (2003) Effects of high-dose furosemide and small-volume hypertonic saline solution infusion in comparison with a high dose of furosemide as bolus in refractory congestive heart failure: Long-term effects. *Am Heart J* **145**:459–66.

Lilly LS, Dzau VJ, Williams GH, Rydstedt L, Hollenberg NK. (1984) Hyponatremia in congestive heart failure: Implications for neurohumoral activation and responses to orthostasis. *J Clin Endocrinol Metab* **59**:924–30.

Mann DL. (1999) Mechanisms and models in heart failure – a combinatorial approach. *Circulation* **100**:999–1008.

McMurray J, Pfeffer MA. (2002a) New therapeutic options in congestive heart failure: part i. *Circulation* **105**:2099–106.

McMurray J, Pfeffer MA. (2002b) New therapeutic options in congestive heart failure – part ii. *Circulation* **105**:2223–8.

Muir WW, Milne DW, Skarda RT. (1976) Acute hemodynamic effects of furosemide administered intravenously in horse. *Am J Vet Res* **37**:1177–80.

Ng CS, Pillans PI, Johnson DW, Sturtevant JM. (2008) Acute renal failure in patients on diuretics and/or NSAID, COX-2 inhibitors, ACEI, ARA. *J Pharmacy Pract Res* **38**:280–2.

Opie LH, Gersh BJ. (2005) *Drugs for the Heart*. Elsevier Saunders.

Paterna S, Di Pasquale P, Parrinello G, et al. (2000) Effects of high-dose furosemide and small-volume hypertonic saline solution infusion in comparison with a high dose of furosemide as a bolus, in refractory congestive heart failure. *Eur J Heart Fail* **2**:305–13.

Peacock WF, Costanzo MR, De Marco T, et al. (2009) Impact of intravenous loop diuretics on outcomes of patients hospitalized with acute decompensated heart failure: Insights from the adhere registry. *Cardiology* **113**:12–19.

Reef VB, Bain FT, Spencer PA. (1998) Severe mitral regurgitation in horses: Clinical, echocardiographic and pathological findings. *Equine Vet J* **30**:18–27.

Schrier RW. (1988a) Pathogenesis of sodium and water retention in high-output and low-output cardiac failure, nephrotic syndrome, cirrhosis, and pregnancy (1). *N Engl J Med* **319**:1065–72.

Schrier RW. (1988b) Pathogenesis of sodium and water retention in high-output and low-output cardiac failure, nephrotic syndrome, cirrhosis, and pregnancy (2). *N Engl J Med* **319**:1127–34.

Sleeper MM, McDonnell SM, Ely JJ, Reef VB. (2008) Chronic oral therapy with enalapril in normal ponies. *J Vet Cardiol* **10**:111–15.

Spital A. (1999) Diuretic-induced hyponatremia. *Am J Nephrol* **19**:447–52.

Swedberg K, Eneroth P, Kjekshus J, Wilhelmsen L. (1990) Hormones regulating cardiovascular function in patients with severe congestive-heart-failure and their relation to mortality. *Circulation* **82**:1730–6.

Szady AD, Hill JA. (2009) Diuretics in heart failure: A critical appraisal of efficacy and tolerability. *Drugs* **69**:2451–61.

Tan LB, Jalil JE, Pick R, Janicki JS, Weber KT. (1991) Cardiac myocyte necrosis induced by angiotensin-ii. *Circ Res* **69**:1185–95.

The RALES Investigators. (1996) Effectiveness of spironolactone added to an angiotensin-converting enzyme inhibitor and a loop diuretic for severe chronic congestive heart failure. *Am J Cardiol* 78:902–7.

Thohan V, Torre-Amione G, Koerner MM. (2004) Aldosterone antagonism and congestive heart failure: A new look at an old therapy. *Curr Opin Cardiol* **19**:301–8.

Valle R, Aspromonte N, Milani L, et al. (2011) Optimizing fluid management in patients with acute decompensated heart failure (ADHF): The emerging role of combined measurement of body hydration status and brain natriuretic peptide (BNP) levels. *Heart Fail Rev* **16**:519–29.

Velavan P, Khan NK, Goode K, et al. (2010) Predictors of short term mortality in heart failure – insights from the euro heart failure survey. *Int J Cardiol* **138**:63–9.

Wargo KA, Banta WM. (2009) A comprehensive review of the loop diuretics: Should furosemide be first line? *Ann Pharmacother* **43**:1836–47.

Weber KT, Brilla CG. (1991) Pathological hypertrophy and cardiac interstitium – fibrosis and renin-angiotensin-aldosterone system. *Circulation* **83**:1849–65.

Wong PS, Davidsson GK, Timeyin J, et al. (2002) Heart failure in patients admitted to hospital: Mortality is still high. *Eur J Int Med* **13**:304–10.

Worth LT, Reef VB. (1998) Pericarditis in horses: 18 cases (1986–1995). *J Am Vet Med Assoc* **212**:248–53.

Yelton SL, Gaylor MA, Murray KM. (1995) The role of continuous-infusion loop diuretics. *Ann Pharmacother* **29**:1010–14.

CHAPTER 18

Fluid therapy during neurologic disease

Yvette S. Nout-Lomas

Assistant Professor – Equine Internal Medicine, Department of Clinical Sciences
College of Veterinary Medicine and Biomedical Sciences Colorado State University, USA

Overview of fluid therapy in neurologic disease

Fluid therapy is indicated in the treatment of neurologic diseases when the patient is (i) unable to maintain appropriate water and/or electrolyte homeostasis in the body, and/or (ii) unable to maintain adequate delivery of oxygen to tissues. Maintaining water and electrolyte homeostasis requires establishing a balance between intake and output such that plasma osmolality remains constant (within approximately 2% of normal). In horses, certain neurologic diseases can cause disturbances in either intake or output, requiring fluid therapy for correction. Tables 18.1 and 18.2 show neurologic disorders in horses that may affect fluid intake and/or output. Delivery of oxygen to tissues is dependent on cardiac output and blood oxygen content. These parameters are not primarily affected by neurologic disease; however, they may be disturbed under certain conditions, such as following brain or spinal cord trauma.

In horses, neurologic disorders that may affect water intake include conditions that affect mental status or mobility resulting in diminished voluntary drinking, and damage to peripheral nerves that are involved in water ingestion and swallowing (Table 18.1). In addition, there are neurologic disorders that disturb transport and absorption of food and water in the gastrointestinal tract, such as equine grass sickness. Finally, excessive losses of water and/or electrolytes can occur through sweating, loss from the gastrointestinal tract, excess obligatory water loss, and third space sequestration. Neurologic conditions in horses that may result in excessive water loss are shown in Table 18.2.

Most equine neurologic conditions that require fluid therapy are those that cause reduced intake. The hydration status of these patients will improve, normalize, or is maintained by providing supportive care. Providing easy access to good quality water, delivering maintenance fluid therapy by nasogastric tube, or administering maintenance fluids intravenously are all examples of supportive care that may be indicated in these cases. However, there are a number of conditions that cause neurologic disease, or are sequelae to neurologic disease, for which more advanced fluid therapy may be indicated. These conditions include central nervous system edema and abnormal serum or plasma concentrations of electrolytes and/or other substrates (Table 18.3).

The central nervous system is unique because two barriers, the blood–brain barrier and the blood–cerebrospinal fluid barrier, provide a high degree of protection. The composition of brain interstitial fluid is determined by active transport of substances through the blood–brain barrier, whereas secretory processes through choroid plexus epithelia determine the composition of the cerebrospinal fluid. The blood–brain and blood–cerebrospinal fluid barriers essentially separate the brain interstitial fluid and cerebrospinal fluid, respectively, from the general circulation. However, in doing so, delivery of therapeutic agents to the central nervous system is also made more difficult.

The brain and spinal cord are protected by the meninges (pia mater, arachnoid, and dura mater), and by the skull and vertebral column, respectively. These structures provide a rigid casing for the central nervous system. Under normal circumstances, when the brain and spinal cord are healthy, the blood–brain and

---

Equine Fluid Therapy, First Edition. Edited by C. Langdon Fielding and K. Gary Magdesian.
© 2015 John Wiley & Sons, Inc. Published 2015 by John Wiley & Sons, Inc.

Table 18.1 Equine neurologic disease that may reduce voluntary water intake and/or absorption.

Affecting	Neuroanatomy	Specific conditions
Intake	Mental status: Cerebral disease: coma, stupor, depression, behavior, seizures	Drugs: sedatives, anesthetics, fluphenazine, reserpine Toxins Toxic neuropathies: hepatoencephalopathy, nigropallidal encephalopathy, leukoencephalomalacia Electrolyte/substrate abnormalities: Na^+, K^+, Mg^{2+}, Ca^{2+}, glucose, ADH (syndrome of ADH) Infection: viral, bacterial, protozoal; encephalitides, meningitis Degeneration Neoplasia Trauma Psychogenic polydipsia
	Mobility/recumbency: Cerebral, brainstem, spinal cord, peripheral	Conditions affecting mental status (see above) Vestibular disease Cerebellar disease Spinal ataxia Peripheral nerve damage
	Prehension and transport to pharynx: Cranial nerves: I, II, V, VII, XII, IX Swallowing: Cranial nerves: IX, X, XI	Blindness, disorders in olfactory or brainstem, otitis media, guttural pouch disease, vestibular disease, peripheral nerve disease Brainstem disorders, peripheral nerve disease
Absorption	Esophageal disorders Gastrointestinal	Cranial nerve X Grass sickness

Table 18.2 Equine neurologic disease that may result in excessive fluid loss.

Affecting	Neuroanatomy	Specific condition
Sweating	Mental status; see Table 18.1	Drugs, toxins, toxic encephalopathies, infection, neoplasia, trauma, behavioral abnormalities
Gastrointestinal	Ileus	Grass sickness
Obligatory losses	Polyuria	Diuretics, glucocorticoids, hypernatremia, hyperglycemia

Table 18.3 Conditions affecting the central nervous system that may require advanced fluid therapy.

Central nervous system edema	Neoplasia Trauma Encephalopathies Inflammatory conditions
Electrolyte/substrate abnormalities	Hyponatremia, hypernatremia Hyperkalemia Hypokalemia Hypocalcemia Hypermagnesemia, hypomagnesemia Hypoglycemia Hyperglycemia ADH
Trauma	Shock, hemorrhage

blood–cerebrospinal fluid barriers, the meninges, and the skull and vertebral column provide superb protection for these vulnerable tissues. However, when brain and/or spinal cord are under duress, this rigid protection can also be damaging. This is explained by the Monro–Kellie doctrine, which states that once the fontanelles and sutures of the skull are closed, the brain is enclosed in a non-expandable case of bone and the volume inside the cranium is fixed. The three

compartments within this rigid encasing are (i) brain parenchyma, (ii) blood volume, and (iii) cerebrospinal fluid volume. A change in volume of any of these three compartments will need to be compensated for by a change in volume, in the opposite direction, by another compartment. For example, if the brain swells (e.g., neoplasia, edema), the pressure within the cranium increases, and the volume of other compartments (other areas of the brain, blood volume) will have to

Table 18.4 Considerations for a fluid therapy plan for horses with neurologic disease.

Safety!	Horse	Protection of animal
		Protection of access sites
		(catheter, administration sets)
	Handlers	Zoonoses
		Animal movements
Route	Oral	Drinking
		Nasogastric intubation
	Intravenous	Through needle
		Permanently placed catheter
Type	Crystalloids	Isotonic (NaCl, balanced
		electrolyte solutions)
		Hypertonic (NaCl, mannitol)
	Colloids	
	Blood substitutes	
	Electrolyte/substrate	Na^+, K^+, Mg^{2+}, Ca^{2+}, glucose/
	additions	dextrose
Volume	Maintenance	60 mL/kg/day is safe
	Losses	Estimate or measure
Rate	Bolus	
	Continuous rate	
	infusion	

decrease in order to prevent a rise in intracranial pressure. In these situations, the primary concern is prevention of secondary (further) brain injury. When the brain is under duress, preventing further swelling and risk of brain herniation is the priority of clinical management. Maintaining sufficient cerebral blood flow and delivery of oxygen to brain tissues to prevent further ischemic injury is crucial.

When devising a fluid therapy plan for a horse with neurologic disease the following considerations should be met (Table 18.4 and Figure 18.1). First, the safety of handlers and the horse needs to be considered. Although horses have been domesticated for thousands of years, they remain "fright and flight" animals. When these animals are moved to an unfamiliar environment (hospital setting) or become debilitated (e.g., disease, pain), behavioral alterations are likely to occur. Horses with neurologic disease can be unpredictable and, therefore, dangerous. In addition, infection control precautions should be undertaken when treating horses with neurologic disease since there is a risk of underlying infectious and/or zoonotic disease (e.g., equine herpes virus-1, rabies). Appropriate precautions such as protective barrier clothing and minimizing human exposure should be undertaken. Second, the route, type, volume, and rate of fluid administration need to be determined (Figure 18.1).

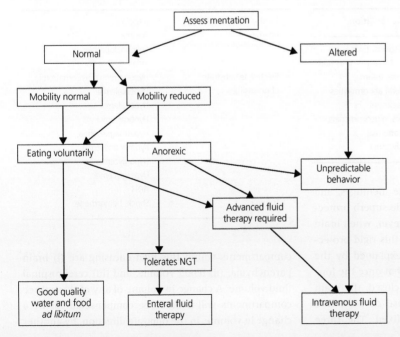

Figure 18.1 Decision tree that can be used for devising a fluid therapy plan for the horse with neurologic disease. NGT, nasogastric tube.

Specific conditions and treatment

Normal mentation with reduced mobility

Treatment of patients with reduced mobility should include supportive therapy that facilitates access to high-quality feed and water. *Ad libitum* hay and water should be available at a site and height that is easily reached. Feed and water intake should be measured. Hydration status should be monitored, for example, through periodic determination of urine specific gravity. A healthy adult horse drinks 44–70 mL/kg/day (Kohn & Hansen, 2010).

Mentation altered – depressed, anorexic, or recumbent horses

Generally speaking, horses that eat will also drink, and horses that do not eat are also unlikely to drink a sufficient amount to maintain hydration. Some horses will be able/willing to drink when access to water is facilitated and water is of high quality (see above). These horses must be able to maintain themselves in a standing or sternal position for long enough periods of time to drink. Horses that are unable (e.g., dysphagia) or unwilling to drink but have a healthy gastrointestinal tract and are amenable to intermittent or indwelling nasogastric intubation can be administered fluids through this route if safe to do so. Since these horses do not have sufficient nutrient intake, electrolytes should be included in orally administered fluids.

An example of a fluid composition for orally administered fluids is: 10 g NaCl, 15 g NaHCO$_3$, 75 g KCl, and 60 g K$_2$HPO$_4$ in 21 L of water. Calcium should be added separately (Hardy, 2010). A healthy adult horse (450 kg) can tolerate up to 10 L of water by nasogastric tube every 30 minutes, for example, during treatment of intestinal tract impactions (Lopes, 2003; Sosa Leon et al., 1997). However, most neurologic horses will not require such large volumes for maintenance, but rather 2–3 mL/kg/h. In addition, if enteral nutrition is provided through a nasogastric tube in the form of gruel or complete liquid diets, volumes of added fluids should be accounted for in the total fluid therapy plan (Nout & Reed, 2005). Delivery of enteral fluids is more safely performed by gravity flow rather than by pump (Ecke et al., 1997).

Hydration and electrolyte status of affected horses should be monitored closely. Urine specific gravity and serum electrolyte concentrations can be measured frequently in these horses.

Mentation altered – unpredictable

Enteral fluid therapy may not be possible if (i) the horse is not amenable to nasogastric intubation, (ii) the horse has, or is at risk for developing, gastrointestinal dysfunction (e.g., ileus, fecal impaction), or (iii) advanced fluid therapy is required. In these situations the intravenous route of delivery of fluids is chosen. Fluid therapy may be administered through any large peripheral vein that is easily and safely accessed, most commonly the jugular and cephalic veins. A catheter may be placed if the insertion site can be protected against damage and contamination. If risk for vessel damage and/or contamination is high due to the circumstances of the case (e.g., persistent movement of recumbent patient), bolus fluids can be delivered through a short-term catheter. Maintenance fluid therapy can be administered as periodic boluses (e.g., 5 L every 4–6 h in a 450-kg horse), so long as rapid bolus administration is not contraindicated (e.g., increased intracranial pressure where any rise in central venous pressure should be avoided). Balanced electrolyte solutions should be used for maintenance fluid therapy except under very specific circumstances as dictated by electrolyte or acid–base derangements. Advanced fluid therapy may be indicated to correct electrolyte abnormalities, to provide dextrose, and/or to treat central nervous system edema. Treatment of sodium disorders is addressed in Chapter 2; this chapter is focused on central nervous system trauma and treating brain and spinal cord edema.

Spinal cord injury

Pathophysiology

Spinal cord injury (SCI) secondary to trauma is a dynamic process where the severity of injury is related to the velocity, degree, and duration of the impact. Primary injury is the initial mechanical damage to the components of the spinal cord that follows an acute insult. With this type of injury, blood vessels may be damaged, axons disrupted, and neuron and glial cell membranes compromised.

The consequences of primary injury are predominantly visible in the central gray matter. Immediately after injury, the gray matter at the region of impact contains disrupted cells and hemorrhage. However, the surrounding white matter, and the gray matter cranial and caudal to the impact region, can appear remarkably intact. The reason for this is not entirely clear. It is most likely related to the rich blood supply and increased metabolic requirements for oxygen and glucose of the nerve cell bodies in the gray matter, and the biomechanical protective properties of the myelin ensheathed axons in the surrounding white matter. Ensuing pathophysiologic processes involving ischemia, release of chemicals from injured cells, and electrolyte shifts alter the metabolic milieu at the level of the lesion.

A secondary injury cascade that substantially compounds initial mechanical damage is triggered. These secondary injury processes do not necessarily coincide with the clinical picture. The pathologic changes may progress in severity for weeks to months, even in the face of clinical improvement.

Acute injury results in immediate hemorrhage within the central gray matter. This early, often progressive, hemorrhage is one of the hallmarks of acute SCI. Loss of microcirculation involving predominantly capillaries and venules subsequently spreads over a considerable distance cranial and caudal to the site of injury. Furthermore, the cord swells within minutes of injury mainly due to hemorrhage and development of edema (Flanders et al., 1999; Mihai et al., 2008). Figure 18.2 shows a magnetic resonance image of the spinal cord after traumatic injury. Swelling, hemorrhage, and edema are visible. This initial hemorrhage, edema, and

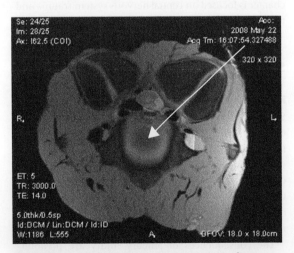

Figure 18.2 T2-weighted magnetic resonance image from a rat spinal cord 8 hours after injury. The arrow points to the hypointense lesion center that is surrounded by a hyperintense ring. The hypointense core is likely blood and blood products, whereas the hyperintense ring surrounding this core is likely edema.

hypoperfusion of the gray matter extends centripetally within minutes to hours of injury and results in central necrosis, white matter edema, and eventually demyelination of axons through secondary injury processes.

Spinal cord ischemia develops over several hours after injury and is considered one of the most important contributors to secondary injury (Kwon et al. 2004; Tator & Fehlings, 1991). The mechanical disruption of the microvasculature causes petechial hemorrhage and intravascular thrombosis, which in combination with vasospasm of intact vessels and edema, leads to profound local hypoperfusion and ischemia. Cord swelling that exceeds venous blood pressure results in secondary ischemia; ischemia is further exacerbated by cessation of autoregulation of spinal cord blood flow, as well as systemic hypotension.

Under normal circumstances, constant local cord hemodynamics are maintained during systolic blood pressure fluctuations between approximately 50 and 130 mmHg through autoregulation of blood flow (Kobrine et al., 1975; Kwon et al., 2004). Loss of autoregulation after SCI makes the cord vulnerable to systemic arterial pressure. In experimental studies of other species it has been demonstrated that immediately after initial SCI a brief period of systemic hypertension is followed by systemic hypotension (Griffiths, 1975; Guha & Tator, 1988; Nout et al. 2011; Sandler & Tator, 1976; Senter & Venes, 1978). Furthermore, acutely traumatized patients can present with systemic hypotension secondary to hypovolemia and/or consequences of loss of sympathetic tone, such as neurogenic shock and bradycardia. SCI can be markedly worsened under ischemic and hypoxic conditions. Systemic hypotension may exacerbate spinal cord hypoperfusion and ischemia. Maintaining normotension after SCI is therefore recommended and has been shown to improve spinal cord perfusion. Unfortunately during conditions of reperfusion, secondary injury may be worsened as a consequence of an increase in oxygen-derived free radicals (Lukacova et al., 1996).

In addition to bradycardia and hypotension, acute SCI often leads to impaired ventilation. These cardiopulmonary derangements are particularly evident in lesions cranial to C5 (respiratory center affected) and cranial to T2 (origin of sympathetic outflow = thoracolumbar spinal cord).

Fluid treatment in spinal cord injury

Volume resuscitation is clearly indicated in shock and for restitution of tissue perfusion. The current recommendation is to maintain euvolemic normotension.

Because of sympathetic outflow disruption after cranial SCI, pressor therapy is commonly indicated in the treatment regimen in addition to fluid therapy. Maintenance of normal mean arterial blood pressure is important to consider during stabilization of the acutely injured horse, and is particularly important when horses are placed under general anesthesia for various diagnostic or therapeutic procedures.

Hypertonic saline has been widely investigated for resuscitation in shock (Dubick et al., 2006; Moore et al., 2004; Pinto et al., 2006; Velasco et al., 1980) and for reducing intracranial pressure to treat cerebral edema after traumatic brain injury (Baker et al., 2008; Forsyth et al., 2008; Pinto et al., 2006; Ziai et al., 2007). Hypertonic saline mobilizes free water from the intracellular into the extracellular space by osmotic force and reduction of peripheral vascular resistance. In shock, the result is a rapid improvement of arterial pressure and cardiac output. In cases with cerebral edema, hypertonic saline lowers intracranial pressure by establishing an osmotic gradient between the intracellular and intravascular space. In addition, improved cerebral blood flow and increased delivery of oxygen cause a compensatory vasoconstriction and a reduction in cerebral blood volume, which further contributes to lowering of intracranial pressure (Forsyth et al., 2008).

There have been a number of investigations into the use of hypertonic saline in SCI (Legos et al., 2001; Nout et al., 2009; Spera et al., 2000; Sumas et al., 2001; Young et al., 1994;), and although most studies report positive effects of hypertonic saline on behavioral, magnetic resonance imaging, and/or histopathologic outcomes, this has not yet led to widespread use of hypertonic saline in human or experimental SCI. Hypertonic saline appears to be a promising addition to a combinatorial treatment strategy in SCI, and further research is required to examine its potential beneficial role in SCI.

In addition to hypertonic saline, a balanced electrolyte solution should be used concurrently or after administration of hypertonic saline to maintain euvolemia and blood pressure. Because calcium plays a role in tissue injury, fluids containing calcium (e.g., lactated Ringer's solution – LRS) may best be avoided when alternatives such as Normosol™-R or Plasma-Lyte®- A are available. The latter contain magnesium rather than calcium, which may be advantageous for acute neurologic injury patients. The goal of these fluids is to maintain hydration and a normal blood pressure, without causing fluid overload that will potentiate tissue edema. Frequent monitoring of hydration and perfusion status is warranted. Monitoring central venous pressure (CVP) is particularly useful in avoiding fluid overload, and serial checking of urine specific gravity can direct fluid rates.

Traumatic brain injury

Pathophysiology

After head trauma, forces are transmitted to the intracranial soft tissues. The brain is consequently shaken within the uneven bony interior of the skull and/or directly damaged by osseous fragments or foreign bodies. Most severe damage generally takes place at the site of impact (coup), and/or opposite to the side of impact (contrecoup). Additionally, the brain is subjected to other forces after trauma, such as rotational and shockwave forces. Traumatic brain injury (TBI) is a result of both (i) direct, immediate mechanical disruption of brain tissue ("primary" injury), and (ii) indirect, delayed ("secondary") injury mechanisms.

The primary damage to the brain is a result of the biomechanical effects of the injury. It is characterized by immediate and often irreversible damage to neuronal cell bodies, dendritic arborizations, axons, glial cells, and brain vasculature. This initial brain injury may be focal, multifocal, or diffuse. Focal brain injury is typically associated with blows to the head leading to cerebral contusions, lacerations, and epidural, subdural, and intracerebral hematomas. In contrast, diffuse brain injury includes traumatic axonal injury that occurs following moderate to severe TBI and results from forces that rapidly rotate and deform the brain (Gennarelli, 1993; Smith et al., 1997). Diffuse axonal injury is a significant component of TBI, and injured axons can display delayed axonal swelling, impairments in axonal transport, and eventual disconnection.

Secondary injury is a complex cascade of molecular, cellular, and biochemical events that can occur for days to months following the initial insult, resulting in delayed tissue damage. In addition, systemic alterations further contribute to the tissue damage. Exacerbation of the initial injury can be due to hypoxia, ischemia, brain swelling, alterations in intracranial pressure, hydrocephalus, infection, breakdown of the blood–brain barrier, impaired energy metabolism, altered ionic homeostasis, changes in gene expression, inflammation, and activation/release of autodestructive molecules.

Vascular damage following head injury can occur in the epidural (between dura mater and the skull), subdural (between the dura mater and arachnoid mater), or subarachnoid (between arachnoid mater and pia mater) spaces; it can also involve superficial (vessels immediately under the pia mater), intraparenchymal, or intraventricular vessels. Subarachnoid hemorrhage, or hemorrhage into the CSF, occurs commonly in horses (Reed, 1987). Hematoma formation is of special concern because of the potential for devastating expansion within the rigid calvarium, similar to what occurs with edema. These processes displace brain tissue with possible sequelae including herniation, pressure necrosis, and brainstem compression. Additionally, hemorrhage around the interventricular foramen or mesencephalic aqueduct may obstruct CSF outflow and lead to hydrocephalus. Increased intracranial pressure is of particular concern after TBI, and may develop from hemorrhage and edema.

Principles of raised intracranial pressure are described in the Monro–Kellie doctrine, which states that once the fontanelles and sutures of the skull are closed: (i) the brain is enclosed in a non-expandable case of bone, (ii) the brain parenchyma is nearly incompressible, (iii) the blood volume in the cranial cavity is therefore nearly constant, and (iv) a continuous outflow of venous blood from the cranial cavity is required to make room for continuous incoming arterial blood (Andrews & Citerio, 2004). Blood flow to the brain is controlled by changes in the diameter of resistance blood vessels. Cerebral blood flow is controlled by autoregulation whereby the perfusion pressure is maintained within a range of mean arterial pressure of approximately 50–150 mmHg (Steiner & Andrews, 2006). Outside this range, cerebral blood flow decreases at pressures below the lower limit and increases at pressures above the upper limit.

Autoregulation occurs in response to changes in cerebral perfusion pressure (mean arterial blood pressure minus intracranial pressure). Cerebral autoregulation is altered unpredictably after TBI, and it appears that the minimum acceptable cerebral perfusion pressure is higher than normal after trauma. Increased intracranial pressure leads to a decrease in cerebral perfusion pressure and subsequently reduces cerebral blood flow. Reduced cerebral blood flow results in areas of ischemia and subsequent restriction of delivery of substrates such as oxygen and glucose to the brain. Reduced cerebral blood flow has been associated with an unfavorable neurologic outcome in human patients and has been implicated in increased susceptibility of the brain to secondary injury (Golding, 2002; Narayan et al., 1981).

The cascade of secondary injury results in necrotic and apoptotic cell death. In addition, concomitant inflammation and endothelial damage cause derangements in normal cerebrovascular reactivity and contribute to a mismatch of oxygen delivery to tissue demand, resulting in local or diffuse ischemia. A major consequence of ischemia is reduced delivery of oxygen and glucose. Blood flow interruption is responsible for disruption in ion homeostasis (especially calcium, sodium, and potassium), and a switch to anaerobic glycolysis resulting in lactic acid production and local acidosis. Cell membrane lipid peroxidation with subsequent prostaglandin and thromboxane synthesis, formation of reactive oxygen species, nitric oxide, and energy failure also ensue. Due to the high metabolic rate and oxygen demands of the brain, disruption of blood flow rapidly compromises the energy-supplying processes and leads to impaired nerve cell function (and even cell death). Impaired mitochondrial function with subsequent energy depletion leads to a loss in maintenance of membrane potentials resulting in abnormal depolarization of neurons and glia (Verweij et al., 2000).

Cytotoxic or intracellular edema develops through the failure of the Na/K-ATPase pump in the presence of hypoxia. Edema forms with an influx of water that passively follows sodium and chloride. This type of edema occurs both in gray and white matter and decreases the extracellular fluid volume (Fishman, 1975). If capillary endothelial cells develop edema, the capillary lumen size will diminish, creating an increased resistance to arterial blood flow. Capillary permeability is usually not directly affected in cytotoxic edema. Major decreases in cerebral function occur with cytotoxic edema, with stupor and coma being common signs (Fishman, 1975). In addition to cytotoxic edema, vasogenic edema develops as a result of disruption of the blood–brain barrier; this includes damage to endothelial cells, degeneration of pericytes, and loss of astrocytes, all of which result in increases in blood–brain barrier permeability. Extravasation of blood components and water occurs resulting in increased extracellular fluid accumulation. This is what is referred to as vasogenic edema (Fishman,

1975). Cerebral white matter is especially vulnerable to vasogenic edema, possibly owing to its low capillary density and blood flow (Fishman, 1975; Golding, 2002). This vasogenic edema displaces cerebral tissue and increases intracranial pressure. Understanding these complex pathophysiologic events that take place after TBI is important for developing effective monitoring and treatment strategies.

Fluid therapy and initial stabilization in TBI

Treatment of TBI is aimed at optimizing delivery of oxygen and substrates in order to salvage tissues that are undamaged or only reversibly damaged. This requires optimizing cerebral blood flow, through maintenance of normal mean arterial blood pressure and hemoglobin concentration, and minimizing increases in intracranial pressure. Emergency surgical treatment (although not commonly performed in horses) is warranted in open cranial fractures and in the face of deteriorating clinical signs despite medical therapy. Once the patient is stabilized, repair of less life-threatening fractures can be considered.

Maintaining the head in an elevated position can reduce intracranial pressure and has been demonstrated in horses (Brosnan et al., 2002). This is a particularly important consideration in horses requiring sedation, where the head should be prevented from dropping. In human neurocritical care units, treatment to reduce intracranial pressure is commenced at pressures of 20–25 mmHg. In the acute setting, human neurointensivists perform a neurologic examination and hyperventilate patients (to a targeted P_aCO_2) at risk for having increased intracranial pressures while awaiting brain imaging. Hyperventilation reduces the partial pressure of carbon dioxide in the blood, and subsequently leads to cerebral vasoconstriction. Reduced cerebral blood volume decreases intracranial pressure. However, cerebral vasoconstriction may also lead to reduction of cerebral blood flow to ischemic levels. Therefore, it is currently recommended that hyperventilation to reduce intracranial pressure is only used if hyperemia is a contributor to increased intracranial pressure. Hyperventilation is also recommended in combination with intensive neuromonitoring (including P_aCO_2) and for only a limited duration.

Limited hyperventilation, and particularly avoidance of hypoventilation, could be considered in cases of increased intracranial pressure in horses. In anesthetized horses proper hyperventilation requires monitoring of arterial blood gases, and may require use of neuromuscular blockers if the horse is not comatose and is resisting the ventilator.

Cerebrospinal fluid drainage is commonly used in humans to reduce intracranial pressure. Drainage is considered a therapeutic option only if there is cerebrospinal fluid outflow obstruction. If these methods are ineffective, repeat imaging is pursued to investigate the presence of mass lesions before medical treatments are commenced such as administration of hyperosmolar substances and induction of barbiturate coma. Hyperosmolar treatment, with mannitol or hypertonic saline, is commonly used in horses with neurologic signs attributable to TBI.

As with spinal cord injury, mean arterial blood pressure should be maintained within normal limits. Following TBI, normal mean arterial blood pressure and euvolemia should be maintained using isotonic crystalloid intravenous fluid therapy. Unlike the treatment of spinal cord injury, where sympathetic outflow often is disrupted, pressor therapy is rarely indicated following TBI. Interestingly, in a study comparing treatment guided by intracranial pressure (<20 mmHg) versus treatment guided by cerebral perfusion pressure (CPP: >70 mmHg), the incidence of acute respiratory distress syndrome was significantly higher when treatment was guided by CPP (Robertson et al., 1999). There were no functional outcome differences between the two treatment regimens (Robertson et al., 1999). A recent study recommends individual tailoring of these treatment strategies depending on the relationship of mean arterial and intracranial pressure responses to treatment (Howells et al., 2005).

Crystalloid fluids are recommended as the intravenous fluid therapy of choice, particularly in light of findings of the serum versus albumin fluid evaluation (SAFE) study (Finfer et al., 2004). The SAFE study did not identify any difference between outcomes when administering albumin versus normal saline in the intensive care unit. A subgroup analysis demonstrated an increased mortality in TBI patients that were treated with albumin (Finfer et al., 2004). However, isotonic crystalloid fluids administered in typical shock doses of 40–90 mL/kg/h may produce worsening of cerebral edema and increased intracranial pressure (Gunnar et al., 1988). Therefore, smaller and serial challenge doses of isotonic crystalloids (10 mL/kg) should be used for fluid resuscitation of the hypovolemic TBI equine patient when isotonic fluids are selected, with frequent reassessment. The decision on fluid rates in TBI patients is an extremely challenging one. Monitoring of CVP, though requiring placement of CVP catheters, can aid in preventing rises in intracranial pressure with fluid therapy.

Comparison of isotonic crystalloid fluids with hypertonic saline solutions has shown hypertonic saline to be the fluid of choice for fluid support of head trauma patients in shock (White et al., 2006). Hypertonic saline is associated with significant decreases in intracranial pressure and cerebral water content compared with isotonic fluid treatment. Furthermore, hypertonic saline has positive effects on cerebral blood flow, oxygen consumption, and inflammatory response at a cellular level (Kempski, 2001). Hypertonic saline can be administered intravenously to head trauma horses in shock as 5% or 7% NaCl solutions (4–6 mL/kg) over 15 minutes. Isotonic fluids can then be used for maintenance if needed. Contraindications to the use of hypertonic saline include significant dehydration, ongoing intracerebral hemorrhage, hypernatremia, renal failure, hyperkalemic periodic paralysis, and hypothermia. Potential systemic side effects include coagulopathies, excessive intravascular volume (particularly relevant if active hemorrhage is present), and electrolyte abnormalities. Monitoring central venous pressure and maintaining it within normal limits (5–7 cmH$_2$O) is therefore important as well as monitoring serum sodium and potassium concentrations if hypertonic saline is used frequently (White et al., 2006). Persistent hypernatremia should be avoided.

Mannitol has been the primary osmotherapeutic drug for the last four decades. Mannitol induces changes in blood rheology and increases cardiac output, leading to improved cerebral perfusion pressure and cerebral oxygenation. Improved cerebral oxygenation induces cerebral artery vasoconstriction and subsequent reduction in cerebral blood volume and intracranial pressure. Mild dehydration after osmotherapy is desirable and may improve cerebral edema; however, severe dehydration can lead to hyperosmolality, tissue hypoperfusion, and renal failure. Mannitol also decreases CSF production by up to 50%, which can lead to prolonged intracranial pressure decreases (White et al., 2006).

In horses, 20% mannitol can be administered at 0.25–2.0 g/kg intravenously over 20 minutes. Horses receiving osmotic diuretics should be adequately hydrated prior to administration of the osmotic agent. The use of osmotic substances is warranted in any horse with: (i) worsening mental status, (ii) abnormal pupillary size or inequality (indicating transtentorial herniation), or (iii) development of paresis. Although mannitol administration is very effective in reducing intracranial pressure, there are several limitations to its use. Persistent hyperosmolality can be associated with renal and central nervous system effects. Furthermore, administration of multiple doses of mannitol may lead to hypovolemia (through diuresis), hypotension, and reduction of cerebral blood flow. Therefore, current research is focused on the use of substitutes for mannitol, of which the most promising is hypertonic saline.

Hypertonic saline has a number of beneficial effects in TBI. The permeability of the blood–brain barrier to sodium is low. Hypertonic saline produces an osmotic gradient between the intravascular and the interstitial/intracellular compartments, leading to shrinkage of brain tissue and subsequent reduction of intracranial pressure. The reflection coefficient of NaCl is greater than that of mannitol, making it potentially a more effective osmotic drug.

As described above, hypertonic saline augments volume resuscitation and increases circulating blood volume temporarily, mean arterial blood pressure, and cerebral perfusion pressure. Other beneficial effects of hypertonic saline include restoration of neuronal membrane potential, maintenance of the blood–brain barrier integrity, and modulation of the inflammatory response (by reducing adhesion of leukocytes to endothelium) (Soustiel et al., 2006; White et al. 2006). Hypertonic saline typically is used as 3%, 5%, or 7.5% solutions, but one study showed beneficial effects of using small-volume 23.4% hypertonic saline to reduce intracranial pressure (Ware et al., 2005)

Animal studies support the use of hypertonic saline in TBI (Walsh et al., 1991; Zornow et al., 1990), but definitive human trials with mortality as endpoint in brain trauma are lacking. Nevertheless, hypertonic saline osmotherapy should be considered a therapeutic adjunct to the multimodal medical management of TBI. An example for an approach to its use for reducing intracranial pressure in humans is intravenous administration of a 4 mL/kg bolus of 3% hypertonic saline that is repeated until intracranial pressure is normalized or until a sodium concentration of 155 mmol/L is achieved. The serum sodium concentration is maintained at this level until intracranial pressure is stabilized and then gradually allowed to decrease. If intracranial pressure is still raised after 3–4 days, furosemide is used in an effort to mobilize tissue sodium (White et al., 2006).

Blood transfusions may be indicated in situations of severe hemorrhage. Hemoglobin deficiency adversely affects oxygen delivery to tissues, and guidelines for traumatic injury traditionally have advocated aggressive treatment of anemia in TBI. However, a human study has demonstrated that, similar to other critical care patients, blood transfusions negatively affected outcome in TBI patients (Carlson et al., 2006). The threshold for transfusion, thus, should be no different than in other critical care patients.

The use of carbohydrate-containing intravenous solutions should be avoided early in the treatment of head trauma patients, unless hypoglycemia is present. Glucose suppresses ketogenesis and may increase lactic acid production by the traumatized brain tissue. This can limit the availability of non-glycolytic energy substrates (Robertson et al., 1991). Furthermore, carbon dioxide liberated from glucose metabolism could cause vasodilation and worsening of cerebral edema. Maintaining blood glucose concentrations at 80–110 mg/dL through intensive insulin therapy has reduced morbidity and mortality in human critical care patients in some studies (van den Berghe et al., 2001). However, more recently, neurointensivists have shown that tight glucose control is associated with increased hypoglycemic episodes and with direct extracellular (microdialysis) evidence of cellular distress and brain energy crisis (Vespa et al., 2006). The currently available clinical and preclinical evidence does not support tight glucose control (maintenance of blood glucose levels below 110–120 mg/dL) during the acute care of human patients with severe TBI (Marion, 2009).

References

Andrews PJ, Citerio G. (2004) Intracranial pressure. Part one: historical overview and basic concepts. *Intensive Care Med* **30**:1730–3.

Baker AJ, Park E, Hare GM, Liu E, Sikich N, Mazer DC. (2008) Effects of resuscitation fluid on neurologic physiology after cerebral trauma and hemorrhage. *J Trauma* **64**:348–57.

Brosnan RJ, Steffey EP, LeCouteur RA, Imai A, Farver TB, Kortz GD. (2002) Effects of body position on intracranial and cerebral perfusion pressures in isoflurane-anesthetized horses. *J Appl Physiol* **92**:2542–6.

Carlson AP, Schermer CR, Lu SW. (2006) Retrospective evaluation of anemia and transfusion in traumatic brain injury. *J Trauma* **61**:567–71.

Dubick MA, Bruttig SP, Wade CE. (2006) Issues of concern regarding the use of hypertonic/hyperoncotic fluid resuscitation of hemorrhagic hypotension. *Shock* **25**:321–8.

Ecke P, Hodgson DR, Rose RJ. (1997) Review of oral rehydration solutions for horses with diarrhoea. *Aust Vet J* **75**: 417–20.

Finfer S, Bellomo R, Boyce N, French J, Myburgh J, Norton R. (2004) A comparison of albumin and saline for fluid resuscitation in the intensive care unit. *N Engl J Med* **350**:2247–56.

Fishman RA. (1975) Brain edema. *N Engl J Med* **293**:706–11.

Flanders AE, Spettell CM, Friedman DP, Marino RJ, Herbison GJ. (1999) The relationship between the functional abilities of patients with cervical spinal cord injury and the severity of damage revealed by MR imaging. *AJNR Am J Neuroradiol* **20**:926–34.

Forsyth LL, Liu-DeRyke X, Parker D Jr, Rhoney DH. (2008) Role of hypertonic saline for the management of intracranial hypertension after stroke and traumatic brain injury. *Pharmacotherapy* **28**:469–84.

Gennarelli TA. (1993) Mechanisms of brain injury. *J Emerg Med* **11**(Suppl. 1): 5–11.

Golding EM. (2002) Sequelae following traumatic brain injury. The cerebrovascular perspective. *Brain Res Brain Res Rev* **38**:377–88.

Griffiths IR. (1975) Vasogenic edema following acute and chronic spinal cord compression in the dog. *J Neurosurg* **42**:155–65.

Guha A, Tator CH. (1988) Acute cardiovascular effects of experimental spinal cord injury. *J Trauma* **28**:481–90.

Gunnar W, Jonasson O, Merlotti G, Stone J, Barrett J. (1988) Head injury and hemorrhagic shock: studies of the blood brain barrier and intracranial pressure after resuscitation with normal saline solution, 3% saline solution, and dextran-40. *Surgery* **103**:398–407.

Hardy J. (2010) Basic procedures in adult equine critical care. In: Reed SM, Bayly WM, Sellon DC (eds) *Equine Internal Medicine*. St Louis, MO: Saunders Elsevier, pp. 249–58.

Howells T, Elf K, Jones PA, et al. (2005) Pressure reactivity as a guide in the treatment of cerebral perfusion pressure in patients with brain trauma. *J Neurosurg* **102**:311–17.

Kempski O. (2001) Cerebral edema. *Semin Nephrol* **21**:303–7.

Kobrine AI, Doyle TF, Martins AN. (1975) Autoregulation of spinal cord blood flow. *Clin Neurosurg* **22**:573–81.

Kohn CW, Hansen B. (2010) Polyuria and polydipsia. In: Reed SM, Bayly WM, Sellon DC (eds) *Equine Internal Medicine*. St Louis, MO: Saunders Elsevier, pp. 126–31.

Kwon BK, Tetzlaff W, Grauer JN, Beiner J, Vaccaro AR. (2004) Pathophysiology and pharmacologic treatment of acute spinal cord injury. *Spine J* **4**:451–64.

Legos JJ, Gritman KR, Tuma RF, Young WF. (2001) Coadministration of methylprednisolone with hypertonic saline solution improves overall neurological function and survival rates in a chronic model of spinal cord injury. *Neurosurgery* **49**:1427–33.

Lopes MAF. (2003) Administration of enteral fluid therapy: methods, composition of fluids and complications. *Equine Vet Educ* **15**:107–12.

Lukacova N, Halat G, Chavko M, Marsala J. (1996) Ischemia-reperfusion injury in the spinal cord of rabbits strongly enhances lipid peroxidation and modifies phospholipid profiles. *Neurochem Res* **21**:869–73.

Marion DW. (2009) Optimum serum glucose levels for patients with severe traumatic brain injury. *F1000 Med Rep* **1**(42).

Mihai G, Nout YS, Tovar CA, et al. (2008) Longitudinal comparison of two severities of unilateral cervical spinal cord injury using magnetic resonance imaging in rats. *J Neurotrauma* **25**:1–18.

Moore FA, McKinley BA, Moore EE. (2004) The next generation in shock resuscitation. *Lancet* **363**:1988–96.

Narayan RK, Greenberg RP, Miller JD, et al. (1981) Improved confidence of outcome prediction in severe head injury. A comparative analysis of the clinical examination, multimodality evoked potentials, CT scanning, and intracranial pressure. *J Neurosurg* **54**:751–62.

Nout YS, Reed SM. (2005) Management and treatment of the recumbent horse. *Equine Vet Educ* **7**:416–32.

Nout YS, Mihai G, Tovar CA, Schmalbrock P, Bresnahan JC, Beattie MS. (2009) Hypertonic saline attenuates cord swelling and edema in experimental spinal cord injury: a study utilizing magnetic resonance imaging. *Crit Care Med* **37**:2160–6.

Nout YS, Beattie MS, Bresnahan JC. (2011) Severity of locomotor and cardiovascular derangements after experimental high-thoracic spinal cord injury is anesthesia dependent in rats. *J Neurotrauma* **29**:990–9.

Pinto FC, Capone-Neto A, Prist R, E Silva MR, Poli-de-Figueiredo LF. (2006) Volume replacement with lactated Ringer's or 3% hypertonic saline solution during combined experimental hemorrhagic shock and traumatic brain injury. *J Trauma* **60**:758–63; discussion 763–4.

Reed SM. (1987) Intracranial trauma. In: Robinson NE (ed.) *Current Therapy in Equine Medicine*. Philadelphia: W.B. Saunders Co., pp. 377–80.

Robertson CS, Goodman JC, Narayan RK, Contant CF, Grossman RG. (1991) The effect of glucose administration on carbohydrate metabolism after head injury. *J Neurosurg* **74**:43–50.

Robertson CS, Valadka AB, Hannay HJ, et al. (1999) Prevention of secondary ischemic insults after severe head injury. *Crit Care Med* **27**:2086–95.

Sandler AN, Tator CH. (1976) Effect of acute spinal cord compression injury on regional spinal cord blood flow in primates. *J Neurosurg* **45**:660–76.

Senter HJ, Venes JL. (1978) Altered blood flow and secondary injury in experimental spinal cord trauma. *J Neurosurg* **49**:569–78.

Smith DH, Chen XH, Xu BN, McIntosh TK, Gennarelli TA, Meaney DF. (1997) Characterization of diffuse axonal pathology and selective hippocampal damage following inertial brain trauma in the pig. *J Neuropathol Exp Neurol* **56**:822–34.

Sosa Leon LA, Hodgson DR, Rose RJ. (1997) Gastric emptying of oral rehydration solutions at rest and after exercise in horses. *Res Vet Sci* **63**:183–7.

Soustiel JF, Vlodavsky E, Zaaroor M. (2006) Relative effects of mannitol and hypertonic saline on calpain activity, apoptosis and polymorphonuclear infiltration in traumatic focal brain injury. *Brain Res* **1101**:136–44.

Spera PA, Vasthare US, Tuma RF, Young WF. (2000) The effects of hypertonic saline on spinal cord blood flow following compression injury. *Acta Neurochir (Wien)* **142**:811–17.

Steiner LA, Andrews PJ. (2006) Monitoring the injured brain: ICP and CBF. *Br J Anaesth* **97**:26–38.

Sumas ME, Legos JJ, Nathan D, Lamperti AA, Tuma RF, Young WF. (2001) Tonicity of resuscitative fluids influences outcome after spinal cord injury. *Neurosurgery* **48**:167–72; discussion 172–3.

Tator CH, Fehlings MG. (1991) Review of the secondary injury theory of acute spinal cord trauma with emphasis on vascular mechanisms. *J Neurosurg* **75**:15–26.

van den Berghe G, Wouters P, Weekers F, et al. (2001) Intensive insulin therapy in the critically ill patients. *N Engl J Med* **345**:1359–67.

Velasco IT, Pontieri V, Rocha e Silva M Jr, Lopes OU. (1980) Hyperosmotic NaCl and severe hemorrhagic shock. *Am J Physiol* **239**:H664–73.

Verweij BH, Muizelaar JP, Vinas FC, Peterson PL, Xiong Y, Lee CP. (2000) Impaired cerebral mitochondrial function after traumatic brain injury in humans. *J Neurosurg* **93**:815–20.

Vespa P, Boonyaputthikul R, McArthur DL, et al. (2006) Intensive insulin therapy reduces microdialysis glucose values without altering glucose utilization or improving the lactate/pyruvate ratio after traumatic brain injury. *Crit Care Med* **34**:850–6.

Walsh JC, Zhuang J, Shackford SR. (1991) A comparsion of hypertonic to isotonic fluid in the resuscitation of brain injury and hemorrhagic shock. *J Surg Res* **50**:284–92.

Ware ML, Nemani VM, Meeker M, Lee C, Morabito DJ, Manley GT. (2005) Effects of 23.4% sodium chloride solution in reducing intracranial pressure in patients with traumatic brain injury: a preliminary study. *Neurosurgery* **57**:727–35; discussion 735–6.

White H, Cook D, Venkatesh B. (2006) The use of hypertonic saline for treating intracranial hypertension after traumatic brain injury. *Anesth Analg* **102**:1836–46.

Young WF, Rosenwasser RH, Vasthare US, Tuma RF. (1994) Preservation of post-compression spinal cord function by infusion of hypertonic saline. *J Neurosurg Anesthesiol* **6**:122–7.

Ziai WC, Toung TJ, Bhardwaj A. (2007) Hypertonic saline: first-line therapy for cerebral edema? *J Neurol Sci* **261**:157–66.

Zornow MH, Oh YS, Scheller MS. (1990) A comparison of the cerebral and haemodynamic effects of mannitol and hypertonic saline in an animal model of brain injury. *Acta Neurochir Suppl (Wien)* **51**:324–5.

CHAPTER 19
Fluid therapy for muscle disorders

Darien J. Feary

Senior Lecturer in Equine Medicine, School of Animal and Veterinary Science, Equine Health and
Performance Centre, The University of Adelaide, Roseworthy, South Australia

Rhabdomyolysis specifically refers to skeletal muscle cell damage and necrosis resulting in the release of toxic intracellular contents from myocytes into the systemic circulation. Rhabdomyolysis is a clinical manifestation common to a wide variety of causes in horses, which may be exertional, genetic, nutritional, metabolic, toxic, traumatic, infectious, anaesthetic-related, or immune-mediated in origin (Table 19.1). The term "rhabdomyolysis" is not synonymous with myopathy, as there are a number of well-recognized equine myopathies that do not result in significant rhabdomyolysis.

The most common factor preceding an episode of acute rhabdomyolysis in horses is exercise, the nature of which is quite variable between and within individuals (Harris, 1998). The term "exertional rhabdomyolysis" refers to sporadic, chronic, and recurrent forms of rhabdomyolysis where physical exertion is clearly the final triggering factor, although the underlying predisposition may be different between horses. In some horses that are presented with obvious clinical signs of acute exertional rhabdomyolysis, the cause may be readily apparent, such as with overexertion or exercising in hot, humid conditions. In other cases, the cause may not be easily identified and further diagnostic investigation is warranted. Although a multitude of theories have been proposed throughout decades of studies of equine exertional rhabdomyolysis, a specific aetiology remains elusive in many cases (Valentine, 2008).

In recent years, there have been significant advances in the recognition and understanding of many exertional and non-exertional causes of rhabdomyolysis in horses. In some cases a specific genetic abnormality of muscle metabolism has been identified (Aleman, 2008),

including glycogen branching enzyme 1 deficiency in quarter horse and paint foals (Ward, 2004), genetic abnormality in the glycogen synthase 1 (*GYS1*) gene responsible for some horses with polysaccharide storage myopathy (PSSM), and mutation in the *RyR1* gene causing malignant hyperthermia in quarter horses (Aleman et al., 2004). Atypical myopathy ("seasonal pasture myopathy") is a severe and frequently fatal myopathy that has been reported to occur in a seasonal pattern in young horses and ponies grazing pasture in the United Kingdom and many other European countries, Canada, and the United States (Votion & Serteyn, 2008). Recently, atypical myopathy has been associated with ingestion of hypoglycin A within seeds of the box elder tree in the United States and of the sycamore maple (*Acer pseudoplatanus*) in Europe (Valberg et al., 2013; Votion et al., 2014). Ingestion of certain toxic plants is an uncommon but often fatal cause of acute, severe rhabdomyolysis in horses. Severe, acute rhabdomyolysis is an uncommon but life-threatening complication of *Streptococcus equi* subsp. *equi* infection (Sponseller et al., 2005), and can also occur in cases of infarctive purpura hemorrhagica. A detailed review of the many causes and diagnosis of acute rhabdomyolysis in horses is beyond the scope of this chapter. The reader is referred to some excellent review articles for further information (Aleman, 2008; Beech 2000a,2000b; Keen, 2011; Valberg, 2009; Valentine, 2008; Votion &Sertayn, 2008).

There is wide variation in the clinical signs of rhabdomyolysis in horses, ranging from mild stiffness in gait or lameness, to inability to move, recumbency, shock, and death. The need for urgent veterinary intervention should be determined by the severity of the clinical

---

Equine Fluid Therapy, First Edition. Edited by C. Langdon Fielding and K. Gary Magdesian.
© 2015 John Wiley & Sons, Inc. Published 2015 by John Wiley & Sons, Inc.

Table 19.1 Causes of acute rhabdomyolysis in horses

Non-exertional rhabdomyolysis	Exertional rhabdomyolysis
Nutritional	Sporadic
Selenium/vitamin E deficiency	Inadequate fitness/training
Metabolic	Overexertion
Polysaccharide storage	Metabolic exhaustion
myopathy	Heat stress
Glycogen branching enzyme	Chronic
deficiency	Recurrent exertional
Mitochondrial myopathy	rhabdomyolysis
Toxic	Polysaccharide storage
Ionophore toxicity	myopathy
White snake root toxicity	Dietary imbalance
Organophosphate toxicity	Idiopathic
Ivermectin	Traumatic
Cantharidin (blister beetle)	Excessive struggling/cast
Traumatic (direct)	
Infectious	
Viral (equine influenza virus,	
equine infectious anemia,	
equine herpesvirus 1)	
Bacterial (*Clostridium* spp.)	
Parasitic (*Sarcocystis* spp.)	
Immune-mediated	
Streptococcus-associated	
myositis	
Anaesthesia-associated	
Malignant hyperthermia	
Compartment myopathy	
Atypical myopathy	

signs, degree of muscle damage, and suspected complications, regardless of the cause. Clinical signs in severe cases often include a stiff gait, reluctance to move or recumbency, hard and painful epaxial and hind limb muscles, excessive sweating, tachycardia, tachypnea, and anxiety. Myoglobinuria is a common finding in most, but not all, severely affected horses. Although rhabdomyolysis can often be readily diagnosed on the basis of the horse's clinical signs and history, confirmation requires determination of abnormally increased serum concentrations of the muscle-derived enzyme creatine kinase (CK), usually in combination with aspartate aminotransferase (AST) or lactate dehydrogenase (LDH) (Valberg, 2009). The magnitude of elevation in the muscle-specific enzyme CK is proportional to the degree of muscle cell necrosis, reaching values greater than tens to hundreds of thousands of international

units per liter in severe rhabdomyolysis cases (Harris, 1989; Valberg, 2009), but this is not always reflected in the severity of clinical signs (Keen, 2011; Valberg, 2009). It is also important to recognize and differentiate acute rhabdomyolysis from conditions that cause similar initial clinical signs including colic, laminitis, severe electrolyte imbalance (e.g., hypocalcemia), tetanus, pleuritis, hyperkalemic periodic paralysis (HYPP), and tick (*Otobius megnini*) myotonia. A thorough history, clinical examination, and assessment of serum biochemistry and urine are extremely valuable in determining if muscle cell necrosis is a predominant feature of a suspected case of acute rhabdomyolysis.

Horses with acute rhabdomyolysis are at risk for developing major complications including myoglobin-induced acute renal failure, electrolyte abnormalities causing cardiac arrhythmia, disseminated intravascular coagulation (DIC), laminitis, and death. The general approach to the management of acute, severe rhabdomyolysis involves minimizing further muscle damage by ceasing to move or exercise the horse, replacement of intravascular volume and diuresis to prevent renal injury, correction of acid–base and electrolyte abnormalities, and managing pain and anxiety.

While many of the therapeutic options for the treatment of acute rhabdomyolysis in horses remain controversial and of unproven benefit, providing early and aggressive intravenous (IV) fluid therapy is, without question, the most important intervention in the prevention and management of the complications of rhabdomyolysis. In order to understand the basis for fluid therapy recommendations it is important to understand, compare, and contrast the pathophysiology of rhabdomyolysis in both humans and horses, and its associated complications.

Pathophysiology and complications of acute rhabdomyolysis

Regardless of the inciting mechanism, an increase in free ionized calcium in muscle cell cytoplasm is central to the pathogenesis of rhabdomyolysis (Chatzizisis et al., 2008; Warren et al., 2002). Normally, in resting muscle the sarcoplasmic Ca^{2+} concentration is strictly maintained within a very low range compared to that of the extracellular fluid; this is accomplished by a series of cell membrane pumps, channels, and exchangers. These mechanisms allow a controlled increase in Ca^{2+} necessary for actin-myosin binding during muscle contraction. Known mechanisms of increased cytosolic Ca^{2+} include direct injury to the myoctye, (e.g., trauma) or depletion of ATP, which results in pump failure and a persistent increase in sarcoplasmic Ca^{2+} (Bosch et al., 2009). Any cause of persistently increased sarcoplasmic Ca^{2+} results in activation of destructive proteolytic enzymes and causes muscle cell membrane lysis, increased permeability, and eventual dissolution of the myocyte. This increase in sarcoplasmic Ca^{2+} appears to be the final common pathway in acute severe rhabdomyolysis, regardless of the underlying cause (Huerta-Alardin et al., 2005).

The etiology of recurrent exertional rhabdomyolysis ("RER") in Thoroughbred horses is believed to be associated with an inability to regulate intracellular calcium concentrations within skeletal muscle (Valberg et al., 1999). Microelectrode studies in horses support the premise that skeletal muscle cytoplasmic Ca^{2+} concentrations are much greater in horses suffering from exertional rhabdomyolysis compared with normal controls (López et al., 1995). However, the exact mechanism by which this increase in cytoplasmic Ca^{2+} occurs in equine exertional rhabdomyolysis has not yet been determined.

Extensive muscle cell injury is accompanied by massive influx of sodium, chloride, and calcium into the cytoplasm, followed by massive efflux of potassium, phosphate, myoglobin, cytosolic enzymes, and organic acids into the systemic circulation. Damaged muscle tissue creates a third space for redistribution of large volumes of intravascular fluid, which results in relative hypovolemia that contributes to coexisting hemodynamic instability (Bagley et al., 2007; Holt & Moore, 2001).

Myoglobin-induced acute kidney injury

Myoglobin-induced renal failure is one of the most serious, life-threatening complications of acute rhabdomyolysis. The incidence of acute kidney injury as a complication of rhabdomyolysis in horses is not reported, but is likely to involve similar mechanisms in humans and horses.

Myoglobin is a heme protein released from damaged muscle cells into circulation and freely filtered by the renal glomeruli, where it is metabolized by tubular epithelial cells. Myoglobinuria only occurs as a consequence of rhabdomyolysis, and appears grossly as a reddish-brown pigment in the urine only when serum myoglobin levels are significantly above the renal threshold. Myoglobin is rapidly eliminated from plasma through renal clearance and has a short half-life (2–3 h in humans) (Huerta-Alardin et al., 2005). Therefore the absence of myoglobinuria does not preclude a diagnosis of rhabdomyolysis, or the possibility of myoglobin-induced kidney injury.

There are three main mechanisms by which rhabdomyolysis is believed to lead to the development of acute kidney injury: renal vasoconstriction, direct and ischemic tubule injury, and tubule obstruction by myoglobin cast formation (Figure 19.1).

Renal vasoconstriction occurs as a result of a combination of various mechanisms and is a characteristic feature of acute kidney injury associated with rhabdomyolysis (Bosch et al., 2009). Initially, intravascular volume depletion due to fluid accumulation within damaged muscle tissues stimulates activation of the RAAS, vasopressin, and the sympathetic nervous system. Renal blood flow is additionally reduced by activation of vascular mediators including endothelin-1, thromboxane A_2, tumor necrosis factor (TNF), and isoprostanes, as well as a reduction in vasodilation by the scavenging of nitric oxide by myoglobin (Holt & Moore, 2001).

Tubule obstruction by myoglobin cast formation occurs principally in the distal tubules. Myoglobin is concentrated along the renal tubules, particularly in the face of volume depletion and renal vasoconstriction. Myoglobin cast formation occurs when myoglobin interacts with Tamm–Horsfall protein from damaged renal tubular cells, which is a process enhanced in acidic urine (Zager, 1989).

Myoglobin is a heme protein and contains iron in the form of ferrous oxide (Fe^{2+}). Reactive oxygen species are generated by the oxidation of ferrous to ferric oxide (Fe^{3+}), which is favored in acidic urine. Oxidant injury and lipid peroxidation of proximal tubule cells results in direct tubule injury in the form of acute tubular necrosis (Zager, 1989).

In the absence of hypovolemia and aciduria, myoglobin appears to have minimal nephrotoxic effects in humans (Huerta-Alardin et al, 2005). However, in the presence of coexisting hypovolemia and aciduria the risk of myoglobin-induced renal failure is much greater. Therefore, the main goals of fluid therapy in human patients have traditionally aimed at large-volume fluid resuscitation, diuresis, and urinary alkalinization.

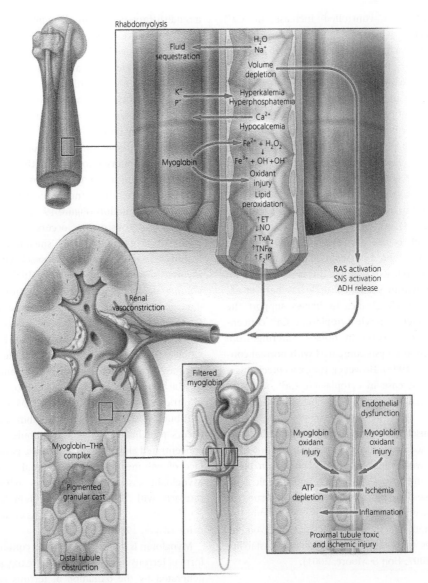

Figure 19.1 Pathophysiologic mechanisms in myoglobin-induced acute kidney injury. Sequestration of fluid in injured muscles results in depletion of circulating blood volume with consequent activation of the sympathetic nervous system (SNS), antidiuretic hormone (ADH), and the renin-angiotensin system (RAS), which favors intrarenal vasoconstriction and sodium and water retention. Myoglobin-induced oxidative injury further increases the activity of vasoconstrictive agents and inhibits vasodilators. Kidney injury results from a combination of ischemia due to renal vasoconstriction, direct tubular toxicity mediated by myoglobin-associated oxidative injury (insert, lower right), tubular damage due to ischemia, and distal tubule obstruction due to precipitation of pigmented granular casts (insert, lower left). As in acute kidney injury due to other causes, endothelial dysfunction and local inflammation contribute to tissue damage and organ dysfunction. ET, endothelin; F_2IP, F2 isoprostanes; NO, nitric oxide; THP, Tamm–Horsfall protein; TNFα, tumor necrosis factor α; TxA_2, thromboxane A_2. Image from Bosch, X., Poch, E., Grau, JM. 2009. Rhabdomyolysis and Acute Kidney Injury: Current Concepts. *New England Journal of Medicine* 361(1):62–72, with permission.

The presence of myoglobinuria in horses can be readily determined by gross red-brown discoloration of urine. This may be further supported by a simple urine dipstick test that is positive for blood, in the absence of erythrocytes in the urine supernatant after centrifugation. Although this test cannot distinguish myoglobin from hemoglobin, if the serum is not hemolysed then further laboratory investigation to distinguish between these proteins is unlikely to be necessary as it requires special tests that are not readily available in most equine practices. Differentiation of myoglobin from hemoglobin in urine can be performed in commercial laboratories, such as with ammonium sulfate precipitation. Horses observed to have myoglobinuria are likely to have significant myonecrosis and would definitely benefit from fluid therapy to prevent the development of renal complications, as well as further assessment of serum biochemistry and urine analytes.

Metabolic acidosis resulting in aciduria is reported to occur commonly in humans with severe rhabdomyolysis and is believed to be a critical factor contributing to the development of myoglobin-induced acute renal failure (Sinert et al., 1994; Watanabe, 2001). In contrast, the most common acid–base and electrolyte abnormality reported in horses with acute rhabdomyolysis is mild hypochloremic metabolic alkalosis (Freestone & Carlson, 1991; Koterba & Carlson, 1982). Although horse urine is normally alkaline, urine pH is reported to range from 6.0 to 8.5 in cases of acute rhabdomyolysis. Paradoxic aciduria has also been reported in horses with metabolic alkalosis that were suffering from rhabdomyolysis (Freestone & Carlson, 1991). Very few reports in the veterinary literature, involving only small numbers of horses, specify the acid–base abnormalities and urine pH in cases of acute rhabdomyolysis. Therefore it is difficult to predict the likely abnormalities in an individual case, as these are greatly influenced by the factors associated with the development of the acute episode.

The development of acute renal failure is a late, rather than immediate complication of acute rhabdomyolysis and may not be readily apparent during the initial evaluation of horses with rhabdomyolysis. Therefore it is critical to be aware of the risks of myoglobin-induced renal failure and perform the necessary diagnostic tests, and to institute fluid therapy to prevent renal injury. Furthermore, applying therapies specifically aimed at combating aciduria indiscriminately may not be an appropriate goal in horses, as it is in human patients.

Electrolyte and acid–base abnormalities

Typical electrolyte changes reported to occur initially in acute rhabdomyolysis in humans include hyperkalemia, hyperphosphatemia, hyperuricemia, and hypocalcemia. The electrolyte abnormalities that occur during the initial stages of rhabdomyolysis are a consequence of massive release of intracellular constituents from damaged myocytes into the systemic circulation. Electrolyte and acid–base abnormalities that occur associated with acute rhabdomyolysis usually precede the development of acute renal failure and should ideally be evaluated as soon as rhabdomyolysis is suspected.

Hyperkalemia is an early manifestation of rhabdomyolysis and can be a life-threatening complication in humans (Bagley et al., 2007) and horses (Perkins et al., 1998). Hyperkalemia is further exacerbated by the presence of metabolic acidosis and the development of renal failure. The hypocalcemia that also occurs in the early stages of rhabdomyolysis contributes to the cardiotoxic effects of hyperkalemia. Potassium concentrations generally peak 12 to 36 hours following muscle injury. Risk of life-threatening cardiac arrhythmias increases when potassium concentrations exceed 6.0 mmol/L and associated ECG changes are observed. There is one report of four foals with severe rhabdomyolysis associated with selenium/vitamin E deficiency in which profound hyperkalemia, hypocalcemia, hyperphosphatemia, and hyponatremia were identified (Perkins et al., 1998). Significant hyperkalemia is more likely to occur in severe cases of acute rhabdomyolysis, and is less likely in horses suffering from rhabdomyolysis associated with prolonged endurance exercise. However, the incidence of hyperkalemia in adult horses and foals with acute rhabdomyolysis is unknown. Hyperkalemia should be identified early and treated aggressively with fluid therapy as outlined in the next section.

Hypocalcemia occurs commonly in humans with severe rhabdomyolysis and it can occur in horses with severe rhabdomyolysis, particularly associated with the exhausted horse syndrome. Initial hypocalcemia is due to the movement of calcium into damaged muscle cells, and also from the precipitation of calcium and phosphate in necrotic muscle tissue (soft tissue calcification) in humans (Criddle, 2003). Initial hypocalcemia is generally followed by gradually developing hypercalcemia as the patient is hydrated and deposited calcium is mobilized from damaged muscle tissue back into the circulation. Soft tissue calcification as a complication of rhabdomyolysis is well recognized in human patients and can be determined by the use of technetium (99Tc) bone scanning (Holt & Moore, 2001). Perkins et al. (1998) reported increased calcium deposition in damaged skeletal muscle evident at post mortem in young foals with severe rhabdomyolysis, but its occurrence and significance in equine patients is otherwise unknown.

Hypocalcemia is rarely symptomatic or important in humans with rhabdomyolysis and generally resolves without treatment. Muscle tetany would be the most obvious clinical sign observed if hypocalcemia was severe. Occasionally ionized hypocalcemia may cause cardiovascular compromise associated with hypotension and poor cardiac performance (Holt & Moore, 2001). Unique to horses, hypocalcemia may manifest as synchronous diaphragmatic flutter, which requires treatment that should include supplemental intravenous calcium.

Metabolic acidosis is the most common acid–base abnormality reported in humans with acute, severe rhabdomyolysis and is due to the release of organic acids, uric acid, phosphate, sulfate, and potassium from damaged muscle cells into the systemic circulation. It is exacerbated by coexisting hyperlactatemia due to hypovolemia and reduced tissue perfusion (Bagley et al., 2007; Criddle, 2003; Luck & Verbin, 2008). As previously mentioned, mild hypochloremic metabolic alkalosis is the most commonly reported abnormality in adult horses with rhabdomyolysis (Freestone & Carlson, 1991; Koterba & Carlson, 1982). Hypochloremia is proposed to occur as a result of excessive or prolonged sweating often associated with severe acute rhabdomyolysis (Koterba & Carlson, 1982).

Considering that most cases of exertional rhabdomyolysis develop following periods of low-intensity or sub-maximal exercise, metabolic acidosis does not appear to be a common feature of horses with acute rhabdomyolysis as it is in humans. However, mixed acid–base abnormalities are likely to be present if an initial hypochloremic metabolic alkalosis progresses to metabolic acidosis with hypovolemia and ensuing shock. Clearly, the presence and specific nature of acid–base and electrolyte abnormalities in equine rhabdomyolysis is unpredictable and will vary with the cause and severity of myonecrosis. Determination of venous blood gas and electrolyte values in horses with severe rhabdomyolysis, regardless of the cause, should be sought as early as possible after presentation to determine if significant abnormalities are present, and to guide optimal therapy.

Fluid therapy recommendations

Acute, severe rhabdomyolysis in horses is a medical emergency. Horses with rhabdomyolysis exhibiting only mild signs of muscle stiffness and normal or near normal vital signs may be effectively managed with oral fluid therapy alone. However, all horses with clinical signs of rhabdomyolysis benefit from some form of fluid therapy and should have at least a minimum biochemical database performed to evaluate renal parameters, electrolytes, and muscle-derived enzyme activities, have their urination observed, and urinalysis performed if possible. Horses with severe signs of rhabdomyolysis, which is often associated with myoglobinuria, require immediate IV fluid therapy, particularly if non-steroidal anti-inflammatory (NSAID) medications are also administered.

The author is unaware of any clinical studies evaluating the use or effectiveness of IV fluid therapy in the management of acute rhabdomyolysis in horses. However, clinical studies in human patients clearly show that early and aggressive IV fluid therapy represents the single most important intervention in preventing the development of complications of rhabdomyolysis (Gunal et al., 2004; Homsi et al., 1997; Shimazu et al., 1997). Traditionally, the main goals of fluid therapy in human patients with rhabdomyolysis are to induce diuresis with large volumes of isotonic crystalloid fluids and diuretics, and to maintain urine pH above 6.5 by urinary alkalinization. As such, the routine addition of mannitol and bicarbonate to the fluid therapy protocol has been considered the standard of care in the management of human patients with acute rhabdomyolysis (Better & Stein, 1997; Gunal et al., 2004; Homsi et al., 1997). While of theoretical benefit, the widespread use of mannitol and bicarbonate has more recently been questioned due to the lack of clinical evidence supporting any significant benefit over large-volume crystalloid fluid replacement alone in the prevention of acute renal failure due to rhabdomyolysis (Hogg, 2010).

The following recommendations for fluid therapy in horses with acute rhabdomyolysis are based on recent human medical literature, with modifications pertaining to the pathophysiology of rhabdomyolysis in equine species.

Fluid replacement

While there is no question that early, large-volume infusion of isotonic crystalloids is the mainstay of therapy in the treatment of severe acute rhabdomyolysis, the optimal fluid composition for volume replacement remains controversial in human patients. Certainly the specific composition of replacement fluids has not received as much attention and debate in the medical literature as has the use of diuretics and urinary alkalinization.

The majority of the human medical literature recommends the use of large volumes of isotonic (0.9%) saline for intravenous volume replacement in the treatment of acute, severe rhabdomyolysis, probably because isotonic 0.9% saline is the most commonly used IV crystalloid for fluid therapy in human critical care medicine (Guidet et al., 2010). Large-volume infusion of isotonic 0.9% saline has the potential to induce dilutional hyperchloremic metabolic acidosis, which is likely to contribute to aciduria and increased risk for myoglobin-induced kidney injury in human patients. Therefore, it seems logical to consider alternative, less acidifying fluid types when treating acute rhabdomyolysis. Cho et al. (2007) concluded that fluid replacement using large volumes of a balanced polyionic fluid (lactated Ringer's solution) was superior to isotonic (0.9%) saline for the treatment of drug-induced rhabdomyolysis in humans because metabolic acidosis and aciduria were less likely to occur.

The optimal crystalloid fluid choice for resuscitation in horses with rhabdomyolysis is unknown, but should ideally be based on acid–base and electrolyte measurements performed on a blood sample collected at the time of presentation. The causative factors of the acute episode are also important. Considering that horses with acute rhabdomyolysis may be more likely to be hypochloremic and alkalotic, the use of isotonic (0.9%) saline would seem an appropriate initial replacement fluid due to the higher chloride concentration. However, coexisting hypovolemia, electrolyte derangements, or acute kidney injury are likely to result in a mixed acid–base disorder.

When the acid–base and electrolyte status is unknown or normal, or if acidemia or aciduria is present, then large volumes of balanced isotonic replacement fluids such as lactated Ringer's solution (LRS), Normosol®-R, Plasma-Lyte® A or Plasma-Lyte® 148 would be appropriate. Focusing on small details, one might consider LRS to be the fluid of choice with rhabdomyolysis, because the acetate salt in Normosol-R and Plasma-Lyte fluids is primarily metabolized by muscle tissue. Fluids should be delivered at high rates of 20–40 mL/kg/h (10–20 L/h for a 500-kg horse) until urination is observed, and diuresis continued at 5–10 mL/kg/h (2.5–5 L/h for a 500-kg horse) until urine is clear, vital signs normalize, and serum creatinine is normal.

In exhausted endurance horses with suspected rhabdomyolysis, and in other cases in which a hypochloremic metabolic alkalosis is documented or suspected, then the use of large volumes of isotonic (0.9%) saline for initial fluid replacement may be appropriate. Acid–base and electrolyte status should be re-evaluated following initial fluid replacement (i.e., after 30–50 L) if possible. If hypochloremia and other electrolyte abnormalities have resolved then continuing fluid therapy with a balanced isotonic crystalloid fluid would be recommended.

Hypertonic (7.2%) saline

There are many potential advantages of including hypertonic (7.2%) saline in the initial resuscitation of horses with severe rhabdomyolysis. Resuscitation with hypertonic saline in humans with acute rhabdomyolysis is an evolving topic of investigation. The multiple potential advantages of hypertonic fluids and small-volume fluid resuscitation over isotonic crystalloids alone in the treatment of shock states in horses have been well demonstrated (Fielding & Magdesian, 2011; Schmall et al., 1990). Hypertonic (7.2%) saline significantly increases plasma volume expansion, as well as improving urine output in dehydrated endurance horses compared with isotonic (0.9%) saline alone (Fielding & Magdesian, 2011). These findings suggest that hypertonic (7.2%) saline may have beneficial effects in preventing renal failure in horses with severe rhabdomyolysis.

The effect of hypertonic (7.2%) saline resuscitation on acid–base status and urine pH, or its effectiveness in the treatment of horses with rhabdomyolysis, have not been reported. However, the judicious use of hypertonic saline in the early resuscitation of horses with acute rhabdomyolysis showing signs of shock should be considered for its beneficial effects on plasma volume expansion, and improved tissue perfusion and renal blood flow. The dose of hypertonic saline should not exceed 4 mK/kg, given as an initial bolus, and must be followed by additional fluid therapy with large volumes

(60–80 mL/kg) of balanced isotonic crystalloid fluids. Acid–base status, urine output, and renal parameters should be closely monitored.

Bicarbonate therapy

Alkalinization of urine with IV sodium bicarbonate has traditionally been a mainstay of fluid therapy for the prevention of myoglobin-induced renal failure in humans with rhabdomyolysis (Better & Stein, 1990; Homsi et al., 1997). The empirical benefits of using alkalinizing agents to prevent acute kidney injury are based on animal models of rhabdomyolysis. These studies show that myoglobin cast formation is favored in acidic urine (Zagar, 1989), and that alkalinization reduces redox cycling of myoglobin and lipid peroxidation (Moore et al., 1998), and renal vasoconstriction is more likely to occur in an acidic medium (Heyman et al., 1997). The main disadvantage of alkalinization is a reduction in ionized calcium, which can exacerbate existing initial hypocalcemia in acute rhabdomyolysis. However, despite its widespread use, a review of the retrospective clinical studies shows that there is no convincing evidence that alkaline diuresis is a superior treatment compared with aggressive, isotonic crystalloid fluid therapy alone in the prevention of myoglobin-induced renal failure in humans (Hogg, 2010).

The urine pH of horses with acute rhabdomyolysis has not been reported in a large enough number of cases to determine if aciduria is an important risk factor in the development of myoglobin-induced kidney injury in this species. Considering that the urine pH of horses is normally alkaline, and that metabolic alkalosis is probably more common in horses with rhabdomyolysis than in humans, the indiscriminate use of bicarbonate therapy for urinary alkalinization in horses is not justified. Bicarbonate therapy is also not recommended in the initial fluid therapy management of horses with documented metabolic acidosis, as in most cases acidosis will resolve following adequate fluid volume replacement with IV isotonic crystalloid fluids. One exception would be in the treatment of severe, life-threatening hyperkalemia when glucose ± insulin therapy fails to lower plasma K^+ concentrations. If severe acidemia persists and/or urine pH is acidic (pH <6.0) despite adequate fluid replacement and diuresis, then bicarbonate therapy should be considered. Indiscriminate administration of bicarbonate-containing solutions may be detrimental, particularly in dehydrated,

hypochloremic, or hypokalemic horses, in which sustained metabolic alkalosis and hypocalcemia may develop (Koterba & Carlson, 1982). If sodium bicarbonate therapy is used, then urine pH and serum bicarbonate, calcium, and potassium concentrations should be monitored.

Mannitol

The use of diuretics in the management of rhabdomyolysis remains controversial in human medicine, although it is clear that adequate fluid replacement must be established before any diuretic agent is administered. Mannitol has several theoretical beneficial effects and continues to be recommended for the prevention of acute kidney injury in human patients with rhabdomyolysis (Better & Rubinstein, 1997; Lameire et al., 2005). The rationale for the use of mannitol mainly relates to its osmotic diuretic properties, although its ability to act as a free-radical scavenger may have some additional benefit (Bosch et al., 2009). The osmotic effects of mannitol cause diuresis and increased urine output, as well as the redistribution of fluid from injured muscle tissue into the extracellular fluid space resulting in a reduction in tissue edema. Despite its theoretical justification and beneficial effects, clinical studies have failed to show significant benefit of mannitol therapy over aggressive large-volume crystalloid fluid resuscitation alone in the prevention of acute renal failure in human patients with rhabdomyolysis (Brown et al., 2004; Homsi et al., 1997). Other literature suggests that the use of mannitol may actually be harmful (Visweswaren et al., 1997).

However, the judicious use of mannitol and/or loop diuretics in the management of persistent anuria/oliguria in horses despite appropriate fluid therapy could be considered in the same manner as recommended for acute renal failure due to other causes (see Chapter 14). If forced diuresis with mannitol is employed in the management of acute rhabdomyolysis it must not be administered until adequate fluid replacement has been achieved, then plasma osmolality and the osmolal gap should be monitored frequently during therapy.

Correction of hyperkalemia

The general approach to the treatment of hyperkalemia in horses with acute rhabdomyolysis is similar to that in the treatment of hyperkalemia due to other causes (see Chapter 3), with the exception of the timing of IV calcium administration. Serum potassium concentrations should be determined early in the initial assessment of horses with acute severe rhabdomyolysis and monitored frequently to detect rapidly rising levels. An ECG should be assessed for cardiac manifestations of hyperkalemia. If the potassium concentration exceeds 6.0 mmol/L and/or ECG abnormalities are detected then potassium-lowering therapies should be instituted. Briefly, IV fluid therapy should be continued using isotonic 0.9% saline combined with standard therapies that result in the movement of potassium from the extracellular fluid (ECF) to the intracellular fluid (ICF) (intravenous glucose, insulin, and/or sodium bicarbonate). If unsuccessful, further therapy is aimed at enhancing potassium elimination through the use of diuretic agents, ion-exchange resins, or dialysis.

Although IV calcium has no direct effect on serum potassium concentrations, it is used to minimize the cardiotoxic effects of hyperkalemia by increasing the cell membrane threshold potential, thereby reducing membrane excitability. Because intravenous calcium administration is not recommended in the treatment of acute rhabdomyolysis (see next section), its use should be reserved for the treatment of hyperkalemia associated with life-threatening ECG changes.

The treatment of life-threatening hyperkalemia was reported to be a major therapeutic challenge in four foals with severe rhabdomyolysis associated with selenium/vitamin E deficiency (Perkins et al., 1998). Treatment to lower serum potassium concentrations was unsuccessful in some of the foals using standard therapies, including IV glucose, insulin, and sodium bicarbonate, necessitating the use of fludrocortisone with mineralocorticoid activity and loop diuretics, as well as anion-exchange resins to enhance elimination of potassium. Balanced polyionic crystalloid fluids contain between 4 and 5 mmol/L of potassium, and although this is only a very small fraction of total body potassium concentration, large-volume infusion of these fluids should ideally be avoided in horses with life-threatening hyperkalemia.

Intravenous calcium administration

The administration of IV calcium is frequently recommended in the veterinary literature to treat hypocalcemia in horses with severe rhabdomyolysis. Supplemental calcium may seem to be a logical choice when the patient is hypocalcemic, particularly considering the importance of ionized calcium in muscle contraction. However, the measured decrease in extracellular calcium observed commonly in acute rhabdomyolysis is due to influx into the damaged muscle cells, where it contributes to further cell damage and death. Administration of additional exogenous calcium is only likely to compound cell damage, and may contribute to soft tissue calcification.

The use of IV calcium to correct hypocalcemia in humans with acute rhabdomyolysis is not recommended unless symptomatic hypocalcemia or life-threatening hyperkalemia is observed (Bagley et al., 2007; Holt & Moore, 2001; Luck & Verbin, 2008). Similarly for horses, calcium supplementation cannot be recommended as part of fluid therapy management for acute rhabdomyolysis unless life-threatening hyperkalemia or symptomatic hypocalcemia (tetany, synchronous diaphragmatic flutter) is observed. One exception may be in the management of exhausted endurance horses with rhabdomyolysis. In this specific subgroup of horses routine intravenous calcium therapy is considered beneficial because of the significant hypocalcemia and whole body electrolyte losses commonly present, although this requires further study.

Dialysis

The inclusion of a brief discussion of dialysis as a potential therapy for the management of myoglobin-induced renal failure in horses is warranted because of its reported success in a small number of equine patients. Renal replacement therapy is recommended in human patients with refractory hyperkalemia, metabolic acidosis, or fluid volume overload associated with oliguric renal failure when other therapies have been unsuccessful. Conventional hemodialysis does not remove myoglobin effectively due to the latter's large molecular size, thus intermittent hemodialysis is usually required (Bosch et al., 2009). The use of hemodialysis in horses is limited by expense and the need for specialized equipment and expertise.

Peritoneal dialysis has been used effectively as a viable therapeutic alternative to hemodialysis in the management of horses with acute renal failure refractory to conventional therapies. Continuous peritoneal dialysis has been reported to be effective in the management of myoglobin-induced acute renal failure in an adult horse, and both intermittent and continuous peritoneal dialysis have been used in the effective management of acute renal failure due to other causes in horses (Gallatin et al., 2005; Han & McKenzie, 2008). These reports suggest that peritoneal dialysis should be considered early in the management of horses with acute renal failure associated with rhabdomyolysis that does not respond adequately to conventional therapies.

Summary

Acute, severe rhabdomyolysis in horses has a wide range of etiologies, exertional and non-exertional in origin. Regardless of the cause, horses with severe clinical signs are at risk of developing life-threatening complications including hyperkalemia and myoglobin-induced renal failure. Administration of large volumes of intravenous isotonic crystalloid fluids to achieve diuresis remains the most important therapeutic intervention in horses and humans with acute rhabdomyolysis. The most commonly reported electrolyte and acid–base abnormality in horses with acute rhabdomyolysis is hypochloremic metabolic alkalosis, although this is likely to be complicated by metabolic acidosis in hypovolemic patients. Therefore IV fluid replacement with large volumes of a balanced isotonic crystalloid such as lactated Ringer's solution or Normosol-R is recommended in most cases if acid–base and electrolyte status is unknown. Fluid replacement with isotonic (0.9%) saline would be more appropriate in the initial treatment of horses that have a hypochloremic metabolic alkalosis (such as exhausted endurance horses) or severe hyperkalemia. The indiscriminate use of sodium bicarbonate and mannitol for the treatment of rhabdomyolysis is not indicated in human or equine patients. Although hypocalcemia is a common finding in acute rhabdomyolysis, the administration of IV calcium is also not recommended unless hypocalcemia is symptomatic (synchronous diaphragmatic flutter, tetany).

There is a need for large retrospective and prospective clinical studies evaluating volume deficits, acid–base and electrolyte, and urinalysis findings in horses with severe acute rhabdomyolysis of various etiologies, and to determine risk factors for the development of myoglobin-induced acute kidney injury. These data would provide useful information on which to base more equine-specific recommendations for optimal fluid therapy.

References

Aleman, Monica R. (2008) A review of equine muscle disorders. *Neuromuscular Disord* **18**:277–87.

Aleman M, Riehl J, Aldridge BM, Lecouteur RA, Stott JL, Pessah IN. (2004) Association of a mutation in the ryanodine receptor 1 gene with equine malignant hyperthermia. *Muscle Nerve* **3093**:356–65.

Bagley WH, Yang H, Shah KH. (2007) Rhabdomyolysis. *Intern Emerg Med* **2**:210–18.

Beech J. (2000a) Equine muscle disorders 1: Chronic intermittent rhabdomyolysis. *Equine Vet Educ* **12**:163–7.

Beech J. (2000b) Equine muscle disorders 2. *Equine Vet Educ* **12**:208–13.

Better OS, Rubinstein I. (1997) Management of shock and acute renal failure in casualties suffering from the crush syndrome. *Renal Failure* **19**:647–53.

Better OS, Stein JH. (1990) Early management of shock and prophylaxis of acute renal failure in traumatic rhabdomyolysis. *N Engl J Med* **322**:825–9.

Bosch X, Poch E, Grau JM. (2009) Rhabdomyolysis and acute kidney injury: Current concepts. *N Engl J Med* **361**:62–72.

Brown CV, Rhee P, Chan L, Evans K, Demetriades D, Velmahos GC. (2004) Preventing renal failure in patients with rhabdomyolysis: do bicarbonate and mannitol make a difference? *J Trauma* **56**:1191–6.

Chatzizisis YS, Misirli G, Hatzitolios AI, Giannoglou GD. (2008) The syndrome of rhabdomyolysis: Complications and treatment. *Eur J Int Med* **19**:568–74.

Cho YS, Lim H, Kim SH. (2007) Comparison of lactated Ringer's solution and 0.9% saline in the treatment of rhabdomyolysis induced by doxylamine intoxication. *Emerg Med J* **24**:276–80.

Criddle LM. (2003) Rhabdomyolysis: pathophysiology, recognition and management. *Crit Care Nurse* **23**:14–30.

Fielding CL, Magdesian KG. (2011) A comparison of hypertonic (7.2%) and isotonic (0.9%) saline for fluid resuscitation in horses: A randomised, double-blinded, clinical trial. *J Vet Int Med* **25**:1138–43.

Freestone JF, Carlson GP. (1991) Muscle disorders in the horse: a retrospective study. *Equine Vet J* **23**:86–90.

Gallatin LL, Couetil LL, Ash SR. (2005) Use of continuous-flow peritoneal dialysis for the treatment of acute renal failure in an adult horse. *J Am Vet Med Assoc* **226**:756–9.

Guidet B, Soni N, Della Rocca G, Kozek S, Vallet B, Annane D, James M. (2010) A balanced view of balanced solutions. *Crit Care* **14**:325–37.

Gunal AI, Celiker H, Dogukan, A, et al. (2004) Early and vigorous fluid resuscitation prevents acute renal failure in the crush victims of catastrophic earthquakes. *J Am Soc Nephrol* **15**:1862–7.

Han JH, McKenzie III HC. (2008) Intermittent peritoneal dialysis for the treatment of acute renal failure in two horses. *Equine Vet Educ* **20**:256–64.

Harris P. (1989) Equine rhabdomyolysis syndrome. *In Practice* **11**: 3–8.

Harris P. (1998) Equine rhabdomyolysis syndrome. In: Watson T (ed.) *Metabolic and Endocrine Problems of the Horse.* W.B. Saunders, pp. 75–99.

Heyman SN, Greenbaum R, Shina A, Rosen S, Brezis M. (1997) Myoglobinuric acute renal failure in the rat: a role for acidosis? *Exp Nephrol* **5**:210–16.

Ho AMH, Karmakar MK, Contardi LH, Ng SS, Hewson JR. (2001) Excessive use of normal saline in managing traumatized patients in shock: a preventable contributor to acidosis. *J Trauma* **51**:173–7.

Hogg K. (2010) Towards evidence based emergency medicine: best BETs from the Manchester Royal Infirmary. *Emerg Med J* **28**:898.

Holt SG, Moore KP. (2001) Pathogenesis and treatment of renal dysfunction in rhabdomyolysis. *Intens Care Med* **27**:803–11.

Homsi E, Barreiro MK, Orlando JM, Higa EM. (1997) Prophylaxis of acute renal failure in patients with rhabdomyolysis. *Renal Failure* **19**:283–8.

Huerta-Alardin AL, Varon J, Marik PE. (2005) Bench-to-bedside review: Rhabdomyolysis – an overview for clinicians. *Crit Care* **9**:158–69.

Keen J. (2011) Diagnosis and management of equine rhabdomyolysis. *In Practice* **33**:68–77.

Koterba A, Carlson GP. (1982) Acid-base and electrolyte alterations in horses with exertional rhabdomyolysis. *J Am Vet Med Assoc* **180**:303–5.

Lameire N, Van Biesen W, Vanholder R. (2005) Acute renal failure. *Lancet* **365**:417–30.

López JR, Linares N, Cordovez G, Terzic CA. (1995) Elevated myoplasmic calcium in exercise-induced equine rhabdomyolysis. *Eur J Physiol* **430**:293–5.

Luck, RP, Verbin S. (2008) Rhabdomyolysis. A review of clinical presentation, etiology, diagnosis, and management. *Pediatr Emerg Care* **24**:262–8.

Moore KP, Holt SG, Patel RP, et al. (1998) A causative role for redox cycling of myoglobin and its inhibition by alkalinisation in the pathogenesis and treatment of rhabdomyolysis-induced renal failure. *J Biol Chem* **273**:31731–7.

Perkins G, Valberg SJ, Madigan JM, Carlson GP, Jones SL. (1998) Electrolyte disturbances in foals with severe rhabdomyolysis. *J Vet Intern Med* **12**:173–7.

Schmall LM, Muir WW, Robertson JT. (1990) Haemodynamic effects of small volume hypertonic saline in experimentally induced haemorrhagic shock. *Equine Vet J* **22**:273–7.

Shimazu T, Yoshioka T, Nakata Y, et al. (1997) Fluid resuscitation and systematic complications in crush syndrome: 14 Hanshin-Awaji earthquake patients. *J Trauma* **42**:641–6.

Sinert R, Kohl L, Rainone T, Scalea T. (1994) Exercise-induced rhabdomyolysis. *Ann Emerg Med* **23**:1301–6.

Sponseller BT, Valberg SJ, Tennent-Brown BS, Foreman JH, Kumar P, Timoney JF. (2005) Severe acute rhabdomyolysis associated with Streptococcus equi infection in four horses. *J Am Vet Med Assoc* **227**:1800–7.

Valberg SJ. (2009) Diseases of muscles. In: Smith BP (ed.) *Large Animal Internal Medicine*, 4th edn. Mosby, Elsevier Inc., pp. 1388–1418.

Valberg SJ, Mickelson JR, Gallant EM, et al. (1999) Exertional rhabdomyolysis in Quarter Horses and Thoroughbreds: one syndrome, multiple aetiologies. *Equine Vet J (Suppl.)* **30**: 533–8.

Valberg SJ, Sponseller BT, Hegeman AD, et al. (2013) Seasonal pasture myopathy/atypical myopathy in North America is associated with ingestion of hypoglycin A within seeds of the box elder tree. *Equine Vet J* **45**:419–26.

Valentine BA. (2008) Understanding exertional rhabdomyolysis. *Equine Vet Educ* **20**:539–41.

Visweswaren P, Massin EK, Dubose TD. (1997) Mannitol-induced acute renal failure. *J Am Soc Nephrol* **8**:1028–33.

Votion DM, Sertayn D. (2008) Equine atypical myopathy: A review. *Vet J* **178**:185–90.

Votion DM, van Galen G, Sweetman L, et al. (2014) Identification of methylencyclopropyl acetic acid in serum of European horses with atypical myopathy. *Equine Vet J* **46**: 146–9.

Ward TL, Valberg SJ, Adelson DL, Abbey CA, Binns MM, Mickelson JR. (2004) Glycogen branching enzyme (GBE1) mutation causing equine glycogen storage disease IV. *Mammal Genome* **15**:570–7.

Warren JD, Blumbergs PC, Thompson PD. (2002) Rhabdomyolysis: A review. *Muscle Nerve* **25**:332–47.

Watanabe T. (2001) Rhabdomyolysis and acute renal failure in children. *Pediatr Nephrol* **16**:1072–5.

Zager RA. (1989) Studies of mechanisms and protective maneuvers in myoglobinuric acute renal injury. *Lab Invest* **60**:619–29.

CHAPTER 20

Perioperative fluid therapy

Julie E. Dechant

Associate Professor, Clinical Equine Surgical Emergency and Critical Care, School of Veterinary Medicine, University of California, USA

Introduction

Perioperative fluid balance should be considered in any horse undergoing general anesthesia and surgery. General anesthesia inevitably compromises the hemodynamic status of the patient, and the significance of that compromise depends on the patient's clinical status and the duration of anesthesia. Supportive therapy to improve the hemodynamic state is indicated in most situations to minimize complications. The mainstay of hemodynamic supportive therapy is fluid therapy. The use of vasopressors or inotropic agents is frequently indicated in concert with intravenous fluid support, and readers are directed to equine anesthesia references for specific information on pharmacological methods of hemodynamic support.

Perioperative fluid therapy should be a component of all but the shortest general anesthetic procedures in the healthiest patients. At a minimum, intraoperative fluid therapy is useful to maintain vascular access throughout the procedure. Fluid replacement is a frequent indication for perioperative fluid therapy. Fluid deficits may be present prior to anesthesia or develop during the anesthetic period. These preoperative deficits can be severe in the context of emergency anesthesia, due to the underlying disease, associated compromise, and limited opportunity to stabilize the patient prior to surgery. However, healthy elective patients may have some pre-existing fluid deficits due to withholding of food and water prior to surgery. Intraoperative fluid losses can arise from surgical hemorrhage, evaporative losses from exposed viscera, third space fluid sequestration, and respiratory losses associated with non-humidified inhalant gases (Kudnig & Mama, 2002).

Preoperative considerations

A complete physical examination, paying particular attention to the cardiovascular and respiratory systems, is essential in any horse undergoing general anesthesia. Fluid balance can be assessed by skin turgor, mucous membrane moistness and color, capillary refill time, pulse quality, and jugular fill. A complete blood count should be considered as a minimum database for general anesthesia of healthy elective patients. Packed cell volume (PCV) and total protein (TP) concentration are useful, but crude, determinants of hydration status. Any compromised or diseased patient should be further assessed by a serum biochemistry panel to better assess electrolyte status and renal function.

Preoperative fluid deficits (dehydration or hypovolemia) should be corrected, if at all possible, prior to anesthesia. If they cannot be corrected preoperatively, the deficits must be addressed during general anesthesia, in addition to meeting the necessary intraoperative fluid support. Strategies for fluid resuscitation will be discussed later in this chapter.

Pre-existing azotemia should prompt special consideration for perioperative fluid management. Impaired renal function has been a documented consequence of anesthesia (Campbell et al., 1990; Steffey et al., 1979, 1993). Horses with pre-existing renal injury are at further risk for additional renal compromise if not adequately perfused during surgery.

Electrolyte and acid–base disturbances can accompany certain disease conditions and should be addressed as part of the perioperative fluid therapy plan. Hyperkalemia, hypocalcemia, and acidemia are the

Equine Fluid Therapy, First Edition. Edited by C. Langdon Fielding and K. Gary Magdesian.
© 2015 John Wiley & Sons, Inc. Published 2015 by John Wiley & Sons, Inc.

most frequently encountered electrolyte disturbances in association with equine anesthesia (Kudnig & Mama, 2002). These and other electrolyte imbalances have been discussed in Section 1 of this book. Common electrolyte abnormalities that may need treatment in anesthetized patients will be discussed in more detail later in this chapter.

Anesthetized patients are less tolerant of anemia due to reduced baroreceptor reflexes, myocardial depression, and anesthesia-associated vasodilation (Kudnig & Mama, 2002; Wilson et al., 2003). Anemia has a profound effect on oxygen-carrying capacity, because hemoglobin is the primary contributor to blood oxygen content and dissolved oxygen is a relatively minor component (Hubbell & Muir, 2009). Anemia may be described as normovolemic or hypovolemic. Hypovolemic anemia is found with hemorrhagic blood loss and requires replacement of the vascular deficit and protein losses, as well as restoring the oxygen-carrying capacity of the blood. Hypovolemic anemia is best addressed by whole blood transfusion (see Chapter 23). Normovolemic anemia is not complicated by decreased vascular volume; however, the impact on oxygen-carrying capacity is equally important. It has been recommended to maintain the PCV ≥25% in anesthetized patients (Kudnig & Mama, 2002; Wagner, 2009), which is a more aggressive transfusion trigger than typically used for awake patients.

Hypoproteinemia affects perioperative fluid decisions due to the reduction in colloid osmotic pressure (COP), predisposing to the development of tissue edema. Colloid osmotic pressure decreases further during anesthesia, primarily due to intraoperative fluid therapy (Boscan & Steffey, 2007; Boscan et al., 2007; Wendt-Hornickle et al., 2011). In healthy horses anesthetized for 2.5 hours, total protein concentration decreased by over 25% and COP decreased by over 30% (Boscan et al., 2007). The use of colloid solutions (see Chapter 24) should be considered as part of the perioperative fluid therapy to ameliorate further dilution of plasma proteins during surgery.

Perioperative catheter considerations

Intravenous catheters should be placed prior to general anesthesia to facilitate redosing of injectable anesthetic agents and to allow intravenous fluid therapy. Intravenous catheters have been discussed in detail in Chapter 9. Intravenous catheters used for perioperative fluid administration must accommodate the fluid needs of the patient under anesthesia and allow for higher flow rates if additional fluid support is given during anesthesia.

Catheter flow rates can be approximated by Poiseuille's law whereby laminar flow of fluids is directly proportional to tube radius and pressure gradient and indirectly proportional to length of the tube and fluid viscosity. This approximation overestimates flow rates that can be achieved with intravenous catheterization, because flow is both laminar and turbulent at clinically relevant flow rates (McPherson et al., 2009). Regardless, catheter internal diameter is the most significant factor affecting flow. Fluid flow is directly related to catheter radius raised to the fourth power (i.e., doubling the catheter diameter increases flow by a multiple of 16) (Hardy, 2009). Although flow is indirectly proportional to the length of the catheter, short catheters risk dislodgement from the vein. Other factors in the fluid administration apparatus that affect fluid flow rates are diameter changes between extension sets and connectors, direction changes within the administration apparatus, and piggybacking fluids (Ash, 2007; Dutky et al., 1989).

Large-diameter, short-term intravenous catheters are recommended for perioperative fluid administration. A 14-gauge, 5¼-inch catheter is generally appropriate for routine surgery in full-sized horses. Larger catheters (12-gauge or 10-gauge) or multiple catheters should be used when aggressive fluid therapy is anticipated or needed. A 16-gauge catheter is often appropriate in foals or miniature horses. Over-the-wire catheters are usually less suitable for perioperative fluid administration, because of greater impedance to flow due to their longer length, reduced lumen diameters (especially with multi-lumen catheters), and decreased rigidity, which predisposes them to lumen collapse (Ash, 2007). The short-term intravenous catheters most appropriate for perioperative fluid therapy can be replaced by extended-use catheters if fluid therapy is continued after surgery.

Higher flow rates are obtained with catheters placed in central veins compared to peripheral veins, because larger vessels have greater capacitance and less turbulence with fluid infusion (Hodge et al., 1986). Other patient factors affecting flow rates include intravascular pressure, vessel tortuosity, and venous valves (Hodge et al., 1986). The jugular vein is recommended for perioperative catheter placement in the horse. The jugular vein has the benefits of being easy to access for anesthesia and a large-diameter vessel in close proximity to the central circulation. The jugular vein is usually not as sensitive to intraoperative positioning of the patient and is less likely to be disrupted during anesthetic recovery compared to alternative catheter sites. If the jugular vein is not accessible or patent for perioperative catheter placement, other vessels that can be used include the lateral thoracic vein, cephalic vein, or saphenous vein, in decreasing order of preference.

Perioperative fluid administration

Replacement balanced electrolyte crystalloid fluids are most appropriate for use during anesthesia because they are isotonic and can quickly expand the intravascular space (Kudnig & Mama, 2002). Hypotonic fluids, such as 5% dextrose or half-strength dextrose-ionic solutions, are less appropriate for the typical perioperative patient, because they may cause hyponatremia and hypo-osmolality, especially with large-volume administration. Most balanced electrolyte solutions include a buffering agent, which is metabolized by the body to produce bicarbonate. A disadvantage of crystalloid fluids is that they rapidly equilibrate with the extravascular space, which means that the intravascular expansion is of short duration.

Lactated Ringer's solution and acetated polyionic fluids (Normosol™-R or Plasma-Lyte®-148) are commonly used for perioperative fluid therapy (Table 20.1). Normal saline may be used, but is a less appropriate choice in most cases because it induces a hyperchloremic acidosis. One argument against acetated polyionic fluids is that vasodilation has been described in a single anesthetized dog with rapid administration of acetate (Pascoe, 2012). A disadvantage of lactated Ringer's solution is that it is mildly hypotonic relative to plasma and therefore promotes interstitial fluid accumulation (Muir, 2009). Other fluids that may be useful in the management of compromised patients include hypertonic saline and colloidal solutions. These will be discussed in more detail later in this chapter.

Perioperative fluid infusion rates are adapted to the horse's clinical condition, length of anesthesia, surgical type, and intraoperative fluid losses (Hardy, 2009).

A fluid administration rate of 10–15 mL/kg/h has been recommended for anesthesia for major surgery (Campbell et al., 1990). These fluid rates support cardiac output (Aida et al., 1996; Taylor, 1998), renal blood flow (Watson et al., 2002), and muscle perfusion (Duke et al., 2006; Raisis, 2005; Stopyra et al., 2010). Hypovolemic or dehydrated patients require replacement of the deficit in addition to meeting recommended administration rates. These infusion rates can result in interstitial fluid accumulation and edema, which may be countered by colloid support if vessel integrity to colloids is intact (Pantaleon et al., 2006).

Perioperative fluid monitoring

Many of the physical examination findings used to assess fluid balance and response to fluid therapy (see Chapter 10) are masked or blunted by general anesthesia. Therefore, other measures are needed to monitor fluid therapy in the perioperative patient and determine its fluid and electrolyte needs.

The primary goal of fluid therapy is to support cardiac output, thereby maintaining organ perfusion and oxygenation. Cardiac output is the ideal parameter to determine the adequacy of fluid therapy (Corley et al., 2003; Hallowell & Corley, 2005, 2006); however, this monitoring equipment is not routinely available for clinical use in most equine hospitals.

Arterial blood pressure is an important parameter for fluid therapy in the anesthetized horse, because arterial blood pressure is directly associated with cardiac output. Despite its value as a monitoring tool, adequate arterial blood pressure does not equate to adequacy of flow and organ perfusion. Systemic vascular resistance, which is increased in vasoconstricted states or manipulated through the use of vasopressors in the anesthetized patient, can maintain blood pressure in the presence of low cardiac output. Arterial blood pressure may be monitored directly using an arterial catheter and a pressure manometer or transducer, or indirectly using Doppler ultrasound or oscillometry and a tail cuff (see Chapter 10). Mean arterial blood pressure should be maintained above 70 mmHg in anesthetized horses, because mean arterial blood pressures below 60 mmHg are associated with anesthetic complications (Duke et al., 2006; Hubbell & Muir, 2009; Raisis, 2005).

Table 20.1 Compositions of commonly used intravenous fluid solutions and compatibility with other drugs that may be used in the perioperative period

Solution	Sodium (mEq/L)	Potassium (mEq/L)	Chloride (mEq/L)	Calcium (mEq/L)	Magnesium (mEq/L)	Buffer (mEq/L)	Osmolality (mOsm/L)	Colloid osmotic pressure (mmHg)	Comments
Lactated Ringer's solution (LRS)	130	4	109	3	–	Lactate: 28	273	0	Contains calcium. Do not administer with blood products or sodium bicarbonate
Acetated polyionic solution	140	5	98	–	3	Acetate: 27 Gluconate: 23	294	0	If no calcium added, may be used with blood products and sodium bicarbonate
0.9% saline	154	–	154	–	–	–	308	0	Compatible with most solutions; may precipitate with mannitol
5% dextrose	–	–	–	–	–	–	252	(<1)	Alkaline solutions may precipitate
1.3% sodium bicarbonate	155	–	–	–	–	Bicarbonate: 155	310	0	Incompatible with catecholamines. Forms calcium carbonate with calcium solutions
7.2% hypertonic saline	1232	–	1232	–	–	–	2464	0	Compatible with most solutions; may precipitate mannitol
Hetastarch in 0.9% NaCl	154	–	154	–	–	–	309	33	Incompatible with some antibiotics (amikacin, tobramycin, selected cephalosporins)
Hextend in LRS	143	3	124	5	0.45	Lactate: 28	307	31	See comment for hetastarch
Blood, plasma	Varies	Varies	Varies	Varies	Varies	Varies	275–312	20–22	Do not administer with calcium

Adapted from Kudnig and Mama (2002), Hardy (2009), Pantaleon (2010), and Pascoe (2012).

Blood volume may be estimated by central venous pressure (CVP). CVP measures right atrial pressure, which relates to preload of the heart. Although CVP is an indicator of blood volume, it can be affected by heart rate, myocardial function, venous tone, intrathoracic pressure, and patient positioning (Hubbell & Muir, 2009). Jugular venous pressure can be used to approximate CVP in laterally recumbent clinical patients (Tam et al., 2011). CVP is not routinely used in most anesthetized patients, but has clinical utility in horses at risk for hypervolemia or hypovolemia.

Pulse pressure variation and systolic pressure variation may useful predictors of fluid responsiveness in mechanically ventilated, anesthetized patients (Fielding &

Stolba, 2012). Mechanical ventilation causes cyclical variation in intrathoracic pressure, which similarly alters preload. This causes cyclical changes in maximum and minimum systolic and pulse pressures over the course of the respiratory cycle. Large variations in maximum and minimum peak pressures indicate inadequate fluid replacement (Hubbell & Muir, 2009).

Assessment of blood composition can be helpful in determining fluid balance, tissue perfusion, and electrolyte and acid–base status. Changes in PCV and TP can reflect alterations to plasma volume in response to fluid therapy. PCV and TP are unreliable indicators in the presence of ongoing loss of blood components, such as hemorrhage or protein exudation, or splenic contraction. Colloid osmotic pressure (COP) is a measure of the oncotic pressure produced by plasma proteins and other colloid solutions. COP is used to monitor the propensity for interstitial fluid accumulation, either due to dilution or loss of colloids from the blood.

Lactate may reflect many physiologic or pathologic processes. Most commonly, lactate is used as an indicator of tissue perfusion and oxygenation. Increased lactate often is interpreted to indicate the presence of anaerobic metabolism. Lactate clearance (change in lactate over time) has been shown to be a prognostic indicator in critically ill foals and horses (Tennent-Brown et al., 2010; Wotman et al., 2009), and can be used in the perioperative period. Lactate increases during anesthesia for elective surgery and colic surgery (Boscan & Steffey, 2007; Boscan et al., 2007). Large increases in lactate during anesthesia may suggest inadequate tissue perfusion and oxygenation.

Acid–base and electrolyte balance should be assessed to determine if electrolytes require supplementation or if bicarbonate replacement is indicated. The acid–base disturbance that usually warrants treatment in perioperative patients is acidemia, and this may be respiratory or metabolic in origin. Metabolic acidemia with a pH less than 7.2 generally indicates a need for treatment with sodium bicarbonate (Hardy, 2009). Electrolyte disturbances most commonly seen during anesthesia include hypokalemia and hypocalcemia (Kudnig & Mama, 2002), and these have been discussed in more detail in earlier chapters. Other electrolyte disturbances that require specific attention in the perioperative patient will be reviewed later in this chapter.

Related to the discussion of electrolyte balance, the electrocardiogram (ECG) is used to monitor electrical activity of the heart. An abnormal ECG may reflect changes in electrolyte status. The nature of the ECG changes correlates with the type and magnitude of serum electrolyte change (Pascoe, 2012). An abnormal ECG should prompt assessment of serum electrolytes; however, a normal ECG does not guarantee normal cardiac function and normal electrolyte status.

Selected perioperative considerations

Colic

Horses with acute abdominal disease are often hemodynamically compromised due to hypovolemia, endotoxemia, and shock. The benefits of preoperative fluid loading in healthy horses have been demonstrated (Dyson & Pascoe, 1990). Preoperative stabilization of colicky horses can be limited by the need for rapid correction of the underlying lesion and the difficulty in safely managing a large, painful patient. Horses undergoing colic surgery are often hypotensive and require fluid resuscitation. Small-volume fluid resuscitation with hypertonic saline and synthetic colloids prior to or during anesthesia can rapidly improve or support the hemodynamic state.

Hypertonic (7.2–7.5%) saline increases plasma volume by three times the infused volume by mobilizing fluid from the interstitium into the intravascular space (Pantaleon, 2010; Schmall et al., 1990). Other hemodynamic benefits include increased cardiac contractility, greater cardiac output, and improved microcirculation (Gasthuys, 1994; Pantaleon, 2010; Schmall et al., 1990). Recommended dosage for hypertonic saline is 3–6 mL/kg administered at a maximum rate of 1 mL/kg/min to avoid hypotension associated with rapid hypertonic saline infusion (Pantaleon et al., 2006). A disadvantage of hypertonic saline is its relatively short-lived effect, which peaks at 20 minutes and decreases thereafter due to redistribution into the interstitial space (Hardy, 2009; Schmall et al., 1990). In a clinical study, hypertonic saline administered prior to anesthesia in horses with surgical colic did not improve the cardiac index compared to colloid administration (Hallowell & Corley, 2006). Hypertonic saline does cause sodium and chloride concentrations to increase, but these are usually tolerated by most patients as fluid resuscitation with isotonic crystalloid fluids continues. Contraindications to hypertonic saline use include pre-existing hypernatremia, severe dehydration, and anuria or oliguria.

Synthetic colloids may be used for plasma volume expansion by increasing plasma oncotic pressure. The duration of the colloid effect depends on the type of colloid administered and the disease state of the patient. If administered alone, synthetic colloids will cause fluid to redistribute from the interstitial space into the vascular space. If administered with crystalloid fluids, colloids will prolong the retention of crystalloid fluid within the vascular space. The degree of vascular expansion associated with colloid administration depends on the colloid osmotic pressure of the specific colloid (Muir, 2009). Typically, plasma volume will expand by 70–100% of the administered colloid volume (Hardy, 2009; Pantaleon, 2010). In a clinical study evaluating preoperative administration of pentastarch in horses undergoing colic surgery, pentastarch was associated with a higher cardiac index for 2.5 hours of anesthesia (Hallowell & Corley, 2006). Disadvantages of colloids include their expense and the coagulopathies associated with higher dosages. Maximum dosages of 10 mL/kg/day for hydroxylethyl starches have been advised in horses (Pantaleon, 2010).

The combined use of colloids and hypertonic saline is more effective than the use of either solution alone (Moon et al., 1991; Pantaleon, 2010; Pantaleon et al., 2006). The rapid volume expansion associated with hypertonic saline is preserved with the administration of the colloid. Highly concentrated hypertonic saline-colloid volume expanders (e.g., 25% saline + 24% dextran 70) should be avoided, because hemolysis and cardiac arrhythmias have been observed with their administration (Moon et al., 1991). The use of 5 mL/kg 7.2% hypertonic saline followed by 5–10 mL/kg of 6% hetastarch has been suggested for small-volume resuscitation in horses (Pantaleon, 2010; Pantaleon et al., 2006, 2007). This strategy could be used preoperatively to rapidly fluid resuscitate patients prior to emergency surgery or it could be used intraoperatively to treat fluid deficits. Small-volume fluid resuscitation has the advantage of supporting hemodynamic status with less risk of causing volume overload (see Figure 20.1) (Pantaleon 2010; Pantaleon et al., 2006).

Hemorrhage

Significant blood loss is best managed by whole blood transfusion to restore oxygen-carrying capacity and plasma volume. Hemoglobin-based oxygen-carrying fluids were previously marketed to improve the oxygen-carrying capacity of the blood and provide colloidal

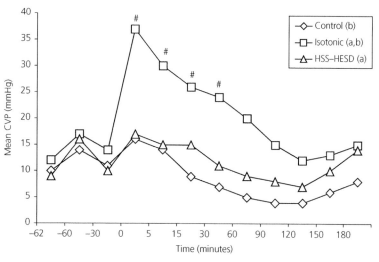

Figure 20.1 Mean central venous pressure (CVP (mmHg)) before (−62 min), during (−60 min), and after (−30 min) lipopolysaccharide infusion; followed by 15 mL/kg isotonic (Control, diamonds), 60 mL/kg isotonic (Isotonic, squares), or 15 mL/kg 7.2% hypertonic saline and 5 mL/kg hetastarch (HSS-HES, triangles) infusion (−30–0 min). Groups with the same letter were significantly different at $P < 0.05$. # indicates significant difference ($P < 0.05$) from baseline Isotonic. From Pantaleon LG et al. Cardiovascular and pulmonary effects of Hetastarch plus hypertonic saline solutions during experimental endotoxemia in anesthetized horses. *J Vet Intern Med* 2006; 20:1422–1428. ©Copyright 2006. American College of Veterinary Internal Medicine – reproduced with permission.

support; however, these products were expensive for use in large animals and are no longer available in the United States. If hemorrhage is anticipated prior to elective surgery, a donor horse can be identified and readied, or preoperative autologous blood collection can be arranged. If unexpected hemorrhage occurs during surgery, initial resuscitation occurs with crystalloids at a rate of 3 mL isotonic crystalloid per milliliter of blood loss (Muir, 2009; Wagner, 2009). Hypertonic saline effectively improves cardiac output in hemorrhagic shock (Schmall et al., 1990); however, it should be used with caution in uncontrolled hemorrhage, because bleeding may increase (Pantaleon, 2010; Trim et al., 1997). Cardiovascular status may be challenging to monitor in the anesthetized, hemorrhaging patient, because hematocrit and heart rate may not change and blood pressure may be artificially supported by ongoing inotrope or vasopressor administration (Trim et al., 1997; Wilson et al., 2003). Due to the conflicting information arising from anesthetic monitoring parameters, it is advisable to gauge intraoperative blood loss by collecting and quantifying hemorrhagic losses in buckets, suction containers, or laparotomy sponges (Wagner, 2009).

Neonates

Fluid therapy in neonatal foals is discussed in Chapter 22. Factors relevant for perioperative fluid therapy are the recognition that the neonatal heart is less compliant and has limited stroke volume reserve compared to adult horses (Klein, 1985; Quandt, 1995). This means that the foal is less tolerant of fluid loading and fluid deficits. The extracellular fluid compartment is larger and capillary permeability is greater in foals than in adults (Driessen, 2012). As a result, foals are more susceptible and sensitive to interstitial fluid accumulation. Fluid infusion rates of 7.5–10 mL/kg/h have been advocated to maintain circulatory volume in healthy, anesthetized foals (Driessen, 2012). Furthermore, neonatal foals have limited glycogen reserves (Driessen, 2012; Quandt, 1996). Glucose levels should be monitored and glucose supplementation initiated as needed to maintain normoglycemia.

Pregnancy

Pregnancy imparts a significant physiologic burden on the dam, which is further exaggerated during anesthesia. Furthermore, anesthesia of the pregnant patient must address the well-being of both dam and fetus.

Physiologic changes associated with pregnancy include expansion of the blood volume. The plasma volume increases to a greater degree than the red cell mass and total protein amount, resulting in relative hemodilution of red cells and total protein (Donaldson, 2006; Taylor, 1997). Cardiac output increases, in part due to a higher heart rate and larger stroke volume (Donaldson, 2006). The extravascular compartment increases and may predispose to edema formation (Taylor, 1997).

The pregnant animal has less cardiovascular reserve to adapt to hypovolemia or hypotension (Taylor, 1997). Hypotension is of particular significance to the pregnancy, because the uterine blood flow is not autoregulated and is directly affected by perfusion pressure (Taylor, 1997). Hypotension in the anesthetized pregnant mare is strongly associated with risk of abortion (Chenier & Whitehead, 2009). Volume support is an important component of the anesthetic management of the pregnant mare, and close attention must be paid to dilutional effects of fluid loading on oxygen-carrying capacity and colloid osmotic pressure (Donaldson, 2006).

Hyperkalemic periodic paralysis (HyPP)

Hyperkalemic periodic paralysis is a channelopathy caused by an autosomal dominant genetic defect in the sodium channel of certain lineages of quarter horses (Aleman, 2008). While the primary effect is on sodium permeability, the clinically relevant consequence is the efflux of potassium out of the cell, leading to hyperkalemia and muscular depolarization signs of HyPP. Anesthesia can potentiate an episode of HyPP.

The mainstay of preventing HyPP episodes in HyPP patients is to reduce the potassium burden through dietary management and potassium-wasting diuretics (Waldridge et al., 1996). Perioperative management also focuses on preventing and countering hyperkalemia. Potassium-free fluids should be used to dilute and minimize hyperkalemia (Waldridge et al., 1996). Close monitoring of the ECG and electrolyte status is necessary to identify early changes that may precipitate an episode (Bailey et al., 1996; Pang et al., 2011). If hyperkalemia develops or an episode is observed, there are multiple strategies to address the problems. Calcium gluconate (23%) may be administered slowly at a dosage of 50–100 mg/kg over 10–20 minutes intravenously (Bailey et al., 1996; Waldridge et al., 1996). While calcium does not improve the hyperkalemia, it is cardioprotective and antiarrhythmic by raising the threshold potential for generating an action potential (Bailey et al., 1996; Pang et al., 2011; Waldridge et al., 1996). Hyperkalemia may be reduced by glucose and insulin infusions. Glucose acts through endogenous stimulation of insulin release. Insulin acts by driving glucose and potassium intracellularly and by activating Na^+/K^+-ATPase pumps, which also causes potassium to move into the cells (Pang et al., 2011; Waldridge et al., 1996). Sodium bicarbonate has been advocated as a treatment, but it appears to have minimal effect on hyperkalemia, especially without concurrent acidemia (Pang et al., 2011).

Uroperitoneum

Uroperitoneum is the most frequent reason to have severe electrolyte derangements in an equine patient requiring surgery. Uroperitoneum is typically observed in neonatal foals, which further complicates the perioperative management. The blood volume deficits and the electrolyte derangements must be addressed prior to anesthesia (Doherty & Valverde, 2006; Quandt, 1996). Hyperkalemia, hyponatremia, hypochloremia, and acidemia develop during uroperitoneum due to the inability to eliminate urine from the body and the equilibration of urine electrolytes and blood electrolytes across the peritoneum (Quandt, 1996). The vasodilatory and cardiotoxic effects of anesthetic drugs are potentiated by hyperkalemia (Hardy, 2009). Hyponatremia can contribute to the obtundation and muscle weakness (Doherty & Valverde, 2006).

Low-potassium or potassium-free fluids are administered to restore the circulating blood volume and reduce the hyperkalemia. Depending on the concurrent electrolyte derangements and acid–base status, this may include isotonic saline, isotonic bicarbonate, balanced electrolyte fluids, or combinations of these fluids. Although the balanced electrolyte fluids (lactated Ringer's solution or acetated polyionic fluids) contain potassium, they are usually of low concentration and may not exacerbate the hyperkalemia, especially if other hyperkalemia management strategies are used (Doherty & Valverde, 2006). The sodium and chloride deficit is typically corrected by the same fluid management that addresses the hyperkalemia. Hypertonic saline has been suggested to support the vascular space and increase sodium levels (Doherty & Valverde, 2006); however, this is not universally advocated due to the rapidity of the fluctuations and the concurrent dehydration in these patients. An important part of the management is to reduce the potassium burden

by draining the abdomen of urine. This should be done slowly and concurrently with intravenous fluid support to minimize the circulatory effects of relieving severe abdominal distention (Quandt, 1996). Other treatments to lower serum potassium levels are dextrose infusions and insulin administration, as mentioned for HyPP. The arrhythmogenic effects of hyperkalemia can be countered with calcium administration to raise threshold potential and by normalizing serum sodium levels (Doherty & Valverde, 2006). A target prior to anesthesia is a potassium level below 6 mEq/L or a significant decrease in potassium levels from presentation (Doherty & Valverde, 2006).

Consequences of perioperative fluid balance

Perioperative fluid administration is important to maintain physiologic functions and replace fluid losses during surgery. The goal is to maintain effective circulating volume while avoiding fluid overload (Lobo et al., 2006). This is easier to achieve in patients with normal electrolyte and fluid balance and with more readily estimated surgical fluid losses. Emergency surgical patients are more likely to have derangements that require aggressive fluid resuscitation to maintain circulating volume and therefore some interstitial fluid overload may be inevitable (Lobo et al., 2006). The goal of maintaining euvolemia and avoiding fluid overload is further complicated in equine anesthesia patients, because of the propensity for developing hypotension with anesthesia and the life-threatening consequences of inadequate perfusion.

Although the importance of the 10 mL/kg/h intraoperative fluid administration rate has been discussed, this rate appears to result in some degree of overhydration and fluid overload. This is supported by studies showing reduced colloid osmotic pressures in elective and colic surgery patients (Boscan & Steffey, 2007; Boscan et al., 2007; Wendt-Hornickle et al., 2011). Experimental studies in endotoxemic anesthetized horses showed edema formation in horses receiving large-volume crystalloid therapy. Other findings associated with large-volume fluid administration include hyperchloremia (Boscan & Steffey, 2007), pulmonary hypertension (Pantaleon et al., 2006), and pulmonary edema (Taylor, 1998).

The perioperative patient is especially susceptible to iatrogenic fluid accumulations from the high fluid infusion rates that are necessary to counter the physiologic challenges of equine anesthesia and any underlying systemic derangements. The patient's ability to tolerate fluid deficits or excesses is indirectly associated with the severity of disease (Hilton et al., 2008). Fluid overload is significant to the surgical patient, because human medical literature has associated fluid overload with increased morbidity, altered pulmonary function, pulmonary edema, postoperative ileus, and impaired wound healing (Figures 20.2 and 20.3) (Brandstrup, 2006, Lobo et al., 2006). Dilutional coagulopathies have been observed in

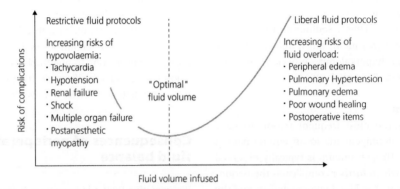

Figure 20.2 Hypothetical curve of the risk of fluid therapy-related complications versus volume of fluid infused. Risk is associated with both persistent hypovolemia and fluid overload, although the actual and relative risks of these two extremes are difficult to quantify in individual patients. Restrictive and liberal fluid protocols aim to minimize the risks of fluid overload and hypovolemia, respectively. However, by not accounting for individual patient differences, these protocols may produce their own complications. From Hilton AK et al. Avoiding common problems associated with intravenous fluid therapy. MJA 2008; 189(9):509–513. ©Copyright 2008. *The Medical Journal of Australia* – reproduced and modified with permission.

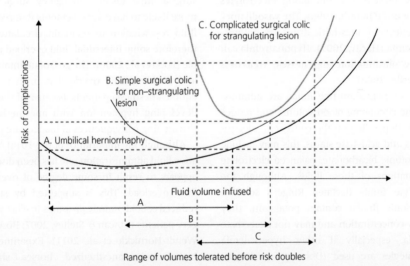

Figure 20.3 Hypothetical risk versus volume replacement curves for an individual patient in different clinical scenarios. Curve A: Low-risk clinical context, such as elective umbilical herniorrhaphy, where optimal fluid requirements are minimal, and the patient can tolerate significant variations in volume replacement. Curve B: The same patient in a slightly higher-risk context, such as simple colic surgery for a non-strangulating lesion. The volume for optimal fluid replacement is higher than in Scenario A, and the tolerance for error slightly lower, given the larger volume of fluid replacement and pathophysiologic changes associated with the underlying condition. Curve C: The same patient in a high-risk clinical context, such as complicated colic surgery for a strangulating lesion. Fluid requirements are expected to be high, and the patient is less likely to tolerate significant deviations from this amount. From Hilton AK et al. Avoiding common problems associated with intravenous fluid therapy. MJA 2008; 189(9):509–513. ©Copyright 2008. *The Medical Journal of Australia* – reproduced and modified with permission.

people, especially with large-volume crystalloid administration associated with surgical bleeding (Innerhofer & Keinast, 2010).

Another potential complication of perioperative fluid overload may be the effect on pharmacokinetics of drugs that are distributed within the extracellular fluid compartment. Expansion of this compartment could cause dilution of drugs administered using dosage recommendations from euvolemic animals. Intravenous fluid administration or peritoneal lavage was not found to have a significant effect on gentamicin pharmacokinetics (Easter et al., 1997; Jones et al., 1998; van der Harst et al., 2005); however, the power to detect differences was limited in these studies and extracellular compartment expansion was not confirmed.

Postoperative fluid considerations

Postoperative fluid considerations will depend on the clinical condition of the patient and the patient's ability to maintain their own fluid homeostasis. Other considerations are the need to correct any electrolyte or acid–base derangements resulting from the preoperative condition, surgery, or postoperative status. Fluid deficits or excesses must be addressed accordingly. In some patients, fluid therapy may be needed to facilitate continuous infusion of medications or counter the side effects of certain treatments. Postoperative fluid therapy will often have similar considerations to the preoperative and operative fluid therapy decisions; however, the progression, and hopefully the resolution, of the patient's clinical problem will necessitate adjustments to the perioperative fluid management.

References

Aida H, Mizuno Y, Hobo S, Yoshida K, Fujinaga T. (1996) Cardiovascular and pulmonary effects of sevoflurane anesthesia in horses. *Vet Surg* **25**:164–70.

Aleman M. (2008) A review of equine muscle disorders. *Neuromusc Disord* **18**:277–87.

Ash SR. (2007) Fluid mechanics and clinical success of central venous catheters for dialysis – answers to simple but persisting problems. *Semin Dialysis* **20**:237–56.

Bailey JE, Pablo L, Hubbell JAE. (1996) Hyperkalemic periodic paralysis episode during halothane anesthesia in a horse. *J Am Vet Med Assoc* **208**:1859–65.

Boscan P, Steffey EP. (2007) Plasma colloid osmotic pressure and total protein in horses during colic surgery. *Vet Anaesth Analg* **34**:408–15.

Boscan P, Watson, Z, Steffey EP. (2007) Plasma colloid osmotic pressure and total protein trends in horses during anesthesia. *Vet Anaesth Analg* **34**:275–83.

Brandstrup B. (2006) Fluid therapy for the surgical patient. *Best Pract Res Clin Anaesthesiol* **20**:265–83.

Campbell IT, Baxter JN, Tweedie IE, Taylor GT, Keens SJ. (1990) I.V. fluids during surgery. *Br J Anaesth* **65**: 726–9.

Chenier TS, Whitehead AE. (2009) Foaling rates and risk factors for abortion in pregnant mares presented for medical or surgical treatment of colic: 153 cases (1993–2005). *Can Vet J* **50**:481–5.

Corley KTT, Donaldson LL, Durando MM, Birks EK. (2003) Cardiac output technologies with special reference to the horses. *J Vet Int Med* **17**:262–72.

Doherty T, Valverde A. (2006) Anesthesia of foals. In: Doherty T, Valverde A (eds) *Manual of Equine Anesthesia and Analgesia*. Ames: Blackwell Publishing, pp. 219–28.

Donaldson L. (2006) Anesthesia and pregnancy. In: Doherty T, Valverde A (eds) *Manual of Equine Anesthesia and Analgesia*. Ames: Blackwell Publishing, pp. 244–52.

Driessen B. (2012) Anesthesia and analgesia in foals. In: Auer JA, Stick JA (eds) *Equine Surgery*, 4th edn. St Louis: Saunders Elsevier, pp. 229–46.

Duke T, Filzek U, Read MR, Read EK, Ferguson JG. (2006) Clinical observations surrounding an increased incidence of postanesthetic myopathy in halothane-anesthetized horses. *Vet Anaesth Analg* **33**:122–7.

Dutky PA, Stevens SL, Maull KI. (1989) Factors affecting rapid fluid resuscitation with large-bore introducer catheters. *J Trauma* **29**:856–60.

Dyson DH, Pascoe PJ. (1990) Influence of preinduction methoxamine, lactated Ringer solution, or hypertonic saline solution infusion or postinduction dobutamine infusion on anesthetic-induced hypotension in horses. *Am J Vet Res* **51**:17–21.

Easter JL, Hague BA, Brumbaugh GW, et al. (1997) Effects of postoperative peritoneal lavage on pharmacokinetics of gentamicin in horses after celiotomy. *Am J Vet Res* **58**:1166–70.

Fielding CL, Stolba DN. (2012) Pulse pressure variation and systolic pressure variation in horses undergoing general anesthesia. *J Vet Emerg Crit Care* **22**:372–5.

Gasthuys F. (1994) The value of 7.2% hypertonic saline solution in anaesthesia and intensive care: myth or fact? *J Vet Anaesth* **21**:12–14.

Hallowell GD, Corley KTT. (2005) Use of lithium dilution and pulse contour analysis cardiac output determination in anaesthetized horses: a clinical evaluation. *Vet Anaesth Analg* **32**:201–11.

Hallowell GD, Corley KTT. (2006) Preoperative administration of hydroxyethyl starch or hypertonic saline to horses with colic. *J Vet Int Med* **20**:980–6.

Hardy J. (2009) Venous and arterial catheterization and fluid therapy. In: Muir WW, Hubbell JAE (eds) *Equine Anesthesia*

Monitoring and Emergency Therapy, 2nd edn. St Louis: Saunders Elsevier, pp. 131–48.

Hilton AK, Pellegrino VA, Scheinkestel CD. (2008) Avoiding common problems associated with intravenous fluid therapy. *Med J Aust* **189**:509–13.

Hodge D, Delgado-Paredes C, Fleisher G. (1986) Central and peripheral catheter flow rates in "pediatric" dogs. *Ann Emerg Med* **15**:1151–4.

Hubbell JAE, Muir WW. (2009) Monitoring anesthesia. In: Muir WW, Hubbell JAE (eds) *Equine Anesthesia Monitoring and Emergency Therapy*, 2nd edn. St Louis: Saunders Elsevier, pp. 149–170.

Innerhofer P, Keinast J. (2010) Principles of perioperative coagulopathy. *Best Pract Res Clin Anaesthesiol* **24**:1–14.

Jones SL, Wilson WD, Milhalyi JE. (1998) Pharmacokinetics of gentamicin in healthy adult horses during intravenous fluid administration. *J Vet Pharmacol Ther* **21**:247–9.

Klein L. (1985) Anesthesia for neonatal foals. *Vet Clin N Am Equine Pract* **1**:77–89.

Kudnig ST, Mama K. (2002) Perioperative fluid therapy. *J Am Vet Med Assoc* **221**:1112–21.

Lobo DN, Macafee DA, Allison SP. (2006) How perioperative fluid balance influences postoperative outcomes. *Best Pract Res Clin Anaesthesiol* **20**:439–55.

McPherson D, Adekanye O, Wilkes AR, Hall JE. (2009) Fluid flow through intravenous cannulae in a clinical model. *Anesthes Analg* **108**:1198–02.

Moon PF, Snyder JR, Haskins SC, Perron PR, Kramer GC. (1991) Effects of a highly concentrated hypertonic saline-dextran volume expander on cardiopulmonary function in anesthetized normovolemic horses. *Am J Vet Res* **52**:1611–18.

Muir W. (2009) Fluid choice for resuscitation and perioperative administration. *Compend Contin Educ Vet* **31**:E1–E10.

Pang DSJ, Panizzi L, Paterson JM. (2011) Successful treatment of hyperkalemic periodic paralysis in a horse during isoflurane anaesthesia. *Vet Anaesth Analg* **38**:113–20.

Pantaleon LG. (2010) Fluid therapy in equine patients: small-volume fluid resuscitation. *Compend Contin Educ Vet* **32**:E1–E7.

Pantaleon LG, Furr MO, McKenzie II HC, Donaldson L. (2006) Cardiovascular and pulmonary effects of hetastarch plus hypertonic saline solutions during experimental endotoxemia in anesthetized horses. *J Vet Int Med* **20**:1422–8.

Pantaleon LG, Furr MO, McKenzie II HC, Donaldson L. (2007) Effects of small- and large-volume resuscitation on coagulation and electrolytes during experimental endotoxemia in anesthetized horses. *J Vet Int Med* **21**:1374–9.

Pascoe PJ. (2012) Perioperative management of fluid therapy. In: Dibartola SP (ed.) *Fluid, Electrolyte and Acid-Base Disorders in Small Animal Practice*, 4th edn. St Louis: Saunders Elsevier, pp. 405–35.

Quandt JE. (1995) Considerations in sedating and anesthetizing foals. *Compend Contin Educ Vet* **17**:1413–16.

Quandt JE. (1996) Anesthetic techniques and considerations in foals. *Compend Contin Educ Vet* **18**:307–12.

Raisis A. (2005) Skeletal muscle blood flow in anaesthetized horses. Part II: effects of anaesthetics and vasoactive agents. *Vet Anaesth Analg* **32**:331–7.

Schmall LM, Muir WW, Robertson JT. (1990) Haemodynamic effects of small volume hypertonic saline in experimentally induced haemorrhagic shock. *Equine Vet J* **22**:273–7.

Steffey EP, Zinkl J, Howland D. (1979) Minimal changes in blood cell counts and biochemical values associated with prolonged isoflurane anesthesia of horses. *Am J Vet Res* **40**:1646–8.

Steffey EP, Giri SN, Dunlop CI, Cullen LK, Hodgson DS, Willits N. (1993) Biochemical and haematological changes following prolonged halothane anaesthesia in horses. *Res Vet Sci* **55**:338–45.

Stopyra A, Jaynski M, Sobiech P, Chyczewski M, Holak P, Lew M. (2010) The effect of isotonic multiple electrolyte infusions during anesthesia on blood gas and enzymatic values in horses. *Pol J Vet Sci* **13**:287–92.

Tam K, Rezende M, Boscan P. (2011) Correlation between jugular and central venous pressures in laterally recumbent horses. *Vet Anaesth Analg* **38**:580–3.

Taylor PM. (1997) Anaesthesia for pregnant animals. *Equine Vet J Suppl* **24**:1–6.

Taylor PM. (1998) Endocrine and metabolic responses to plasma volume expansion during halothane anaesthesia in ponies. *J Vet Pharmacol Ther* **21**:485–90.

Tennent-Brown BS, Wilkins PA, Lindborg S, Russell G, Boston RC. (2010) Sequential plasma lactate concentrations as prognostic indicators in adult equine emergencies. *J Vet Int Med* **24**:198–205.

Trim CM, Eaton SA, Parks AH. (1997) Severe nasal hemorrhage in an anesthetized horse. *J Am Vet Med Assoc* **210**:1324–7.

van der Harst MR, Bull S, Laffont CM, Klein WR. (2005) Influence of fluid therapy on gentamicin pharmacokinetics in colic horses. *Vet Res Commun* **29**:141–7.

Wagner AE. (2009) Complications in equine anesthesia. *Vet Clin N Am Equine Pract* **24**:735–52.

Waldridge BM, Lin H-C, Purohit RC. (1996) Anesthetic management of horses with hyperkalemic periodic paralysis. *Compend Contin Educ Vet* **18**:1030–8.

Watson ZE, Steffey EP, VanHoogmoed LM, Snyder JR. (2002) Effect of general anesthesia and minor surgical trauma on urine and serum measurements in horses. *Am J Vet Res* **63**:1061–5.

Wendt-Hornickle EI, Snyder LBC, Tang R, Johnson RA. (2011) The effects of lactated Ringer's solution (LRS) or LRS and 6% hetastarch on the colloid osmotic pressure, total protein and osmolality in healthy horses under general anesthesia. *Vet Anaesth Analg* **38**: 336–41.

Wilson DV, Rondenay Y, Shance PU. (2003) The cardiopulmonary effects of severe blood loss in anesthetized horses. *Vet Anaesth Analg* **30**:80–6.

Wotman K, Wilkins PA, Palmer JE, Boston RC. (2009) Association of blood lactate concentration and outcome in foals. *J Vet Int Med* **23**:598–605.

CHAPTER 21

Enteral fluid therapy

Marco A.F. Lopes

Department of Veterinary Medicine and Surgery, College of Veterinary Medicine, University of Missouri, USA

Enteral fluid therapy (EFT) is the administration of fluids into the gastrointestinal (GI) tract using a tube to bypass the mouth. Oral fluid therapy, the natural route for fluid uptake, is commonly used in human medicine (Al-Benna, 2011; Atia & Buchman, 2009, 2010; Hartling et al., 2006; Kenefick et al., 2006; Rouhani et al., 2011) but not in sick horses. The lack of patient cooperation limits use of oral fluid therapy in horses. Clinically ill horses commonly reduce their fluid intake and it is usually impossible to stimulate drinking of sufficient amounts to restore and/or maintain hydration status and electrolyte balance.

Forced oral administration of fluids in horses is not practical, is stressful for the horse, and is likely to result in fluid aspiration. The most practical route for EFT in horses is through a nasoesophageal or nasogastric tube. Alternative routes for EFT do exist, but cannot be used in the vast majority of cases. These include the following:

- Through an esophagostomy – this involves a surgical procedure that can lead to life-threatening complications (such as periesophageal infection and septic mediastinitis) and can only be justified if the esophagostomy will help to resolve an esophageal obstruction or will also be used as the route for nutrition (Lopes et al., 2001).
- Through a fistula in the large intestine – which is an invasive approach with potential for life-threatening complications (e.g., septic peritonitis), and has only been used experimentally in healthy horses (Ferreira et al., 2011; Mealey et al., 1995).
- Into the rectum (i.e., enema) – which can effectively hydrate the content of the rectum and small colon but has limited systemic effects, produces discomfort for

the horse, and can cause life-threatening injury to the rectum (Hjortkjaer, 1979).

The focus of this chapter is the most practical form of EFT – via a nasoesophageal or nasogastric tube.

Most relevant physiologic aspects relative to EFT

The gastrointestinal (GI) tract is the natural route for the uptake of water and electrolytes. It is capable of handling large volumes of fluids ingested or administered enterally and is an effective route for rehydration. The stomach functions as a reservoir that regulates the delivery of nutrients to the intestine in order to optimize digestion and absorption (Tack, 2006). In human athletes, gastric emptying can be a limitation for using the enteral route for rapid rehydration (Gisolfi, 2000; Murray 2006; Ryan et al., 1998). The effect of gastric emptying on EFT has not been extensively studied in the horse, but there is evidence that despite its relatively small capacity (8–20 L) (Pfeiffer & MacPherson, 1990) the equine stomach is very effective at handling large volumes of fluids. Average-sized horses deprived of food and water drank 66 mL/kg (about 32 L) during the first hour of free access to water (Carlson et al., 1979). Ponies subjected to water deprivation drank more than 50 mL/kg in the first 30 min of free access to water (Sufit et al., 1985). Horses treated with 8 L of fluids via nasogastric tube at rest and 2 min after submaximal exercise until exhaustion were able to empty 90% of their gastric fluid in 15 min (Sosa-León et al., 1997).

After ingestion or administration into the esophagus or stomach, fluids rapidly pass through the pylorus and

Equine Fluid Therapy, First Edition. Edited by C. Langdon Fielding and K. Gary Magdesian.
© 2015 John Wiley & Sons, Inc. Published 2015 by John Wiley & Sons, Inc.

move aborally to reach the large intestine (Alexander & Benzie, 1951; Argenzio et al., 1974) and change the composition of ingesta throughout the equine GI tract (Figure 21.1) (Avanza et al., 2009; Freeman et al., 1992; Lopes et al., 2004). Distention produced by fluids ingested or administered into the stomach can also activate the gastrocolic response and increase motility of the large intestine (Freeman et al., 1992) further contributing to speed GI transit. Water and electrolytes administered enterally can rapidly produce significant changes in plasma composition (Figure 21.2) (Avanza et al., 2009; Lopes et al., 2001, 2002, 2004).

The GI mucosa functions as a barrier separating intra-luminal content from the intravascular space. Mucosal permeability to water and electrolytes varies throughout the different segments of the GI tract (Barrett & Dharmsathaphorn, 1994; Johnson, 2007). Maximal permeability to water occurs in the duodenum, which functions as an equilibration chamber where there is little resistance to movement of water in either direction (from the lumen to the extracellular space or vice versa) depending on the osmotic gradient (Barrett & Dharmsathaphorn, 1994; Johnson, 2007). Water absorption is passive following the osmotic gradient generated by active absorption of water-soluble solutes such as electrolytes, carbohydrates, amino acids, and vitamins.

Specialized carriers or gates located in the membrane of the epithelial cells of the intestine have the function

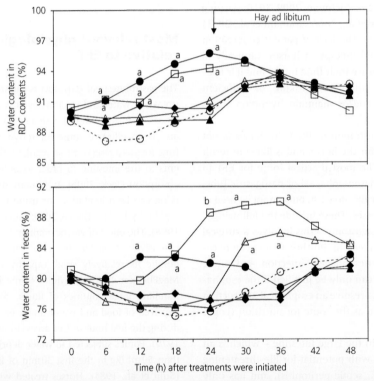

Figure 21.1 Mean water content in the right dorsal colon (RDC) contents and feces obtained during a 48-h observation period from six horses with fistulas in the RDC receiving six treatments in a crossover design: No treatment (control; open circles); IV fluid therapy with lactated Ringer's solution (5 L/h for 12 h; closed triangles); enteral administration of magnesium sulfate (1 g/kg in 1 L of water; open triangles); enteral administration of sodium sulfate (1 g/kg in 3 L of water; open squares); enteral administration of water (5 L/h for 12 h; closed diamonds); enteral administration via a nasogastric tube of an electrolyte solution (5 L/h for 12 h; closed circles) containing 135 mmol/L of Na^+, 5 mmol/L of K^+, 95 mmol/L of Cl^-, and 45 mmol/L of bicarbonate. Food was withheld for the initial 24 h and all treatments were started or administered at time 0. Within a time point, values with different letters were significantly ($P \le 0.05$) different from control values and between treatments. From Lopes MAF, White NA, Donaldson L, Crisman MV, Ward DL. Effects of enteral and intravenous fluid therapy, magnesium sulfate, and sodium sulfate on colonic contents and feces in horses. Am J Vet Res. 2004 May;65(5):695–704; with permission.

of promoting or facilitating absorption of solutes. The main route for water absorption is thought to be the intercellular spaces of the epithelium (Barrett & Dharmsathaphorn, 1994; Johnson, 2007). Absorption of fluid and electrolytes by the GI tract is not only affected by the volume and composition of ingesta (Lopes et al., 2002, 2004) but is also controlled by several mechanisms triggered by the body's physiologic status. For instance, absorption of sodium and water by the GI mucosa is enhanced when the animal is dehydrated and the renin-angiotensin-aldosterone system is

activated (Argenzio, 1990; Clarke et al., 1992; Garg et al., 2012; Johnson, 2007; Muñoz et al., 2010). Conversely, absorption of water by the GI mucosa is inhibited when the animal is overhydrated (Duffy et al., 1978). Horses use their GI tract as a large reservoir of water and electrolytes, which can be effectively retrieved whenever necessary (Danielsen et al., 1995; Kasirer-Izraely et al., 1994; Warren et al., 1999). Therefore, it is no surprise that, particularly in the horse, EFT is a very effective way to restore systemic hydration and electrolyte balance.

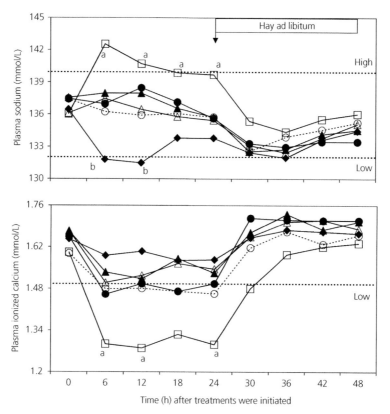

Figure 21.2 Mean concentrations of sodium and ionized calcium in plasma obtained during a 48 h observation period from six horses with fistulas in the right dorsal colon (RDC) receiving six treatments in a crossover design: No treatment (control; open circles); IV fluid therapy with lactated Ringer's solution (5 L/h for 12 h; closed triangles); enteral administration of magnesium sulfate (1 g/kg in 1 L of water; open triangles); enteral administration of sodium sulfate (1 g/kg in 3 L of water; open squares); enteral administration of water (5 L/h for 12 h; closed diamonds)); enteral administration via a nasogastric tube of an electrolyte solution (5 L/h for 12 h; closed circles) containing 135 mmol/L of Na^+, 5 mmol/L of K^+, 95 mmol/L of Cl^-, and 45 mmol/L of bicarbonate. Food was withheld for the initial 24 h and all treatments were started or administered at time 0. Dotted lines within the graphs indicate the laboratory normal ranges for the concentrations of sodium and chloride in plasma. Within a time point, values with different letters are significantly ($P \leq 0.05$) different from control values and between treatments. From Lopes MAF, White NA, Donaldson L, Crisman MV, Ward DL. Effects of enteral and intravenous fluid therapy, magnesium sulfate, and sodium sulfate on colonic contents and feces in horses. Am J Vet Res. 2004 May;65(5):695–704; with permission.

Indications for EFT

Treat and/or prevent dehydration and electrolyte and acid–base imbalances

Enteral fluid therapy is an effective treatment to restore and/or maintain hydration as well as electrolyte and acid–base balance. It has been shown that plasma electrolyte composition (Figure 21.2) and acid–base balance can be effectively changed by EFT (Lopes et al., 2001, 2004; Waller & Lindinger, 2007). In extreme cases, when immediate expansion of plasma volume and/or immediate changes in plasma composition are indicated, it is best to bypass the GI tract since EFT cannot produce the immediate changes achieved with IV fluid therapy (Kenefick et al., 2006). However, even in these extreme situations, EFT may still be used simultaneously with IV fluid therapy or after part of the water and electrolyte deficits have been replaced with IV fluids.

Enteral fluid therapy may also be used in horses that do not have obvious signs of dehydration or electrolyte imbalance yet have reduced intake of food and water or have increased fluid losses. Two of the most common causes of increased losses of water and electrolytes are exercise and diarrhea. Oral administration of electrolytes to replenish electrolytes and stimulate water intake has been extensively used in exercising horses. Such treatments are known to contribute to the maintenance and restoration of hydration status and electrolyte balance and to contribute to a speedier recovery and better performance (Geor & McCutcheon, 1998; Hyyppä et al., 1996, Marlin et al., 1998; Monreal et al., 1999; Rose et al., 1986, Sosa León et al., 1995, Waller et al., 2009).

Enteral fluid therapy can also be used to restore/maintain hydroelectrolytic and acid–base balance in horses with diarrhea. In severe cases EFT may not be sufficient and IV fluid therapy is indicated (McKenzie, 2008). Theoretically mucosal damage associated with diarrhea can be severe enough to compromise absorption of solutes and water and limit the systemic effects of EFT. However, the surface area of the intestinal epithelium is so large that EFT may still be at least partially effective. In humans EFT is recommended not only for cholera and other forms of secretory diarrhea, but also for diarrhea caused by microorganisms that produce mucosal damage such as *Salmonella*, *Shigella*, and rotavirus (Atia & Buchman,

2009, 2010; Guarino et al., 2012; Varavithya et al., 1991). This issue has not been investigated in horses, but even if diarrhea is associated with extensive damage of the intestinal mucosa, EFT may still help to partially restore and maintain hydroelectrolytic balance and minimize the volume of fluids required intravenously. EFT may increase the volume and/or make feces more watery in horses with diarrhea, which should not be considered signs of worsening of the GI disease if the horse is simultaneously showing signs of clinical improvement.

Promote diuresis

In horses with conditions such as aminoglycoside nephrotoxicity and exertional rhabdomyolysis, over-hydration is thought to be beneficial since it will increase glomerular filtration, which minimizes kidney damage. Traditionally IV fluid therapy has been used for these conditions but EFT is also effective to promote diuresis (Avanza et al., 2009; Lopes et al., 2001, 2002, 2003, 2004).

Promote hydration of the GI content and catharsis

Enteral fluid therapy has been shown to produce a marked increase in hydration of ingesta and feces (Figure 21.1) (Lester et al., 2013; Lopes et al., 2001, 2002, 2004). EFT has been successfully used to treat impactions of the stomach, cecum, and colon (Hallowell, 2008; Lopes et al., 1999, 2003; Monreal et al., 2010; Vainio et al., 2011). EFT can also be used to soften feces and facilitate defecation after surgical treatment of rectal prolapse (Lopes et al., 2003) and perineal laceration.

Fill the GI tract with fluid and facilitate ultrasonographic evaluation

Studies of transcutaneous ultrasonography in horses have shown that GI filling produced by EFT can facilitate the evaluation of the small intestine (Lopes et al., 2009; Norman et al., 2010).

Only the first three of the above indications are also valid for IV fluid therapy. Controlled studies have shown that IV fluid therapy, even if combined with a full dose of $MgSO_4$ (1 g/kg) given enterally, is not as effective as an isotonic electrolyte solution given enterally for increasing the water content of ingesta or feces (Lopes et al., 2002). In addition to being less expensive than IV fluid therapy (Hallowell, 2008; Lopes et al., 2003; Monreal et al., 2010), EFT has the unique ability to rapidly hydrate and soften the GI contents (e.g., in horses with gastric or large intestinal impaction, and in horses submitted for surgical procedures of the rectum). In horses with an experimental fistula of the large colon, the administration of an isotonic electrolyte solution (20 mL/kg/h for 6 h) was more effective in promoting hydration of the colonic content and feces than the combination of IV lactated Ringer's solution (20 mL/kg/h for 6 h) and enteral administration of the full dose of $MgSO_4$ (1 mg/kg) (Lopes et al., 2002). EFT has also been successfully used in horses with other clinical conditions such as gastric impaction (Banse et al., 2011; Lopes et al., 2003; Vainio et al., 2011), large colon displacements (Lindegaard et al., 2011; Monreal et al., 2010), acute kidney failure (Lopes et al., 2003), and postoperative treatment in horses submitted to colic surgery (Lopes et al., 2006). More experimental studies and clinical reports of the use of EFT are needed to better define the indications of this approach for fluid administration in horses.

Contraindications for EFT

The only absolute contraindication for EFT is complete intestinal obstruction or ileus. If this is the case, parenteral fluid therapy is the only option. Several other conditions may be considered relative contraindications for EFT (i.e., EFT should not be administered unless there is a very strong reason to do so such as financial constraints). Such conditions are considered below.

Inability to utilize a nasogastric tube

When a nasogastric tube cannot be passed (e.g., esophageal obstruction that cannot be resolved by flushing the esophagus), the only way to administer EFT is through an esophagostomy. This is an invasive procedure to create a route to the esophagus and can have serious complications (Lopes, 2001). An esophagostomy should only be performed as a last resort and when it will also serve other purposes (i.e., relieve an esophageal obstruction, enable nutritional support). If neither a nasoesophageal nor an esophagostomy tube can be passed (e.g., due to an obstruction in the thoracic esophagus), it is not possible to administer EFT. Creation of a cecal fistula for fluid administration has been used

experimentally but it is an invasive and risky approach (Ferreira et al., 2011; Mealey et al., 1995). An enema is not recommended since its effects would be limited to promoting hydration of the contents of the rectum and small colon (Hjortkjaer, 1979).

Recumbency

When horses are recumbent, there may be a higher risk of complications of EFT such as gastroesophageal reflux, fluid aspiration, and abdominal discomfort. Abdominal discomfort was observed in a normal horse experimentally treated with EFT while fasted for 12 h. The horse preferred to lay in lateral recumbency when muzzled (Lopes et al., 2004). In addition, abdominal distention produced by EFT (Figure 21.3) is more likely to compromise lung ventilation in a recumbent horse than in a standing horse. If EFT is used in a recumbent horse, support should be provided to maintain the horse in sternal recumbency (e.g., with hay bales).

Pre-existing abdominal distention

If pronounced abdominal distention is present due to conditions such as advanced pregnancy, additional abdominal distention produced by EFT may cause discomfort, compromise splanchnic perfusion, or compromise ventilation and should be used with caution. Pronounced pre-existing abdominal distention in a horse with colic suggests that the horse has a disease that typically is treated surgically (e.g., large colon displacement, small colon impaction with complete luminal obstruction). However, EFT has been successfully used to treat large colon displacements (Lindegaard et al., 2011; Monreal et al., 2010).

Intolerance of enteral fluid therapy

If the horse is intolerant to small volumes of fluids administered by the nasoesophageal tube (i.e., shows signs of abdominal discomfort during fluid administration and does not respond to analgesics), it is not possible to administer EFT. This was reported in a horse that was later found to have extensive gastric ulceration and a large enterolith wedged in the transverse colon (Lopes, 1999).

Decision to initiate EFT

Intravenous fluid therapy is by far the most common approach for fluid and electrolyte administration in horses. However, in many cases treated with IV fluids,

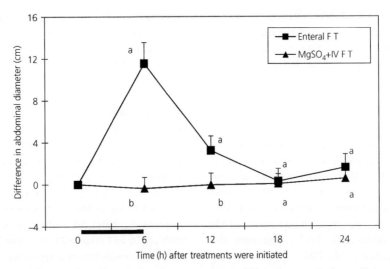

Figure 21.3 Means of the changes (difference from time 0) in abdominal circumference of four horses with fistulas in the right dorsal colon (RDC) receiving two treatments in a crossover design: an electrolyte solution containing 135 mmol/L of Na^+, 5 mmol/L of K^+, 95 mmol/L of Cl^-, and 45 mmol/L of bicarbonate (10 L/h for 6 h) administered via nasogastric tube; $MgSO_4$ (1 g/kg in 1 L of water) administered via nasogastric tube and IV fluid therapy with lactated Ringer's solution (10 L/h for 6 h). The horizontal bar below the graph indicates the period when the horses were receiving fluid therapy. Whiskers denote standard error. Within one time, means with different letters are significantly different at alpha = 0.05 according to the Bonferroni corrected multiple comparisons. From Lopes MA, Walker BL, White A, Ward DL. Treatments to promote colonic hydration: enteral fluid therapy versus intravenous fluid therapy and magnesium sulphate. *Equine Vet J.* 2002 Jul;34(5):505–9; with permission.

there is no definitive indication for bypassing the GI tract. This issue has been raised previously (Lopes et al., 2002, 2003; Schott, 1998) and practices appear to be changing. Recent publications reporting the use of EFT in horses demonstrate significant progress in this area, but equine veterinarians still are not using EFT as often as they could.

In human medicine, there is evidence that the indiscriminate use of parenteral fluid therapy is not beneficial (Hartling et al., 2006; Kenefick et al., 2006; Taniguchi et al., 2009). In horses, no well-designed studies of a large series of cases comparing IV and EFT have been published. There is no reason to believe that bypassing the GI tract is advantageous for horses with many clinical conditions routinely treated with IV fluids exclusively. Perhaps one of the most important reasons to avoid the unnecessary use of parenteral fluid therapy in horses whenever possible is cost: large volumes of fluids for IV administration, commonly needed in horses, are expensive compared to fluids for EFT. Although the labor associated with administration of EFT may not be very different than that required for the administration of IV fluids, sterile and commercially prepared fluids are

not required for EFT. The cost of medication is often a major limitation for treatment of sick horses and a major contributor to the decision to perform euthanasia. Even when the initial estimate of treatment cost is compatible with the budget established by the owner or insurance company, treatment expenses may unexpectedly rise due to complications and ultimately the horse may be euthanized due to financial constraints. Therefore, the use of the most expensive fluid therapy (i.e., IV fluid therapy) when not absolutely necessary can be a contributing factor for the decision to perform euthanasia in horses with reasonable chances of recovery if treatment is not interrupted due to financial constraints.

Enteral fluid therapy is often considered a last resort by many veterinarians (i.e., when IV fluid therapy is not economically viable or did not produce the expected effects). Some possible reasons for this approach include the following:

1 Traditionally veterinarians have been taught that IV fluid therapy is always the safest and most effective route for fluid therapy in horses.
2 Many veterinarians may not be familiar with EFT using a small-bore tube, which is a relatively new

approach that requires some learning (e.g., how to properly insert a small-bore nasoesophageal tube and secure it in place).

3 Due to the lack of experience with EFT, veterinarians may presume that placement of an IV catheter and administering IV fluids is much faster and easier to do than passing and securing a small bore nasoesophageal tube and administering EFT.

4 Veterinarians may fear complications of EFT, such as abdominal discomfort and rupture of the GI tract, which can be prevented by patient selection and judicious administration of EFT.

In human medicine, EFT is considered the standard of care for many clinical conditions. In athletes, ingestion of electrolyte solutions is known to be the best method to restore and/or maintain hydration except in cases of extreme dehydration (Kenefick et al., 2000, 2006). For the last few decades, fluid administration through the enteral route has also been the standard of care for most types of diarrhea (Atia & Buchman, 2009; Goodgame, 2001; Guarino et al., 2012; Hill & Beeching, 2010; WHO, 2005). The use of oral rehydration solutions for diarrhea is considered one of the most significant medical advances of the twentieth century because it has saved millions of lives (Guarino et al., 2012). In children with dehydration, oral fluid therapy is the first choice in terms of route of delivery; when oral rehydration is not possible, nasogastric and IV rehydration have similar outcomes even in cases with moderate to severe dehydration (Rouhani et al., 2011).

Intravenous fluid therapy is still considered the gold standard for fluid resuscitation (McSwain et al., 2011). However, there is growing evidence that oral and nasogastric fluid therapy are viable alternatives for resuscitation in humans with extensive burns and other severe wounds and hemorrhage when the ideal conditions for intensive care are not readily available (e.g., in war zones, after a disaster with many casualties). In these circumstances, EFT should be used at least as a complement to parenteral fluid therapy (Cancio et al., 2006; Kramer et al., 2010; Thomas et al., 2003). These recommendations are based on evidence gathered from clinical cases and experimental studies in laboratory animals (Cancio et al., 2006; Kramer et al., 2010; Michell et al., 2006; Thomas et al., 2003). Despite the relative scarcity of publications about EFT in horses, there is already substantial evidence that EFT is beneficial and can be safely used in horses (Lester et al., 2013; Lopes et al., 2002,

2004). Unless a definitive contraindication to EFT is identified, EFT should be considered as a less expensive option than IV fluid therapy for many types of cases. It is also a more effective route of fluid therapy for some clinical disorders, especially impactions of the large intestine, where it can be considered more effective than IV fluid therapy (Lester et al., 2013; Lopes et al., 2002, 2004).

Instituting EFT

Patient assessment before and during EFT (e.g., for planning and adjusting EFT)

The same principles recommended for assessing the horse's condition before and during IV fluid therapy are valid for EFT. The calculations of water and electrolyte needs should be based on estimated deficits, maintenance requirements, and ongoing losses as conducted for IV fluid therapy. These principles are reported elsewhere in this book.

Supplies: tube, fluid line, and container for EFT

Any commercial nasogastric tube designed for horses can be used for EFT. The large-bore tubes commonly used during clinical evaluation of horses with colic are the most common type utilized. Because of its large internal diameter, this kind of tube has the advantage of allowing rapid drainage of gastric contents in case the horse manifests abdominal discomfort during EFT. However, its large external diameter makes this type of tube more likely to produce nasal irritation and motivate the horse to interfere with the tube. A large-bore tube is also more likely to compromise swallowing and transit of ingesta through the esophagus. Whenever a large-bore tube is indwelling, it is advisable to keep the horse nil per os (NPO). As a result, large-bore tubes may be less appropriate for continuous EFT over prolonged periods. It is possible to intermittently remove the tube to allow the horse to eat; however, the risk of causing damage to the nasal passages, pharynx, and esophagus will likely be increased due to repeated intubation.

In the author's experience the optimal tube for EFT are small-bore tubes such as those designed for enteral nutrition (e.g., Nasogastric Tube – 18-Fr × 250 cm; Mila International Inc., 12 Price Avenue, Erlanger, KY 41018, USA). These tubes are less likely to cause nasal irritation and discomfort, and do not compromise swallowing or transit of ingesta through the esophagus (Lopes et al., 2003). Therefore, the small-bore tube is the best option for prolonged EFT because the horse can be allowed to eat while receiving fluids. There is evidence that fasting delays GI transit (Freeman et al., 1989; Lopes et al., 2004), which is not desirable in many instances such as in horses with large colon impactions. The small-bore tube comes with a guide wire to make it less pliable and facilitate placement. There are two disadvantages of the small-bore tube relative the large bore tube:

1 The small-bore tube cannot be used to drain gastric contents; drainage may be desirable if the horse becomes uncomfortable during EFT.

2 While inserting this type of tube, it is not very easy to feel the advancement of the tube by digital palpation of the dorsolateral aspect of the trachea. It is also more difficult to feel the resistance to tube advancement through the esophagus that is often felt when passing larger diameter tubes. Therefore, it is more difficult to confirm esophageal location of the tube. However, after some training and experience, it is possible to detect a slight resistance to tube advancement, which is indicative of successful esophageal insertion.

Regardless of the type of tube used for EFT, it is probably best to leave the tube tip within the esophagus rather than in the stomach. Nasogastric intubation with a large-bore tube delays gastric emptying (Cruz et al., 2006; Lammers et al., 2005) and it is possible that this also happens when a small-bore tube is used. Another potential problem with leaving the tube tip in the stomach is that tube occlusion with solid ingesta becomes more likely. This complication is more common when the small-bore tube is used, in horses that are fed while intubated, and when EFT is temporarily discontinued (e.g., when the horse is taken for a walk).

Following placement of the tube, it should be securely attached to the halter (e.g., with tape or cable ties). A muzzle can be used to prevent damage or removal of the tube by the horse; the muzzle can be intermittently removed to allow the horse to eat.

For continuous administration of EFT, any coiled fluid line marketed for IV fluid therapy in horses (e.g., STAT Large Animal I.V. Set; International WIN, Ltd., 340 North Mill Road, Suite 6, Kennett Square, PA 19348, USA) can be used. This type of setting allows the horse to move freely in the stall while receiving EFT (Figure 21.4). The fluid container can be a large (10- or

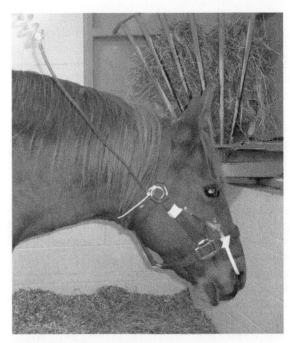

Figure 21.4 Unrestrained horse in a stall receiving enteral fluid therapy through a small-bore nasoesophageal tube.

20-L) plastic carboy, which can be hung in the stall on the same hook used for hanging IV fluid bags. EFT can also be administered intermittently as multiple boluses. For this approach, fluids can be administered through a funnel when a large-bore tube is used; or boluses can be administered with the coiled fluid line adjusted for maximum rate. The tube, fluid line, and carboy used for EFT can be reused multiple times for the same horse because sterility is not required. However, disinfection is necessary as a prophylactic measure against transmission of infectious diseases between patients. When EFT is administered to horses known to have a contagious disease (e.g., salmonellosis) the tube and fluid line should not be reused for other horses.

Fluid composition

While fluids for EFT do not have to be sterile, they must be devoid of significant amounts of toxins and microorganisms capable of causing disease when ingested. Water that is considered to be safe for drinking (e.g., tap water, water from a non-polluted lake or creek, rain water) (Carson, 2000) can be used to make fluids for EFT.

Fluids administered as part of EFT should contain electrolytes in order to avoid development of free water overload (e.g., hyponatremia). The ideal composition of fluids for enteral administration in horses may vary depending on the clinical condition. Unless relatively large volumes of fluids with extreme composition are administered, a horse that does not have severe kidney disease is likely to maintain a normal plasma electrolyte composition. Feed intake also likely minimizes the risk of inducing severe electrolyte imbalances during EFT. Conversely, a horse with severe kidney disease that is not eating will require fluids with a well-adjusted electrolyte composition, because the patient's ability to regulate plasma electrolyte content may be severely compromised.

Similar to parenteral fluid therapy, it is not possible to precisely predict the best fluid composition for the duration of treatment. Therefore, the type of enteral fluids administered should be based on electrolyte and acid–base status measured just prior to starting fluid therapy. Subsequently, the composition of fluids can be adjusted based on measurement of plasma electrolyte concentrations at least once daily.

Ingestion of fluids with a low electrolyte content is well tolerated because normal horses concurrently ingest electrolytes within feeds. Normal kidneys can excrete an excess of free water that is ingested (McKenzie, 2007). However, administration of large volumes of fluids with a very low concentration of sodium by any route is dangerous and can cause severe dilution of the body fluids (e.g., hyponatremia) (Figure 21.2) and reduced plasma osmolarity, even in normal individuals (Byramji et al., 2008; Geor & McCutcheon, 1998; Lester et al., 2013; Lopes et al., 2004; Monreal et al., 1999). Electrolyte derangements produced by water overload may lead to hyponatremic encephalopathy, which can lead to permanent brain damage or fatality even when appropriate treatment is promptly instituted (Fraser & Arieff, 1997; Moritz & Ayus, 2007). A case of cerebral edema manifested as altered mental status and seizures has been reported in a horse with kidney disease that received a limited volume of water enterally (Lopes, 1999). The risk of hyponatremic encephalopathy is increased when the plasma concentration of arginine vasopressin (AVP) is increased. This condition may be present in critically ill humans (Fraser & Arieff, 1997; Moritz & Ayus, 2007). Increased AVP concentrations are also found in horses commonly treated with fluid therapy, such as those with colic (Ludders et al., 2009), sepsis, and post-exercise dehydration (Muñoz et al., 2010).

As observed with the voluntary intake of water by horses, administration of limited volumes of water through the enteral route is safe. The maximum volume of water that can be safely administered enterally to normal horses is not known. Experimental administration of 5 L/h of tapwater for 12 h (total 121.6 mL/kg/12 h) to normal horses that were fasted for 24 h produced mild hyponatremia (no lower than 126 mmol/L); this was not associated with signs of encephalopathy (Lopes et al., 2004). In a recent study investigating nasogastric administration of water at slower rates than used in the previous study (50, 100, and 150 mL/kg/24 h), normal horses deprived of water for 24 h but not fasted developed even milder hyponatremia than reported in the previous study (Lester et al., 2013). Sick horses may be considerably less tolerant of the administration of hyponatremic fluids than healthy horses. Therefore, plain water should not be used for EFT.

Inexpensive salts such as sodium chloride, sodium bicarbonate, and potassium chloride can be added to water to produce electrolyte solutions for EFT. Few studies investigating the effects of fluid composition in horses treated with EFT have been published. An electrolyte solution containing Na^+, K^+, and Cl^- in concentrations similar to those of equine plasma (5.27, 0.37, and 3.78 g/L of NaCl, KCl, and $NaHCO_3$, respectively; 135, 5, and 95 mmol/L of Na^+, K^+, and Cl^-, respectively; calculated osmolarity = 280 mOsm/L) seems to be safe even when large volumes are administered (Lopes et al., 2002, 2004, 2006). Electrolyte solutions containing a larger ratio of chloride to sodium relative to plasma composition in normal horses have also been used. An isotonic solution containing 103, 40, and 143 mmol/L of Na^+, K^+, and Cl^- and with calculated osmolarity of 286 mOsm/L (6.03 and 2.98 g/L of NaCl and KCl) was used for horses with experimentally induced dehydration (Monreal et al., 1999) and large colon obstructions (Monreal et al., 2010). In both studies, this electrolyte solution produced a mild increase in plasma Cl^- concentration and a mild decrease in strong ion difference. Normal saline (0.9% NaCl) – a solution with calculated concentrations of 154 mmol/L for Na^+ and Cl^- and calculated osmolarity of 308 mOsmol/L – seems to have a pronounced laxative effect, which is beneficial for horses with impactions. However, 0.9% NaCl can lead to hyperchloremia and a decreased strong ion difference if large volumes are administered (Lopes et al., 2001). Hyperchloremic metabolic acidosis

(HCMA) has been receiving much attention in human critical care in recent years, as it has detrimental physiologic effects.

A hypotonic solution containing 63, 24.5, 87, 3.4, and 3.4 mmol/L of Na^+, K^+, Cl^-, Mg^{2+}, and SO_4^{2-}, respectively – and calculated osmolarity of 181 mOsmol/L (3.67, 1.83, and 0.83 g/L of NaCl, KCl, and $MgSO_4$) – was successfully used to treat 18 out of 20 horses with gastric impaction. Theoretically, this solution could lead to plasma dilution of sodium; however, the authors did not report its effects on plasma electrolyte concentrations (Vainio et al., 2011). A single 8-L dose of a hypertonic solution containing 762.2, 53.6, 53.6, 1291.9, and 208.3 mmol/L of Na^+, K^+, Cl^-, acetate, and glucose, respectively, and calculated osmolarity of 2369.6 mOsmol/L (62.5, 4, 37.5, and 31.25 g/L of sodium acetate, KCl, glucose, and pure acetate) produced a marked increase in strong ion difference and alkalosis in well-conditioned horses both at rest and 24 h after exercise (Waller & Lindinger, 2007).

The laxative effect of enteral fluids appears to be directly proportional to the electrolyte content of the administered fluid. Addition of less absorbable electrolytes (such as divalent cations) to the solution, or the concurrent administration of a saline cathartic, also increases the laxative effect (Avanza et al., 2009). Magnesium sulfate ($MgSO_4$) is an example of a means of increasing the laxative effect of enteral fluids; the large amounts of Mg^{2+} and SO_4^{2-} provided with the recommended dose of $MgSO_4$ (1 g/kg) can affect plasma electrolyte content. At this dose, it is unlikely to cause clinical signs of electrolyte imbalance if the horse does not have severe kidney disease and is simultaneously receiving large volumes of alternative fluids (Avanza et al., 2009; Lopes et al., 2002, 2004).

In humans it is well established that the addition of simple carbohydrates (monomers or very short polymers) to fluids administered enterally increases the absorption of sodium and water because of sodium-glucose cotransporters and secondary water passive absorption (Gisolfi & Duchman, 1992; Gregorio et al., 2009; Wright et al., 2007). Although the same cotransporters are found in the equine small intestine (Benders et al., 2005; Cehak et al., 2009; Dyer et al., 2002), no benefit of adding carbohydrate monomers or short polymers was observed in the few published studies conducted in horses submitted to experimental dehydration (Avanza et al., 2009; Ecke et al., 1998; Monreal

et al., 1999; Sosa León et al., 1995). In the most recent study, horses were kept on·a diet low in hydrolyzable carbohydrates (tropical grass hay) for several weeks prior to the study. The diet may have contributed to minimizing the expression of the sodium-glucose cotransporter (SGLT1), the intestinal concentration of which is known to be directly proportional to the content of hydrolyzable carbohydrates in the diet (Dyer et al., 2009). Additional limitations of study design (e.g., small number of horses, administration of fluids as a few boluses over a short period of time) may explain at least in part why no benefit of adding glucose to the electrolyte solution could be found in these four studies. In one of these studies, maltodextrin (average molecular weight 1800 daltons, which translates to an average glucose polymer length of 10 glucose molecules) was added to the electrolyte solution instead of dextrose; the aim was to minimize the osmotic load of simple carbohydrates in the fluid. However, this approach did not seem to have any benefit (Avanza et al., 2009).

Considering the well-documented fluid-absorptive effects of carbohydrates in humans (Gisolfi & Duchman, 1992; Gregorio et al., 2009; Wright et al., 2007), the few studies with negative results conducted in horses should not necessarily be taken as definitive evidence for a lack of benefit of adding carbohydrates to electrolyte solutions in horses. Addition of amino acids or short peptides can also promote sodium absorption through specific cotransporters. However, no benefit of replacing carbohydrate with amino acids was found in humans with diarrhea (Bhan et al., 1994; Gutiérrez et al., 2007). Furthermore, amino acids are less stable than glucose and are potentially toxic (Schedl et al., 1994).

Temperature of fluids for EFT

In humans, gastric emptying is faster after ingestion of cold water (5 °C) than water at room temperature (20–25 °C) (Ritschel & Erni, 1977). In the only published study about the effect of temperature of fluids administered enterally to horses, temperature (5, 21, and 37 °C) did not affect absorption or elimination of fluids (Sosa Léon et al., 1995). In most equine cases it is likely that fluids can be administered at room temperature. Administration of a large volume of cold fluids produces heat loss and increases energy expenditure (Carlson, 1971), which may be undesirable in sick horses. In horses with malnutrition or hypothermia, it may be best to administer fluids at body temperature (i.e., 38 °C). Conversely, the administration of cold fluids may be beneficial in horses with hyperthermia.

Fluid rates

The magnitude of the clinical effects of EFT (gastrointestinal and systemic) is proportional to fluid rate, as it is for parenteral fluid therapy. Higher fluid rates maximize the effects on GI contents, plasma volume, and plasma electrolyte concentrations. However, aggressive EFT increases the likelihood of undesirable effects such as abdominal discomfort. As with any other form of fluid therapy, serial adjustment of the rate of administration is crucial to maximize the benefits and minimize the risks of EFT.

Fluid rates that do not exceed 15 mL/kg/h (7.5 L/h for a 500-kg horse) are well tolerated by most horses (Avanza et al., 2009; Lopes et al., 2006), but this is a relatively high rate of fluid administration. EFT administered at this rate for 24 h will provide 360 mL/kg/day, which is approximately six times the requirement of water for maintenance in adult horses (Fonnesbeck, 1968; Tasker, 1967). Fluid rates as high as 20 mL/kg/h (480 mL/kg/day, or approximately eight times the maintenance water requirement; i.e., 10 L/h for a 500-kg horse) can be tolerated by some horses but are certainly not needed in most clinical situations (Lopes et al., 2002). The administration of EFT at 20 mL/kg every 30 min, for a total of three boluses, has been reported in horses with experimentally induced diarrhea. The only observed complication produced by EFT in these horses was transient and mild colic signs after administration of the last bolus (Ecke et al., 1998). In cases where a horse needs such large volumes of fluids administered rapidly, it is advisable to combine EFT with IV fluid therapy in order to minimize the risks of GI overload and abdominal discomfort (Emmanuel et al., 2011).

Horses that initially may not be tolerant of high enteral fluid rates sometimes become more tolerant after a few hours. This increased tolerance over time may be explained by the following effects of EFT:

1 Restoration of hydration status and electrolyte balance may contribute to increased GI motility and enhanced aboral transit of fluids, thereby preventing excessive gastric dilation.

2 Gradual softening of feed impactions, which may reduce the pain produced by the increase in colonic motility secondary to gastric filling with enteral fluids(i.e., the gastrocolic response).

3 An increase in the capacity of the GI tract due to accommodation (i.e., relaxation of the smooth muscle of the GI tract); this relaxation may increase GI compliance and minimize the increase in intraluminal pressure produced by EFT.

Because of these effects, it is preferable to start EFT with a relatively slow rate of fluid administration (e.g., 5–10 mL/kg/h) and, if necessary, gradually increase the rate after a few hours.

As is recommended for parenteral fluid therapy, it is appropriate to taper the fluid administration rate over several hours rather than suddenly discontinuing EFT. However, a gradual interruption of fluid therapy seems to be less important when the enteral route is used because the increased water and electrolyte content within the GI tract produced by EFT functions as a reservoir for gradual absorption. The rebound effects after sudden termination of EFT are not as dramatic as those produced after abrupt discontinuation of IV fluid therapy (Figure 21.5) (Lopes et al., 2002).

Potential complications of EFT

Complications of EFT are preventable and/or can be resolved before causing any serious harm to the horse. Nasoesophageal intubation can lead to nasal mucosal trauma and bleeding. These complications are less likely to occur when a small-bore tube is used. It is also crucial that the outer surface of the tube is smooth. When a small-bore enteral feeding tube is used, it is also important to make sure that the guide wire is shorter than the tube and will not protrude beyond the tip of the tube.

Regardless of the tube chosen for EFT, it is essential to insert the tube very carefully. It should be introduced gently and under appropriate restraint of the horse. A lubricant gel should be used to minimize friction. The tip of the tube should be gently touched to the back of the pharynx until the horse swallows. Air should be blown through the tube as it is passed to encourage dilation of the esophagus, a maneuver that is particularly important when a small-bore tube is used to prevent retroflexion of the tube during tube insertion.

As with any kind of indwelling nasal tube, irritation of the nasal passages will occur with prolonged use of a nasoesophageal tube. Tolerance to these indwelling tubes is highly variable, with some horses beginning to rub the tube after hours to days. When maintaining an

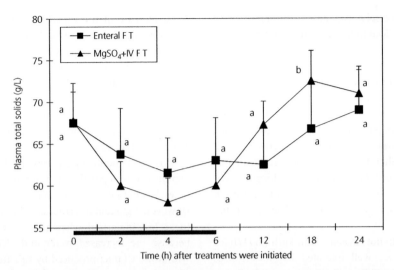

Figure 21.5 Plasma total solids obtained during a 24 h observation period of four horses with fistulas in the RDC receiving two treatments in a crossover design: an electrolyte solution containing 135 mmol/L of Na^+, 5 mmol/L of K^+, 95 mmol/L of Cl^-, and 45 mmol/L of bicarbonate (10 L/h for 6 h) administered via nasogastric tube; and $MgSO_4$ (1 g/kg in 1 L of water) administered via nasogastric tube and IV fluid therapy with lactated Ringer's solution (10 L/h for 6 h). The horizontal bar below the graph indicates the time when the horses were receiving fluid therapy. Vertical whiskers denote standard error. Within one time, means with different letters are significantly different at alpha = 0.05 according to the Bonferroni corrected multiple comparisons. From Lopes MA, Walker BL, White A, Ward DL. Treatments to promote colonic hydration: enteral fluid therapy versus intravenous fluid therapy and magnesium sulphate. *Equine Vet J*. 2002 Jul;34(5):505–9; with permission.

indwelling tube for several days, it is helpful to intermittently remove the tube and reinsert it into the opposite nostril every 24 h in order to minimize nasal irritation. Even when this recommendation is followed, some horses may be particularly sensitive to the presence of the tube in their nasal passage and may require the use of a muzzle between meals to protect the tube. When using the small-bore feeding tube described above, maintaining the guide wire within the tube lumen may make tube removal by the horse less likely to occur. Although the manufacturer recommends removing the guide wire after the tube is successfully inserted, keeping the guide wire in place does not interfere with fluid administration and is not harmful to the horse because the wire is protected within the tube.

Interruption of fluid flow is a sign of tube obstruction by gastric contents filling the tip of the tube. This may be more common if the tube tip is left in the stomach rather than in the esophagus, if the horse is being fed while receiving EFT, and if fluid is administered intermittently rather than continuously. In most cases, flushing the tube with water using a large syringe may be enough to resolve the obstruction. If this maneuver fails, however, the tube will need to be removed for the obstruction to

be cleared. Kinking of the tube would be another explanation for flow interruption. Tube advancement while the guide wire is not in place is a likely cause of tube kinking. Therefore, it is important to reinsert the guide wire before advancing the tube. Gently blowing air through the tube while advancing it through the esophagus can also help to prevent tube kinking.

Accidental insertion of the tube into the trachea is relatively common; this usually induces vigorous coughing unless the horse is severely depressed or sedated. Whenever there is evidence of tracheal intubation, the tube should be removed immediately and reinserted. Palpation of the neck in the region of the cervical esophagus aids in determining the location of the tube. If the horse is not coughing, and if palpation of the neck is inconclusive (i.e., the location of the tube cannot be determined), administration of a small volume of water or isotonic electrolyte solution (e.g., 100 mL when a small enteral feeding tube is used, 500 mL when a large-bore tube is used) usually will demonstrate if the tube is in the esophagus or trachea. This small volume of fluid would not be harmful if administered into the trachea but would certainly induce coughing unless the horse is severely depressed or sedated. Cervical ultrasonography

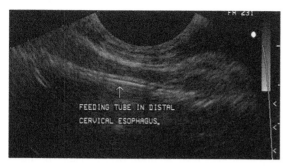

Figure 21.6 Ultrasonographic image (longitudinal view) of the neck of a horse with an enteral feeding tube in the esophagus. The tube is indicated by the arrow. From Lopes MAF, Hepburn RJ, McKenzie HC, Sikes BW. Enteral fluid therapy for horses. Compend Cont Educ. 2003;25(5):390–7, with permission.

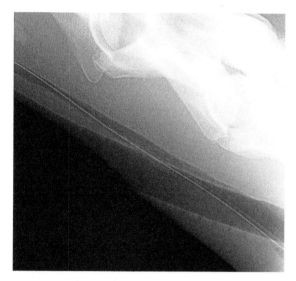

Figure 21.7 Radiographic image of the neck (lateral view) of a horse with a small-bore tube in the esophagus. The radiopaque line in the tube can be seen. There is no superposition of the tube with the trachea throughout the neck, indicating that the tube had been correctly placed in the esophagus. From Lopes MAF, Hepburn RJ, McKenzie HC, Sikes BW. Enteral fluid therapy for horses. Compend Cont Educ. 2003;25(5):390–7, with permission.

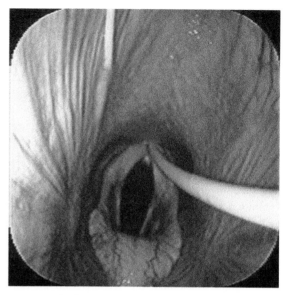

Figure 21.8 Endoscopic image of the pharynx of a horse with an enteral feeding tube in the esophagus. From Lopes MAF, Hepburn RJ, McKenzie HC, Sikes BW. Enteral fluid therapy for horses. Compend Cont Educ. 2003;25(5):390–7, with permission.

(Figure 21.6), cervical radiography (Figure 21.7), or pharyngeal endoscopy (Figure 21.8) can be used to document that tracheal intubation has not occurred (Lopes et al., 2003).

Signs of mild to moderate abdominal discomfort during administration of enteral fluids do not necessarily indicate total intolerance of EFT. In horses with large colon obstruction (e.g., impaction), signs of colic may be induced simply by the increase in colonic motility that occurs secondary to filling of the stomach with fluid (Freeman et al., 1992; Lopes et al., 1999). If the clinician is confident about the diagnosis of a condition amenable to EFT, a short-acting analgesic (e.g., scopolamine, xylazine) can be used to control pain (Monreal et al., 2010). When signs of mild discomfort are present, EFT may be temporarily interrupted and reinitiated after 30 to 60 minutes at half the initial fluid rate.

If the horse does not respond to short-acting analgesics and temporary interruption of fluid administration, tube removal and insertion of a large-bore tube should be performed to evaluate for the presence of gastric dilation. Persistent pain after emptying the stomach indicates that the cause of the discomfort was not gastric filling with fluids. Mild to moderate abdominal discomfort is not uncommon in the beginning of EFT and horses seem to gradually become more tolerant to faster rates of fluid administration. Therefore, starting EFT with a lower fluid rate (5–10 mL/kg/h) for the first few hours and gradually increasing the fluid rate to the desired level is the most prudent approach.

Persistent pain during EFT may also be a sign that a surgical lesion is present such as an impacted enterolith

(Lopes, 1999) or intussusception (Albanese et al., 2011). In these cases EFT would not resolve the obstruction but might contribute to the decision to perform surgery sooner. It may not be possible to distinguish animals that are transiently intolerant to EFT from those that will never tolerate or respond to EFT. Therefore, when there are no financial constraints and the horse is showing pain when treated with EFT, the clinician may choose to interrupt EFT and switch to IV fluid therapy.

Severe electrolyte imbalances can be caused by EFT. Life-threatening hyponatremia may occur if fluids with very low sodium concentration (e.g., tapwater) are administered. A case of cerebral edema manifested as altered mental status and seizures in a horse with kidney disease has been reported; this horse received a limited volume of water but was later found to have extensive kidney disease (Lopes, 1999). Conversely, excessive concentrations of sodium in the electrolyte solution can lead to life-threatening hypernatremia. A case of inadvertent administration of 9% NaCl to one horse leading to severe hypernatremia, hyperchloremia, and neurologic signs (altered mental status followed by seizures) has also been reported (Lopes, 2008). Subclinical hypo- and hypernatremia have been experimentally produced in horses treated with fluids with very low sodium content (Lester et al., 2013; Lopes et al., 2004; Monreal et al., 1999) and 0.9% NaCl (Lopes et al., 2001), respectively. Administration of 0.9% NaCl also led to hyperchloremia and a reduced strong ion difference (Lopes et al., 2001). Severe hypermagnesemia has also been reported after large doses (1.67–2 g/kg) of $MgSO_4$ were administered as a hypertonic solution via nasogastric tube to normal (Scarratt & Swecker, 1999) and dehydrated horses (Henninger & Horst, 1997). In normal horses, even a regular dose (1 g/kg) of $MgSO_4$ administered enterally as a hypertonic solution can produce an increase in plasma magnesium concentration within the reference range (Lopes et al., 2004). An increase in plasma SO_4^{2-} concentration and hypocalcemia were produced in six normal horses experimentally treated with 1 g/kg of Na_2SO_4 while clinical signs of hypocalcemia (i.e., muscular fasciculations, diaphragmatic flutter, and colic) were produced in only one of the horses (Lopes et al., 2004). These observations highlight the importance of using an electrolyte solution with the appropriate composition; this should be based on clinical findings, particularly plasma electrolyte content and acid–base status, measured before

and during EFT. If there is no evidence of a pre-existing electrolyte imbalance (e.g., hypochloremia) and if repeated assessment of plasma electrolyte concentration is not possible, it is prudent to use a balanced, isotonic electrolyte solution with concentrations of sodium, potassium, and chloride similar to equine plasma (Lopes et al., 2002, 2004).

Severe overhydration is another potential complication of EFT. Experimental administration of a large volume of electrolyte solution over a relatively short period of time (administration rate up to 20 mL/kg/h) caused a marked drop in plasma total solids concentration and packed cell volume (PCV), as well as plasma volume expansion, hyposthenuria, pollakiuria, and polyuria. However, none of the horses had any clinical sign of complications due to severe fluid overload (Avanza et al., 2009; Lopes et al., 2001, 2002, 2004). The findings of these studies demonstrate that EFT can produce overhydration. In contrast to IV fluid therapy, the systemic effects of EFT depend on the absorption of fluids from the intestinal lumen, which is reduced during overhydration (Duffy et al., 1978). Thus, EFT is less likely to produce severe systemic overhydration than is IV fluid therapy.

Rupture of the GI tract triggered by EFT is a potential concern in horses with very large impactions. The increased colonic motility produced by gastric filling with fluids may result in excessive tension on the walls of the cecum or colon already compromised by the primary disease. The author is not aware of any reports or cases of GI rupture in horses with colon impaction treated with EFT. In three case series of large colon impactions treated with EFT, GI rupture was not observed in any horse (Hallowell, 2008; Lopes et al., 1999; Monreal et al., 2010). The author has administered EFT to a horse initially diagnosed with simple ingesta impaction and later found to have a large enterolith wedged in the transverse colon. Enteral fluid therapy did not resolve the obstruction but it did not lead to colonic rupture either (Lopes, 1999). A case of cecal rupture in one horse with cecal impaction treated exclusively with EFT and pain medication has been documented (Lopes, 1999). A high occurrence of cecal rupture (23 cases, or 40.4%) was observed in a series of 57 horses with cecal impaction. Aggressive IV fluid therapy (3–4 L/h) combined with nasogastric administration of 6–8 L of water every 2 h was the standard treatment used in these cases. All ruptures occurred within 24 h of diagnosis or admission but the authors did not report how many cases were treated with EFT before rupture occurred (Collatos & Romano, 1993). If indeed in all cases EFT was initiated before the occurrence of cecal rupture, the prevalence of cecal rupture in the horses treated simultaneously with IV and EFT (Collatos & Romano 1993), was significantly higher (Fisher's exact p-value = 0.004 calculated with the proc freq of SAS; SAS Institute Inc., Cary, NC) than the 18.4% prevalence of cecal rupture observed in a recent series of 103 cases of cecal impaction that did not receive EFT (Plummer et al., 2007). However, the pitfalls in comparing results from two different studies, especially retrospective studies, must be pointed out. Gastric rupture was presumptively diagnosed in 1 out of 20 horses with gastric impaction treated with EFT (Vainio et al., 2011). Gastric rupture was also observed in a horse that received a small volume of fluids via nasogastric tube (Hogan et al., 1995). Therefore, EFT should be used with great caution in horses with gastric or cecal impactions.

Abdominal distention and increase in abdominal pressure are expected and often harmless consequences of the filling effects of EFT on the GI tract (Figure 21.3) (Barrett et al., 2013; Lopes et al., 1999, 2002, 2004). Abdominal distention produced by EFT may only be a problem in horses with pre-existing abdominal distention (e.g., due to advanced pregnancy or tympany). Diarrhea is also commonly seen in horses treated with EFT (Lopes et al., 1999, 2001, 2002, 2003, 2004; Monreal et al., 2010) and should not be considered a complication, but rather a normal response to treatment. Reduction of the administration rate should be expected to make feces more consistent and defecation less frequent and voluminous. Diarrhea should subside shortly after interrupting EFT. There is no reason to believe that EFT-induced diarrhea can lead to colitis.

EFT in foals

Enteral fluid therapy can also be used in foals. Due to their smaller body size, the financial benefits of using inexpensive electrolyte solutions for EFT in foals are less significant than in adult horses. Foals can tolerate EFT well, and a small-bore nasoesophageal tube used for fluid administration does not interfere with nursing (Figure 21.9). The same principles mentioned in the

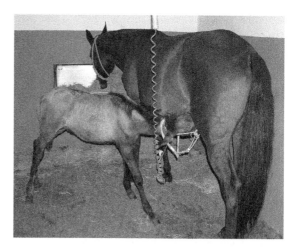

Figure 21.9 Unrestrained foal receiving enteral fluid therapy through a small-bore nasoesophageal tube while nursing.

previous sections of this chapter also apply for foals. Commercial small-bore tubes designed for foals are also available (e.g., Nasogastric Tube – 14-Fr × 125 cm, Mila International Inc., 12 Price Avenue, Erlanger, KY 41018, USA).

References

Albanese V, Credille B, Ellis A, Baldwin L, Mueller POE, Woolums A. (2011) A case of a colocolic intussusception in a horse. *Equine Vet Educ* **23**:281–5.

Al-Benna S. (2011) Fluid resuscitation protocols for burn patients at intensive care units of the United Kingdom and Ireland. Ger Med Sci 9:Doc14.

Alexander F, Benzie D. (1951) A radiological study of the digestive tract of the foal. *Quart J Exper Physiol Cogn Med Sci* **36**:213–17.

Argenzio RA. (1990) Physiology of digestive, secretory and absorptive processes. In: White NA II (ed.) *The Equine Acute Abdomen*. Philadelphia: Lea & Febiger, pp. 25–35.

Argenzio RA, Lowe JE, Pickard DW, Stevens CE. (1974) Digesta passage and water exchange in the equine large intestine. *Am J Physiol* **226**:1035–42.

Atia AN, Buchman AL. (2009) Oral rehydration solutions in non-cholera diarrhea: a review. *Am J Gastroenterol* **104**: 2596–604.

Atia A, Buchman AL. (2010) Treatment of cholera-like diarrhoea with oral rehydration. *Ann Trop Med Parasitol* **104**:465–74.

Avanza MFB, Filho JDR, Lopes MAF, Ignacio FS, Carvalho TA, Guimarães JD. (2009) Enteral fluid therapy in horses – electrolyte solution associated or not with glucose, maltodextrine and magnesium sulphate. *Ciência Rural* **39**: 1126–33.

Banse HE, Gilliam LL, House AM, et al. (2011) Gastric and enteric phytobezoars caused by ingestion of persimmon in equids. *J Am Vet Med Assoc* **239**:1110–16.

Barrett EJ, Munsterman AS, Hanson RR. (2013) Effects of gastric distension on intraabdominal pressures in horses. *J Vet Emerg Crit Care (San Antonio)* **23**:423–8.

Barrett KE, Dharmsathaphorn K. (1994) Transport of water and electrolytes in the gastrointestinal tract: Physiological mechanisms, regulation, and methods of study. In: Narins RG (ed.) *Maxwell and Kleeman's Clinical Disorders of Fluid and Electrolyte Metabolism*, 5th edn. New York: McGraw-Hill, pp. 493–519.

Benders NA, Dyer J, Wijnberg ID, Shirazi-Beechey SP, van der Kolk JH. (2005) Evaluation of glucose tolerance and intestinal luminal membrane glucose transporter function in horses with equine motor neuron disease. *Am J Vet Res* **66**:93–9.

Bhan MK, Mahalanabis D, Fontaine O, et al. (1994) Clinical trials of improved oral rehydration salt formulations: a review. *Bull World Health Org* **72**:945–55.

Byramji A, Cains G, Gilbert JD, Byard RW. (2008) Hyponatremia at autopsy: an analysis of etiologic mechanisms and their possible significance. *Forensic Sci Med Pathol* **4**:149–52.

Cancio LC, Kramer GC, Hoskins SL. (2006) Gastrointestinal fluid resuscitation of thermally injured patients. *J Burn Care Res* **27**:561–9.

Carlson GP. (1971) Energy loss in fluid therapy. *N Engl J Med* **285**:1328–9.

Carlson GP, Rumbaugh GE, Harrold D. (1979) Physiologic alterations in the horse produced by food and water deprivation during periods of high environmental temperatures. *Am J Vet Res* **40**:982–5.

Carson TL. (2000) Current knowledge of water quality and safety for livestock. *Vet Clin N Am Food Anim Pract* **16**:455–64.

Cehak A, Burmester M, Geburek F, Feige K, Breves G. (2009) Electrophysiological characterization of electrolyte and nutrient transport across the small intestine in horses. *J Anim Physiol Anim Nutr (Berl)* **93**:287–94.

Clarke LL, Roberts MC, Grubb BR, et al. (1992) Short-term effect of aldosterone on Na-Cl transport across equine colon. *Am J Physiol* **262**:R939–46.

Collatos C, Romano S. (1993) Cecal impaction in horses: causes, diagnosis and medical treatment. *Comp Cont Educ Pract Vet* **15**:976–81.

Cruz AM, Li R, Kenney DG, Monteith G. (2006) Effects of indwelling nasogastric intubation on gastric emptying of a liquid marker in horses. *Am J Vet Res* **67**:1100–4.

Danielsen K, Lawrence LM, Siciliano P, et al: (1995) Effects of diet on weight and plasma variables in endurance exercised horses. *Equine Vet J Suppl* **18**:372–7.

Duffy PA, Granger DN, Taylor AE. (1978) Intestinal secretion induced by volume expansion in the dog. *Gastroenterol* **75**:413–18.

Dyer J, Fernandez-Castaño Merediz E, Salmon KS, Proudman CJ, Edwards GB, Shirazi-Beechey SP. (2002) Molecular characterisation of carbohydrate digestion and absorption in equine small intestine. *Equine Vet J* **34**:349–58.

Dyer J, Al-Rammahi M, Waterfall L, et al. (2009) Adaptive response of equine intestinal Na+/glucose co-transporter (SGLT1) to an increase in dietary soluble carbohydrate. *Pflugers Arch* **458**:419–30.

Ecke P, Hodgson DR, Rose RJ. (1998) Induced diarrhoea in horses. Part 2: Response to administration of an oral rehydration solution. *Vet J* **155**:161–70.

Emmanuel H, Casa DJ, Beasley KN, et al. (2011) Appearance of D2O in sweat after oral and oral-intravenous rehydration in men. *J Strength Cond Res* **25**:2092–9.

Ferreira FPP, Nicoletti JLM, Hussni CA, et al. (2011) Equine intracecal fluid therapy. *Vet e Zootec* **18**: 481–9.

Fonnesbeck PV. (1968) Consumption and excretion of water by horses receiving all hay and hay-grain diets. *J Anim Sci* **27**:1350–6.

Fraser CL, Arieff AI. (1997) Epidemiology, pathophysiology, and management of hyponatremic encephalopathy. *Am J Med* **102**:67–77.

Freeman DE, Ferrante PL, Kronfeld DS, Chalupa W. (1989) Effect of food deprivation on D-xylose absorption test results in mares. *Am J Vet Res* **50**:1609–12.

Freeman DE, Ferrante PL, Palmer JE. (1992) Comparison of the effects of intragastric infusions of equal volumes of water, dioctyl sodium sulfosuccinate, and magnesium sulfate on fecal composition and output in clinically normal horses. *Am J Vet Res* **53**:1347–53.

Garg M, Angus PW, Burrell LM, Herath C, Gibson PR, Lubel JS. (2012) Review article: the pathophysiological roles of the renin-angiotensin system in the gastrointestinal tract. *Aliment Pharmacol Ther* **35**:414–28.

Geor RJ, McCutcheon LJ. (1998) Hydration effects on physiological strain of horses during exercise-heat stress. *J Appl Physiol* **84**:2042–51.

Gisolfi CV. (2000) Is the GI system built for exercise? *News Physiol Sci* **15**:114–19.

Gisolfi CV, Duchman SM. (1992) Guidelines for optimal replacement beverages for different athletic events. *Med Sci Sports Exerc* **24**:679–87.

Goodgame RW. (2001) Viral causes of diarrhea. *Gastroenterol Clin North Am* **30**:779–95.

Gregorio GV, Gonzales ML, Dans LF, Martinez EG. (2009) Polymer-based oral rehydration solution for treating acute watery diarrhoea. *Cochrane Database Syst Rev* Apr 15;(2):CD006519; doi: 10.1002/14651858.CD006519.pub2.

Guarino A, Dupont C, Gorelov AV, et al. (2012) The management of acute diarrhea in children in developed and developing areas: from evidence base to clinical practice. *Expert Opin Pharmacother* **13**:17–26.

Gutiérrez C, Villa S, Mota FR, et al. (2007) Does an L-glutamine-containing, glucose-free, oral rehydration solution reduce stool output and time to rehydrate in children with acute diarrhoea? A double-blind randomized clinical trial. *J Health Popul Nutr* **25**:278–84.

Hallowell GD. (2008) Retrospective study assessing efficacy of treatment of large colonic impactions. *Equine Vet J.* Jun;**40** (4):411–413.

Hartling L, Bellemare S, Wiebe N, Russell K, Klassen TP, Craig W. (2006) Oral versus intravenous rehydration for treating dehydration due to gastroenteritis in children. Cochrane Database Syst Rev Jul 19;(3):CD004390.

Henninger RW, Horst J. (1997) Magnesium toxicosis in two horses. *J Am Vet Med Assoc* **211**:82–5.

Hill DR, Beeching NJ. (2010) Travelers' diarrhea. *Curr Opin Infect Dis* **23**:481–7.

Hjortkjaer RK. (1979) Enema in the horse. Distribution and rehydrating effect. *Nord Vet Med* **31**:508–19.

Hogan PM, Bramlage LR, Pierce SW. (1995) Repair of a full-thickness gastric rupture in a horse. *J Am Vet Med Assoc* **207**:338–40.

Hyyppä S, Saastamoinen M, Pösö AR. (1996) Restoration of water and electrolyte balance in horses after repeated exercise in hot and humid conditions. Equine Vet J Suppl Jul;(22):108–12.

Johnson LR. (2007) Fluid and electrolyte absorption. In: Johnson LR (ed.) *Gastrointestinal Physiology*, 7th edn. Philadelphia: Mosby Elsevier, pp. 127–36.

Kasirer-Izraely H, Choshniak I, Shkolnik A. (1994) Dehydration and rehydration in donkeys: the role of the hind gut as a water reservoir. *J Basic Clin Physiol Pharmacol* **5**:89–100.

Kenefick RW, Maresh CM, Armstrong LE, et al. (2000) Plasma vasopressin and aldosterone responses to oral and intravenous saline rehydration. *J Appl Physiol* **89**:2117–22.

Kenefick RW, O'Moore KM, Mahood NV, Castellani JW. (2006) Rapid IV versus oral rehydration: responses to subsequent exercise heat stress. *Med Sci Sports Exerc* **38**:2125–31.

Kramer GC, Michell MW, Oliveira H, et al. (2010) Oral and enteral resuscitation of burn shock the historical record and implications for mass casualty care. *Eplasty* **10**:e56.

Lammers TW, Roussel AJ, Boothe DM, Cohen ND. (2005) Effect of an indwelling nasogastric tube on gastric emptying rates of liquids in horses. *Am J Vet Res* **66**:642–5.

Lester GD, Merritt AM, Kuck HV, Burrow JA. (2013) Systemic, renal, and colonic effects of intravenous and enteral rehydration in horses. *J Vet Intern Med* **27**:554–66.

Lindegaard C, Ekstrøm CT, Wulf SB, Vendelbo JM, Andersen PH. (2011) Nephrosplenic entrapment of the large colon in 142 horses (2000–2009): analysis of factors associated with decision of treatment and short-term survival. *Equine Vet J* **43**(Suppl 39):63–8.

Lopes MAF. (1999) Efficiency and risks of enteral fluid therapy for horses with large intestine obstruction. In: *Proceedings 11th Annual Research Symposium, Blacksburg, VA, USA*. Blacksburg, VA: Virginia-Maryland Regional College of Veterinary Medicine, p. 14.

Lopes MAF. (2001) How to provide nutritional support via esophagostomy. *Proceedings American Association of Equine Practitioners* **47**:252–6. Available at: http://www.ivis.org/proceedings/AAEP/2001/91010100252.pdf

Lopes MAF. (2008) Intraluminal obstruction of the large colon. In: Robinson NE, Sprayberry KA (eds) *Current Therapy in Equine Medicine*, 6th edn. St Louis, MO: Saunders Elsevier, pp.407–12.

Lopes MAF, Moura DS, Filho JDR. (1999) Treatment of large colon impaction with enteral fluid therapy. In: Proceedings 45th Annual Convention of the America Association of Equine Practitioners (AAEP), Albuquerque, New Mexico, In: pp. 99–102.

Lopes MAF, Johnson S, White NA, Ward DL. (2001) Enteral fluid therapy: slow infusion versus boluses. *In: Proceedings ACVS Veterinary Symposium – Equine Proceedings*. Chicago, IL, USA, 2001, p. 13.

Lopes MA, Walker BL, White A, Ward DL. (2002) Treatments to promote colonic hydration: enteral fluid therapy versus intravenous fluid therapy and magnesium sulphate. *Equine Vet J* **34**:505–9.

Lopes MAF, Hepburn RJ, McKenzie HC, Sikes BW. (2003) Enteral fluid therapy for horses. *Compend Cont Vet Educ* **25**:390–7.

Lopes MAF, White NA, Donaldson L, Crisman MV, Ward DL. (2004) Effects of enteral and intravenous fluid therapy, magnesium sulfate, and sodium sulfate on colonic contents and feces in horses. *Am J Vet Res* **65**:695–704.

Lopes MAF, Aristizabal FA, Avanza MFB, Silva AGA. (2006) Immediate post-operative enteral fluid therapy in horses submitted to intestinal surgery. In: *Proceedings ACVS Veterinary Symposium, Washington, DC, USA, October 2006*. Rockville, MD: American College of Veterinary Surgeons.

Lopes MAF, Pessin AE., Lopes BL. (2009) Ultrasonographic assessment of small intestine distension in horses administered enteral fluids. In: *Proceedings ACVS Veterinary Symposium, Washington, DC, October 2009*. Germantown, MD: American College of Veterinary Surgeons, p. xxxviii.

Ludders JW, Palos HM, Erb HN, Lamb SV, Vincent SE, Gleed RD. (2009) Plasma arginine vasopressin concentration in horses undergoing surgery for colic. *J Vet Emerg Crit Care (San Antonio)* **19**:528–35.

Marlin DJ, Scott CM, Mills PC, Louwes H, Vaarten J. (1998) Rehydration following exercise: effects of administration of water versus an isotonic oral rehydration solution (ORS). *Vet J* **156**:41–9.

McKenzie EC. (2007) Polyuria and polydipsia in horses. *Vet Clin North Am Equine Pract* **23**:641–53.

McKenzie H. (2008) Diagnosis and treatment of enteritis and colitis in the horse. In: White NA, Moore JN, Mair TS. *The Equine Acute Abdomen*, 2nd edn. Jackson, WY: Teton NewMedia, pp. 355–79.

McSwain NE, Champion HR, Fabian TC, et al. (2011) State of the art of fluid resuscitation 2010: prehospital and immediate transition to the hospital. *J Trauma* **70**(5 Suppl):S2–10.

Mealey RH, Carter GK, Roussel AJ, Ruoff WW. (1995) Indwelling cecal catheters for fluid administration in ponies. *J Vet Intern Med* **9**:347–52.

Michell MW, Oliveira HM, Kinsky MP, Vaid SU, Herndon DN, Kramer GC. (2006) Enteral resuscitation of burn shock using World Health Organization oral rehydration solution: a potential solution for mass casualty care. *J Burn Care Res* **27**:819–25.

Monreal, L, Garzon, N, Espada, Y, et al: (1999) Electrolyte vs. glucose-electrolyte isotonic solutions for oral rehydration therapy in horses. *Equine Vet J Suppl* **30**:425–9.

Monreal L, Navarro M, Armengou L, José-Cunilleras E, Cesarini C, Segura D. (2010) Enteral fluid therapy in 108 horses with large colon impactions and dorsal displacements. *Vet Rec* **166**:259–63.

Moritz ML, Ayus JC. (2007) Hospital-acquired hyponatremia – why are hypotonic parenteral fluids still being used? *Nat Clin Pract Nephrol* **3**:374–82.

Muñoz A, Riber C, Trigo P, Castejón-Riber C, Castejón FM. (2010) Dehydration, electrolyte imbalances and renin-angiotensin-aldosterone-vasopressin axis in successful and unsuccessful endurance horses. *Equine Vet J* **42**(Suppl 38):83–90.

Murray R. (2006) Training the gut for competition. *Curr Sports Med Rep* **5**:161–4.

Norman TE, Chaffin K, Schmitz DG. (2010) *Contrast enhancement for ultrasonographic evaluation of the equine small intestine.* Proceedings AAEP, p. 248. Available at: http://ivis.org/proceedings/aaep/2010/z9100110000248.pdf

Pfeiffer CJ, MacPherson BR. (1990) Anatomy of the gastrointestinal tract and peritoneal cavity. In: White NA II (ed.) *The Equine Acute Abdomen.* Philadelphia: Lea & Febiger, pp. 2–24.

Plummer AE, Rakestraw PC, Hardy J, Lee RM. (2007) Outcome of medical and surgical treatment of cecal impaction in horses: 114 cases (1994–2004). *J Am Vet Med Assoc* **231**:1378–85.

Ritschel WA, Erni W. (1977) The influence of temperature of ingested fluid on stomach emptying time. *Int J Clin Pharmacol Biopharm* **15**:172–5.

Rose RJ, Gibson KT, Suann CJ. (1986) An evaluation of an oral glucoseglycine-electrolyte solution for the treatment of experimentally induced dehydration in the horse. *Vet Rec* **119**:522–5.

Rouhani S, Meloney L, Ahn R, Nelson BD, Burke TF. (2011) Alternative rehydration methods: a systematic review and lessons for resource-limited care. *Pediatrics* **127**:e748–57.

Ryan AJ, Lambert GP, Shi X, Chang RT, Summers RW, Gisolfi CV. (1998) Effect of hypohydration on gastric emptying and intestinal absorption during exercise. *J Appl Physiol* **84**:1581–8.

Scarratt WK, Swecker WS. (1999) Administration of therapeutic dosages of magnesium sulphate to clinically normal horses. In: *Proceedings of the 11th Annual Research Symposium*, Virginia-Maryland Regional College of Veterinary Medicine, Blacksburg, Virginia, 1999, p. 24.

Schedl HP, Maughan RJ, Gisolfi CV. (1994) Intestinal absorption during rest and exercise: implications for formulating an oral rehydration solution (ORS). *Med Sci Sports Exerc* **26**:267–80.

Schott HC 2nd. (1998) Oral fluids for equine diarrhoea: an underutilized treatment for a costly disease? *Vet J* **155**:119–21.

Sosa León LA, Davie AJ, Hodgson DR, Rose RJ. (1995) The effects of tonicity, glucose concentration and temperature of an oral rehydration solution on its absorption and elimination. *Equine Vet J Suppl Nov* **(20)**:140–6.

Sosa León, LA, Hodgson, DR, Rose, RJ. (1997) Gastric emptying of oral rehydration solutions at rest and after exercise in horses. *Res Vet Sci* **63**:183–7.

Sufit E, Houpt KA, Sweeting M. (1985) Physiological stimuli of thirst and drinking patterns in ponies. *Equine Vet J* **17**:12–16.

Tack J. (2006) Neurophysiologic mechanisms of gastric reservoir function. In: Barrett KE, Ghishan FK, Merchant JL, Said HM, Wood JD, Johnson LR (eds) *Physiology of the Gastrointestinal Tract*, 4th edn, vol. **1**. Burlington: Elsevier Academic Press, pp. 927–34.

Taniguchi H, Sasaki T, Fujita H, et al. (2009) Preoperative fluid and electrolyte management with oral rehydration therapy. *J Anesth* **23**:222–9.

Tasker JB. (1967) Fluid and electrolyte studies in the horse. III. Intake and output of water, sodium, and potassium in normal horses. *Cornell Vet* **57**:649–57.

Thomas SJ, Kramer GC, Herndon DN. (2003) Burns: military options and tactical solutions. *J Trauma* **54**(5 Suppl):S207–18.

Vainio K, Sykes BW, Blikslager AT. (2011) Primary gastric impaction in horses: A retrospective study of 20 cases (2005–2008). *Equine Vet Educ* **23**:186–90.

Varavithya W, Sunthornkachit R, Eampokalap B. (1991) Oral rehydration therapy for invasive diarrhea. *Rev Infect Dis* **13**(Suppl 4):S325–31.

Waller A, Lindinger MI. (2007) The effect of oral sodium acetate administration on plasma acetate concentration and acid-base state in horses. *Acta Vet Scand* **49**:38.

Waller AP, Heigenhauser GJ, Geor RJ, Spriet LL, Lindinger MI. (2009) Fluid and electrolyte supplementation after prolonged moderate-intensity exercise enhances muscle glycogen resynthesis in Standardbred horses. *J Appl Physiol* **106**:91–100.

Warren LK, Lawrence LM, Brewster-Barnes T, et al. (1999) The effect of dietary fibre on hydration status after dehydration with frusemide. *Equine Vet J Suppl* **30**:508–13.

WHO. (2005) The treatment of diarrhoea – A manual for physicians and other senior health workers. Available at: http://whqlibdoc.who.int/publications/2005/9241593180.pdf/ [accessed 9 September 2014].

Wright EM, Hirayama BA, Loo DF. (2007) Active sugar transport in health and disease. *J Intern Med* **261**:32–43.

CHAPTER 22

Fluid therapy for neonatal foals

K. Gary Magdesian

Professor in Critical Care and Emergency Medicine, School of Veterinary Medicine, University of California, Davis, CA, USA

Unique aspects of fluid balance in neonatal foals

The neonatal foal has a proportionally greater body water content than the adult horse. Studies in healthy neonatal foals have shown a body water content of 71–83% of body weight during the first week of life as compared to 60–70% in adult horses (Andrews et al., 1997; Doreau & Dussap, 1980; Fielding et al., 2011; Forro et al., 2000; Judson et al., 1983; Julian et al., 1956; Oftedal et al., 1983). The extracellular fluid (ECF) compartment is also larger in foals than in adult horses (0.36 ± 0.0001 to 0.39 ± 0.03 L/kg, as compared to 0.21–0.29 L/kg in the adult horse) (Carlson et al., 1979a, 1979b; Evans, 1971; Fielding et al., 2003, 2011; Kohn et al., 1978; Muir et al., 1978).

The intracellular fluid (ICF) compartment is smaller in foals than in adult horses (0.38 ± 0.02 L/kg in foals vs 0.46 ± 0.02 L/kg in adult horses) (Fielding et al., 2003, 2011). Therefore, the ECF volume (ECFV) represents approximately 49–50% of total body water in young foals, as compared to 32% in the adult. Healthy foals have higher plasma (0.10 ± 0.02 L/kg) and blood volumes (0.16 ± 0.03 L/kg) than adult horses (0.05–0.06 L/kg and 0.08–0.10 L/kg, respectively) (Fielding et al., 2011; Marcilese et al., 1964).

This greater body water content, along with a higher metabolic rate, growth, and increased insensible losses (higher surface area to body mass ratio), results in a greater water requirement for neonatal foals as compared to adult horses. Insensible losses mean that urinary, cutaneous, and respiratory losses are greater

than in older horses; neonatal foals appear to have a reduced ability to concentrate urine as compared to adult animals (Brewer et al., 1991; Edwards et al., 1990). Healthy, nursing, neonatal pony foals were found to produce 6 mL/kg/h of urine (Brewer et al., 1991). This is high when compared to the urine production of adult horses, which varies with water intake and losses, but ranges from 0.4 to 2 mL/kg/h in adult horses on feed (Groenendyk et al., 1988; Rumbaugh et al., 1982). The primary reason for this high urine output in foals is a high water intake; healthy foals nurse between 15 and 30% of their body weight in milk per day, leading to a high water intake (Martin et al., 1992; Oftedal et al., 1983). Because mare's milk is approximately 89% water, coupled with the high intake, the urine specific gravity of newborn foals (with the exception of the first 24 h post partum) is usually hyposthenuric (<1.008) and is reported to range from 1.001 to 1.027 at 2 days of age (mean 1.009 ± 0.01) (Brewer et al., 1991). In a study of eight healthy foals, urine specific gravity varied with age as follows (Edwards et al., 1990):

0–6 hours: 1.025 ± 0.008 (range: 1.008–1.035)

12 hours: 1.026 ± 0.018 (range: 1.003–1.041)

24 hours: 1.007 ± 0.01 (range: 1.001–1.031)

48 hours to 42 days: average 1.004–1.007 (range: 1.000–1.016)

58 days: 1.010 ± 0.0013 (1.001–1.038)

Neonatal foal urine is more concentrated during the first 12–24 h of life because of the presence of fetal urine and also proteinuria (peak excretion occurs at 6–12 h post partum). This proteinuria occurs due to filtration of small, low-molecular-weight milk and colostral protein

---

Equine Fluid Therapy, First Edition. Edited by C. Langdon Fielding and K. Gary Magdesian.

fragments (Edwards et al., 1990; Jeffcott, 1974; Jeffcott & Jeffcott, 1974). During the initial 48 hours of life, foals can have marked (up to 2–4+ on urine dipstick) proteinuria. After the first 2 days, this proteinuria should resolve and foal urine should be negative for protein. It should be noted that the first urination in healthy foals occurs at 6 and 10 hours for colts and fillies, respectively, and healthy foals urinate every 1–2 hours during the first 2 weeks of life (Jeffcott, 1972; Kownacki et al., 1978; Tyler, 1969).

Shock fluid therapy ("replacement") in the neonatal foal

Clinical signs of shock

Clinical signs of shock in the foal include abnormalities in the clinical perfusion parameters: obtundation, poor pulse quality, cool to cold extremities, prolonged capillary time, pale mucous membranes, poor jugular refill, and reduced urine output. Heart rate is quite variable in the hypovolemic foal; it may not be reflective of hypovolemia and is therefore considered a somewhat unreliable indicator. Causes of shock are varied in the neonatal foal, but hypovolemia is among the most common. Others include septic or systemic inflammatory response syndrome (SIRS) shock. These are often associated with a combination of hypovolemia, reduced cardiac contractility (late in disease process), and vasodilation (reduced peripheral vascular resistance). Each of these is treated, at least in part, with replacement fluid therapy. Fluid therapy should be particularly cautious in foals with cardiogenic shock, such as those with complex cardiac defects or nutritional myodegeneration (white muscle disease), because fluid overload may be pre-existing along with pulmonary edema.

Dehydration, in the author's experience, is more difficult to detect than hypovolemia in the neonatal foal. Dehydration refers to extravascular fluid deficits, in contrast to the intravascular losses associated with hypovolemia. The signs of dehydration include reduced skin turgor, tacky mucous membranes, and reduced corneal moisture, and are relatively insensitive in adult horses and may be even less sensitive indicators of dehydration in foals (Pritchard et al., 2008). Foals have a relatively compliant interstitium as compared to adult horses, and therefore skin turgor is fairly insensitive and likely represents significant dehydration when abnormal. In addition, the skin turgor can be unreliable

in the opposite direction as well. That is, even in hydrated foals the turgor can appear falsely reduced especially in the regions of the neck and eyelid. Therefore, skin turgor should not be relied upon in the neonate as the sole indicator of dehydration.

Laboratory and monitoring tools in shock

The laboratory evidence of shock in foals includes hyperlactatemia (and sometimes lactic acidosis) and increased oxygen extraction ratio. Serial measurement of packed cell volume (PCV), total protein (TP) concentration, and organ function indicators (especially creatinine) may be adjunctive as well. Each of these is associated with some pitfalls, but should be interpreted in the context of clinical signs and monitoring tools.

Blood or plasma lactate concentration

Lactate is one of the laboratory tests that can be useful as a guide to fluid therapy. However, it must be remembered that lactate may be increased in foals for a number of reasons. Hyperlactatemia refers to persistent, mild to moderate increases (2–5 mmol/L) in blood lactate concentration without a concurrent metabolic acidosis. Persistent moderate to marked increases in blood lactate concentration (usually >5 mmol/L), often (but not always) in association with metabolic acidosis, is termed lactic acidosis. Causes of high lactate concentration include type A hyperlactatemia, in which there is poor tissue perfusion or oxygen delivery. Examples of causes of an absolute decrease in oxygen delivery include hypoperfusion (including hypovolemia and hypotension), low oxygen content of blood, and carbon monoxide poisoning. Relative decreases in oxygen delivery (i.e., relative to an increased demand) include exercise, seizures, and muscle activity. Type B hyperlactatemia is associated with disorders that are not tied to poor tissue perfusion or oxygen delivery. Type B disorders include impaired oxygen utilization, as occurs with SIRS, malignancy, thiamine deficiency, decreased metabolism of lactate due to hepatic or renal failure, and mitochondrial dysfunction. Drug induced-hyperlactatemia (e.g., due to salicylates, iron, acetaminophen, propylene glycol, beta-adrenergic agonists, cyanide, propofol, strychnine, sulfasalazine, lactulose, sodium bicarbonate, and valproic acid) represents another form of type B hyperlactatemia. Foals commonly have increased lactate due to hypoperfusion, but also caused by SIRS, sepsis, and mitochondrial dysfunction. Although the presence of hyperlactatemia on admission appears to be associated with mortality and morbidity in foals in some studies, significant overlap between survivors and non-survivors means that non-survivors cannot be predicted from admission lactate measurement alone (Borchers et al., 2012).

Blood lactate concentrations vary with age in the neonatal foal, being highest at birth and decreasing over time. In one study of 14 healthy foals the blood lactate concentration decreased from 2.38 ± 1.03 mmol/L at birth up to 2 hours of age, to 1.24 ± 0.33 at 24 hours, and to 1.08 ± 0.27 mmol/L at 48 hours of age (Magdesian, 2003). Another study ($n=60$) found a median lactate concentration of 3.60 mmol/L (interquartile range: 2.3–4.99) at birth, with an umbilical vein lactate of 4 mmol/L (3.2–4.65), and umbilical artery lactate of 4.6 mmol/L (3.95–5.35). Blood lactate concentrations decreased temporally and were statistically decreased by 24 h of age and beyond (Pirrone et al., 2012).

Arterial blood pressure

In the clinical setting, indirect blood pressure is easily measured in the neonatal foal, most commonly using a blood pressure cuff over the coccygeal artery of the tail. In critically ill, recumbent foals direct blood pressure can be measured through an arterial catheter in the great metatarsal artery or auricular arteries. Normal blood pressure values vary with gestational age, size, and breed. Pony foals have a lower blood pressure than similarly aged Thoroughbred foals (Franco et al., 1986). Healthy pony foals had systolic, diastolic, and mean pressures of 128 ± 17, 64 ± 10, and 85 ± 10 mmHg, respectively, whereas Thoroughbred foals had pressures of 144 ± 15, 74 ± 9, and 95 ± 13 mmHg, respectively (Franco et al., 1986). Another study found direct mean arterial pressure (MAP) to range from 84.1 ± 4.4 to 101.3 ± 4.4 mmHg from 2 hours to 14 days of age (Thomas et al., 1987). This variability with breed and age may complicate interpretation of mean blood pressure values in neonatal foals. A general guideline of 65 to 120 mmHg can be regarded as the normal mean blood pressure range, and the values should be interpreted in light of perfusion parameters, blood lactate, urine output, and other indicators of perfusion status.

Premature foals may have lower pressures than term foals, which may be ample for organ perfusion. Premature human infants have normal blood pressures that are lower than those of full-term babies, due to low-resistance arteriolar vessels. Therefore, the blood pressure number must be interpreted in light of clinical status. For example, a premature foal with a mean arterial pressure of 55 mmHg may not require intervention if urine output and blood lactate concentrations are normal.

Central venous pressure

Central venous pressure (CVP) is a controversial goal of fluid therapy in humans, because it alone does not reflect blood volume; CVP can be affected by cardiac function, pleural pressure, and venous tone. It is regarded by many to be a component of the early goal-directed therapy bundle in the treatment of sepsis-induced tissue hypoperfusion in humans (Dellinger et al., 2012). With this protocol, sepsis-induced hypoperfusion is treated with specific goals in mind during the first 6 hours of resuscitation. These goals include all of the following (Dellinger et al., 2012):

1 CVP 8–12 mmHg.
2 Mean arterial pressure (MAP) $\geq$65 mmHg.
3 Urine output $\geq$0.5 mL/kg/h.
4 Cranial vena cava oxygen saturation ($S_{cv}O_2$) of 70% or mixed venous oxygen saturation (S_vO_2) of 65%.
5 Normalization of lactate in patients with increased lactate levels.

Whether CVP can be used as a goal of fluid therapy in horses and foals remains to be determined. Although there are limitations to CVP as a marker of intravascular volume status, a subnormal CVP generally is a reliable indicator of the need for fluid loading. Whether normalization of CVP indicates adequacy of intravascular volume in horses is unknown. However, despite the controversy of its utility as a goal of fluid loading, CVP is a reasonable limit or ceiling to resuscitative fluid therapy. In other words, when a high normal CVP is reached, additional bolus fluid administration should not continue.

Central venous pressure can be easily measured in neonatal foals through the use of a 20- to 30-cm catheter inserted through the jugular vein but which terminates in the cranial vena cava (Figure 22.1). Placement can be confirmed through use of radiopaque catheters (such as those from Arrow International, Reading, PA) and thoracic radiographs (Figure 22.2). Central venous pressures in healthy neonatal foals range from 2.8 to 12 cmH_2O (2.1 to 8.9 mmHg) (Thomas et al., 1987). CVP can be measured with a water manometer (Figure 22.3) or a pressure transducer. The CVP should be measured at end expiration; if a pressure transducer is used (rather than a disposable manometer), the CVP is the mean of

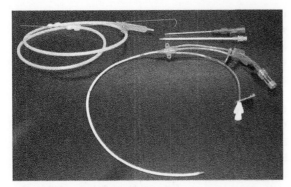

Figure 22.1 A 20-cm triple-lumen polyurethane catheter, used for central venous measurement in foals.

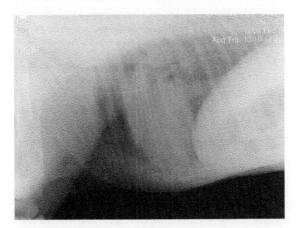

Figure 22.2 Thoracic radiograph demonstrating tip of an IV catheter within the cranial vena cava.

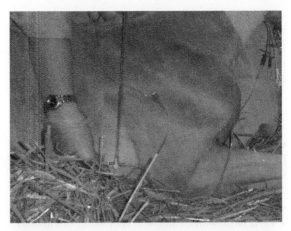

Figure 22.3 Measurement of central venous pressure (CVP) using a water manometer.

the 'a' wave at the end of expiration. The a wave represents atrial contraction, which starts during the PR interval if a concurrent ECG is recorded. Once a CVP of 10–12 cmH$_2$O (7.35–8.9 mmHg) is reached, fluid volume loading should cease. At this point if hypoperfusion is still evident, then inotrope (e.g., dobutamine) and pressor (e.g., norepinephrine) infusions should be instituted.

Urine output

Urine production is a key goal and endpoint to the resuscitative phase of fluid therapy. The initiation of urine flow in a previously anuric or oliguric foal is a reasonable indicator of establishment of renal perfusion. As noted above, healthy newborn foals produce relatively dilute urine (SG 1.001–1.041 during first 24 h, but 1.000–1.016 thereafter) and once a dilute urine is produced (SG <1.020–1.025) then fluid boluses can cease. The one

potential complicating circumstance is renal failure, where isosthenuric, or near isosthenuric, urine will be produced regardless of fluid status; however, even with renal failure the presence of urine flow with fluid therapy is a positive sign.

Urine output is best measured in critically ill foals through the use of urinary catheterization. This can be accomplished through the use of human infant feeding tubes (polyurethane, Figure 22.4) (e.g., 8–10-Fr, 36–42 inch Infant Feeding Tube from Mallinckrodt Medical, St Louis, MO) or Foley catheters (10–12-Fr, 33 cm long for fillies and 64 cm long for colts; e.g., Foley Catheter, Kendall, Mansfield, MA). A closed system, with a sterile urine collection bag (e.g., Mono-Flo® Drainage Bag, Kendall, Mansfield, MA) should be used. In general, once maintenance fluid therapy is initiated, urine output should equal or exceed 50–60% of fluid input, unless excessive gastrointestinal or insensible (cutaneous or respiratory) losses are present.

Development of a fluid plan

The development of a fluid plan consists of four components: (i) type of fluid; (ii) rate; (iii) objectives or goals; and (iv) limits or potential complications.

Types

Crystalloids, colloids, or a combination can be used for fluid resuscitation of the hypovolemic foal. Crystalloids contain electrolytes and/or glucose dissolved in solution,

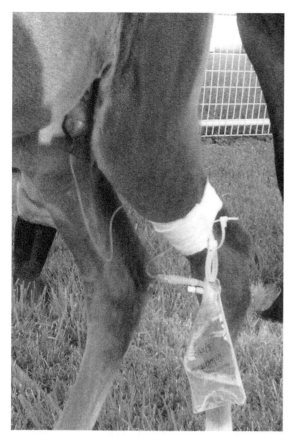

Figure 22.4 Infant feeding tube used as a urinary catheter in a colt.

while colloids contain large molecular weight (>5000 Da) particles, such as proteins or polysaccharides, which cannot freely cross the capillary endothelium. Fluids categorized as "replacement" crystalloids include hypertonic and isotonic crystalloids, as well as colloids such as hetastarch.

Hypertonic solutions, primarily referring to hypertonic saline, are not commonly used in foals, because foals may not be as tolerant of large sodium loads (Buchanan et al., 2005); their kidneys physiologically are not designed to eliminate large sodium loads under normal circumstances, as mare's milk is very low in sodium (7.3 ± 3.1 mEq/L) (Csapo et al., 2009). Therefore, there is potential for acute and marked hypernatremia and hyperchloremia to develop in response to hypertonic saline. This may be of particular concern in foals with renal disease or CNS injury. Therefore, balanced isotonic (or near isotonic) crystalloids are likely most

physiologic for foals during the resuscitation or replacement phase of fluid therapy.

"Maintenance" fluid therapy in foals is meant to maintain hydration, provide for abnormal ongoing losses such as diarrhea, or provide for diuresis as with azotemia. For maintenance, fluids must sustain hydration in both the ECF and ICF; free water is a necessity to ensure hydration of the ICF through osmolarity-induced distribution. Fluids available for maintenance fluid therapy include isotonic or hypotonic crystalloids. Isotonic fluids can be used as maintenance fluids when foals have an alternate free water source; this means that they are either nursing or being fed milk (or milk replacer) as milk is a free water source. In addition, isotonic crystalloids may be appropriate to use when ongoing losses are rich in sodium or electrolytes, such as with diarrhea or enteritis. Otherwise, in foals without access to oral milk, hypotonic fluids are often selected as maintenance fluids in order to prevent development of hypernatremia and interstitial edema, and to allow for hydration of the ICF.

Currently crystalloids are preferred over colloids as the resuscitative fluid type in human patients because of ease of administration, reduced expense, and concerns over safety with synthetic colloids. Recently, studies published by a particular author evaluating the use of hydroxyethyl starch (HES, hetastarch) in human patients have been retracted due to questions over the integrity of data (Boldt et al., 2009). A recent meta-analysis of fluid resuscitation with hydroxyethyl starch (HES) in humans found that published studies are of poor quality and report too few events to reliably estimate the benefits or risks of using 6% HES, regardless of whether the retracted studies were included or excluded (Gattas et al., 2012). A recent Cochrane review found no evidence from randomized controlled trials that colloids reduce the risk of death in human patients with critical illness or following surgery, when compared to resuscitation with crystalloids (Roberts, 2011). The conclusion was that since colloids are not associated with an improvement in survival and are more expensive than crystalloids, their continued use outside of randomized clinical trials cannot be justified (Roberts, 2011). A 2013 Cochrane Review of colloids versus crystalloids for fluid resuscitation in critically ill patients found that there is no evidence from randomized controlled trials that resuscitation with colloids reduces the risk of death as compared to crystalloids in patients with trauma, burns, or following surgery (Perel et al., 2013).

In addition, the review found suggestions that the use of hydroxyethyl starch might increase mortality (Perel et al., 2013). Another recent meta-analysis found similar mortality and renal failure concerns about hetastarch in humans (Zarychanski et al., 2013).

There are no published studies evaluating hetastarch in foals, and the number in adult horses is limited (Jones PA et al., 2001; Jones PH et al., 1997; Schusser et al., 2007). In adult horses, as in humans, hetastarch produces dose-dependent effects on hemostasis (Jones PH et al., 1997). These effects are repeatable at doses at or exceeding 10 mL/kg in adult horses. Other side effects of hetastarch described in humans include renal failure and hypersensitivities, though these appear to be uncommon (Hartog et al., 2011). Until further research of synthetic colloids documenting efficacy or safety is available in foals, the author prefers crystalloids for fluid resuscitation in foals. As for colloids, plasma is the author's preference for the neonatal foal until further research is available regarding synthetic colloids.

Plasma is commonly used in foals for failure of passive transfer and colloid support (especially when foals are hypoalbuminemic). However, it is not conducive to bolus administration as a resuscitative fluid because it must be thawed slowly and can be associated with adverse effects, especially if administered rapidly (Hardefeldt et al., 2010; Wilson et al., 2009). In a study of adult horses administered plasma, the incidence of adverse effects was 10%, and they included urticaria, tachycardia, tachypnea, pyrexia, pruritus, and swollen eyes (Wilson et al., 2009). In a retrospective study of 107 horses and foals that received plasma, 6/62 (9.7%) foals aged under 7 days experienced adverse reactions. The most common reactions included pyrexia, tachycardia, tachypnea, and colic (Hardefeldt et al., 2010). No animals died as a result of reactions to plasma. In light of these studies, foals administered plasma should be monitored for signs of systemic inflammation (fever, tachycardia, and tachypnea) and colic.

In human infants and pediatric patients, colloids have also failed to demonstrate a clear benefit over crystalloids (So et al., 1997). A systematic review of choice of fluids for resuscitation of children with severe sepsis and septic shock found that the current evidence on choice of fluids was weak (Akech et al., 2010). Eight clinical trials were reviewed, the majority of which involved children with malaria or dengue hemorrhagic shock.

Three of these studies (out of six that reported mortality) showed better survival in children resuscitated with colloids compared to crystalloids. However, because of limitations in methodology, caution in interpreting data was advised. Data regarding resuscitation of children with pediatric sepsis are even more limited. The conclusion was that definitive recommendations over choice of resuscitative fluid could not be made from available data (Akech et al., 2010). In a randomized controlled trial of 5% albumin versus isotonic saline for treatment of hypotension in mechanically ventilated preterm infants, there was no difference in the volume of the test solutions required between groups (So et al., 1997). In addition, the mortality rate, the number of infants requiring inotrope support, and the number with chronic lung disease did not differ between groups. In fact, the albumin group required significantly more volume than the saline group, in order to maintain normal blood pressure. The albumin group also had a higher percentage of weight gain by 48 h of age, indicating greater fluid retention (So et al., 1997). Another randomized open-label trial compared resuscitation of pediatric septic shock patients with normal saline or a gelatin polymer colloid solution (Upadhyay et al., 2005). Boluses of 20 mL/kg were used until either hemodynamic stabilization or a maximum (10 mmHg) CVP was reached. Approximately 110 mL/kg of saline and 70 mL/kg of gelatin polymer solution were required to successfully fluid resuscitate these patients. At the end of 1 hour the plasma, ECF, interstitial, and total body water volumes achieved were similar, indicating that both fluids were equally effective as resuscitation fluids. The need for inotropes, incidence of organ dysfunction, and case fatality were similar in the two groups (Upadhyay et al., 2005).

Rate

The rate of fluid delivery in foals is highly variable among clinicians and dependent on the degree of hypovolemia or hypoperfusion. Conventional approaches to fluid delivery have included estimation of the percentage of dehydration of the patient through clinical signs of dehydration and hypovolemia (5–12%). Five percent dehydration (i.e., loss of 5% of body weight in water) is regarded as the earliest that clinical signs of dehydration can be detected. Severe hypovolemic shock is thought to occur at 10–12% dehydration, which is associated with marked clinical and laboratory derangements including significant tachycardia and hemoconcentration. This method of estimating fluid deficits may not be highly accurate and potentially associated with error. The error may be compounded when attempting to estimate the degree of fluid loss from the various body water compartments.

An alternate fluid delivery plan, the "fluid challenge" method adapted from human critical care, circumvents these estimations (Vincent & Weil, 2006). Because it does not rely on estimations from clinical signs and laboratory data, this method of fluid therapy may be associated with reduced chances for error and fluid overloading.

In human critical care the fluid challenge method of resuscitative fluid delivery consists of the administration of sequential boluses of 6–18 mL/kg of replacement (isotonic) crystalloids over 30 minutes (Corley, 2002b; Palmer, 2002; Vincent & Weil, 2006). In foals an isotonic crystalloid dose of 10 mL/kg over 10–15 min has been recommended for foals with hypotension, followed with serial reassessment for the need for additional boluses (Corley, 2002b). The author commonly uses a dose of 10–20 mL/kg over 20–60 min for crystalloids (Box 22.1). Foals with mild to moderate hypovolemia may receive 10 mL/kg whereas foals with moderate to marked hypovolemic shock receive 20 mL/kg. In general the first bolus is administered rapidly (20–30 min) whereas each subsequent bolus is administered more slowly (30–60 min, or longer as signs of shock improve). Foals may require one to four of these boluses, with the majority requiring two to three challenges. Isotonic fluid challenges of 20 mL/kg are used in human pediatrics, with serial boluses administered until hemodynamic stabilization or a CVP limit of 10 mmHg is achieved (Upadhyay et al., 2005). Fluid volume and rates should be more conservative in foals at risk for tissue edema, particularly those with central nervous system disease (e.g., hypoxic-ischemic encephalopathy) or those with acute respiratory distress syndrome or anuric/oliguric renal failure.

Bolus administration of colloids, at a smaller dose of 3–10 mL/kg, may be used in addition to or instead of crystalloid fluids; if used, the colloid bolus should replace one or more of the crystalloid boluses in order to avoid hypervolemia. However, synthetic colloids require study in the neonatal foal, and currently there is no clear benefit in using colloids over crystalloids in human patients (Perel et al., 2013).

Serial reassessment of clinical response to fluid challenges

Serial and close reassessment of the hypovolemic patient is a critical component of the "fluid challenge" method of fluid administration. Reassessment is important for two reasons: (i) to target goals and (ii) to prevent fluid overload and overhydration. Clinical perfusion and hydration parameters should be evaluated at the completion of each fluid bolus in order to determine the need for further fluids. For perfusion, these parameters include extremity temperature, mentation, pulse quality, capillary refill time (CRT), and mucous membrane color. The production of urine is a positive sign that end organ perfusion (in this case renal) has been established, and rapid fluid boluses can be stopped or slowed. For hydration status, skin turgor, corneal texture, and globe position are assessed as indicators of extravascular fluid status.

This fluid challenge protocol of fluid resuscitation is meant to be conservative, with frequent reassessment of the foal's clinical signs, in order to avoid rapid alterations in central venous pressure and subsequent edema formation. Critically ill foals may have altered microvascular permeability and hypoproteinemia, both of which increase the risk of edema formation with increases in hydrostatic pressure after bolus administration of fluids. Reassessment of clinicopathologic indicators of perfusion status should also be performed, including measurement of serial lactate concentration, PCV, and TP concentration. Serial monitoring of arterial blood pressure and urine output should also be part of the reassessment.

Most recumbent and hypovolemic foals require two to three of these 10–20 mL/kg boluses administered over the first to several hours after presentation. A foal with persistent hypoperfusion, after having received 60–80 mL/kg of isotonic fluids, should be considered a candidate for inotrope therapy, followed by pressor therapy if blood pressure remains low.

Objectives

The goals of fluid therapy often include replacement of lost fluids (plasma and interstitial volume for correction of hypovolemia and dehydration, respectively); maintenance of hydration in a foal with water (i.e., milk) input that is below its requirements and losses; or diuresis for renal failure or urinary-excreted toxin removal. "Replacement fluid therapy" refers to fluid

---

Box 22.1 Replacement fluid therapy for the hypovolemic foal

1 Administer 10–20 mL/kg isotonic crystalloid over 20–60 minutes (time depending on degree of hypovolemia).
2 Reassess perfusion parameters and monitoring tools.
3 Each subsequent bolus administered more slowly (i.e., over 1 hour).
4 Continue until perfusion parameters normalize or stop improving.
5 Urine flow is an indicator of volume replacement with renal perfusion.
6 Maximal CVP is a limit to fluid boluses (10–12 cmH$_2$O or 7.4–9 mmHg).
7 If hypoperfusion is still evident, begin dobutamine infusion as an inotrope, followed by a pressor (norepinephrine or vasopressin).

---

resuscitation and is the administration of fluids to correct hypovolemia and dehydration. Dehydration refers to extravascular fluid loss, whereas hypovolemia is loss of intravascular fluids. The priority of replacement fluid therapy is correction of hypovolemia (volume resuscitation) first, followed by addressing interstitial deficits, and finally reversal of intracellular deficits. In "maintenance fluid therapy" the goal is to provide fluids necessary to maintain hydration status and fluid balance.

Specific goals of the fluid resuscitation phase (i.e., treatment of hypovolemia) include improvement of clinical, clinicopathologic, and monitoring criteria. One goal is to resolve abnormal perfusion parameters: improved mentation, pulse quality, extremity temperature, mucous membrane color, CRT, and urine production. A foal that previously was obtunded or stuporous in a recumbent state that now begins to struggle and require increased physical restraint after fluid bolus administration likely has improved cerebral hemodynamics. Urine production is one of the top goals of fluid resuscitation. It is an indirect indicator of organ perfusion, and is a reliable marker of enhanced perfusion in a previously anuric or oliguric foal. While urine production is best quantified with an indwelling urinary catheter, serial ultrasonographic examination of the bladder diameter during the resuscitative fluid phase is an effective means to monitor urine production if a urinary catheter is not in place. A bladder that increases in diameter during fluid therapy is a positive response

to fluid therapy. Packed cell volume and plasma or blood lactate concentrations are additional indirect means of detecting improved circulating volume, especially when they are evaluated serially. It should be noted that lactate concentrations may not normalize with fluid therapy in foals with SIRS states such as sepsis, even with re-establishment of perfusion. Hyperlactatemia in foals is multifactorial; causes include hypoperfusion, inflammation (cytokines may inhibit pyruvate dehydrogenase activity), activation of the sympathetic nervous system (catecholamine surges), liver or kidney dysfunction, and mitochondrial dysfunction, among others (see "Laboratory and monitoring tools in shock" above). Oxygen extraction ratio (or venous oxygen saturation) can be used to assess tissue perfusion. With reduced oxygen delivery the oxygen extraction ratio increases ($=S_aO_2$-S_vO_2/S_aO_2). A small study found an oxygen extraction ratio of $18\pm0.02\%$ in five healthy foals (Corley, 2002a). Optimally a central venous oxygen saturation would be measured rather than a jugular venous oxygen tension. Though mixed venous samples would be even more representative of global tissue oxygenation than central venous oxygen, they require a pulmonary arterial catheter, which is rarely used. Normal mixed venous oxygen tension in neonatal foals is 40.5 ± 0.4 mmHg in recumbent foals, and 35.9 ± 0.4 mmHg in standing foals (Madigan et al., 1992). Improvement in arterial blood pressure, including indirect blood pressure measured with a tail cuff, is another goal of fluid resuscitation. Blood pressure is highly variable among normal foals. Though it has been suggested that a blood pressure equal to or exceeding 65 mmHg should be targeted, premature and small foals may perfuse normally with lower pressures (Corley, 2002b).

Limits (endpoints)

Termination of the resuscitation phase of fluid therapy occurs when either goals are reached (urine flow, normalization of perfusion parameters, improvement in lactate, arterial blood pressure, and oxygen extraction ratios) or when limits are reached (maximum normal CVP, edema). For example, if dilute urine flow has been established in a neonatal foal, it is likely that the bolus fluid rate can be stopped or at least slowed.

Limits to resuscitative fluid boluses include a high normal CVP. A negative CVP and values below 2 cmH$_2$O are indicative of hypovolemia. CVP values within the normal range (2.3–12 cmH$_2$O, or 2.1–8.9 mmHg) do not rule out hypovolemia because they can be increased by raised pleural pressure, cardiac dysfunction, and venous tone as well; however, values above 12 cmH$_2$O (8.9 mmHg) represent a clear indication to stop rapid fluid administration. A risk of edema is present once CVP is above high normal. A decrease in arterial oxygen saturation as measured with pulse oximetry or arterial blood gas analyses, as well as an increase in respiratory rate or character, during fluid therapy also warrant decreases or discontinuation of fluid boluses, because these could be indicators of developing pulmonary edema.

Maintenance fluid therapy of the foal

Fluid administration rates

Maintenance fluid therapy of the neonatal foal is challenging, because every foal has unique requirements. In one study evaluating healthy nursing foals, it was found that consumption of milk was 24.6% of body weight per day in 11–18-day-old foals (Martin et al., 1992). Approximately 12.8 kg of milk was required per day for 1 kg of weight gain (Martin et al., 1992). Another study found a similar milk intake in 11-day-old foals, which was 27.0 ± 0.66% of body weight (Oftedal et al., 1983). In that study, daily water intake (through milk) was 25.5% of body weight. This is equivalent to a water intake of 10.6 mL/kg/h (Oftedal et al., 1983). Foals consumed 10–15% of body weight in milk replacer and water combined, equivalent to 100–150 ml/kg/day (4.2–6.3 mL/kg/h) (Cymbaluk et al., 1993). This suggests that the actual basal daily water requirements of the neonatal foal are closer to 4–6 mL/kg/h rather than 10 mL/kg/h.

Critically ill foals have wide variations in individual fluid requirements, likely dependent on metabolic rate, gestational age, ambient temperature, breed, surface area:mass ratio, growth rate, and underlying disease process. Foals with abnormal gastrointestinal fluid losses, such as those with diarrhea, have higher fluid requirements than those without significant losses; foals without excessive fluid losses, and particularly those at risk for developing tissue edema, have lower fluid requirements. Examples of the latter are foals with perinatal asphyxia syndrome, which are often challenging to provide maintenance fluids for; dehydration and hypovolemia should be avoided, in order to prevent further brain injury; however, excessive fluid administration risks edema formation.

In human pediatric medicine the Holliday–Segar formula is used to calculate maintenance fluid requirements in infants (Holliday & Segar, 1957). Some equine clinicians have adopted this formula for use in developing maintenance fluid plans for foals (Palmer, 2002):

(a) 100 mL/kg/day for the first 10 kg of the foal's body weight (i.e., 1–10 kg)

(b) +50 mL/kg/day for the second 10 kg of the foal's body weight (i.e., 11–20 kg)

(c) +25 mL/kg per day for the remainder of body weight (i.e., for weight in excess of 20 kg).

Based on this formula, a 50-kg foal would receive approximately 1000 mL/day for the first 10 kg of body weight + 500 mL/day for the second 10 kg of body weight + 750 mL for the remaining 30 kg of weight (25 mL/kg/day × 30 = 750 mL) = 2250 mL total per day. The hourly rate of fluid administration based on this formula is approximately 100 mL/h (or 2 mL/kg/h). This is considerably less than the rate of 4–6 mL/kg/h described above. This is a relatively *fluid restrictive* rate, also referred to as a "dry maintenance rate" (Palmer, 2002). Because of the wide discrepancy in these two fluid rates, foals on either protocol should be monitored for adequacy of fluid provision (with the lower rate) as well as fluid overload (with the higher rate). For foals that are not nursing or are intolerant of enteral feeding, where fluid provision is entirely through the parenteral route, the author usually starts with 4–6 mL/kg/h as the "maintenance rate" after the replacement phase of fluid therapy has been completed, and in foals without excessive fluid losses (Box 22.2). Foals that are nursing or being fed enterally usually require lower rates of IV fluid administration.

The variability in fluid needs of the newborn foal, compounded by the effects of specific illnesses, warrants frequent monitoring of the foal receiving IV fluids. Serial physical examinations and measurements of CVP, arterial blood pressure, urine output, and blood lactate concentrations are useful in monitoring the adequacy of fluid therapy and helping to protect from overload. Foals with high normal CVP values (12 cmH$_2$O, or 8.9 mmHg) should be especially monitored in order to prevent fluid overload; exceeding these CVP values would place the foal at risk for edema.

Additional laboratory monitoring includes measurement of serial hematocrit and TP concentrations.

Box 22.2 Maintenance fluid therapy in foals

1 Administer hypotonic maintenance fluids (osmolarity 112–150 mOsm/L) if access to oral water or milk is not available.
2 Isotonic fluids may be used if access to milk or water is available.
3 Begin with a rate of 4–6 mL/kg/h with frequent reassessment.
4 Monitor serum sodium closely.
5 If foal is nursing or being fed enterally, this rate may be decreased.
6 If abnormal ongoing losses are present, such as diarrhea or polyuria, the rate must be increased.
7 Abnormal losses should be replaced with isotonic fluids only.
8 Urine output is an excellent indicator of response to fluid therapy
   • Specific gravity should be 1.003–1.016 (unless foal is in renal failure, in which case it will be isosthenuric)
   • Frequency of urination should be 1–2 times per hour
9 Monitor closely for edema.

A single hematocrit or TP value should not necessarily define adequate hydration, because these can be misleading in that they may be artificially altered. These may be decreased due to anemia and protein loss, respectively, yet be in the normal range because of dehydration. Serial measurements of body weight (accounting for growth), blood urea nitrogen (BUN) and creatinine concentrations, and urine specific gravity are important monitoring tools for maintenance fluid therapy. Normal foals urinate every 1–2 hours until about 2 weeks of age (Kownacki et al., 1978; Tyler, 1969). This would seem a logical goal in foals being treated with fluid therapy. Light breeds of foals (Thoroughbreds and Standardbreds) gain 1.14 ± 0.041 kg per day (2.5 lb/day) (Oftedal et al., 1983). Weight gain markedly above this rate should warrant reassessment of fluid balance.

Electrolyte considerations with fluid therapy

Sodium

Neonatal foals have a relatively low requirement for sodium as indicated by the low sodium content of mare's milk ($\leq$20 mEq/L and $\leq$15 mEq/L on days 0–2 and

$\geq$3 days of lactation, respectively) (Csapo et al., 2009). They have been suspected of not eliminating large sodium loads, although this requires confirmation (Brewer et al., 1991). Therefore, a foal nursing 20% of its body weight in milk receives approximately 1.5–2.8 mEq/kg/day of sodium (Csapo et al., 2009).

A commercial isotonic replacement fluid (Normosol™-R) was evaluated as a maintenance fluid in healthy foals not allowed to nurse (Buchanan et al., 2005). It was administered at a rate of 3.3 mL/kg/h for 24 hours (Buchanan et al., 2005). As a result of administration of this fluid, serum sodium and osmolarity increased with fluid administration, as did urine sodium and osmolarity and the urine-to-serum osmolarity ratio. The rise in serum sodium concentration was one indication that this fluid was not an ideal maintenance fluid for foals. In addition, the decrease in urinary fractional excretion of potassium suggested that total body potassium stores decreased; the decrease was likely because foals were not allowed to nurse and they were not supplemented with potassium except for that contained in Normosol-R (5 mEq/L). Urine output (2.2–3.8 mL/kg/h) matched fluid input. The increases in urine specific gravity (1.015) and osmolarity (476 mOsm/L) and urine sodium concentration (162 mEq/L) by the end of the study suggest that the fluid input of 3.3 mL/kg/h was not physiologic; it appeared to be inadequate to maintain the normally hyposthenuric quality of neonatal foal urine. The urinary fractional excretion of sodium and chloride increased over time, indicating that foals were administered excessive amounts of sodium and chloride. The results of this study suggest that isotonic balanced electrolyte solutions, which are meant to be used as replacement fluids, are inappropriate for use as maintenance fluids in neonatal foals because of excessive sodium and inadequate provision of potassium (Buchanan et al., 2005). The study also suggested that the rate of 3.3 mL/kg/h may not be optimal for maintenance of hydration in foals that are not nursing (Buchanan et al., 2005).

Sodium derangements occur in neonatal foals. Both hyponatremia and hypernatremia should be corrected slowly in foals as in adult horses and other species. Hyponatremia should be corrected at a rate not exceeding 0.5 mEq/h in order to avoid central pontine myelinolysis associated with more rapid correction. If hyponatremia-induced seizures are present, hyponatremia can be partially corrected by increasing the plasma sodium concentration by 2–4 mEq/L rapidly (not to exceed 125 mEq/L) in order to abolish seizure activity. For example, if a foal is presented with seizures and a plasma sodium concentration of 110 mEq/L, increasing the sodium concentration to 112–114 mEq/L fairly rapidly may resolve the clinical signs of seizures. For the remainder of the correction (from 112–114 up to 130 mEq/L), the increase should approximate 0.5 mEq/h.

Hypernatremia should be corrected at a similarly slow rate of 0.5 mEq/h in terms of serum concentration of sodium, in order to avoid development of cerebral edema. Acute hypernatremia (developed over no more than a few hours) can be corrected more rapidly (up to 1–2 mEq/h) if it is well established that it indeed developed acutely. Otherwise, if the duration is unknown, the conservative rate should be used.

Potassium

Mare's milk is relatively high in potassium content (23.8 ± 1.9, 18.2 ± 3.5, and 13.3 ± 1.1 mEq/L on days 0–2, 3–5, and 8–45 days of lactation, respectively (Csapo et al., 2009). Many commercial mare's milk replacers have an even higher potassium concentration; in the author's experience use of milk replacers can result in higher baseline plasma potassium concentrations in foals (as high as 5–5.8 mEq/L). Because the normal intake of potassium is relatively high in foals, sick foals that are not consuming milk have little to no potassium ingestion and require supplemental potassium in IV fluids. Supplementation of fluids is usually empiric as it is for adult horses, with 10–40 mEq/L of potassium chloride usually supplemented depending on the existing plasma potassium concentration. For foals with hyperchloremia, potassium phosphate can be used for a portion of the supplementation (up to 10 mEq/L as potassium phosphate depending on plasma phosphorus concentrations). Potassium phosphate contains 4.4 mEq/mL of potassium and 3 mmol/mL of phosphate. Phosphorus can be safely supplemented at 0.01 mmol/kg/h, and at higher rates if hypophosphatemia present. A maximum safe dose of potassium supplementation is 0.5 mEq/kg/h. This should not be exceeded under normal circumstances, and without very careful and frequent monitoring.

Hyperkalemia may be present in critically ill foals, especially those with uroperitoneum (e.g., ruptured bladder, urachus, or ureter), acute renal failure (especially anuria or oliguria), hyperkalemic periodic paralysis (HYPP), severe rhabdomyolysis (e.g., white muscle disease), and

adrenal insufficiency. Hyperkalemia can be treated with administration of 20 mL/kg of 0.9% sodium chloride containing calcium (e.g., 0.4–1 mL/kg of 23% calcium gluconate depending on plasma calcium concentration) and 4–8 mg/kg/min of dextrose, with the fluid rate depending on the degree of hypovolemia. This can be followed by an additional 10–20 mL/kg of 0.9% sodium chloride containing 1 mEq/kg sodium bicarbonate and dextrose. Alternatively, isotonic sodium bicarbonate (150 mEq each of sodium and bicarbonate per liter; total osmolarity = 300 mOsm/L) can be used with added dextrose. Sodium bicarbonate and calcium should not be mixed in the same bag. Insulin may be required in cases of severe or refractory hyperkalemia or when hyperglycemia is already present (starting with 0.005–0.01 unit/kg/h IV of regular insulin). Cation exchange resins (sodium polystyrene sulfonate) can be administered as enemas or orally to absorb potassium. It should be noted that often the hyperkalemia is difficult to resolve until the source of the derangement is corrected. For example, foals with uroperitoneum are difficult to treat until the urine is drained from the abdomen. In the case of renal failure, hyperkalemia is difficult to resolve until urine production is initiated.

Calcium

Ionized calcium is the active form of calcium in plasma. Significant ionized hypocalcemia is uncommon in neonatal foals except in cases of prolonged anorexia or those with hypoparathyroidism or parathyroid dysfunction. Mild hypocalcemia is common among septic or endotoxemic foals. Alkalosis or rapid administration of sodium bicarbonate can reduce the ionized calcium fraction by increasing binding of calcium to albumin. Calcium supplementation of fluids is usually empiric and similar to that of potassium supplementation. The cut-offs for supplementation vary with clinician, but in general ionized calcium concentrations of 1.1–1.3 mmol/L are used as cut-offs to begin supplementation. Fluids are supplemented with 23% calcium gluconate at 0.2–1 mL/kg diluted in 1 L of fluid once (or as dictated by serial measurements of ionized calcium). The total volume of administered 23% calcium gluconate should not exceed 1 mL/kg unless warranted by ionized calcium concentrations.

Dextrose

Foals that have not been nursing or do not tolerate an adequate level of enteral nutrition require dextrose supplementation. Parenteral nutrition, consisting of dextrose, amino acids, and possibly lipids, is indicated if neonatal foals continue to be intolerant of enteral feeding within 12–24 hours. Foals with ileus or those with severe diarrhea, where they are intentionally withheld from nursing, are examples of foals requiring dextrose supplementation. The dextrose requirement of the late-term fetus has been determined to be 4–8 mg/kg/min (Silver & ComLine, 1976). Most foals maintain euglycemia with a dose rate of 4 mg/kg/min; however, foals with severe hypoglycemia or those with depletion of glycogen stores from prolonged lack of nursing may require up to 8 mg/ kg/min or more (to effect). The administration of 4 mg/ kg/min in fluids is equivalent to 5% dextrose in fluids when they are administered at a maintenance rate of 4–6 mL/kg/h; the percent dextrose varies with the administration rate. For example, a twice maintenance rate of 8 mL/kg/h would require 2.5% dextrose to yield this same rate of dextrose supplementation.

During bolus fluid administration (resuscitative phase) in foals with hypoglycemia or those that have been anorexic, fluids should contain only 0.6–1.2% dextrose if fluids are bolused at a rate of 20 mL/kg over 30 minutes in order to avoid hyperglycemia. Alternatively, the dextrose should be administered through a separate syringe pump at a rate of 4–8 mg/kg/min. Foals with marked hypoglycemia (<40 mg/dL) should receive at least 8 mg/kg/min, and to effect. Foals with hyperglycemia should not be administered dextrose until values decrease, and those with euglycemia (70–110 mg/dL) should be administered dextrose only if not nursing or being fed enterally.

Fluid types available for use in foals

Replacement crystalloids (Table 22.1)

Commercial balanced electrolyte solutions
These are isotonic or near isotonic crystalloids meant to be administered during the resuscitation phase of fluid therapy as a treatment for hypovolemia and/or dehydration. These include balanced electrolyte solutions such as lactated Ringer's solution, Plasma-Lyte A, Plasma-Lyte 148, and Normosol R, as well as physiologic saline, which is not a balanced solution as it only contains sodium and chloride.

The balanced electrolyte solutions have a number of similarities (Table 22.1), including near physiologic concentrations of sodium, chloride, and potassium. Plasma-Lyte A, Plasma-Lyte 148, and Normosol-R

have the same fluid composition. Plasma-Lyte A and Plasma-Lyte 148 are from Baxter Healthcare Corp. (Deerfield, IL) and Normosol-R is from Abbott Laboratories (North Chicago, IL). The difference between Plasma-Lyte A and Plasma-Lyte 148 lies solely with the *in vitro* pH. The pH of Plasma-Lyte 148 has a pH adjusted to 5.5 (range: 4.0–8.0). Plasma-Lyte A pH is adjusted to 7.4 (range: 6.5–8.0). While the pH of 7.4 sounds optimal, the *in vitro* pH has little effect on the overall pH of the patient. The titratable acidity contained within the bags is very little. However, there may be an advantage of a pH of 7.4 in Plasma-Lyte A in terms of endothelial integrity in the catheterized veins, especially with long-term fluid therapy, although this remains to be studied. Exposure of the endothelium to high flow rates of a fluid with a pH of 7.4 is likely to be more physiologic than to one with an acidic pH.

The potassium content of these fluids is similar; Plasma-Lyte 148 and A have a potassium concentration of 5 mEq/L and lactated Ringer's solution (LRS) has a concentration of 4 mEq/L. This should be a consideration in foals with significant hyperkalemia such as oliguric renal failure, severe rhabdomyolysis, or HYPP. Plasma-Lyte 148/A and Normosol-R fluids contain a sodium concentration of 140 mEq/L, whereas LRS has a sodium content of 130 mEq/L. The chloride content is 98 and 109 mEq/L, respectively. Therefore, the electrolyte contents of Plasma-Lyte and Normosol are more similar to normal equine plasma than is LRS. The chloride content of LRS (109 mEq/L) is relatively high compared to that of equine plasma (90–100 mEq/L), while the sodium content is at the low end of the normal range; this can potentially produce a mild hyperchloremia in foals administered large volumes of LRS. This gives a sodium–chloride difference of 42 for the Plasma-Lyte/ Normosol fluids and a difference of 21 for LRS. The former fluids are more physiologic in this regard, as the normal sodium–chloride difference in equine plasma is approximately 40. This provides a neutral to alkalinizing effect from an electrolyte (simplified strong ion difference) content, whereas LRS may be acidifying when considered purely from an electrolyte standpoint, although it is alkalinizing once the lactate is metabolized. There is a larger strong ion difference (SID) in Plasma-Lyte 148 or A (effective SID = 50 mEq/L as opposed to approximately 28 mEq/L in LRS), which is preferred in patients with metabolic acidosis. In addition, the sodium and chloride contents of these

Table 22.1 Comparison of the fluid composition of commercial replacement crystalloids

	Lactated Ringer's solution	Normal saline	Plasma-Lyte® A	Plasma-Lyte® 148	Normosol™-R
Sodium (mEq/L)	130	154	140	140	140
Potassium (mEq/L)	4	0	5	5	5
Chloride (mEq/L)	109	154	98	98	98
Calcium (mEq/L)	3	0	0	0	0
Magnesium (mEq/L)	0	0	3	3	3
Base (mEq/L)	28L[a]	0	27A23G[a]	27A23G[a]	27A23G[a]
Osmolality (mOsm/kg)	272	308	295	295	295
Calories (kcal/L)	9	0	21	21	21
pH in bag	6.5	5.5	7.4	5.5	6.6

[a] L, lactate; A, acetate; G, gluconate.

acetated fluids are the closest to equine plasma of all the commercially available fluids.

Differences among these fluids include the alkalinizing salt as well as the divalent cation included. Plasma-Lyte and Normosol contain acetate (27 mEq/L) and gluconate (23 mEq/L), whereas LRS contains sodium lactate (28 mEq/L). These salts are metabolized to sodium bicarbonate (consuming hydrogen ions) and are therefore alkalinizing. Acetate is metabolized primarily by muscle tissue, but also by the kidneys, liver, and other tissues; gluconate is metabolized by many tissues. Lactate is metabolized primarily by the liver, where it ultimately undergoes gluconeogenesis or is oxidized to carbon dioxide and water, leading to a minor contribution of base through consumption of hydrogen ions. These alkalinizing salts have indications in certain circumstances. Lactate metabolism is reduced in horses with liver dysfunction and therefore the acetated fluids are optimal. It should be noted that the lactate in LRS is the sodium lactate form, which is not acidifying as is lactic acid. In dogs with lymphosarcoma, lactate metabolism is reduced as well (Vail et al., 1990). The accumulation of lactate within plasma, even independent of acidifying effects, is detrimental to myocardial function, and therefore avoidance of LRS in foals with liver failure is optimal when other fluid choices are available.

In terms of differences in divalent cations, LRS contains calcium (3 mEq/L) whereas the acetated fluids (Plasma-Lyte 148/A and Normosol-R) contain magnesium (3 mEq/L). The calcium in LRS precludes its use in the same lines as blood products, because calcium binds citrate and other calcium antagonists. In addition, sodium bicarbonate should not be directly added to LRS, because microprecipitation of calcium and bicarbonate may occur. Because calcium participates in the pathophysiology of cell necrosis, LRS may be best avoided where tissue necrosis is ongoing, especially that of the myocardium and central nervous system. In addition, magnesium, as in Normosol or Plasma-Lyte, may be beneficial to foals with cardiac disease, severe rhabdomyolysis, and central neurologic disease (head trauma, peripartum asphyxia), as it has antiarrhythmic properties and serves to antagonize calcium, which plays a role in the pathophysiology of muscle and nerve cell necrosis. LRS may be preferred to the acetated fluids in cases where magnesium is to be avoided, namely neuromuscular diseases such as botulism.

Lactated Ringer's solutions traditionally have been available as racemic mixtures of D- and L-lactate. Currently most brands of LRS contain only L-lactate. L-Lactate is optimal because D-lactate in racemic fluids is not metabolized by mammalian tissues, does not contribute to alkalinity, requires renal elimination, and may be inflammatory. Another advantage of LRS for neonates specifically is that lactate may be preferentially utilized over glucose as a metabolic fuel by the neonatal brain, at least as demonstrated in dogs (Young et al., 1991). Nuclear magnetic resonance spectroscopy has shown that during lactate infusion the metabolism of lactate could account for most of the metabolic fuel in neonates. Whether this applies to foals remains to be studied.

The acetated fluids can be administered with blood products as well as sodium bicarbonate. Because muscle tissue is heavily involved with acetate metabolism these fluids are good choices for animals with liver disease.

Sodium chloride (0.9% sodium chloride)

Physiologic saline (0.9% sodium chloride, normal saline) is a near isotonic (308 mEq/L) fluid containing sodium and chloride ions. Because saline lacks other electrolytes it is not considered a balanced polyionic fluid; it is not an optimal first-line crystalloid for general use. Its primary indications include:

1 Severe hyperkalemia – it is the only readily available fluid that is free of potassium. Hyperkalemia occurs with oliguric renal failure, severe rhabdomyolysis, HYPP, uroperitoneum, and adrenal dysfunction.
2 Metabolic alkalosis due to hypochloremia.
3 As a drug diluent.

Because of its high chloride content, saline has a sodium-to-chloride ratio of 154:154 or 1:1, which is greater than that of equine plasma, which has approximately 130–140 mEq/L sodium and 90–102 mEq/L of chloride. This relative increase in chloride causes saline to produce a mild strong ion acidosis – hyperchloremic metabolic acidosis (HCMA). Saline would be useful in foals with primary metabolic alkaloses; however, these are uncommon. Because acidoses are more common in the acutely ill foal, saline is not routinely indicated. In laboratory species, HCMA has been shown to be proinflammatory (Kellum et al., 2006). In human patients undergoing abdominal surgery, patients who received 0.9% saline had a higher mortality rate and increased rate of complications, including renal failure and postoperative infection, than those patients administered Plasma-Lyte 148 or A (Shaw et al., 2012).

Isotonic sodium bicarbonate

Sodium bicarbonate is commercially available as 8.4% and 5% solutions. These solutions are hypertonic and not meant for direct administration except under special circumstances because the hypertonicity can have adverse effects on the vascular endothelium. If diluted to a 1.3% solution in water, sodium bicarbonate is isotonic, similar to the commercial replacement fluids. Isotonic sodium bicarbonate can be made by adding 150 mEq of "sodium bicarbonate" (150 mEq of sodium, 150 mEq of bicarbonate) per liter of sterile water. However, in most instances it is not bolused in shock doses because of the potential adverse effects of bolus administration of sodium bicarbonate (see below). It is most often indicated as a replacement fluid (often as one part of the replacement plan) in foals with inorganic acidoses, such as those with hyperchloremia or hyponatremia. Examples of equine diseases with these electrolyte derangements include enteritis, renal tubular acidosis, and uroperitoneum where acidosis is present. It is often utilized in conjunction with other fluids because the amount of sodium bicarbonate administered should not exceed the bicarbonate deficit of the foal (see calculation below); for example, it may be co-administered with 0.9% saline to a foal with uroperitoneum if the foal has some degree of acidemia.

It should be noted that rapid bolus administration of sodium bicarbonate is potentially associated with adverse effects and should be avoided unless the low pH is life threatening; it should be bolused only until the pH equals or exceeds 7.2. Foals administered sodium bicarbonate should be monitored for hypokalemia, decreases in ionized calcium, metabolic alkalosis, and hypercapnia (especially if hypoventilation is present). It should be used with extreme caution in foals with hypoventilation. Rapid alkalinization may also result in left shift in the oxygen dissociation curve, which can decrease offloading of oxygen from hemoglobin in the periphery. Theoretically, rapid administration of sodium bicarbonate can also result in paradoxical intracellular acidosis.

A safe means of administration of sodium bicarbonate is to calculate half of the estimated bicarbonate deficit (body weight in kg × base deficit × 0.4). This can be administered after replacement of fluid deficits, and once the base deficit has been reassessed.

Maintenance fluids (Table 22.2)

Maintenance fluids are designed to maintain hydration in all fluid compartments. This refers to the phase that occurs after the "replacement" phase of fluid therapy has been completed; these are distinct phases of fluid therapy – replacement and maintenance. True "maintenance fluids" are hypotonic and provide free water (solute free) in addition to electrolytes for distribution into the intracellular and extracellular spaces. The tonicity of these fluids is generally in the 110–150 mOsm/L range. The hypotonicity allows for distribution of water into the cells, as osmotic gradient is the primary determinant of fluid movement between the

Table 22.2 Composition of maintenance fluids

Crystalloid	Sodium	Chloride	Potassium	Calcium	Magnesium	Anion	Osm
Normosol™-M	40	40	13	0	3	16 Acetate	112
Plasma-Lyte® 56	40	40	13	0	3	16 Acetate	112
0.45% NaCl/2.5% dextrose	77	77	0	0	0	0	280 (140 *in vivo*)
5% dextrose	0	0	0	0	0	0	252 (0 *in vivo*)
Plasma-Lyte® A mixed with sterile water (1:1 ratio)	70	49	2.5	0	1.5	13.5 Acetate 11.5 Gluconate	148

ECF and ICF. Because of this hypotonicity, maintenance fluids must not be administered as a bolus.

Replacement fluids (isotonic) are commonly used as maintenance fluids in equine practice. This is acceptable in foals that are nursing or tolerant of milk feeding and that have reasonably normal renal function, but that may require additional fluids. True hypotonic maintenance fluids are indicated in neonatal foals that are intolerant of enteral feeding due to ileus, reflux, diarrhea, colic, or prematurity and need alternate sources of fluid input; in such foals continued use of replacement fluids without some amount of free water often results in hypernatremia (Buchanan et al., 2005). Neonatal foals produce hyposthenuric urine (urine specific gravity of 1.001–1.010) with a low sodium concentration because milk contains very little sodium (7–13 mEq/L). In the absence of milk ingestion, the sodium load provided by long-term use of replacement fluids may be excessive when used as maintenance fluids in foals (Buchanan et al., 2005).

One concern with the use of hypotonic fluids in humans is the potential for development of hyponatremia associated with the lower sodium content (Alves et al., 2011; Rey et al., 2011; Saba et al., 2011). Randomized clinical trials have demonstrated significantly greater decreases in plasma sodium concentrations among human patients receiving hypotonic solutions as compared to those on isotonic fluids (Brazel & McPhee, 1996; Kannan et al., 2010; Montanana et al., 2008; Neville et al., 2009). Therefore, there is considerable debate as to whether isotonic or hypotonic fluids should be utilized for maintenance purposes in hospitalized children (Alves et al., 2011; Rey et al., 2011; Saba et al., 2011). Iatrogenic hyponatremia may result in neurologic cell injury or death (Arieff et al., 1992; McJunkin et al., 2001; McRae et al., 1994; Paut et al., 2000; Playfor, 2003; Soroker et al., 1991).

However, in many of these reported cases of hyponatremia associated with hypotonic fluids, the fluids were administered at rates well above those recommended for maintenance fluid therapy in children, and this may be the reason for the adverse effects. Many studies had potential confounders or special circumstances that make direct comparison of isotonic replacement and hypotonic maintenance fluids difficult. They were either limited to critically ill children who may have required further isotonic fluids than they had received or had derangements in antidiuretic hormone, or they included intraoperative study periods, which are quite distinct physiologically from patients presented in hypovolemic shock. Finally, some of the studies compared 0.9% saline with 0.18% saline, the latter of which is rarely used because of a clear risk of hyponatremia (Brazel & McPhee, 1996; Kannan et al., 2010; Montanana et al., 2008; Neville et al., 2009). Saline with 0.18% sodium chloride would have an osmolarity of 62 mOsm/L, which is below that of commercial maintenance fluids (112 mOsm/L), and would therefore have greater risk of inducing hyponatremia. A recent randomized controlled clinical trial in children (both medical and postoperative patients, aged 3 months to 18 years) compared 0.45% saline and 0.9% saline infused as a maintenance fluid for 12 hours (Saba et al., 2011). In this study the sodium concentration significantly increased in the 0.9% group, and also increased, though not significantly, in the 0.45% group. Hyponatremia was not a problem in that study, which compared actual maintenance and replacement fluids as they would be used in neonatal foals, but additional studies are required.

Until further information about the use of fluids in foals is available, plasma sodium concentration should be monitored closely in critically ill foals receiving fluids, regardless of fluid type used. Foals with cerebral disease, such as neonatal encephalopathy or traumatic or hypoxic brain injury, should be monitored especially closely as rapid decreases in plasma sodium concentration can cause or potentiate cerebral edema.

Hypotonic fluids may be particularly indicated for maintenance fluid purposes in foals that do not receive enteral milk or other sources of free water because of ileus, abdominal distention, or colic. Even healthy foals prevented from nursing their dams demonstrated an increase in plasma sodium and chloride concentrations in response to isotonic fluids (Normosol-R) used for maintenance purposes at a rate of 3.3 mL/kg/h (Buchanan et al., 2005). It is important, however, to note that hypotonic fluids should never be administered at a rate greater than that calculated for maintenance requirements (especially as boluses) in order to avoid development of hyponatremia. If higher rates of fluids are required then isotonic fluids should be used to provide the balance, particularly because most abnormal fluid losses are from the ECF, not the ICF. For example, if a foal requires a "twice maintenance" rate for fluid therapy because of diarrhea, then only the baseline maintenance rate (4–6 mL/kg/h) should be provided as hypotonic maintenance fluids. The balance should be provided as isotonic fluids. This is physiologically most appropriate, because most foals requiring rates above a maintenance rate are losing fluids from the ECF, as with diarrhea, reflux, or polyuria, which are electrolyte rich; in such cases an isotonic fluid is most appropriate for replacement of that portion of the fluid loss.

Plasma-Lyte® 56 or Normosol™-M

Commercial maintenance fluids have included Plasma-Lyte 56 (Baxter Healthcare Corporation, Deerfield, IL) and Normosol-M (Abbott Laboratories, North Chicago, IL), which are essentially the same fluid in terms of composition, just manufactured by different companies. However, these products are currently off the market. The osmolarity of these fluids is 111–112 mEq/L. The sodium concentration is lower (40 mEq/L) and the potassium concentration is higher (13 mEq/L) than their replacement counterparts (140 and 5 mEq/L, respectively, in Plasma-Lyte 148 or A and Normosol-R). They also contain magnesium (3 mEq/L), but lack calcium, similar to the replacement fluids.

These fluids contain acetate (16 mEq/L) as the alkalinizing salt, but lack the gluconate found in Plasma-Lyte 148 or A and Normosol-R. Another notable difference between these maintenance fluids and their counterpart replacement fluids is the sodium-to-chloride ratio, which is 1:1 in the maintenance versions (40 mEq/L of each), whereas it is 1.4:1 in the replacement versions (140 mEq/L of sodium and 98 mEq/L of chloride). A narrow sodium:chloride difference represents a slight disadvantage for acidotic patients with hyperchloremia or hyponatremia.

0.45% Saline and 2.5% dextrose

This is a solution of half-strength saline and half-strength dextrose. It is near iso-osmolar *in vitro* (280 mOsm/L); however, once the dextrose is metabolized after administration the fluid is essentially half-iso-osmolar because only the sodium chloride remains (154 mOsm/L). The sodium:chloride ratio of this fluid is 1:1 (77 mEq/L of each), which is slightly disadvantageous from an acid–base point of view because the sodium–chloride difference is 0. This solution lacks potassium, calcium, and other electrolytes, as well as alkalinizing agents. The advantage of this solution is that it is ready to use without having to add dextrose.

Additional formulations of maintenance fluids (not commercially available)

If commercial maintenance fluids are unavailable or a balanced solution is preferred, similar versions can be developed from dilution of replacement fluids. This consists of the administration of one-half the desired fluid rate as 5% dextrose in water (D5W) and one-half as replacement fluid (such as Normosol-R, Plasma-Lyte 148 or A, or LRS). The osmolarity of this mixture is approximately half iso-osmolar *in vivo*. For example, if the fluid administration target is 300 mL/h, this would comprise 150 mL of Plasma-Lyte A and 150 mL of 5% dextrose in water. Sterile water can replace the D5W if dextrose is not desired for the specific case; however, it is imperative that the sterile water be mixed with the isotonic fluid **prior to** entering the foal's vein to prevent entry of water with an osmolarity of 0. Hemolysis and potential endothelial damage may occur with exposure to plain water and a sudden decrease in osmolarity. As with any other maintenance fluids, these mixtures should not be used in a bolus manner.

Intravenous catheterization in foals

Veins available for catheterization in foals include the jugular, cephalic, lateral thoracic, and saphenous veins. The jugular vein is used most often, and a central venous catheter can be placed into the cranial vena cava with a 20–30 cm jugular catheter inserted into the jugular vein, depending on the size of foal. For foals that have a compromised jugular vein (thrombosis, thrombophlebitis, phlebitis), catheters should be placed in other veins to prevent bilateral jugular disease. The author's preferred alternative site is the cephalic vein in foals; triple lumen 7-Fr catheters (e.g., Arrow Central Venous Catheterization Kit, 20 or 30 cm) can be placed in the cephalic vein.

Consideration of catheter material should be made, particularly in foals with sepsis that have hypercoagulation. A study in adult horses suggested that silastic and polyurethane catheters were the least reactive for long-term jugular vein catheterization (2–4 weeks) (Spurlock et al., 1990). Polytetrafluoroethylene catheters caused marked reactions (Spurlock et al., 1990). However, a study of adult horse colic cases demonstrated no difference in the incidence of thrombophlebitis between polytetrafluoroethylene and polyurethane catheters (Lankveld et al., 2001). Despite these conflicting study results, polyurethane should be used whenever available.

Complications of fluid therapy

Complications of fluid therapy of the neonatal foal include fluid overload, electrolyte disturbances, and catheter-related adverse effects. Fluid overload is more likely to occur in foals than in adult horses, as the interstitium in neonatal foals is relatively more compliant and edema may not be noted until late. These foals look and feel "jelly like". Fluid overload causes tissue edema, with particular concern over pulmonary and CNS edema, and increasing oxygen diffusion distance within organs.

Prevention of fluid overload and edema is dependent on close and frequent monitoring of the foal receiving fluid therapy. Serial measurement of CVP, serial body weight measurements (accounting for growth), and serial arterial blood gas analyses or oxygen saturation are all means of preventing fluid overload.

The normal CVP in neonatal foals ranges from 2.1 to 8.9 mmHg (2.8–12 cmH$_2$O), and supranormal values can be markers of fluid overload (in addition to other rule outs such as cardiac dysfunction) (Thomas et al., 1987). Though there is controversy as to the reliability of CVP as an indicator of the adequacy of plasma volume status, it is a reasonable limit to fluid bolus administration (Madger & Bafaqeeh, 2007). If CVP approaches 10–12 cmH$_2$O (7.5–9 mmHg) or if serial arterial oxygen saturation (as measured with serial pulse oximetry or arterial blood gas analyses) decreases during bolus fluid resuscitation, then the rate of fluid administration should be re-evaluated as these changes could signify potential for fluid overload. Decreases in oxygen saturation during bolus fluid administration can signify developing pulmonary edema. If clinical signs and markers of hypoperfusion (e.g., poor pulse quality, cold extremities, poor urine output, high lactate concentrations) persist at the point of a high normal CVP measurement, then inotrope and pressor therapy should be considered instead of continuing fluid boluses.

Urine production in a neonatal foal receiving IV fluid therapy is a reliable indicator of end organ perfusion and in most cases signifies that the fluid boluses can be slowed or discontinued and the maintenance fluid plan can be developed. Normal foals urinate every 1–2 hours until about 2 weeks of age, and foals receiving IV fluids should be doing the same as an indicator of provision of adequate fluid volume (Kownacki et al., 1978; Tyler, 1969). On the other hand, a foal that is urinating every 15–30 minutes may be receiving a higher fluid rate than is necessary, unless diuresis is desired.

Electrolyte derangements, namely sodium and chloride disorders, can occur with large-volume fluid resuscitation or prolonged maintenance fluid administration, particularly in foals with renal dysfunction or those that are intolerant of milk feeding. Administration of hypertonic saline boluses can lead to hypernatremia in neonatal foals and should be used judiciously and cautiously in the neonatal foal. The use of isotonic fluids for maintenance fluid purposes in foals not receiving enteral milk can lead to hypernatremia over time as well (Buchanan et al., 2005). In addition, administration of hypertonic saline or large volumes of isotonic saline can lead to hyperchloremic metabolic acidosis in foals.

Hyponatremia may result from inappropriate bolus or excessive administration of hypotonic maintenance fluids, and therefore the maintenance phase of fluid therapy should be distinct from that of replacement. Also, foals on hypotonic IV maintenance fluids should be serially monitored for hyponatremia.

References

Akech S, Ledermann H, Maitland K. (2010) Choice of fluids for resuscitation in children with severe infection and shock: systematic review. *Brit Med J* **341**:c4416.

Alves JTL, Troster EJ, de Oliveira CAC. (2011) Isotonic saline solution as maintenance intravenous fluid therapy to prevent acquired hyponatremia in hospitalized children. *Jornal de Pediatria* **87**:478–86.

Andrews FM, Nadeau JA, Saabye L, et al. (1997) Measurement of total body water content in horses, using deuterium oxide dilution. *Am J Vet Res* **58**:1060–4.

Arieff AI, Ayus JC, Fraser CL. (1992) Hyponatraemia and death or permanent brain damage in healthy children. *Brit Med J* **304**:1218–22.

Boldt J, Suttner S, Brosch C, Lehmann A, Rohm K, Mengistu A. (2009) Cardiopulmonary bypass priming using a high dose of a balanced hydroxyethyl starch versus an albumin-based priming strategy. *Anesth Analg* **109**:1752–62.

Borchers A, Wilkins PA, Marsh PM, et al. (2012) Association of admission L-lactate concentration in hospitalized equine neonates with presenting complaint, periparturient events, clinical diagnosis and outcome: a prospective multicentre study. *Equine Vet J Suppl* **41**:57–63.

Brazel PW, McPhee IB. (1996) Inappropriate secretion of anti-diuretic hormone in postoperative scoliosis patients: the role of fluid management. *Spine (Phila Pa 1976)* **21**:724–7.

Brewer BD, Clement SF, Lotz WS. (1991) Renal clearance, urinary excretion of endogenous substances, and urinary diagnostic indices in healthy neonatal foals. *J Vet Int Med* **5**:28–33.

Buchanan BR, Sommardahl CS, Rohrbach BW, Andrews FM. (2005) Effect of a 24-hour infusion of an isotonic electrolyte replacement fluid on the renal clearance of electrolytes in healthy neonatal foals. *J Am Vet Med Assoc* **227**:1123–9.

Carlson GP, Harold D, Rumbaugh GE. (1979a) Volume dilution of sodium thiocyanate as a measure of extracellular fluid volume in the horse. *Am J Vet Res* **40**:587–9.

Carlson GP, Rumbaugh GE, Harrold DR. (1979b) Physiologic alterations produced by food and water deprivation during periods of high environmental temperatures. *Am J Vet Res* **40**:982–5.

Corley KTT. (2002a) Monitoring and treating haemodynamic disturbances in critically ill neonatal foals. Part 1: haemodynamic monitoring. *Equine Vet J* **14**:270–9.

Corley KTT. (2002b) Monitoring and treating haemodynamic disturbances in critically ill neonatal foals. Part 2: assessment and treatment. *Equine Vet J* **14**:328–36.

Csapo J, Salamon Sz, Loki K, Csapo-K Zs. (2009) Composition of mare's colostrum and milk II. Protein content, amino acid composition and contents of macro- and micro-elements. *Acta Univ Sapientiae, Alimentaria* **2**:133–48.

Cymbaluk NF, Smart ME, Bristol FM, Pouteaux VA. (1993) Importance of milk replacer intake and composition in rearing orphan foals. *Can Vet J* **34**:479–86.

Dellinger RP, Levy MM, Rhodes A, et al. (2013) Surviving sepsis campaign: international guidelines for management of severe sepsis and septic shock: 2012. *Crit Care Med* **41**:580–637.

Doreau M, Dussap G. (1980) Estimation de la production laitière de la jument allaitante par marquage de l'eau corporelle du poulain. *Reprod Nutr Develop* **20**:1883–92.

Edwards DJ, Brownlow MA, Hutchins DR. (1990) Indices of renal function: values in eight normal foals from birth to 56 days. *Aust Vet J* **67**:251–4.

Evans JW. (1971) Effect of fasting, gestation, lactation and exercise on glucose turnover in horses. *J Anim Sci* **33**:1001–4.

Fielding CL, Magdesian KG, Elliott DA, Craigmill AL, Wilson WD, Carlson GP. (2003) Pharmacokinetics and clinical utility of sodium bromide (NaBr) as an estimator of extracellular fluid volume in horses. *J Vet Intern Med* **17**:213–17.

Fielding CL, Magdesian KG, Edman JE. (2011) Determination of body water compartments in neonatal foals by use of indicator dilution techniques and multifrequency bioelectrical impedance analysis. *Am J Vet Res* **72**:1390–6.

Ford N, Hargreaves S, Shanks L. (2012) Mortality after fluid bolus in children with shock due to sepsis or severe infection: a systematic review and meta-analysis. *PLoS One* **7**:e43953; doi: 10.1371/journal.pone.0043953.

Forro M, Cieslar S, Ecker GL, et al. (2000) Total body water and ECFV measured using bioelectrical impedance analysis and indicator dilution in horses. *J Appl Physiol* **89**:663–71. Franco RM, Ousey JC, Cash RS, et al. (1986) Study of arterial blood pressure in newborn foals using an electronic sphygmomanometer. *Equine Vet J* **18**:475–8.

Gattas DJ, Dan A, Myburgh J, Billot L, Lo S, Finfer S, The CHEST Management Committee. (2012) Fluid resuscitation with 6% hydroxyethyl starch (130/0.4) in acutely ill patients: an updated systematic review and meta analysis. *Anesth Analg* **114**:159–69.

Groenendyk S, English PB, Abetz I. (1988) External balance of water and electrolytes in the horse. *Equine Vet J* **20**:189–93.

Hardefeldt LY, Keuler N, Peek SF. (2010) Incidence of transfusion reactions to commercial equine plasma. *J Vet Emerg Crit Care* **20**:421–5.

Hartog CS, Bauer M, Reinhart K. (2011) The efficacy and safety of colloid resuscitation in the critically ill. *Anesth Analg* **112**:156–64.

Holliday MA, Segar WE. (1957) The maintenance need for water in parenteral fluid therapy. *Pediatrics* **19**:823–32.

Jeffcott L. (1972) Observations on parturition in crossbred pony mares. *Equine Vet J* **4**:209–13.

Jeffcott LB. (1974) Some practical aspects of the transfer of passive immunity to newborn foals. *Equine Vet J* **6**:109.

Jeffcott LB, Jeffcott TJ. (1974) Studies on passive immunity in the foal. III. The characterization and significance of neonatal proteinuria. *J Comp Path* **84**:455–65.

Jones PA, Bain FT, Byars TD, David JB, Boston RC. (2001) Effect of hydroxyethyl starch infusion on colloid oncotic pressure in hypoproteinemic horses. *J Am Vet Med Assoc* **218**:1130–5.

Jones PH, Tomasic M, Gentry PA. (1997) Oncotic, hemodilutional, and hemostatic effects of isotonic saline and hydroxyethyl starch solutions in clinically normal ponies. *Am J Vet Res* **58**:541–8.

Judson GJ, Frauenfelder HC, Mooney GJ. (1983) Plasma biochemical changes in Thoroughbred racehorses following submaximal and maximal exercise. In: Snow DH, Persson SGB, Rose RJ (eds) *Equine Exercise Physiology*. Cambridge: Granta Editions, pp. 408–15.

Julian LM, Lawrence JH, Berlin NI, et al. (1956) Blood volume, body water and body fat of the horse. *J Appl Physiol* **8**:651–3.

Kannan L, Lodha R, Vivekanandhan S, Bagga A, Kabra SK, Kabra M. (2010) Intravenous fluid regimen and hyponatraemia among children: a randomized controlled trial. *Pediatr Nephrol* **25**:2303–9.

Kellum JA, Mingchen S, Almasri E. (2006) Hyperchloremic acidosis increases circulating inflammatory molecules in experimental sepsis. *Chest* **130**:962–7.

Kohn CW, Muir WW, Sams R. (1978) Plasma volume and extracellular fluid volume in horses at rest and following exercise. *Am J Vet Res* **59**:871–4.

Kownacki M, Sasimowski E , Budzynski M, et al. (1978) Observations of the twenty-four hour rhythm of natural behavior of Polish primitive horse bred for conservation of genetic resources in a forest reserve. *Genet Pol* **19**:61–77.

Lankveld DPK, Ensink JM, van Dijk P, Klein WR. (2001) Factors influencing the occurrence of thrombophlebitis after postsurgical long-term intravenous catheterization of colic horses: a study of 38 cases. *J Vet Med* **48**:545–52.

Madger S, Bafaqeeh. (2007) The clinical role of central venous pressure measurements. *J Intensive Care Med* **22**:44–51.

Madigan JE, Thomas WP, Backus KQ, et al. (1992) Mixed venous blood gases in recumbent and upright positions in foals from birth to 14 days of age. *Equine Vet J* **24**:399–401.

Magdesian KG. (2003) Blood lactate levels in neonatal foals: normal values and temporal effects in the post-partum period. *J Vet Emerg Crit Care* **13**:174.

Marcilese NA, Valsecchi RM, Figueiras HD, Camberos HR, Varela JE. (1964) Normal blood volumes in the horse. *Am J Physiol* **207**:223–7.

Martin RG, McMeniman NP, Dowsett KF. (1992) Milk and water intakes of foals sucking grazing mares. *Equine Vet J* **24**:295–9.

McJunkin JE, de los Reyes EC, Irazuzta JE, et al. (2001) La Crosse encephalitis in children. *N Engl J Med* **344**:801–7.

McRae RG, Weissburg AJ, Chang KW. (1994) Iatrogenic hyponatremia: a cause of death following pediatric tonsillectomy. *Int J Pediatr Otorhinolaryngol* **30**:227–32.

Montanana PA, Modesto i Alapont V, Ocon AP, Lopez PO, Lopez Prats JL, Toledo Parreno JD. (2008) The use of isotonic fluid as maintenance therapy prevents iatrogenic hyponatremia in pediatrics: a randomized, controlled open study. *Pediatr Crit Care Med* **9**:589–97.

Muir WW, Kohn CW, Sam SR. (1978) Effects of furosemide on plasma volume and extracellular fluid volumes in horses. *Am J Vet Res* **39**:1688–91.

Neville KA, Sandeman DJ, Rubinstein A, Henry GM, McGlynn M, Walker JL. (2009) Prevention of hyponatremia during maintenance intravenous fluid administration: a prospective randomized study of fluid type versus fluid rate. *J Pediatr* **156**:313–19.

Oftedal OT, Hintz HF, Schryver HF. (1983) Lactation in the horse: milk composition and intake by foals. *J Nutr* **113**:2196–206.

Palmer J. (2002) Practical approach to fluid therapy in neonates. In: *2002 Scientific Proceedings, 8th International Veterinary Emergency and Critical Care Symposium*. San Antonio, TX. Veterinary Emergency and Critical Care Society, pp. 665–8.

Paut O, Remond C, Lagier P, Fortier G, Camboulives J. (2000) Severe hyponatremic encephalopathy after pediatric surgery: report of seven cases and recommendations for management and prevention [in French]. *Ann Fr Anesth Reanim* **19**: 467–73.

Perel P, Roberts I, Ker K. (2013) Colloids versus crystalloids for fluid resuscitation in critically ill patients. Cochrane Database Syst Rev CD000567; doi: 10.1002/14651858.CD000567. pub6.

Pirrone A, Mariella J, Gentilini F, Castagnetti C. (2012) Amniotic fluid and blood lactate concentrations in mares and foals in the early postpartum period. *Theriogenology* **78**:1182–9.

Playfor S. (2003) Fatal iatrogenic hyponatraemia. *Arch Dis Child* **88**:646–7.

Pritchard JC, Burn CC, Barr ARS, Whay HR. (2008) Validity of indicators of dehydration in working horses: a longitudinal study of changes in skin tent duration, mucous membrane dryness, and drinking behavior. *Equine Vet J* **40**:558–564.

Rey C, Los-Arcos M, Hemandez A, Sanchez A, Diaz JJ, Lopez-Herce J. (2011) Hypotonic versus isotonic maintenance fluids in critically ill children: a multicenter prospective randomized study. *Acta Pediatrica* **100**:1138–43.

Roberts PP I. (2011) Colloids versus crystalloids for fluid resuscitation in critically ill patients (Review). *Cochrane Database Syst Rev Issue* **3**:CD000567; doi: 10.1002/14651858. CD000567.pub6.

Rumbaugh GE, Carlson GP, Harrold D. (1982) Urinary production in the healthy horse and in horses deprived of feed and water. *Am J Vet Res* **43**:735–7.

Saba TG, Fairbairn J, Houghton F, Laforte D, Foster BJ. (2011) A randomized controlled trial of isotonic versus hypotonic maintenance intravenous fluids in hospitalized children. *BMC Pediatrics* **11**:1–9.

Schusser GF, Rieckhoff K, Ungemach FR, Huskamp NH. Scheidemann W. (2007) Effect of hydroxyethyl starch solution in normal horses and horses with colic or acute colitis. *J Vet Med A Physiol Pathol Clin Med* **54**:592–8.

Shaw AD, Bagshaw SM, Goldstein SL, et al. (2012) Major complications, mortality, and resource utilization after open abdominal surgery. *Ann Surg* **255**:821–9.

Silver M, ComLine RS. (1976) Feral and placental O2 consumption and the uptake of different metabolites in the ruminant and horse during late gestation. *Adv Exp Med Biol* **75**:731–6.

So K, Fok T, Ng P, Wong W, Cheung K. (1997) Randomised controlled trial of colloid or crystalloid in hypotensive preterm infants. *Arch Dis Child Fetal Neonatal Ed* **76**:F43–F46.

Soroker D, Ezri T, Lurie S, Feld S, Savir I. (1991) Symptomatic hyponatraemia due to inappropriate antidiuretic hormone secretion following minor surgery. *Can J Anaesth* **38**:225–6.

Spurlock SL, Spurlock GH, Parker G, Ward MV. (1990) Long-term jugular vein catheterization in horses. *J Am Vet Med Assoc* **196**:425–30.

Thomas WP, Madigan JE, Backus KQ, et al. (1987) Systemic and pulmonary haemodynamics in normal neonatal foals. *J Reprod Fertil Suppl* **35**:623–8.

Tyler SJ. (1969) *The Behaviour of a Population of New Forest Ponies.* Cambridge, UK: Cambridge University Press.

Upadhyay M, Singhi S, Murlidharan J, et al. (2005) Randomized evaluation of fluid resuscitation with crystalloid (saline) and colloid (polymer from degraded gelatin in saline) in pediatric septic shock. *Indian Pediatr* **42**:223–31.

Vail DM, Ogilvie GK, Fettman MJ, et al. (1990) Exacerbation of hyperlactatemia by infusion of lactate Ringer's solution. *J Vet Int Med* **4**:228–32.

Vincent J-L, Weil MH. (2006) Fluid challenge revisited. *Crit Care Med* **34**:1333–7.

Wilson EM, Holcombe SJ, Lamar A, Hauptman JG, Brooks MB. (2009) Incidence of transfusion reactions and retention of procoagulant and anticoagulant factor activities in equine plasma. *J Vet Int Med* **23**:323–8.

Young RS, Petroff OA, Chen B, Aquila WJ Jr, Gore JC. (1991) Preferential utilization of lactate in neonatal dog brain: in vivo and in vitro proton NMR study. *Biol Neonat* **59**:46–53.

Zarychanski R, Abou-Setta AH, Turgeon AF, et al. (2013) Association of hydroxyethyl starch administration with mortality and acute kidney injury in critically ill patients requiring volume resuscitation: a systematic review and meta-analysis. *JAMA* **309**:678–88.

SECTION 3
Special topics

CHAPTER 23

Blood and blood product transfusions in horses

Margaret Mudge

The Ohio State University, Department of Veterinary Clinical Sciences, Columbus, OH, USA

Blood product transfusion is an integral part of equine practice, both in referral institutions and in ambulatory practice. Blood products may be administered for conditions ranging from life-threatening acute hemorrhage to failure of transfer of passive immunity (FPT). The available equine blood products and indications for transfusion will be discussed in this chapter. Practical considerations for donor selection and collection and administration of blood will also be covered. As with other aspects of fluid therapy, the clinician should weigh the potential risks and benefits of blood and plasma transfusions.

Indications for blood transfusion

Whole blood (WB) transfusions are most often indicated for horses that have suffered acute blood loss due to trauma, surgery, or other conditions such as splenic rupture or uterine artery hemorrhage. In cases of blood loss, the transfusion serves to restore blood volume as well as oxygen-carrying capacity. While there are no set variables that serve as "transfusion triggers", a combination of physical examination and clinicopathologic parameters can be used to guide the decision to transfuse (Hurcombe et al., 2007). Physical examination parameters, such as pale mucous membranes, tachycardia, tachypnea, sweating, colic, and lethargy may indicate a need for blood transfusion, especially when blood loss is estimated to be greater than 30% of blood volume. Acute blood loss can result in hypovolemic shock in addition to loss of red cell mass, so findings may also include cold extremities, hypotension, and increased blood lactate concentrations.

It is important to remember that the packed cell volume (PCV) can still be normal during severe, acute hemorrhage. The PCV and total protein (TP) will decrease as fluid redistributes from the interstitial to the intravascular space over the first 12 hours after hemorrhage. If intravenous fluids are given for resuscitation, the PCV and TP will decrease more rapidly. TP will decrease before PCV decreases substantially, since splenic contraction initially increases the PCV. Blood transfusion is likely needed if the PCV drops below 20–25% during an acute bleeding episode, although in acute, severe cases, transfusion may be needed before there is a significant drop in PCV. In cases of acute hemorrhage, whole blood (WB) or packed red blood cells (PRBC) and plasma, often in conjunction with crystalloid or colloid intravenous fluids, are most commonly used to restore oxygen-carrying capacity and circulating volume.

Estimation of blood loss can be used to guide the decision to transfuse, with loss of more than 30% of blood volume generally requiring transfusion (Garrioch, 2004). The American College of Surgeons' Advanced Trauma Life Support guidelines provide estimates of blood loss based on physical exam and monitoring parameters (Table 23.1). Anesthetized horses may have very stable heart rates and PCV despite massive blood loss; pale mucous membranes with prolonged capillary refill time (CRT), decreasing TP, hypotension, and hypoxemia are better indicators of blood loss in horses (Wilson et al., 2003).

Oxygenation status can help to determine the need for blood transfusion in cases of both acute hemorrhage and chronic anemia. A rise in blood lactate concentration despite volume replacement with crystalloid or colloid

---

Equine Fluid Therapy, First Edition. Edited by C. Langdon Fielding and K. Gary Magdesian.
© 2015 John Wiley & Sons, Inc. Published 2015 by John Wiley & Sons, Inc.

Table 23.1 Estimated blood loss (adapted from American College of Surgeons Advance Trauma Life Support (ATLS) Shock Categories)

Shock category	Percent blood loss	Heart rate	Respiratory rate	Capillary refill time	Blood pressure	Urine output	Other physical exam findings
Stage I	Up to 15%	Normal to minimal increase	Normal	Normal	Normal	Normal	Possible mild anxiety
Stage II	15–30%	Increased	Increased	Mildly prolonged	Normal	Mildly decreased	Mild anxiety
Stage III	30–40%	Moderate to severely increased	Increased	Prolonged	Decreased	Decreased	Altered mentation; cool extremities
Stage IV	>40%	Severely increased	Increased	Absent, very pale mucous membranes	Severe hypotension	Negligible	Obtunded; cool extremities

---

Box 23.1 Oxygen extraction ratio formula

$O_2ER \approx (S_aO_2 - S_vO_2)/S_aO_2$

where:
O_2ER = oxygen extraction ratio
S_aO_2 = arterial oxygen saturation
S_vO_2 = mixed venous oxygen saturation

---

fluids may indicate continued tissue hypoxia and a need for blood transfusion (Greenburg, 1995; Magdesian et al., 2006). Oxygen extraction ratios are also useful measures; a ratio greater than 40% in the context of blood loss may indicate a need for blood transfusion (Box 23.1)(Magdesian, 2008).

In patients with chronic and hemolytic anemias, PCV and TP can be more useful indicators of the need for blood transfusion. While there is no set transfusion trigger in veterinary medicine, in chronic anemia cases, a PCV of less than 12–15%, especially in conjunction with previously mentioned physical examination findings (pale mucous membranes, tachycardia, tachypnea, and lethargy), represents an indication for blood transfusion. Transfusions may need to be given to patients with a higher PCV if they have concurrent disease such as respiratory conditions or sepsis. Since animals with hemolytic or chronic anemia are normovolemic, PRBCs are indicated for transfusion, although WB may also be used. For both acute and chronic anemias, the primary goal of blood transfusion is to increase the oxygen-carrying capacity of the blood. While the blood transfusion will temporarily increase oxygen-carrying capacity, it is essential to diagnose and treat the underlying cause of the anemia.

Transfused red blood cells (RBCs) have been reported to have a very short half-life; however, recent studies indicate that autologous transfused red blood cells have longer survival than originally reported, and allogeneic (donor) transfused RBCs also have a longer half-life than was reported in the original chromium-label studies (Kallfelz et al., 1978; Mudge et al., 2012; Owens et al., 2010; Smith et al., 1992). Red blood cells from allogeneic transfusions do have a much shorter half-life than autologous red cells, so transfusion should still be considered a temporary measure to restore oxygen-carrying capacity, relying on the horse's erythropoietic response or improvement of the underlying disease to provide long-term resolution. There is a 20-day half-life for fresh, crossmatched, blood-typed, allogeneic transfused blood.

Hemoglobin-based oxygen carriers (HBOCs)

Hemoglobin-based oxygen carriers are blood substitutes consisting of polymerized hemoglobin that are given to increase oxygen-carrying capacity in patients with moderate to severe anemia. Oxyglobin® (Biopure Corp., Boston, MA), an HBOC produced with hemoglobin of bovine origin, has been used experimentally in ponies with normovolemic anemia (Belgrave et al., 2002). Oxyglobin improved hemodynamic and oxygen transport parameters; however, one pony did have an anaphylactic reaction. The use of Oxyglobin was also reported for treatment of a pony mare with chronic hemorrhage and a history of acute transfusion reactions (Maxson et al., 1993). Oxyglobin is currently available in 125-mL infusion bags (Dechra Veterinary Products, Shropshire, UK).

Indications for plasma product transfusion

Plasma transfusion is indicated for the treatment of clotting factor deficiency, hypoalbuminemia, decreased colloid osmotic pressure, and failure of transfer of passive immunity. Fresh and fresh frozen plasma (FFP) contain immunoglobulins, coagulation factors (fibrinogen and factors II, VII, IX, X, XI, and XII), and cofactors (factors V and VIII), as well as the anticoagulant proteins antithrombin, protein C, and protein S. Plasma has also been used for treatment of disseminated intravascular coagulation in horses (Welch et al., 1992).

Plasma can be used for colloid support when the TP concentration is less than 4.0 g/dL, serum albumin concentration is less than 2.0 g/dL, or colloid oncotic pressure is less than 14 mmHg acutely. If clotting factors and albumin are not needed, synthetic colloids such as hydroxyethyl starch may be preferred for colloid support.

FPT in neonatal foals over 12 hours of age is best treated by plasma transfusion, as colostrum absorption is greatly diminished after 12 hours (Jeffcott, 1975). An IgG concentration of less than 200 mg/dL is considered complete FPT, and IgG between 400 and 800 mg/dL is considered partial FPT. Although plasma transfusion is not always needed for foals with partial FPT, it is recommended for foals that have pre-existing infection or exposure to pathogens. Commercially available fresh frozen hyperimmune plasma is most commonly used for treatment of neonatal foals (Box 23.2).Equine FFP is a USDA-licensed product, and most products have a minimum guarantee for IgG concentration and a 2 to 3-year shelf-life when frozen. Although commercially available hyperimmune plasma has very high IgG

Box 23.2 Commercial sources of fresh frozen equine plasma

Veterinary Immunogenics (Penrith, Cumbria, UK)
www.veterinaryimmunogenics.com
Lake Immunogenics, Inc. (Ontario, NY)
www.lakeimmunogenics.com
Mg Biologics (Ames, IA)
www.mgbiologics.com
PlasVacc (Templeton, CA)
www.plasvaccusa.com

---

concentrations (1500–2500 mg/dL), plasma from local donor horses may provide better protection against specific local pathogens.

There are multiple hyperimmune plasma products with bacterial- or viral-specific antibodies. There is some evidence for the efficacy of *E. coli* (J5) and *Salmonella typhimurium* hyperimmune plasma for the treatment of equine endotoxemia; however, there are also reports that dispute the efficacy of such products (Durando et al., 1994, Peek et al., 2006, Southwood, 2004, Spier et al., 1989). The use of *Rhodococcus equi* hyperimmune plasma for the prevention of *R. equi* has also been controversial (Caston et al., 2006 Giguère et al., 2002; Hurley & Begg, 1995; Madigan et al., 1991; Perkins et al., 2002). Other plasma products available for specific disease treatment include botulism antitoxin, West Nile virus antibody, and *Streptococcus equi* antibody.

For animals with von Willebrand disease, cryoprecipitate may be used since it contains more concentrated von Willebrand factor (as well as factor VIII, fibrinogen, factor XIII, and fibronectin). Cryoprecipitate would typically be administered to a patient with known deficiency that needs to undergo a surgical procedure or is having life-threatening bleeding associated with primary hemostatic dysfunction. Equine cryoprecipitate is not a commercially available product.

Indications for platelet transfusion

Platelet transfusions are indicated for patients with severe thrombocytopenia and life-threatening hemorrhage or a need for surgical intervention. There is no consensus on a platelet "transfusion trigger" in horses, but platelet transfusion should be considered with a platelet count of less than 20,000/μL in the presence of risk factors for bleeding (Abrams-Ogg, 2003). Platelet transfusion may be less beneficial for patients with immune-mediated thrombocytopenia since the transfused platelets will be rapidly destroyed, and so are reserved for use as a stop-gap measure in extreme circumstances. Often the platelet count does not improve, although the active hemorrhage may temporarily stop.

Fresh WB can also provide platelets, and may be the ideal choice for patients that require RBCs and platelets. WB will not generally provide platelet concentrations high enough to treat severe thrombocytopenia, and may provide excess RBCs for patients that require chronic platelet therapy. For patients with primary thrombocytopenia or thrombocytopathia, platelet concentrates can be given. Platelet concentrates can be obtained by plateletpheresis or by centrifugation using a slow-spin technique (see "Blood and plasma processing" below).

Blood donor selection

There are eight recognized equine blood groups, and 30 different factors identified within seven of these groups (International Society for Animal Blood Group Research, 1987). Because of the large number of blood groups and factors, there are no true universal donors for horses. The ideal equine blood donor is a healthy young gelding weighing at least 500 kg. Donor horses should be up to date on vaccinations, including rhinopneumonitis, tetanus, Eastern and Western encephalitis, rabies, and West Nile virus. Donors should be tested annually for equine infectious anemia. Donors that are used for USDA-licensed plasma products must also be tested for piroplasmosis, dourine, glanders, and brucellosis.

The RBC antigens Aa and Qa are the most immunogenic and have been commonly associated with neonatal isoerythrolysis, so the ideal donor should lack the Aa and Qa alloantigens. There are breed-specific blood factor frequencies, so a donor of the same breed as the recipient may be preferable, especially when blood typing is not available. Horses that have received blood or plasma transfusions and mares that have had foals are not suitable as donors because they have a higher risk of carrying RBC alloantibodies. Donkeys have a RBC antigen known as "donkey factor", which is not present in horses; therefore, donkeys or mules should not be used as donors for horses, as the transfused horses can develop anti-donkey factor antibodies (McClure et al., 1994). Horses with anti-donkey factor antibodies cannot be used as donors for donkeys and mules. For foals with neonatal isoerythrolysis, the mare can be used as a blood donor, but the RBCs must be washed prior to transfusion.

In the referral practice setting, it may be practical to establish a group of blood donor horses. These donor horses should be blood typed and should also be tested for alloantibodies (see below). An alternative to fresh blood from donor horses is commercially available WB or PRBCs (see Box 23.2: PlasVacc).

When a surgical procedure is planned in advance and there is a high risk of substantial blood loss, preoperative autologous donation should be considered, as the horse would be its own ideal blood donor (Mudge, 2005). The life span of transfused autologous RBCs after 28 days of storage is approximately 30 days, compared to a 20-day half-life for fresh, crossmatched, blood-typed, allogeneic blood (Owens et al., 2010; Mudge et al., 2012). Intraoperative or post-hemorrhage cell salvage is also an option for autotransfusion, and its use has been reported in a horse with post-castration hemorrhage (Waguespack et al., 2001). RBC recovery can be performed with specialized cell salvage equipment, which washes and filters collected blood, but cell salvage can also be performed with simple anticoagulation and filtration (Waters, 2005). The technique of cell salvage is limited to cases in which the salvaged blood is not in an area of infection or malignancy, unless specialized washing and filtering equipment is used.

Pretransfusion testing

In an emergency situation, an immediate blood transfusion may be given for the first time with a very minor risk of serious transfusion reaction. Horses can develop alloantibodies within 1 week of transfusion, so blood typing and crossmatching are recommended before a second transfusion is performed (Wong et al., 1986). However, a second blood transfusion may be performed safely within 2 to 3 days of the first transfusion without a blood crossmatch. In non-emergency situations (or when testing is readily available), blood typing and crossmatching are recommended to limit the risk of transfusion reaction and ensure the optimal survival of transfused red blood cells.

Blood typing

Blood typing and alloantibody screening can be used to help find the most appropriate donor horse for the patient requiring transfusion. Blood typing involves the use of antisera to detect specific RBC antibodies. Unfortunately, since blood typing is time-consuming and laboratories performing blood typing are very limited, this is not often a practical method of donor selection (Box 23.3).Blood typing and antibody screening prior to initial transfusion are more important for horses for which subsequent blood transfusions are

Box 23.3 Equine blood typing laboratories in the United States

Hematology Laboratory
Room 1012, Veterinary Teaching Hospital
One Garrod Drive
University of California, Davis
Davis, CA 95616
Phone: 530-752-1303

University of Kentucky
Equine Parentage Testing and Research Lab
102 Animal Pathology Building
Lexington, KY 40546-0076
Phone: 859-257-3656
www.ca.uky.edu/gluck/ServEPVL.asp

Rood and Riddle Veterinary Laboratory
2150 Georgetown Rd
Lexington, KY 40511
Phone: 859-233-0331
www.roodandriddle.com

Hagyard Equine Medical Institute
4250 Iron Works Pike
Lexington, KY 40511-8412
Phone: 859-259-3685
www.hagyard.com

anticipated, and for broodmares that may produce foals with neonatal isoerythrolysis (NI) if sensitized to other blood group factors (Wong et al., 1986). A rapid agglutination method for detection of equine RBC antigens Ca and Aa has been developed that, if it becomes commercially available, may be more practical than full blood typing for pretransfusion testing (Owens et al., 2008).

Antibody screening

Donor animals should ideally be screened for alloantibodies yearly. Naturally occurring anti-Aa and anti-Ac antibodies can be found in horses, and are usually agglutinin antibodies; mares that have been previously sensitized may have anti-Aa hemolysins as well. Recipients may also be tested for RBC antibodies; however, such testing is not widely available, so this is not usually practical in the emergency setting. Antibody screens are routinely performed in mares that may be at risk of having anti-RBC antibodies to the foal's blood type and therefore at risk of causing NI.

Crossmatch

A blood crossmatch is recommended prior to blood transfusion, especially for any horse that may have previously been exposed to RBC antigens. Hemagglutination crossmatching is widely available and rapidly performed; however, it will not predict all transfusion reactions, namely the hemolytic reactions. The major crossmatch detects agglutination reactions between the donor's RBCs and the recipient's plasma (Figure 23.1). The minor crossmatch detects agglutination reactions between the donor's plasma and the recipient's RBCs. Equine crossmatches may be difficult to interpret due to the rouleaux formation of equine RBCs. Normal rouleaux should disperse when a small amount of saline is mixed with the blood, whereas agglutination will not disperse. Crossmatching can also be difficult to interpret in animals with immune-mediated hemolytic anemia, due to the autoagglutination of patient RBCs. The procedure for performing a hemagglutination crossmatch is described in Box 23.4.

The routine crossmatch evaluates agglutination reactions, but does not test for hemolytic reactions. Rabbit complement can be added to the reaction mixture for hemolytic testing, but this is not routinely performed as part of the crossmatch except in some laboratories (Becht et al., 1983). Crossmatch testing also does not accurately predict the lifespan of the transfused red cell or the development of antibodies to the transfused RBCs, and transfusion reactions have been reported even with a compatible crossmatch (Hurcombe et al., 2007). If the minor crossmatch is incompatible,

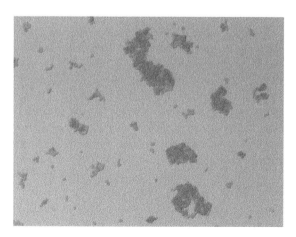

Figure 23.1 Agglutination reaction between donor RBCs and recipient plasma.

but the major crossmatch is compatible, the transfusion can still be performed after washing the donor red blood cells and providing packed red blood cells.

Blood collection technique

When a transfusion is anticipated and fresh whole blood will be used, the donor horses should be weighed and have PCV/TP measured prior to blood collection. Donor PCV should ideally be greater than 35%. The maximum volume to be collected is 20% of blood volume, or approximately 16 mL/kg body weight, and the volume should be calculated based on lean body weight (Malikides et al., 2001). Blood is collected from the jugular vein of the donor horse, either through direct needle cannulation or catheterization. When a large volume of blood is needed, a 10- or 12-gauge catheter is recommended, although a 14-gauge catheter is also sufficient. Blood flow may be improved by placing the catheter opposite the venous blood flow (catheter directed toward the head). Both jugular veins may be used if a large volume of blood is needed immediately. When 15% or more of the donor's blood volume is collected, volume replacement with intravenous crystalloid fluids is recommended. The donor horse's heart rate, respiratory rate, and attitude should be monitored

during the blood collection. Vital parameters should normalize within 1 hour of collection.

Vacuum canisters may be used to speed the collection, but glass bottles with vacuum are not recommended as the glass inactivates platelets and can damage the RBCs (Mudge et al., 2004, Sasakawa & Tokunaga, 1976). Commercially available 450-mL blood collection bags may be used in horses (Baxter Fenwal, Deerfield, IL; MWI Veterinary Supply, Meridian, ID). There are also commercially available 2-L bags with sodium citrate (Plasvacc USA, Templeton, CA), and collections can also be made by the addition of anticoagulant to an empty sterile collection bag.

There are several anticoagulant options for blood collection. When blood is collected for immediate transfusion, anticoagulation with 3.2% sodium citrate is adequate (1:9 anticoagulant to blood ratio). However, when blood is stored for later transfusion, optimal pH and support of RBC metabolism are necessary to sustain RBC viability. If the blood is going to be stored, citrate-phosphate-dextrose (CPD) or citrate-phosphate-dextrose-adenine (CPDA) should be used. When shed blood is collected from cavitary hemorrhage (e.g., abdomen or thorax), less anticoagulant is needed since the blood is already defibrinated. There are commercially available devices that will collect, wash, and filter shed blood. Blood may also be collected into a blood bag with a reduced amount of anticoagulant and then filtered prior to administration. Recommendations for the ratio of anticoagulant to shed blood range from 1:7 to 1:20.

To achieve optimal RBC viability during storage, the blood bags should be weighed to ensure adequate fill (proper blood to anticoagulant ratio). Sterility is very important during the collection and processing of blood for storage, since contamination and bacterial growth may cause significant transfusion reaction. A closed collection system is used, and tube sealer is used to seal the collection tubing. The tubing can be sealed in several increments for later testing or crossmatching.

Biochemical and hematologic parameters suggest that WB stored in CPDA-1 bags may be acceptable for transfusion after 3 weeks of storage (Mudge et al., 2004). A post-transfusion viability study on equine blood stored for 28 days demonstrated a 24-hour labeled RBC survival of 73%, and a half-life of 29 days for autologous blood (Owens et al., 2010). RBC concentrates stored in saline-adenine-glucose-mannitol solution may be

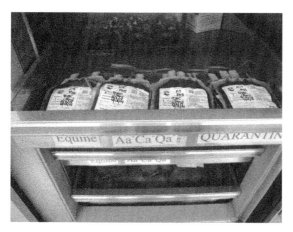

Figure 23.2 Appropriate storage and labeling in a blood bank refrigerator.

suitable for transfusion for up to 35 days after collection (Niinistö et al., 2008). Whole blood and PRBCs are refrigerated at 1–6°C, ideally in a dedicated blood bank refrigerator with an alarm system that signals temperature breaches. The name of donor, date of collection, blood type, and intended recipient (if known) should be clearly indicated on each blood bag. Blood from different species should be stored in separate refrigerators, or at least on separate shelves, with clear labeling (Figure 23.2).

Blood and plasma processing

Whole blood can be given directly or can be processed to make PRBCs and plasma. Due to the rapid sedimentation of equine RBCs, the RBC component can be administered without specialized processing; however, the PRBCs will still contain plasma components unless centrifugation and repeated washing are performed. Washing of RBCs is the preferred technique when a transfusion is given to an NI foal using the mare as a donor. When RBC washing or other processing is planned, blood should be collected into bags rather than bottles due to ease of centrifugation and sterile transfer. In order to separate the components, blood is centrifuged (at 4°C) at 5000 × g for 5 min. Plasma is transferred to the satellite bag using a plasma extractor, and an additive solution is mixed with the PRBCs. For RBC washing, the RBC component is mixed with saline and centrifuged, supernatant removed, and this process is repeated twice more.

Plasma can be prepared by gravity sedimentation, centrifugation, or plasmapheresis (Wilson et al., 2009). When larger volumes of plasma are desired without RBCs, plasmapheresis is the preferred technique as it is more rapid than WB collection and processing, and results in plasma with minimal RBCs and leukocytes (Feige et al., 2003). Plasmapheresis of 4 to 11 L can be performed every 30 days on donor horses (Magdesian et al., 1992). Plasma that is used within 8 hours of collection is considered fresh plasma, and if placed in a freezer within 8 hours of collection is considered to be fresh frozen plasma (FFP). FFP is stored at −18°C or lower, with temperatures of less than −70°C resulting in better preservation of coagulation factors. FFP should be used within 1 year of freezing to ensure optimal clotting factor activity. If plasma is thawed but not needed, it can be refrozen within 1 hour of thawing, and will maintain coagulation factor activity (Yaxley et al., 2010). Plasma that is frozen more than 8 hours after collection, or is more than 1 year old, is considered to be frozen plasma (FP). The labile clotting factors, factor V and factor VIII, will be decreased in FP as compared to FFP. Equine hyperimmune plasma is a USDA-regulated product, and the shelf life for immunoglobulin efficacy is 2–3 years.

Platelets will be present in WB as long as the blood is stored at room temperature and transfused within 8 hours. Plasma is centrifuged in a "soft spin" to create platelet-rich plasma (PRP). Platelet concentrate (PC) is created by further centrifugation of PRP, or by plateletpheresis. The process of plateletpheresis has not been described for the collection of equine platelets in the clinical setting. Platelet concentrate must be stored at room temperature and should be used within 5 to 7 days. Cryopreservation has been described for human and canine platelets, but in practice, room temperature PRP or PC are used most often (Appleman et al., 2009).

Blood product administration

Volumes for transfusion
The volume of blood to be transfused depends on estimated blood loss, estimated total blood volume, and donor PCV. For normovolemic anemia, recipient PCV can be used, as shown in Box 23.5.

In situations of acute hemorrhage, an estimate of blood loss is based on clinical parameters (see Table 23.1). Between 25% and 50% of the total blood lost should be

---

> **Box 23.5 Transfusion equations**
>
> **Blood transfusion volume (mL)**
>
> Body weight in kg × 80 mL/kg ×[(desired PCV –
> actual PCV)/donor PCV]
>
> **Plasma transfusion volume (mL)**
>
> Body weight in kg × 45 mL/kg × [(desired TP –
> actual TP)/donor TP]
>
> PCV, packed cell volume; TP, total protein.

replaced by transfusion since much of the circulating volume will be replaced by fluid shifts. The PCV may not increase after transfusion in cases of hemorrhagic anemia, likely due to endogenous fluid shifts, IV fluid resuscitation, and possibly continued hemorrhage (Hurcombe et al., 2007). It is important to remember that up to 75% of RBCs lost into a body cavity (e.g., hemoperitoneum) are autotransfused back into circulation within 24 to 72 hours (Sellon, 2010). Therefore, lower percentages of blood volume replacement may be needed in cases of intracavitary hemorrhage.

Volumes of plasma needed for treatment of hypoproteinemia can be estimated by total protein or albumin concentrations, although the use of plasma to normalize severe hypoproteinemia can be prohibitively expensive in the adult horse (see Box 23.5). Using the equation for volume of plasma transfusion, a 450-kg horse would need a transfusion of 3–5 L of plasma to raise the total protein by 1 g/dL. However, in practice the volumes required to raise total protein appear to be much greater. Some authors have suggested that 8–10 L of plasma is needed to raise total protein by 1 g/dL in a 450-kg horse (Collatos & Morris, 1999). This discrepancy is likely due to redistribution of albumin in the interstitial space and ongoing loss of protein related to the underlying disease (e.g., protein-losing enteropathy). The volume of plasma given for treatment of hypoproteinemia or coagulopathy is often determined by the clinical and clinicopathologic response. A starting point for treatment of coagulopathy is approximately 4 to 5 mL/kg plasma. Follow-up monitoring with hemostatic testing is recommended to help determine the endpoint of treatment.

The volume of plasma needed in a foal with FPT can be determined if the IgG concentrations of the foal and the plasma are known. A dose of 20 mL/kg of plasma (IgG approximately 1200 mg/dL) will generally raise the foal's IgG concentration by 200–300 mg/dL. A larger volume of plasma may be needed to achieve a similar rise in IgG in clinically ill foals (Wilkins & Dewan-Mix, 1994).

Transfusion technique

Prior to transfusion, blood should be inspected for signs of contamination (dark, discolored, or visible clots). Refrigerated blood can be transfused directly, as warming may cause further deterioration of RBCs. In hypothermic patients, or those receiving large volumes of blood, the blood should be warmed at least to room temperature (22°C) and no warmer than body temperature (37°C). FFP should be thawed in a water bath at 30–37°C. Blood products (including plasma) are administered using a commercial blood delivery set with in-line filter. Standard filters are 170–260 μm, and the filter or administration set should be changed every 2–4 units of blood. Blood should not be given concurrently with hyper- or hypotonic solutions, and should not be given with calcium-containing solutions (such as LRS) as the citrate anticoagulant will bind calcium in the fluids, and will no longer be an effective anticoagulant.

Blood products should be given slowly for the first 10–20 minutes so that the animal can be monitored closely for signs of transfusion reaction (see below), and the transfusion can be stopped, if needed. Approximately 0.3 mL/kg (over 10–20 min) is given initially, and the rate can then be increased, if needed. The rate of transfusion will depend on the patient's volume status, and can be as high as 20–40 mL/kg/h if volume resuscitation is needed. It is not recommended to exceed 2–4 mL/kg/h in patients with significant cardiac disease. The transfusion should be completed within 4 hours to prevent bacterial growth and ensure functional platelets (in the case of fresh whole blood).

Monitoring and adverse reactions

Heart rate, temperature, respiratory rate, and attitude should be monitored every 15 minutes during a transfusion, with particular attention during the first 15 minutes of the transfusion. The incidence of adverse reactions with plasma transfusion ranges from 0% to 10%, and the incidence for blood transfusion reactions has been reported as 16%, with 1 of 44 horses (2%) having a fatal anaphylactic reaction (Hardefeldt et al., 2010; Hurcombe et al., 2007; Wilson et al., 2009). Compatibility on crossmatch does not guarantee a lack of transfusion reaction and does not accurately predict RBC lifespan.

Acute hemolytic transfusion reactions occur when there is incompatibility between donor and recipient blood, resulting in rapid destruction of the transfused RBCs. These reactions can appear during the transfusion or within hours of transfusion. This process typically requires pre-existing antibodies and is classified as a cytotoxic (type II) hypersensitivity. Clinical signs include hemoglobinemia, hemoglobinuria, and progressive anemia or lack of increase in PCV. In addition, the highly inflammatory nature of this reaction can lead to signs of systemic inflammatory response, disseminated intravascular coagulation (DIC), shock, cardiovascular collapse, and death. Severity of signs is directly related to the volume of transfused blood. Acute kidney injury may result from hemoglobinuria, and IV fluid therapy is indicated to protect the kidneys. With acute reactions the transfusion should be stopped immediately and supportive care initiated. Delayed hemolytic transfusion reactions can occur more than 24 hours after transfusion, and also result in RBC lysis. This reaction may be recognized by an unexpected decline in PCV following transfusion, hyperbilirubinemia, and possibly fever. Hemolysis of transfused blood may also occur prior to transfusion due to improper handling of the blood. Improper storage, excessive warming of the blood, administration with hypertonic solutions, and administration using pumps can all lead to RBC destruction (Patterson et al., 2011). Suspected hemolytic transfusion reactions should be investigated by performing post-transfusion crossmatch, monitoring bilirubin, and performing blood cultures.

Non-hemolytic reactions such as fever and allergic reactions may also occur with blood or plasma transfusion and constitute the most common reactions seen in veterinary patients (Hardefeldt et al., 2010; Hurcombe et al., 2007; Prittie, 2003). Fever may be related to donor leukocytes and accumulation of pyrogenic cytokines in the blood over time. As such, older units of blood products are more likely to cause this response. Leukoreduction of stored PRBCs eliminated the inflammatory response to transfusion in experimental dogs (McMichael et al., 2010). Transfusion reactions

from acute allergic (type I) hypersensitivity can include muscle fasciculation, urticaria, pruritus, anaphylaxis, sweating, and piloerection. If an allergic reaction is suspected, the transfusion should be stopped immediately (if severe) or slowed (if mild). Most mild reactions will resolve on their own; however, some will require the administration of a corticosteroid or antihistamine (tripelennamine, 1.1 mg/kg IV), and severe anaphylactic reactions may require the administration of epinephrine (0.01–0.02 mL/kg IV of 1:1000 solution). Allergic reactions can also occur with plasma transfusions, likely due to reaction to a protein in the plasma product to which the recipient has been previously sensitized. These signs usually occur in the first 15 minutes of the transfusion, and treatment is the same as for allergic reactions related to blood transfusions. Although plasma transfusions are not commonly associated with serious adverse reactions, serum hepatitis (Theiler's disease) has been reported in association with transfusions of commercial plasma (Aleman et al., 2005).

Other potential complications of blood transfusion include transmission of infectious disease, bacterial contamination, citrate toxicity with massive transfusion (leading to ionized hypocalcemia and hypomagnesemia and metabolic acidosis), and circulatory overload. Circulatory overload is unlikely in the adult horse, but should be considered in the neonatal foal, especially when large volumes are needed to treat FPT or NI.

The changes that occur to blood during storage, called the "storage lesion", include hyperkalemia, hyperlactatemia, decreased 2,3-diphosphoglycerate (2,3-DPG), and change in RBC shape and membrane. These changes are unlikely to cause clinical problems in the transfusion recipient, except in cases of massive transfusion; there is some evidence of the superiority of fresh whole blood over stored blood from human studies (van de Watering, 2011).

In addition to monitoring for adverse reactions, it is important to assess the clinical response to transfusion. Physical examination, PCV, blood lactate, and oxygen extraction are among the parameters that should be monitored. It is important to remember that with acute or ongoing hemorrhage, the PCV may not increase after transfusion. The primary goal of blood transfusion is to improve oxygen delivery to the tissues, so all of the information from physical examination and blood work should be considered before performing an additional transfusion.

References

Abrams-Ogg ACG. (2003) Triggers for prophylactic use of platelet transfusions and optimal platelet dosing in thrombocytopenic dogs and cats. *Vet Clin North Am Small Anim Pract* **33**:1401–18.

Aleman M, Nieto JE, Carlson GP. (2005) Serum hepatitis associated with commercial plasma transfusion in horses. *J Vet Int Med* **19**:120–2.

Appleman EH, Sachais BS, Patel R, et al. (2009) Cryopreservation of canine platelets. *J Vet Int Med* **23**:138–45.

Becht JL, Page EH, Morter RL. (1983) Evaluation of a series of testing procedures to predict neonatal isoerythrolysis in the foal. *Cornell Vet* **73**:390–402.

Belgrave RL, Hines MT, Keegan RD, et al. (2002) Effects of a polymerized ultrapurified bovine hemoglobin blood substitute administered to ponies with normovolemic anemia. *J Vet Int Med* **16**:396–403.

Caston SS, McClure SR, Martens RJ, et al. (2006) Effect of hyperimmune plasma on the severity of pneumonia caused by Rhodococcus equi in experimentally infected foals. *Vet Ther* **7**:361–75.

Collatos C, Morris DD. (1999) Fluid therapy. In: Auer J, Stick J (eds) *Equine Surgery*. Philadelphia: WB Saunders, pp. 33–9.

Durando MM, MacKay RJ, Linda S, et al. (1994) Effects of polymyxin B and Salmonella typhimurium antiserum on horses given endotoxin intravenously. *Am J Ver Res* **55**:921–7.

Feige K, Ehrat FB, Kästner SB, et al. (2003) Automated plasmapheresis compared with other plasma collection methods in the horse. *J Vet Med A* **50**:185–9.

Garrioch MA. (2004) The body's response to blood loss. *Vox Sanguinis* **87**:S74–S76.

Giguère S, Gaskin JM, Miller C, et al. (2002) Evaluation of a commercially available hyperimmune plasma product for prevention of naturally acquired pneumonia caused by Rhodococcus equi in foals. *J Am Vet Med Assoc* **220**:59–63.

Greenburg AG. (1995) A physiologic basis for red blood cell transfusion decisions. *Am J Surg* **170**:44S–48S.

Hardefeldt LY, Keuler N, Peek SF. (2010) Incidence of transfusion reactions to commercial equine plasma. *J Vet Emerg Crit Care* **20**:421–5.

Hurcombe SD, Mudge MC, Hinchcliff KW. (2007) Clinical and clinicopathologic variables in adult horses receiving blood transfusions: 31 cases (1999–2005). *J Am Vet Med Assoc* **231**:267–74.

Hurley JR, Begg AP. (1995) Failure of hyperimmune plasma to prevent pneumonia caused by Rhodococcus equi in foals. *Aust Vet J* **72**:418–20.

International Society for Animal Blood Group Research. (1987) 20th International Conference on Animal Blood Groups and Biochemical Polymorphisms. *Anim Genet* **18**(Suppl. 1):1–145.

Jeffcott LB. (1975). The transfer of passive immunity to the foal and its relation to immune status after birth. *J Reprod Fertil* **23**:727–33.

Kallfelz FA, Whitlock RH, Schultz RD. (1978) Survival of 59Fe-labeled erythrocytes in cross-transfused equine blood. *Am J Vet Res* **39**:617–20.

Madigan JE, Hietala S, Muller N. (1991) Protection against naturally acquired Rhodococcus equi pneumonia in foals by administration of hyperimmune plasma. *J Reprod Fertil Suppl* **44**:571–8.

Magdesian KG. (2008) Acute blood loss. *Compend Equine* **3**:80–90.

Magdesian KG, Brook D, Wickler SJ. (1992) Temporal effects of plasmapheresis on serum proteins in horses. *Am J Vet Res* **53**:1149–53.

Magdesian KG, Fielding CL, Rhodes DM, et al. (2006) Changes in central venous pressure and blood lactate concentration in response to acute blood loss in horses. *J Am Vet Med Assoc* **229**:1458–62.

Malikides N, Hodgson JL, Rose RJ, et al. (2001) Cardiovascular, hematological and biochemical responses after large volume blood collection in horses. *Vet J* **162**:44–55.

Maxson AD, Giger U, Sweeney CR, et al. (1993) Use of bovine hemoglobin preparation in the treatment of cyclic ovarian hemorrhage in a miniature horse. *J Am Vet Med Assoc* **203**:1308–11.

McClure JJ, Kock C, Traub-Dargatz J. (1994) Characterization of a red blood cell antigen in donkeys and mules associated with neonatal isoerythrolysis. *Anim Genet* **25**:119–20.

McMichael MA, Smith SA, Galligan A, et al. (2010) Effect of leukoreduction on transfusion-induced inflammation in dogs. *J Vet Int Med* **24**:1131–7.

Mozzarelli A, Ronda L, Faggiano S, et al. (2010) Haemoglobin-based oxygen carriers: research and reality towards an alternative to blood transfusions. *Blood Transfus* **8**:S59–S69.

Mudge MC. (2005) How to perform pre-operative autologous blood donation in equine patients. In: *Proceedings of 51st Forum of the American Association of Equine Practitioners*, Seattle, WA. AAEP, pp. 263–4.

Mudge MC, Macdonald MH, Owens SD, et al. (2004) Comparison of 4 blood storage methods in a protocol for equine pre-operative autologous donation. *Vet Surg* **33**:475–86.

Mudge MC, Borjesson DL, Walker NJ, et al. (2012) Post-transfusion survival of biotin labeled allogeneic RBCs in adult horses. *Vet Clin Pathol* **41**:56–62.

Niinistö K, Raekallio M, Sankari S. (2008) Storage of equine red blood cells as a concentrate. *Vet J* **176**:227–31.

Owens SD, Snipes J, Magdesian KG, et al. (2008) Evaluation of a rapid agglutination method for detection of equine red cell surface antigens (Ca and Aa) as part of pretransfusion testing. *Vet Clin Pathol* **37**:49–56.

Owens SD, Johns JJ, Walker NJ. (2010) Use of an in vitro biotinylation technique for determination of posttransfusion survival of fresh and stored autologous red blood cells in Thoroughbreds. *Am J Vet Res* **71**:960–6.

Patterson J, Rousseau A, Kessler RJ, et al. (2011) In vitro lysis and acute transfusion reactions with hemolysis caused by inappropriate storage of canine red blood cell products. *J Vet Int Med* **25**:927–33.

Peek SF, Semrad S, McGuirk SM, et al. (2006) Prognostic value of clinicopathologic variables obtained at admission and effect of antiendotoxin plasma on survival in septic and critically ill foals. *J Vet Int Med* **20**:569–74.

Perkins GA, Yeager A, Erb HN, et al. (2002) Survival of foals with experimentally induced Rhodococcus equi infection given either hyperimmune plasma containing R. equi antibody or normal equine plasma. *Vet Ther* **3**:334–46.

Prittie JE. (2003) Triggers for use, optimal dosing, and problems associated with red cell transfusions. *Vet Clin North Am Small Anim Pract* **33**:1261–75.

Sasakawa S, Tokunaga E. (1976) Physical and chemical changes of ACD-preserved blood: a comparison of blood in glass bottles and plastic bags. *Vox Sanguinis* **31**:199–210.

Sellon DC. (2010) Disorders of the hematopoietic system. In: Reed SM, Bayly WM, Sellon DC (eds) *Equine Internal Medicine*, 3rd edn. St Louis: Saunders Elsevier, pp. 730–76.

Smith JE, Dever M, Smith J, et al. (1992) Post-transfusion survival of 50Cr-labeled erythrocytes in neonatal foals. *J Vet Int Med* **6**:183–5.

Southwood LL. (2004) Postoperative management of the large colon volvulus patient. *Vet Clin North Am Equine Pract* **20**:167–97.

Spier SJ, Lavoie JP, Cullor JS, et al. (1989) Protection against clinical endotoxemia in horses by using plasma containing antibody to an Rc mutant E. coli (J5). *Circ Shock* **28**:235–48.

Van de Watering L. (2011) Red cell storage and prognosis. *Vox Sanguinis* **100**:36–45.

Waguespack R, Belknap J, Williams A. (2001) Laparoscopic management of postcastration haemorrhage. *Equine Vet J* **33**:510–13.

Waters JH. (2005) Red blood cell recovery and reinfusion. *Anesthesiology* **23**:283–94.

Welch RD, Watkins JP, Taylor TS, et al. (1992) Disseminated intravascular coagulation associated with colic in 23 horses (1984–1989). *J Vet Int Med* **6**:29–35.

Wilkins PA, Dewan-Mix S. (1994) Efficacy of intravenous plasma to transfer passive immunity in clinically healthy and clinically ill equine neonates with failure of passive transfer. *Cornell Vet* **84**:7–14.

Wilson DV, Rondenay Y, Shance PU. (2003) The cardio-pulmonary effects of severe blood loss in anesthetized horses. *Vet Anaesth Analg* **30**:80–6.

Wilson EM, Holcombe SJ, Lamar A, et al. (2009) Incidence of transfusion reactions and retention of procoagulant and anti-coagulant factor activities in equine plasma. *J Vet Int Med* **23**:323–8.

Wong PL, Nickel LS, Bowling AT, et al. (1986) Clinical survey of antibodies against red blood cells in horses after homologous blood transfusion. *Am J Vet Res* **47**:2566–71.

Yaxley PE, Beal MW, Jutkowitz LA, et al. (2010) Comparative stability of canine and feline hemostatic proteins in freeze-thaw-cycled fresh frozen plasma. *J Vet Emerg Crit Care* **20**: 472–8.

CHAPTER 24

Colloids

Lucas Pantaleon

Board Certified Large Animal Internal Medicine Specialist, Industry Consultant,
Director Technical Services, Ogena Solutions, Versailles, KY, USA

Introduction

Fluid resuscitation is a mainstay for the management of critically ill patients (Perel & Roberts, 2007). A major dilemma facing medical professionals regarding fluid therapy is the choice between crystalloid and colloid solutions (Boldt et al., 1996b; Choi et al., 1999; Khandelwal et al., 2002; Oliveira et al., 2002b). Despite years of human and animal research, the question of which is the optimal fluid for resuscitation in a given clinical situation remains unanswered in both horses and humans (Bedenice, 2007; Choi et al., 1999; Marik & Eglesias, 2000). In a meta-analysis of findings in humans, no evidence of improved survival in critically ill patients treated with crystalloid versus colloid fluid resuscitation was found for either fluid type (Perel & Roberts, 2007). A recent Cochrane review found no evidence from randomized controlled trials that colloids reduce the risk of death in human patients with critical illness or in the postoperative period following surgery, when compared to resuscitation with crystalloids (Perel & Roberts, 2011). However, it is possible that there are certain subgroups where the use of a specific fluid type could be more effective (Boluyt et al., 2006; Hollenberg et al., 2004). Selection of intravenous fluid on an individual basis is very important as the efficacy of fluid administration depends on the type of fluid administered (Niemi et al., 2010).

Colloid solutions can be of two types: natural – plasma, whole blood, and albumin – or synthetic – hydroxyethyl starch solutions (i.e., hetastarch, Hextend®, Voluven®, VetStarch™, pentastarch), dextran, gelatin, and polymerized hemoglobin (de Jonge & Levi, 2001; Jones et al., 2001; McFarlane, 1999). There are a variety of colloid solutions that vary in molecular size, half-life, colloid osmotic pressure, side effects, and cost (Traylor & Pearl, 1996). The most commonly used colloids for fluid resuscitation in human medicine are albumin and hydroxyethyl starch (HES) (Boldt et al., 1998; Hollenberg et al., 2004). In horses, hydroxyethyl starches and fresh frozen plasma are most commonly used for resuscitation and/or correction of hypoproteinemia (Box 24.1).

Artificial colloids

Hydroxyethyl starches

Hydroxyethyl starches (HES) are highly polymeric glucose compounds, manufactured through hydrolysis and subsequent hydroxyethylation from the highly branched starch amylopectin, originating initially as thin boiling waxy corn or sorghum starch (Marik & Iglesias, 2000; Traylor & Pearl, 1996; Treib & Haass, 1997; Treib et al., 1999; Warren & Durieux, 1997). HES consists of D-glucose units that are connected within the chain through α-1,4 glycosidic bonds and occasional α-1,6 glycosidic branching linkages (Figure 24.1) (Marik & Iglesias, 2000; Treib & Haass, 1997; Treib et al., 1997, 1999). The degree of branching is approximately 1:20, that is, one 1–6 branch for every 20 glucose monomer units.

The blood volume expansion effects and rate of degradation of the colloids depends on three chemical attributes: (i) molecular weight; (ii) degree of substitution;

Equine Fluid Therapy, First Edition. Edited by C. Langdon Fielding and K. Gary Magdesian.
© 2015 John Wiley & Sons, Inc. Published 2015 by John Wiley & Sons, Inc.

and (iii) C2/C6 ratio. The molecular weight (MW) can be regarded as the average molecular weight or as weight average molecular weight (Treib et al., 1999). Average molecular weight is the arithmetic mean of the molecular weights in the solution; it assigns equal weight to all molecules regardless of size. The weight average MW assigns higher relative significance to larger molecules, being a weighted MW. The latter is used most commonly in clinical medicine (Treib et al., 1999). Lower molecular weight solutions exert a greater oncotic pressure (greater number of particles), but have a lower half-life in the circulation as they are more rapidly degraded and eliminated.

1 *Molecular weight:* Depending on the distribution of the weight average molecular weight of the particles, colloids can be categorized as either monodisperse or polydisperse (Warren & Durieux, 1997). Monodisperse colloids consist of molecules of one molecular weight only (e.g., albumin), while polydisperse (e.g., HES) contain a range of molecules with different MWs (Jones et al., 2001; Marik & Iglesias, 2000; Treib et al., 1999; Warren & Durieux, 1997). The MW determines the colloidal activity of HES (Treib et al., 1999).

Box 24.1 Colloids or crystalloids?

- Fluid resuscitation protocols remain controversial in horses and humans.
- Meta-analysis to date has failed to demonstrate an improvement in survival between administration of colloids vs crystalloids.

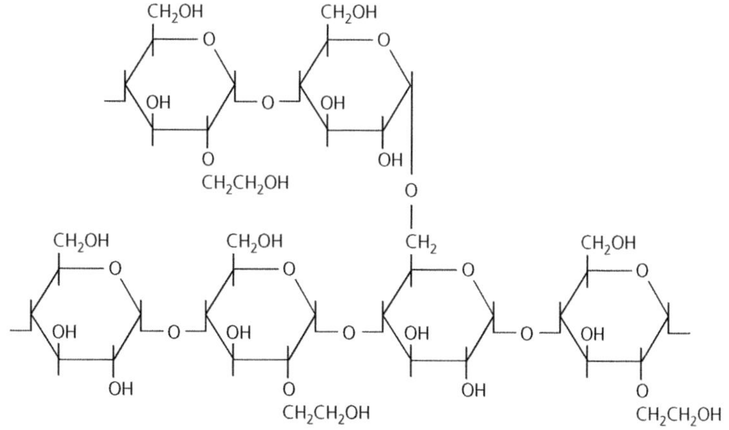

Moreover, a higher MW will result in a slower elimination rate.

2 *Degree of substitution (DS):* The degree of substitution of HES (expressed as a number between 0 and 1) indicates the average number of hydroxyethyl groups per glucose unit (Marik & Iglesias, 2000; Traylor & Pearl, 1996; Treib & Haass, 1997; Treib et al., 1997, 1999; Warren & Durieux, 1997). The importance of the degree of substitution is that α-amylase can only degrade unsubstituted glucose units (Marik & Iglesias, 2000; Traylor & Pearl, 1996; Treib & Haass, 1997). Thus by changing the degree of substitution, it is possible to influence the degree of enzymatic breakdown and control the extent and duration of the volume effect (Marik & Iglesias, 2000; Treib & Haass, 1997; Treib et al., 1997). A higher degree of substitution results in slower breakdown and elimination of the molecule (Traylor & Pearl, 1996).

3 *C2/C6 ratio:* HES hydroxyethylation can occur at carbon positions C2, C3, or C6 of the glucose molecule, depending on manufacturing (Treib et al., 1997, 1999). The substitution type is identified by the C2/C6 hydroxyethylation ratio (Treib et al., 1999). The higher the ratio (i.e., the greater the number of glucose molecules hydroxyethylated at the C2 atom compared to the C6 atom), the slower the starch is metabolized (de Jonge & Levi, 2001; Treib et al., 1997; Warren & Durieux, 1997). The reason for this slow metabolism is that hydroxyethyl residues bound at the C2 position of glucose inhibit plasma amylase, therefore increasing the intravascular half-life of HES. Thus, the hydroxyethylation pattern greatly influences the

Figure 24.1 Chemical structure of hydroxyethyl starch (HES) molecule.

in vivo characteristics of HES, even if they have the same MW (Treib et al., 1999). Importantly, renal function has been shown to decrease after administration of HES with a degree of substitution of more than 0.62 in humans undergoing surgery, as well with the administration of 10% solutions.

The pharmacokinetic profile of HES is directly related to its particle size (MW), which determines colloidal activity, and to its degree of substitution and hydroxyethylation pattern (C2/C6 ratio), which are the major determinants of metabolism and circulating half-life (de Jonge & Levi, 2001; Traylor & Pearl, 1996; Treib et al., 1999). For example, a high molecular weight range (450 kDa vs 200 kDa) and a more extensive degree of substitution (0.7 vs 0.5) will result in slower elimination. Plasma-expanding capacity on a low molecular weight and degree of substitution HES (i.e., 130 kDa; DS: 0.38–0.45), is achieved by increasing the C2/C6 ratio (Niemi et al., 2010) (Box 24.2).

HES is removed from circulation by two main mechanisms: renal excretion and redistribution (Warren & Durieux, 1997). The most important mechanism is renal elimination, which removes 70–80% of the molecules, and it consists of two phases (Marik & Iglesias, 2000; McFarlane, 1999; Meister et al., 1992; Warren & Durieux, 1997). The first phase occurs almost immediately after administration and consists of the elimination, by glomerular filtration, of polymers with a MW of less than 50 kDa (Marik & Iglesias, 2000; Traylor & Pearl, 1996; Treib et al., 1999; Warren & Durieux, 1997). A second phase of glomerular filtration is more prolonged and occurs as the HES molecules are metabolized (Marik & Iglesias, 2000; Traylor &

Pearl, 1996). Metabolism due to hydrolysis by α-amylase results in an average *in vivo* MW that is significantly lower than the average MW of the infused solution (de Jonge & Levi, 2001). Once the product of α-amylase digestion is smaller than 72 kDa, it can be renally excreted (Traylor & Pearl, 1996; Warren & Durieux, 1997). Some of these molecules, metabolized by α-amylase, are also excreted in the bile; however, this is a much less important elimination route (Traylor & Pearl, 1996).

The second mechanism of removal from the circulation is redistribution, which accounts for 20–30% of the elimination and consists of uptake and temporary storage of HES in tissues (McFarlane, 1999; Warren & Durieux, 1997). The extravasated molecules are stored in phagocytic cells of the liver, lymph nodes, and spleen and degradation by lysosomal enzymes occurs over time (McFarlane, 1999). After 24 hours, 23% of the total dose of HES is extravasated into the interstitial space (Warren & Durieux, 1997). As a result of these processes, only 38% of the initial dose remains in the intravascular space 24 hours post-administration, whereas 39% is excreted in urine and 23% is sequestered in tissues (Warren & Durieux, 1997). The duration of volume expansion with HES is approximately 24 hours, although trace amounts can be detected in the circulation for up to 17–26 weeks (Hollenberg et al., 2004; Marik & Iglesias, 2000; McFarlane, 1999; Treib et al., 1999; Warren & Durieux, 1997) (Box 24.3).

The elimination rate of HES varies both over time and among species (McFarlane, 1999). Variation in the elimination of larger molecules may reflect species differences in serum α-amylase concentrations (Jones et al., 2001; McFarlane, 1999). Serum α-amylase concentration and activity are less in horses compared with humans (Jones et al., 2001; McFarlane, 1999). The enzyme α-amylase, due to intravascular hydrolysis of large polymers of HES, yields a greater number of osmotically active molecules and serves to sustain the increases in plasma colloid osmotic pressure (COP)

Box 24.2 Pharmacokinetics of hydroxyethyl starch (HES)

The pharmacokinetics of HES are determined by:

- Particle size (MW). This determines colloidal activity – the higher the MW the slower the elimination.
- Degree of substitution – the higher the value, the greater the substitution, and the slower are breakdown and elimination.
- Hydroxyethylation pattern (C2/C6 ratio). This is a major determinant of metabolism and half-life. A higher C2/C6 ratio means slower degradation.

Box 24.3 Elimination of HES

- Renal excretion (70–80%):
  ○ Glomerular filtration of small particles
  ○ Glomerular filtration post α-amylase metabolism
- Redistribution (20–30%)

Table 24.1 Properties of commonly available hydroxyethyl starches (HES)

Product (HES)	Concentration and solvent	MW (kDa)	Molar substitution	C2/C6 ratio	Classification	Tradenames
670/0.75	6%, balanced	670	0.75	4.5:1	Hetastarch	Hextend®
450/0.7	6%, saline	450	0.7	5:1		Hespan®
200/0.62	6%, saline	200	0.62	9:1	Hexastarch	Elohes®
200/0.5	6% and 10%, saline	200	0.5	5:1	Pentastarch	Pentaspan®
130/0.4	6%, saline	130	0.4	9:1	Tetrastarch	Voluven® VetStarch™
130/0.42	6% or 10%, balanced	130	0.42	6:1	Tetrastarch	Tetraspan®

associated with hetastarch administration (Jones et al., 1997).

Different HES solutions are listed in Table 24.1; these products vary in the concentration of colloid particles, MW, degree of substitution, and C2/C6 ratio (Marx, 2003; Treib et al., 1999). These differences allow varying effects on plasma volume expansion, COP, coagulation, and rheology (Marx, 2003). However, it should be noted that data from different studies concerning the extent and duration of volume expansion of various HES solutions are difficult to compare (Marx, 2003; Treib et al., 1999).

There are three HES products available in the United States:

- hetastarch (0.7 degree substitution);
- pentastarch (0.5 degree substitution);
- tetrastarch (0.4 degree substitution).

The most widely used HES solution in human and veterinary medicine in the United States is hetastarch 450/0.7 (Hespan®, B. Braun Medical); this solution has an average MW of 450 kDa and degree of substitution of 0.7 (i.e., 70 % of its glucose units have a hydroxyethyl group) (Traylor & Pearl, 1996). It is composed of a heterogeneous population of molecules, with 80% of the molecules having MWs between 300 and 2400 kDa (McFarlane, 1999; Traylor & Pearl, 1996). The advantage of this type of HES is its relatively prolonged volume effect because of the larger MW colloid particles and the high degree of substitution. However, it has been associated with dose-dependent coagulation abnormalities (Treib et al., 1999). Hetastarch in Hespan is suspended in a 0.9% sodium chloride solution. Hextend (BioTime, Inc.) has a MW of 670 kDa and the same degree of substitution as Hespan, but it is suspended in a calcium-containing lactated Ringer's solution (LRS) similar to commercial LRS, although electrolyte concentrations are slightly different (Na, 143 mEq/L; Cl, 124 mEq/L; K, 3 mEq/L; lactate, 28 mEq/L). The dilution in a balanced electrolyte solution may be advantageous in reducing the amount of chloride delivered as compared to saline (which is the diluent for Hespan), which could contribute to a hyperchloremic metabolic acidosis. Hextend also contains very small amounts of magnesium and dextrose (0.99%).

Tetrastarches have a 0.4 degree substitution. In 2008, the Food and Drug Administration also approved the use of a third-generation HES, Voluven. Voluven® (Hospira) is also diluted in 0.9% sodium chloride. VetStarch™ (Abbott Laboratories) is a relatively new HES product available for use in small animals. Like hetastarch these tetrastarches are a 6% HES solution in 0.9% sodium chloride. However, their molecular weight is lower (130) and the range of MW is much narrower than in hetastarch, at 110–150 kDa, and therefore the solution is fairly homogenous. The low molar substitution (0.4) is the main reason for the benefits of VetStarch on the pharmacokinetics, intravascular volume expansion, and hemodilution effects. The C2/C6 ratio is 9:1, which increases the half-life compared to hetastarch. The recommended dose for small animals is 20 mL/kg/day. Contraindications include fluid overload, especially pulmonary edema and congestive heart failure, renal failure with oliguria or anuria, and severe hypernatremia. The elimination of VetStarch is faster than pentastarch, with lower persistence in tissue. Because of the lower MW and degree of substitution these tetrastarches may be associated with fewer renal side effects.

A pentastarch (Pentaspan®; Bristol-Myers Squibb) is available in the United States for leukapheresis in humans, but not for fluid therapy. It is available as a

10% solution with a MW of 264 kDa. Pentastarch is used for treatment of hypovolemia in Europe.

Hemoglobin-based oxygen-carrying solutions (HBOCs)

Hemoglobin-based oxygen-carrying solutions (HBOCs) were developed to provide an alternative to whole blood transfusions. Only one commercial product (Oxyglobin®) was available in veterinary medicine and was labeled for the treatment of canine anemia[1]. This product was an acellular, ultrapurified, polymerized hemoglobin solution. The polymerization of the hemoglobin lengthened the half-life of the product and decreased the renal toxicity (Hohenhaus, 2002).

HBOCs have oxygen-carrying properties, are excellent colloids, and decrease blood viscosity. The decrease in blood viscosity improves tissue perfusion (Hollis, 2011). The large polymers exert a strong plasma oncotic effect, comparable to or greater than HES (Hohenhaus, 2002; Magdesian, 2003). In a hemorrhagic model in sheep, an HBOC showed greater colloidal activity than HES (Posner et al., 2003). In anemic ponies, an HBOC caused a greater increase in the central venous pressure than HES, thus suggesting that the colloid effects were superior to those of HES (Belgrave et al., 2002). While HBOCs vary in their colloid osmotic pressure, the most widely described product in veterinary medicine is reported to have a COP of approximately 40 mmHg (Day, 2003)

Purified hemoglobin is used in horses principally for the treatment of acute life-threatening anemia. Due to the cost of the commercially available products, HBOCs have been used primarily in newborn foals with neonatal isoerythrolysis (Hollis, 2011). Doses of 5 mL/kg in neonatal foals and 2 mL/kg in adult horses have been described (Hollis, 2011). No adverse effects and a good clinical response for the treatment of anemia were described (Hollis, 2011) (Box 24.4).

Box 24.4 Beneficial effects of Oxyglobin

- Oxygen-carrying capacity
- Strong colloid activity
- Lowers blood viscosity

---

[1]Oxyglobin is currently unavailable in the United States (http://www.oxyglobin.com/) but is available in the EU through Dechra.

Colloid use in equine critical care

A decrease in colloid osmotic pressure (COP) is one of the clinical effects associated with the administration of large volumes of intravenous crystalloids to horses (Boscan et al., 2007). However, the intravenous administration of colloids may result in an increase in the COP, therefore potentially increasing plasma volume (through Starling's law) (Jones et al., 1997; McFarlane, 1999). Based on Starling's law, COP is one important determinant of fluid distribution between the intravascular and extravascular spaces (Boscan et al., 2007). One liter of HES solution produced a 36% increase in the COP, 1 L of albumin increased the COP by 11%, and 1 L of saline decreased the COP by 12% in humans (Treib et al., 1999).

Increased circulating volume increases cardiac preload, arterial blood pressure, cardiac contractility, and cardiac output, thereby improving perfusion and oxygen delivery (Jones et al., 1997; McFarlane, 1999). The currently accepted and long-standing view in human critical care is that maintenance of colloid osmotic pressure is of secondary importance to maintenance of circulating volume (Webb, 1999). The use of colloids may prevent further reductions in COP, but very few human and veterinary intensive care units measure COP (Boscan & Steffey, 2007; Webb, 1999).

In contrast to crystalloids, resuscitation with colloids preserves COP, thereby mitigating transcapillary fluid movement and potentially resulting in a more effective volume expansion than with crystalloids per equivalent volume of fluid administration (Jones et al., 2001). Resuscitation with colloids requires smaller volumes and shorter infusion times to restore hemodynamic stability and improve tissue oxygen transport (Choi et al., 1999; Jones et al., 1997, 2001). The infusion of 1 L of HES expands the plasma volume by between 700 mL and 1 L in humans (Hollenberg et al., 2004). It has been shown that colloids improve myocardial contractility and cardiac output (Choi et al., 1999). In experimental studies with endotoxemic rats resuscitated with a crystalloid (0.9% saline) or a colloid (Hextend), the investigators found longer survival times and less metabolic acidosis, and that smaller amounts of fluid were needed in the colloid group (Kellum et al., 2002). In a porcine sepsis model, HES-infused animals showed improved systemic oxygenation, higher cardiac output and systemic oxygen delivery, and lower oxygen extraction ratio compared to crystalloid-treated animals (Marx, 2003). In horses, an improvement in global perfusion (increased cardiac index and stroke volume index) was observed when hydroxyethyl starch (pentastarch, MW 200 kDa) was used prior to colic surgery. These effects lasted for up to 195 minutes (Hallowell & Corley, 2006). However, meta-analysis and several studies comparing crystalloids versus colloids, could not demonstrate differences in mortality, pulmonary edema, or length of hospital stay (Choi et al., 1999; Hartog et al., 2011; Perel & Roberts, 2007; Rizoli, 2003). Moreover, a meta-analysis found no evidence that one colloid was safer than another in critically ill patients; however, it could not rule out clinically significant differences (Bunn et al., 2008).

Hydroxyethyl starch may have the ability to seal endothelial "pores" or gaps that develop in the microvessels after different forms of endothelial injury, including sepsis and endotoxemia (Warren & Durieux, 1997). By this means, HES may prevent the leakage of plasma proteins (especially albumin) from the intravascular space, thus preventing secondary fluid extravasation (Warren & Durieux, 1997). The medium MW particles, between 100 and 300 kDa, may act as plugs at these endothelial "pores" (Hughes, 2001; Jones et al., 2001; McFarlane, 1999). It has been postulated that there are two different-sized pores in the capillaries, small pores through which only water and electrolytes can flow and large pores through which large molecules such as albumin can extravasate (Conhaim et al., 1999; Marik & Iglesias, 2000). According to this theory, it is the number of the pores rather than the size, that increases in patients with capillary leak syndrome (Marik & Iglesias, 2000). The oncotic pressure exerted by HES would not affect flow through the large pores, but it would decrease flow through small pores, which are assumed to account for the major porosity of the capillaries, both in health and sepsis (Conhaim et al., 1999; Marik & Iglesias, 2000). Unfortunately, there are no clinically applicable techniques for measuring the magnitude of microvascular changes during vascular leak states; one clinical suggestion of increased permeability would be an unexpectedly short duration of action (volume expansion) of the infused colloid (Hughes, 2001). An *in vivo* study found that HES of medium MW and low degree of substitution had a retention rate, within the blood vessels, comparable with high MW HES in rat tissue (Hitosugi et al., 2007). Low molecular weight HES (200/0.5) has a

larger portion of molecules that are smaller than albumin, yet they do not freely extravasate. The likely reasons why these molecules do not escape to the interstitial space are the presence of surface binding proteins, the charge of the subendothelial matrix, and the surface charge (Marx, 2003).

Evidence suggests that HES has the ability to modulate the endothelial inflammatory response and by this mechanism attenuate the permeability increase associated with sepsis (Jones et al., 2001). In one of the few long-term studies (5 days) involving human septic patients, those treated with HES solution had a significant reduction in plasma concentrations of adhesion molecules, including soluble endothelial leukocyte adhesion molecule 1 (ELAM-1), soluble intercellular cell adhesion molecule 1 (ICAM-1), and soluble vascular cell adhesion molecule 1 (VCAM-1) (Boldt et al., 1996a). This could also explain why this therapy produces less tissue edema and injury (Marik & Iglesias, 2000; Boldt et al., 1996a). This reduction in circulating concentration of adhesion molecules may indicate diminished endothelial damage or represent decreased endothelial activation (Marik & Iglesias, 2000). It has been suggested that HES inhibits P-selectin expression (Boldt et al., 1996a; Marik & Iglesias, 2000). Because leukocyte–endothelial cell interactions are a prerequisite for transendothelial migration and infiltration of leukocytes into tissues, attenuation of this pathway could reduce tissue injury (Marik & Iglesias, 2000). Thus by binding to surface receptors HES molecules could alter the expression of adhesion molecules by the endothelium (Marik & Iglesias, 2000). Another mechanism by which HES could decrease the expression of adhesion molecules is by acting as a scavenger for oxygen free radicals and possibly by decreasing the release of cytokines, such as interleukin 6 (IL-6) (Boldt et al., 1996a, 1996b; 1998; Marik & Iglesias, 2000). The effect on the reduction of IL-6 is important because this cytokine exerts detrimental effects at the microcirculatory level (Boldt et al., 1996a, 1998). HES also improves macro and microcirculatory flow, resulting in less expression or release of adhesion molecules in the circulation, thereby reducing leukocyte adhesion (Boldt et al., 1996b; Marik & Iglesias, 2000). In an *in vitro* study the addition of HES to plasma from septic patients decreased neutrophil aggregation and adhesion (Khan et al., 2011).

In humans HES is administered at much higher doses and for longer periods of time compared to horses.

In horses, recommended doses for high molecular weight HES are 5 to 10 mL/kg. In humans the dose of HES varies between 20 and 50 mL/kg, depending on the type of HES administered (Niemi et al., 2010). This same dose in adult horses would be cost prohibitive in many cases and could lead to adverse effects on coagulation. Most often HES is used in critically ill horses for initial resuscitation concurrent with or followed by infusion of balanced crystalloid solutions. By using HES during initial resuscitation, the risks of volume overload with massive amounts of crystalloid fluids may be minimized; assuming permeability to colloids is not altered (Box 24.5).

Adverse effects

Plasma viscosity is determined by the number and physical properties of macromolecules in plasma (Treib et al., 1999). Plasma viscosity is an important contributor to the microcirculatory disturbances that characterize shock (Treib et al., 1999). Highly substituted HES is less desirable in this regard because it increases plasma viscosity (Treib et al., 1999). Medium MW HES, with low C2/C6 ratios, and low MW starches decrease plasma viscosity and have better rheological properties (Treib et al., 1999).

A major concern regarding the use of HES in horses relates to its effects on hemostasis (Jones et al., 1997). All colloids induce dilution of red blood cells, platelets, and coagulation factors; in cases of extreme hemodilution these abnormalities become clinically significant (Niemi et al., 2010). However, there is conflicting and controversial information in the literature regarding the effects of HES solutions on coagulation in humans (de Jonge & Levi, 2001; Warren & Durieux, 1997). In addition, the true risk for bleeding complications of patients treated with HES solutions is difficult to predict, unless the patient has a known underlying coagulopathy in which case HES should not be used (Treib et al., 1999; Stump et al., 1985; Warren & Durieux, 1997). The risk of clinical bleeding is influenced by the quantity of HES infused, the preparation selected, whether single or multiple infusions are given, the nature of other fluids infused, and the medical condition of the patient (e.g., underlying coagulation abnormality or thrombocytopenia) (de Jonge & Levi, 2001; Stump et al., 1985; Treib et al., 1999). The release of inflammatory mediators – tumor necrosis factor (TNF) and IL-1 – may have additional effects on coagulation (Boldt et al., 1998). Patients with septic shock are in a procoagulant state and are at risk of developing disseminated intravascular coagulation and thrombocytopenia (Falk et al., 1988).

HES causes dose-dependent decreases in factor VIII and von Willebrand factor (vWf) activity and prolongation of partial thromboplastin time (PTT) (Hollenberg et al., 2004; Marik & Iglesias, 2000; Stump et al., 1985). These abnormalities may only be relevant in patients with baseline low concentrations of clotting factors and or in patients undergoing surgery (Marik & Iglesias, 2000). Factor VIII is an important factor for maintaining a normal activated PTT (aPTT) (Stump et al., 1985). HES 480/0.7 (hetastarch) produces a decrease in factor VIII that is beyond those effects attributed to hemodilution, and presumably is due to additional mechanisms (Stump et al., 1985). It also has been shown that the bleeding complications associated with HES are due to an acquired von Willebrand syndrome (Treib et al., 1997).

Furthermore, HES can affect platelet function by adhering to the platelet membranes and decreasing the number of binding sites (glycoprotein IIb/IIIa) for fibrinogen and von Willebrand factor (Wierenga et al., 2007). Molecular weight and degree of substitution are correlated with greater platelet dysfunction, with higher values inducing greater defects.

With HES 480/0.7, bleeding complications were reported in humans after the use of high doses for several days (Stump et al., 1985; Treib et al., 1997). However, HES 480/0.7 produces only minor effects on clotting when infused to human or animals in moderate amounts (not exceeding 20 mL/kg, or 1500 mL total volume, to a person over 24 hours) (Strauss, 1981; Strauss et al., 1988; Stump et al., 1985). Platelet counts either remained normal or decreased transiently, always remaining above the levels required for normal hemostasis (>100,000/mL) (Strauss, 1981). Even when the clotting parameters were abnormal, specific clotting proteins were present in amounts thought to be sufficient to ensure effective hemostasis (Strauss, 1981). Therefore the coagulation effects of small to moderate doses of HES 480/0.7 were transient and trivial, whereas administration of massive infusions resulted in a wide variety of laboratory abnormalities and even clinical hemorrhage (Strauss, 1981).

It has been reported that after a single administration of HES the concentration of fibrinogen decreases (Treib et al., 1997). This effect is probably due to an acceleration of fibrin polymerization, and its effects on hemostasis are considered irrelevant (Treib et al., 1997). In a study with healthy human volunteers, HES 480/0.7 decreased fibrinogen concentration immediately after infusion, an alteration that was attributed to dilutional effects (Stump et al., 1985).

Thus the major effects of HES on coagulation are dilution of plasma clotting factors, an additional decrease in factor VIII, and accelerated fibrin clot formation in the last stages of clotting. In addition, platelet dysfunction associated with coating of their surface occurs.

An equine study was carried out to investigate the effects of HES in normal ponies (Jones et al., 1997). Ponies were divided into three groups: those infused at a dose of 10 mL/kg of HES or 20 mL/kg of HES, and a control group administered 80 mL/kg of saline. All infusions were done within a 2-hour period. In the HES groups dose-dependent alterations in vWf and factor VIII were observed over time. The effects on these coagulation proteins were beyond the dilutional effects of HES. The maximal decrease in factor VIII activity was coincidental with the maximal reduction in vWf activity, suggesting the role of vWf as a carrier protein for factor VIII, and that direct effects of HES on factor VIII could have been responsible (Jones et al., 1997). A difference from other human and animal studies is that the aPTT and partial thrombin time (PTT) values were not prolonged, as would be expected based on the decrease in factor VIII concentration. Therefore it can be assumed that the reduction in factor VIII was not great enough to have a clinical effect. The primary hemostasis in this study was evaluated by measuring cutaneous bleeding time (Jones et al., 1997). Bleeding time is considered the most physiologically and clinically relevant test of the platelet response to vascular injury (Harker et al., 1972; Jones et al., 1997). Minimal effects were seen on this parameter in ponies treated with HES (Jones et al., 1997). A reduction in platelet count attributed to the dilutional effect was observed in the group with the highest HES dose.

Hextend (HES 670/0.7) is a calcium-containing balanced polyionic HES solution. This product could have the ability to improve platelet function due to its calcium content. However, an *in vitro* study assessing platelet function in dogs found no beneficial effect of the calcium-containing HES over HES in saline (Wierenga et al., 2007). The effects on coagulation of Hextend (in balanced solution) were less than those of slowly degradable HES in normal saline; however, these differences were clinically insignificant (Martin et al., 2002). Another advantage of balanced HES solutions (Hextend) is the lack of acid–base disturbances that may be caused by administration of large volumes of 0.9% saline, namely hyperchloremic metabolic acidosis.

Tetrastarches are third-generation hydroxyethyl starches and reportedly are much safer than standard hetastarches. They have fewer adverse effects on coagulation and bleeding as well as on renal function. In humans, tetrastarches seem to have minimal effects on coagulation and renal function; however, these remain to be studied in horses.

It should be pointed out that an investigator (Joachim Boldt, MD) has been found to have committed scientific misconduct (Editors-in-Chief, 2011). Therefore, several of his published research trials (88 of 102) have been retracted, and this has called the safety of HES into doubt.

The adverse effects of hydroxyethyl starches have recently attracted renewed interest in human medicine. A recent meta-analysis evaluated critically ill patients requiring acute volume resuscitation (Zarychanski et al., 2013). The meta-analysis included 38 trials and 10,880 patients. Hetastarch did not decrease mortality. When seven trials (590 patients) were excluded due to retraction of these studies because of scientific misconduct, hydroxyethyl starch was found to be associated with increased mortality among the remaining 10,290 patients (RR 1.90; 95% CI: 1.02–1.17). In addition, there was increased renal failure among patients who received HES (Zarychanski et al., 2013). How this increase in mortality and incidence of renal failure relate to equine medicine is unknown. There are no reports of renal failure secondary to HES administration in horses, and no studies have evaluated mortality in horses receiving colloids versus those that only received crystalloids. However, the results of this meta-analysis raise concern.

Natural colloids

Plasma is the liquid component of the blood and constitutes approximately 55–65% of the blood volume in horses (Marcilese, 1965). It is 95% water; the remaining

5% is composed of electrolytes, hormones, cytokines, and proteins. Albumin is the main protein component of plasma; it has a molecular weight of 69 kDa. Albumin has multiple vital functions such as the maintenance of COP, transport of endogenous and exogenous substances, mediation of coagulation, and inhibition of oxidative damage (Mazzaferro, 2002). Albumin also plays an important role in maintaining the integrity, function, and repair of the gastrointestinal tract (Mazzaferro, 2002). Albumin is synthesized by hepatocytes and degraded by the reticuloendothelial system. Plasma COP at the hepatic interstitial space is one of the strongest stimuli for albumin synthesis; thus supranormal administration of colloids suppresses albumin synthesis (Mazzaferro, 2002). Albumin accounts for approximately 70–80% of the plasma COP, while other plasma proteins such as globulins collectively account for the rest of the oncotic pressure (Mazzaferro, 2002; Warren & Durieux, 1997). The total body albumin (in humans) is 4.5–5.0 g/kg, one-third of which is intravascular (Warren & Durieux, 1997). The interstitial space contains 60–70% of the total albumin (Mazzaferro, 2002). The extravascular pool of albumin acts as a reservoir and serves as a source to replenish the intravascular pool in cases of acute albumin loss (Mazzaferro, 2002).

Colloid osmotic pressure is an important force that regulates transvascular fluid flow, and it is one of the forces opposing fluid escape from the vasculature. Another phenomenon that contributes to water's attraction to colloids is the Gibbs–Donnan effect. The negative charges of albumin molecules attract sodium cations, this in turn causes water to follow across the semipermeable endothelial membrane (Mazzaferro, 2002).

Critically ill patients can develop hypoalbuminemia secondary to the systemic inflammatory response syndrome, hepatic failure, protein-losing enteropathies, and nephritic/nephrotic syndrome. Hypoalbuminemia in turn results in further complications such as organ dysfunction, pulmonary and tissue edema, enteral feeding intolerance, poor wound healing, and hypercoagulability. In humans and animals, hypoalbuminemia has been correlated with increased morbidity and mortality (Mazzaferro, 2002).

To date, there are no commercially available concentrated equine or canine albumin products (Cohn et al., 2007). Plasma transfusions are the only source of equine specific albumin replacement. Equine plasma contains approximately 2.6–3.7 g/dL of albumin, and canine plasma contains 2.5–3.0 g/dL of albumin. Therefore, treatment of severely hypoproteinemic horses would require large volumes of plasma. Cost, availability, potential for adverse reactions, and volume overload are all considerations with large-volume plasma transfusions in horses (Cohn et al., 2007). In dogs treated with human serum albumin, severe life-threatening reactions were detected post-administration (Cohn et al., 2007).

Plasma contains other proteins besides albumin that are beneficial. Plasma immunoglobulins are used for the treatment of foals with partial or complete failure of passive transfer. Other important plasma proteins include macroglobulins, coagulation proteins (II, VII, IX, and X), antithrombin III, elastase, and proteinase inhibitors among others.

It has been suggested that adult horses would require large volumes of plasma, in the range of 6–8 L/day, in order to increase and maintain plasma protein concentration (Jones, 2004). There are no published guidelines for plasma therapy for albumin replacement in critically ill horses. It has been suggested that 10–15 mL/kg of plasma would raise the plasma albumin by 0.1 g/dL in horses, while in small animals 22.5 mL/kg of plasma is required to increase the plasma albumin by 0.5 g/dL (Mazzaferro, 2002). The following formula can be used to estimate the amount (mL) of plasma needed to increase the concentration of recipient plasma total solids; this assumes there are no interstitial deficits or ongoing losses (Mazzaferro, 2002).

$$
\begin{aligned}
\mathrm{Plasma\,(mL)} =\, & \mathrm{desired\,recipient\,TS\,(g\,/\,dL)} \\
& -\mathrm{recipient\,TS\,(g\,/\,dL)} \times \mathrm{weight\,(kg)} \\
& \times 50\,/\,\mathrm{donor\,TS\,(g\,/\,dL)}
\end{aligned}
\tag{24.1}
$$

where TS = total solids.

Each gram of albumin can hold 18 mL of water within the intravascular space (Mazzaferro, 2002). Assuming that albumin content in equine plasma averages 3.0 g/dL, each liter of plasma should be able to retain 540 mL of water within the intravascular space. Furthermore, it can be assumed that the administration of 8 L of equine plasma could expand the intravascular space by approximately 4 L, thus the plasma volume expansion of exogenous plasma is less than that of artificial colloids. The administration or coadministration of synthetic colloids to critically ill patients that are hypoalbuminemic may be more effective in restoring and maintaining plasma volume and COP. Synthetic colloids may reduce the risks of volume overload and edema formation that large volumes of plasma administration could potentially produce.

Given that 60% of the total body albumin is located extravascularly, administration of albumin can replenish the extravascular interstitial pool as well as the intravascular concentration. Consequently in critically ill hypoalbuminemic patients with leaky vasculature, the administration of an albumin source will not result in increases in the COP if most of the administered albumin moves into the interstitium (Mazzaferro, 2002). This can potentiate pulmonary edema in patients with acute respiratory distress syndrome. In humans and small animals, the aim is to maintain the plasma albumin concentration at 2.0 g/dL (Mazzaferro, 2002). Since the use of plasma alone to maintain COP is expensive and there is the risk of volume overload, combination therapy with synthetic colloids may be a better alternative, although potential adverse effects of synthetic colloids listed above should be considered. Addition of colloids will help to maintain COP, prevent formation of interstitial edema, and maintain plasma volume.

The addition of albumin to serum from septic patients resulted in decreased platelet and neutrophil activation and decreased formation of platelet-neutrophil aggregates (Khan et al., 2011). Moreover, neutrophil–endothelial cell interactions were minimized if endothelial cells were incubated with albumin, and endothelial E-selectin expression was reduced (Khan et al., 2011).

References

Bedenice D. (2007) Evidence-based medicine in equine critical care. *Vet Clin North Am Equine Pract* **23**:293–316.

Belgrave RL, Hines MT, Keegan RD, et al. (2002) Effects of a polymerized ultrapurified bovine hemoglobin blood substitute administered to ponies with normovolemic anemia. *J Vet Intern Med* **16**:396–403.

Boldt J, Muller M, Heesen M, et al. (1996a) Influence of different volume therapies and pentoxifylline infusion on circulating soluble adhesion molecules in critically ill patients. *Crit Care Med* **24**:385–91.

Boldt J, Mueller M, Menges T, et al. (1996b) Influence of different volume therapy regimens on regulators of the circulation in the critically ill. *Br J Anaesth* **77**:480–7.

Boldt J, Muller M, Mentges D, et al. (1998) Volume therapy in the critically ill: is there a difference? *Intensive Care Med* **24**:28–36.

Boluyt N, Bollen CW, Bos AP, et al. (2006) Fluid resuscitation in neonatal and pediatric hypovolemic shock: a Dutch Pediatric Society evidence-based clinical practice guideline. *Intensive Care Med* **32**:995–1003.

Boscan P, Steffey EP. (2007) Plasma colloid osmotic pressure and total protein in horses during colic surgery. *Vet Anaesth Analg* **34**:408–15.

Boscan P, Watson Z, Steffey EP. (2007) Plasma colloid osmotic pressure and total protein trends in horses during anesthesia. *Vet Anaesth Analg* **34**:275–83.

Bunn F, Trivedi D, Ashraf S. (2008) Colloid solutions for fluid resuscitation. Cochrane Database Syst Rev CD001319; doi: 10.1002/14651858.CD001319.pub2.

Choi PT, Yip G, Quinonez LG, et al. (1999) Crystalloids vs. colloids in fluid resuscitation: a systematic review. *Crit Care Med* **27**:200–10.

Cohn LA, Kerl ME, Lenox CE, et al. (2007) Response of healthy dogs to infusions of human serum albumin. *Am J Vet Res* **68**:657–63.

Conhaim RL, Watson KE, Potenza BM, et al. (1999) Pulmonary capillary sieving of hetastarch is not altered by LPS-induced sepsis. *J Trauma* **46**:800–8; discussion 808–10.

Consensus conference. (1985) Fresh-frozen plasma. *Indications and risks. JAMA* **253**:551–3.

Day TK. (2003) Current development and use of hemoglobin-based oxygen-carrying (HBOC) solutions. *J Vet Emerg Crit Care* **13**:77–93.

de Jonge E, Levi M. (2001) Effects of different plasma substitutes on blood coagulation: a comparative review. *Crit Care Med* **29**:1261–7.

Editors-in-Chief. (2011) Editors-in-Chief statement regarding published clinical trials conducted without IRB approval by Joachim Boldt. Available at: http://www.aaeditor.org/EIC. Joint.Statement.on.Retractions.pdf.

Falk JL, Rackow EC, Astiz ME, et al. (1988) Effects of hetastarch and albumin on coagulation in patients with septic shock. *J Clin Pharmacol* **28**:412–15.

Hallowell GD, Corley KT. (2006) Preoperative administration of hydroxyethyl starch or hypertonic saline to horses with colic. *J Vet Intern Med* **20**:980–6.

Harker LA, Slichter SJ. (1972) The bleeding time as a screening test for evaluation of platelet function. *N Engl J Med* **287**:155–9.

Hartog CS, Bauer M, Reinhart K. (2011) The efficacy and safety of colloid resuscitation in the critically ill. *Anesth Analg* **112**:156–64.

Hitosugi T, Saito T, Suzuki S, et al. (2007) Hydroxyethyl starch: the effect of molecular weight and degree of substitution on intravascular retention in vivo. *Anesth Analg* **105**:724–8.

Hohenhaus AE. (2002) Oxyglobin: a transfusion solution? *J Vet Intern Med* **16**:394–5.

Hollenberg SM, Ahrens TS, Annane D, et al. (2004) Practice parameters for hemodynamic support of sepsis in adult patients: 2004 update. *Crit Care Med* **32**:1928–48.

Hollis ACK. (2011) Initial experience of ultrapurified bovine haemoglobin use in horses. *Equine Vet Education* **23**:562–8.

Hughes D. (2001) Fluid therapy with artificial colloids: complications and controversies. *Vet Anaesth Analg* **28**:111–18.

Jones PA, Tomasic M, Gentry PA. (1997) Oncotic, hemodilutional, and hemostatic effects of isotonic saline and hydroxyethyl starch solutions in clinically normal ponies. *Am J Vet Res* **58**:541–8.

Jones PA, Bain FT, Byars TD, et al. (2001) Effect of hydroxyethyl starch infusion on colloid oncotic pressure in hypoproteinemic horses. *J Am Vet Med Assoc* **218**:1130–5.

Jones SL. (2004) Inflammatory diseases of the gastrointestinal tract causing diarrhea. In: Reed B, Bayly W, Sellon D (eds) *Equine Internal Medicine*, 2nd edn. St Louis, MO: Elsevier, pp. 884–913.

Kellum JA. (2002) Fluid resuscitation and hyperchloremic acidosis in experimental sepsis: improved short-term survival and acid-base balance with Hextend compared with saline. *Crit Care Med* **30**:300–5.

Khan R, Kirschenbaum LA, Larow C, et al. (2011) The effect of resuscitation fluids on neutrophil-endothelial cell interactions in septic shock. *Shock* **36**:440–4.

Khandelwal P, Bohn D, Carcillo JA, et al. (2002) Pro/con clinical debate: do colloids have advantages over crystalloids in paediatric sepsis? *Crit Care* **6**:286–8.

Magdesian K. (2003) Colloid replacement in the ICU. *Clin Tech Equine Pract* **2**:130–7.

Marcilese NA, Valsecchi RM, Figueiras HD, et al. (1965) Normal blood volumes in the horse. *Am J Physiol* **207**:223–7.

Marik PE, Iglesias J. (2000) Would the colloid detractors please sit down! *Crit Care Med* **28**:2652–4.

Martin G, Bennett-Guerrero E, Wakeling H, et al. (2002) A prospective, randomized comparison of thromboelastographic coagulation profile in patients receiving lactated Ringer's solution, 6% hetastarch in a balanced-saline vehicle, or 6% hetastarch in saline during major surgery. *J Cardiothorac Vasc Anesth* **16**:441–6.

Marx G. (2003) Fluid therapy in sepsis with capillary leakage. *Eur J Anaesthesiol* **20**:429–42.

Mazzaferro EM. (2002) The role of albumin replacement in the critically ill veterinary patient. *J Vet Emerg Crit Care* **12**:113–24.

McFarlane D. (1999) Hetastarch: A synthetic colloid with potential in equine patients. *Comp Contin Educ Pract Vet* **21**:867–77.

Meister D, Hermann M, Mathis GA. (1992) Kinetics of hydroxyethyl starch in horses. *Schweiz Arch Tierheilkd* **134**:329–39.

Niemi TT, Miyashita R, Yamakage M. (2010) Colloid solutions: a clinical update. *J Anesth* **24**:913–25.

Oliveira RP, Velasco I, Soriano F, et al. (2002a) Clinical review: Hypertonic saline resuscitation in sepsis. *Crit Care* **6**:418–23.

Oliveira RP, Weingartner R, Ribas EO, et al. (2002b) Acute haemodynamic effects of a hypertonic saline/dextran solution in stable patients with severe sepsis. *Intensive Care Med* **28**:1574–81.

Perel P, Roberts I. (2007) Colloids versus crystalloids for fluid resuscitation in critically ill patients. *Cochrane Database Syst Rev Oct* **17**(4): CD000567.

Perel P, Roberts I. (2011) Colloids versus crystalloids for fluid resuscitation in critically ill patients (Review). *Cochrane Database Syst Rev Issue* **3**:CD000567; doi: 10.1002/14651858. CD000567.pub4.

Posner LP, Moon PF, Bliss SP, et al. (2003) Colloid osmotic pressure after hemorrhage and replenishment with Oxyglobin Solution, hetastarch, or whole blood in pregnant sheep. *Vet Anaesth Analg* **30**:30–6.

Rizoli SB. (2003) Crystalloids and colloids in trauma resuscitation: a brief overview of the current debate. *J Trauma* **54**:S82–88.

Strauss RG, Stansfield C, Henriksen RA, et al. (1988) Pentastarch may cause fewer effects on coagulation than hetastarch. *Transfusion* **28**:257–60.

Strauss RG. (1981) Review of the effects of hydroxyethyl starch on the blood coagulation system. *Transfusion* **21**:299–302.

Stump DC, Strauss RG, Henriksen RA, et al. (1985) Effects of hydroxyethyl starch on blood coagulation, particularly factor VIII. *Transfusion* **25**:349–54.

Traylor RJ, Pearl RG. (1996) Crystalloid versus colloid versus colloid: all colloids are not created equal. *Anesth Analg* **83**:209–12.

Treib J, Haass A. (1997) Hydroxyethyl starch. *J Neurosurg* **86**:574–5.

Treib J, Haass A, Pindur G. (1997) Coagulation disorders caused by hydroxyethyl starch. *Thromb Haemost* **78**:974–83.

Treib J, Baron JF, Grauer MT, et al. (1999) An international view of hydroxyethyl starches. *Intensive Care Med* **25**:258–68.

Warren BB, Durieux ME. (1997) Hydroxyethyl starch: safe or not? *Anesth Analg* **84**:206–12.

Webb AR. (1999) Crystalloid or colloid for resuscitation. Are we any the wiser? *Crit Care (Lond)* **3**:R25–R28.

Wierenga JR, Jandrey KE, Haskins SC, et al. (2007) In vitro comparison of the effects of two forms of hydroxyethyl starch solutions on platelet function in dogs. *Am J Vet Res* **68**:605–9.

Zarychanski R, Abou-Setta AH, Turgeon AF, et al. (2013) Association of hydroxyethyl starch administration with mortality and acute kidney injury in critically ill patients requiring volume resuscitation: a systematic review and meta-analysis. *JAMA* **309**:678–88.

CHAPTER 25

Parenteral nutrition

Harold C. McKenzie, III

Associate Professor of Large Animal Medicine, Department of Veterinary Clinical Sciences, Virginia-Maryland Regional College of Veterinary Medicine, Virginia Polytechnic and State University, USA

Introduction

During the course of their illness, many equine patients suffer from some degree of malnutrition, either due to decreased voluntary intake or the withholding of food as part of the treatment protocol. In most cases the degree of malnutrition experienced will be minor and transient, and not require intervention on the part of the clinician. In patients with severe, prolonged illness, malnutrition can become clinically significant and may result in cachexia, metabolic disturbances, impaired immunity, and impaired wound healing. Healthy adult horses in normal body condition can endure 2–3 days of feed withholding without serious consequences (Carr & Holcombe, 2009; Magdesian, 2003). However, there is good evidence from human medicine that early nutritional support can be beneficial in minimizing the development of secondary complications and improving outcomes (Dan et al., 2006; Scurlock & Mechanick, 2008; Seron-Arbeloa et al., 2011).

Certain subsets of the equine patient population are less capable of tolerating periods of malnutrition, and these include: foals, ponies, miniature horses, donkeys, and obese individuals. In these groups, early nutritional support is critical in order to avoid complications such as hypoglycemia in neonates, and hypertriglyceridemia and hyperlipemia in ponies, miniature horses, donkeys, and obese horses. The introduction of nutritional support is often delayed due to the difficulty in determining which patients are likely to suffer from longer periods of malnutrition. In order to avoid these unanticipated periods of malnutrition, the clinician needs to consider early provision of nutritional support.

While enteral nutrition should always be the primary means of supplying nutrients to adult horses or foals, there are many situations in which voluntary enteral intake will be insufficient or contraindicated. Under those circumstances the clinician will be faced with two choices: assisted enteral feeding or parenteral feeding. Assisted enteral feeding is preferred in situations in which the gastrointestinal tract is functional, but in situations where there is reason to doubt the functionality of the gastrointestinal tract, it is best to use the parenteral route. The use of parenteral nutrition (PN) could be of benefit in ensuring adequate nutritional intake for many patients, particularly during the early stages of disease or recovery from surgery. In some cases, the simultaneous use of both enteral and parenteral nutrition could allow for the use of more conservative administration rates through both routes. This approach may decrease the risk of complications that may be encountered during more aggressive supplementation by either route alone.

Some veterinarians are reluctant to implement PN; this reluctance can be attributed not only to the complexities of formulation, administration, and clinical monitoring, but also to concerns regarding the possibility of complications and the expense to the client. While these concerns are valid, recent advances in formulations of PN have decreased their complexity. Also, there is a new appreciation that the patient's true energy needs are likely to be somewhat less than was previously believed. As a result the rates of administration for PN can be reassessed and potentially decreased, which may allow for a decrease in the cost of treatment and the frequency of complications.

Parenteral nutrition theory

The evidence-based scientific literature regarding the application of parenteral nutrition in an equine patient is limited and consists mostly of conference proceedings, individual case reports, retrospective studies, and review articles (Bercier, 2003; Dunkel & McKenzie, 2003; Furr, 2002; Greatorex, 1975; Hansen, 1986; Hoffer et al., 1977; Lopes & White, 2002; Magdesian, 2010; McKenzie & Geor, 2009; Myers et al., 2009; Ousey, 1994; Spurlock & Donaghue, 1990; Spurlock & Ward, 1991; Suann, 1982). There are only a few published controlled studies (Durham et al., 2003, 2004; Hansen et al., 1988; Ousey et al., 1997). For this reason much of the available information regarding PN in equine medicine has been extrapolated from the vast body of literature regarding human parenteral nutrition. This presents challenges for the equine clinician, as PN in human patients often varies drastically from PN in horses. In humans, PN is used both as a short-term intervention and as a long-term nutritional strategy. In horses PN is usually limited to relatively short-term use, due to both practical and financial concerns, typically for a maximum of 4–5 days (Bercier, 2003; Lopes & White, 2002).The prolonged administration of PN has been associated in human patients with increased risk of bloodstream infections, catheter complications, metabolic disorders, abnormal liver function tests, intestinal atrophy, and loss of gut mucosal barrier function (Finck, 2000).

When human patients are maintained on PN for long periods of time (months to years), it is critical that the formulations used address 100% of the patient's nutritional needs, as is reflected in the concept of total parenteral nutrition (TPN). TPN must contain all of the major macronutrients (carbohydrates, protein, and lipids) as well as micronutrients (vitamins, minerals). Care must also be taken that the formulations used contain the essential amino acids and essential fatty acids. These considerations are less critical when PN is used as a form of short-term nutritional support, particularly if the patient can simultaneously receive even small amounts of enteral nutrition (Hays et al., 2006).

Most instances of equine parenteral nutritional support will comprise "partial parenteral nutrition" (PPN) rather than TPN, for a variety of medical, practical, and financial reasons. Some confusion exists in the literature as to the meaning of the term PPN, but for this discussion PPN will refer to intravenous nutritional support that does not provide for 100% of the patient's nutritional requirements in terms of either caloric needs and/or specific nutrients (lipids). The most common use of PPN in equids is as a bridge to enteral support by providing nutritional support until such time as the enteral route becomes viable. Traditionally the goal of PN in this situation was to supply as close to complete nutritional support as possible. It has become clear that this approach is unnecessary in most cases, and may actually be deleterious in some circumstances. Complicating the clinician's task is the fact that defining the actual nutritional requirements of sick, hospitalized horses and foals has proven to be difficult.

Historically, it was believed that critical illness created a hypermetabolic state (Barton, 1994; Lunn & Murray, 1998), where patients had increased caloric requirements caused by increased tissue energy consumption; high rates of caloric supplementation were therefore recommended.

It has become clear that the energy requirements of sick horses are not as great as once thought (Ousey, 1994), likely as a result of a reduction in activity level. In foals there is also a temporary reduction in growth rate during critical illness, resulting in decreased caloric requirements. Indeed, one study using indirect calorimetry testing of clinically ill foals revealed that the resting energy requirement was approximately one-third that of active, normal foals (Paradis, 2001). In adult horses, an episode of anesthesia and surgery did not induce a hypermetabolic state, as it only resulted in a 10% increase in resting energy expenditure (Cruz et al., 2006).

As it is difficult to determine the actual nutrient requirements of hospitalized animals, clinicians must rely on reasonable estimations of energy requirements, rather than direct assessments. The rate of administration for PN solutions is dependent upon the energy density of the solution used, as the requirements for amino acids and lipids (if included) will be addressed in the formulation of the solution. The estimated daily resting energy requirement represents the most logical starting point. As PN is rarely administered to horses for a prolonged period of time, the primary goal of PN support is prevention of severe malnutrition and entry into a severely catabolic state during the time period prior to full resumption of enteral feeding. Full caloric support is rarely required to achieve this goal (Tillotson et al., 2002). The validity of this approach is reinforced by increasing evidence supporting hypocaloric nutrition in critical illness in humans (Boitano, 2006; Eve & Sair, 2008). This approach addresses the fact that aggressive nutritional support can result in overfeeding, the risks of which may outweigh the benefits of providing nutritional support.

In contrast to the risks of overfeeding, there is little evidence in human patients that short-term (i.e., several days' duration) hypocaloric nutritional support results in worsened outcomes as compared to those regimes designed to meet metabolic needs (Boitano, 2006). Recent evidence indicates that the hypocaloric approach is associated with decreased rates of complications and improved outcomes (Pichard et al., 2009), especially in regards to maintaining stringent control of blood glucose levels (Dandona et al., 2005). While little research has been done to address this question in horses, one of the earliest indicators of malnutrition is an increase in serum triglyceride concentrations (Gomma et al., 2009). Hypertriglyceridemia is an indicator of fat mobilization as a source of energy. The provision of as little as 5–10 kcal/kg/day in the form of dextrose-containing solutions has been shown to aid in the correction of hypertriglyceridemia in clinically ill horses (Dunkel & McKenzie, 2003; Hardy, 2003).

Short-term parenteral caloric support

Carbohydrate-containing solutions are the simplest means of providing intravenous caloric support. This is particularly true in patients withheld from feed for only a short period of time. A 5% dextrose solution can be used, and there are several commercially available options including: 5% dextrose in water; lactated Ringer's solution with 5% dextrose; 0.45% saline with 5% dextrose; and hypotonic maintenance electrolyte solutions containing 5% dextrose. Alternatively, one can compound a 5% dextrose solution by adding 100 mL of 50% dextrose solution per liter of isotonic polyionic fluids used for routine fluid support. Fluids containing dextrose should not be used for initial large-volume fluid resuscitation (i.e., they should not be bolused). This would almost certainly result in the delivery of

excessive amounts of dextrose to a dehydrated patient, and lead to profound hyperglycemia. However, following initial fluid resuscitation, it may be reasonable to use dextrose-supplemented polyionic fluids as the primary maintenance fluids.

Dextrose 5% in water should not be used as a maintenance solution because of the absence of electrolytes (Table 25.1). This solution is primarily useful in providing electrolyte-free water to patients suffering from hyperosmolar conditions. The caloric content of a 5% dextrose solution is 0.17 kcal/mL, so an infusion rate of 10 mL/kg/h would be required to deliver approximately 40 kcal/kg/day (0.17 kcal/mL × 10 mL/kg/h × 24 h/day = 40.8 kcal/kg/d). This rate is over twice that considered to be a maintenance fluid rate for neonatal foals (4–5 mL/kg/h), and five to ten times greater than a maintenance fluid rate for adult horses (1–2 mL/kg/h). At maintenance rates of 5 mL/kg/h, a 5% dextrose-containing solution would provide 20.4 kcal/kg/day to a foal. A maintenance rate of 1 mL/kg/h would provide 4 kcal/kg/day to an adult horse. Because 5 mL/kg/h (20 kcal/kg/day) is typically the limit for administering these solutions, a 5% dextrose solution cannot be used as the primary form of PN. In addition, care must always be taken when adjusting the infusion rates of dextrose-containing solutions in response to changes in the patient's fluid status, in order to prevent inadvertent hyperglycemia.

As an alternative to adding dextrose to the primary fluids, a 50% dextrose solution can be delivered using an infusion pump. Additional isotonic fluids must be administered concurrently through the same intravenous line to provide dilution and avoid endothelial injury caused by the hypertonic nature of this solution. Use of 50% dextrose solutions in this manner should be avoided if an infusion pump is not available, because it is very easy to inadvertently administer an excessive amount of dextrose, leading to hyperglycemia. The caloric content of 50% dextrose solution is 1.7 kcal/mL (Table 25.1). An infusion rate of 1 mL/kg/h of this solution would deliver approximately 40 kcal/kg/day (1.7 kcal/kg/h × 24 h/day = 41 kcal/kg/day). This low rate of infusion means that the primary fluid needs of the patient can be met with dextrose-free isotonic polyionic fluids. The infusion rate of the primary fluids can then be altered in response to changes in patient fluid status without concerns related to the dextrose infusion rate.

Table 25.1 Composition of various solutions that can be used to provide nutritional support by the parenteral route. Volumes of dextrose, amino acids, and lipids are given as component parts of a ratio, rather than specific volumes, in order to allow for compounding any given formula in different final volumes

Parenteral nutrition solution	Dextrose 50%	Amino acids 8.5%	Lipids 20%	kcal/mL	Final dextrose concentration (%)	Dextrose (g/mL)	Amino acid (g/mL)	Lipid (g/mL)	Osmolarity (mOsm/L)
Dextrose 50%	1	0	0	1.7	50	0.5	0	0	2525
Dextrose 5% in water	1	0	0	0.17	5	0.05	0	0	253
Lipid-free PN	1	1	0	1.02	25	0.25	0.0425	0	1685
Lipid-containing PN 1	3	4	1	1.08	18.75	0.1875	0.0425	0.025	1435
Lipid-containing PN 2	2	3	1	1.07	16.7	0.1667	0.0425	0.033	1345

Because dextrose-containing fluids are an incomplete nutritional source, they should not be used as the primary nutritional source for more than 24 hours in foals or 48–72 hours in adult horses. At the end of these time periods, the fluid therapy and nutritional plans should be revisited in order to determine whether the patient can tolerate enteral nutrition. Continued PN support at this juncture requires a more complete formulation that also provides amino acids and possibly lipids.

Parenteral nutrition components

The primary components of PN are carbohydrates, protein, and lipids. Carbohydrates and proteins are the basic components of all PN solutions, with lipids being added to the formulation in some instances. Dextrose is the most commonly used carbohydrate, and is typically used in the form of a 50% solution. This solution contains 1.7 kcal/mL of energy and represents the most cost-effective source of energy for parenteral administration. Dextrose solutions contain only water and dextrose and provide no other nutrients. Fifty percent dextrose solutions are very hypertonic, with an osmolarity of 2550 mOsm/L. The osmolarity of this solution is typically reduced when the dextrose is combined with amino acids and/or lipid solutions that have lower tonicities, or when dextrose is delivered by piggybacking onto the primary intravenous fluid line. Excessive administration of dextrose-containing solutions will result in hyperglycemia, which is considered a proinflammatory stimulus and has been associated with

worsened outcomes in human critical illness (Dandona et al., 2005; Klein et al., 1998). Because PN solutions always contain substantial concentrations of carbohydrates, great care should be taken when introducing PN. Patients must be closely monitored to prevent hyperglycemia.

Protein supplementation, provided in the form of amino acid solutions, is used in PN formulations to provide both essential and non-essential amino acids. Amino acid supplementation during critical illness is important, as the metabolic response to injury and sepsis is to increase muscle protein degradation. This catabolic response can be reduced by supplying a source of both amino acids and calories. The generally recommended ratio for non-protein calories to nitrogen is 100–200 non-protein calories per gram of nitrogen. In foals, the non-protein nitrogen calories to grams nitrogen ratio was negatively correlated with the rate of weight gain, which demonstrates that lower rates of protein supplementation are correlated with decreased growth (Spurlock & Donaghue, 1990). Excessive administration of amino acids should be avoided, however, as this may contribute to azotemia (Klein et al., 1998). Amino acid solutions are readily available as 8.5% and 10% solutions, which supply 0.085 and 0.010 g/mL of amino acids, respectively. The caloric content of these solutions is 0.313 and 0.4 kcal/mL for the 8.5% and 10% solutions, respectively.

The energy contribution from protein in the PN formula is controversial. In some situations, the caloric contribution of amino acids in the solution will be excluded from calculation of the total caloric content of the solution. This recommendation is based on the concept of "protein sparing", wherein the energy needs of the patient are met using non-protein energy sources only (carbohydrates and lipids) in order to "spare" protein for anabolism. In reality, this is an arbitrary concept, as the supplied nutrients will be utilized as needed. It is likely that some amino acids will be used for energy, particularly where total energy requirements are not being met (Klein et al., 1998). Omitting protein calories from the calculation of the total energy content of PN solutions results in an underestimate of the caloric content of the solution by 15–20% (Skipper & Tupesis, 2005), which could potentially result in caloric overfeeding and hyperglycemia.

There has been much discussion in both the human and veterinary literature about the potential benefits of including the "conditionally essential" amino acid glutamine in enteral and parenteral feeding formulations. Glutamine has an impact on antioxidant capacity, immune function, tissue protection, and metabolic functions and is an important fuel, particularly for enterocytes (Mok & Hankard, 2011). Recent research has demonstrated that intestinal mucosal atrophy is a theoretical concern in human patients on PN only, but it did not occur even after 1 month of complete intravenous nutritional support without glutamine (Pichard et al., 2009).

Glutamine supplementation of PN has been shown to reduce the incidence of bloodstream infections in certain subsets of adult human patients on PN. These include critically ill postoperative and ventilator-dependent patients, burns patients, and those with acute pancreatitis (Vanek et al., 2011). At this time, there is not enough information to support specific recommendations regarding glutamine supplementation of PN in human neonatal and pediatric patients (Vanek et al., 2011). No studies have investigated this question in horses or foals. There is no evidence that glutamine supplementation is harmful, however, and it is used in the management of many human patients, particularly outside the United States (Wernerman, 2011). From a practical standpoint glutamine can be difficult to obtain, as there are no commercially available glutamine products for PN supplementation available in the United States at this time (Vanek et al., 2011). Glutamine solutions can be compounded, but the solutions are fairly unstable and even under refrigeration cannot be used after 30 days. Glutamine also can contribute to instability of the PN solution, which may complicate clinical

use of these solutions. Due to these concerns, glutamine supplementation of PN solutions is not performed at the author's institution.

The inclusion of lipids in parenteral nutrition formulations allows for the provision of a slightly larger number of calories per unit volume compared with solutions containing only dextrose. A 20% lipid solution has a caloric content of 2.0 kcal/mL, as opposed to 1.7 kcal/mL for 50% dextrose. Krause and McKenzie (2007) reported that the use of lipid-containing parenteral nutrition solutions allowed for the provision of 40–92 kcal/kg/day (mean = 63 kcal/kg/day) to foals, as opposed to 25–66 kcal/kg/day (mean = 41 kcal/kg/day) with a dextrose-based, lipid-free solution. In short-term situations, the primary benefit of including lipids in the PN formulation is that it allows for a decrease in the amount of carbohydrates being administered for any given level of caloric support. This can be helpful when managing patients with insulin resistance (Dan et al., 2006). Another advantage of lipid emulsions is that they are isotonic, thereby moderating the hypertonicity of the PN formulation and potentially decreasing the risk of thrombophlebitis.

Unfortunately, formulating PN solutions with lipids increases the cost and may increase the risk of complications (Hansen, 1986). Hyperlipidemia can occur in association with lipid administration to foals, but this does not appear to result in adverse effects (Hansen, 1986; Krause & McKenzie, 2007). Lipid emulsions are also susceptible to contamination and promote bacterial growth (Kuwahara et al., 2010). Due to these risks, the IV lines through which lipid-containing solutions are administered should be changed daily, as opposed to every 72 hours, thereby substantially increasing client cost.

Micronutrients can be included in PN formulations, although this is not critical for patients receiving short-term parenteral support. Micronutrients can include electrolytes as well as vitamins and trace minerals. Most equine patients receiving PN will be receiving concurrent intravenous fluid therapy, and these fluids represent the most practical route for addressing electrolyte supplementation. It has become common practice to supplement maintenance intravenous fluids with potassium chloride (KCl) solution in order to ensure adequate potassium intake. KCl supplementation for maintenance fluids is typically provided at 20–40 mEq/L. Care should be taken in patients receiving large-volume IV fluid therapy, as administering potassium at rates above 0.5 mEq/kg/h should be avoided due to the risk of toxicity (Corley, 2008). Calcium can be added to maintenance IV fluids using 23% calcium gluconate at the rate of 25–50 mL/L, and this should be delivered at a rate of 1 mEq/kg/day (1 mL of 23% calcium gluconate solution/kg/day) (Magdesian, 2010). Some IV fluid formulations contain magnesium at 3 mEq/L[1,2], or magnesium can be added to the intravenous fluids at the same concentration by adding 1.5 ml/L of a 25% $MgSO_4$ solution (Magdesian, 2010).

B-vitamin supplementation is indicated for animals on PN, as they likely have decreased intestinal production during this period of time (Stratton-Phelps, 2008). B-vitamin supplementation can be performed by adding 1–2 mL of B-vitamin complex per liter of PN (Stratton-Phelps, 2008). Alternatively, B-vitamins can be provided at the rate of 1–2 mL/45 kg/day (Magdesian, 2010). Supplementation with fat-soluble vitamins (A, D, and K) and trace minerals should be considered in patients with severe malnutrition or those that are expected to require PN for a prolonged period of time without any enteral support. The multivitamin products marketed for PN supplementation have been difficult to obtain in the United States in recent years. For these reasons, the inclusion of multivitamins in PN solutions should not be considered mandatory, particularly for short-term PN administration.

Parenteral nutrition formulation

There are two basic approaches to the formulation of PN. The first involves the exact determination of the anticipated metabolic needs of the patient. A formulation is developed to meet those needs using a mixture of dextrose, amino acids, and possibly lipids. This approach is fairly complex and is best performed using a computerized spreadsheet to aid in performing the various calculations. A second approach, which is more practical in a clinical setting, consists of using two basic PN formulas. The following formulas have been used for both foals and adults in the author's institution for over 10 years, and it is very rare that these formulas are deviated from for individual patients.

The two basic PN formulas are lipid-free and lipid-containing solutions (see Table 25.1). Lipid-free PN solutions are intended for short-term use and are typically formulated using equal volumes (1:1) of 50% dextrose[3] and 8.5% amino acids[4] (Krause & McKenzie, 2007). The final composition of this lipid-free PN solution is 25% dextrose and 4.25% amino acids, with a caloric density of 1.02 kcal/mL. The ratio of non-protein calories to nitrogen is 125 non-protein calories per gram of nitrogen (NPC/gN).

The second basic formula incorporates lipids, and is preferred for long-term administration or for administration to patients that are poorly tolerant of infused dextrose (lipid-containing PN). There are various ways to formulate such a solution. One formulation is to use three parts of 50% dextrose, one part of 20% lipids[5], and four parts of 8.5% amino acids (lipid-containing solution 1 in Table 25.1) (Krause & McKenzie, 2007). This solution contains 18.75% dextrose, 2.5% lipids, and 4.25% amino acids, has a caloric content of 1.08 kcal/mL, and a non-protein calorie to nitrogen ratio of 131 NPC/gN. Reducing the dextrose content and increasing the lipid content will lower the osmolarity of the solution and further decrease the infused carbohydrate load (Table 25.1). It can be appreciated that the primary benefit of adding lipids to the PN formulation for patients on short-term support is not to dramatically increase the caloric density of the solution, but rather to deliver roughly the same calories using a solution lower in carbohydrate content. In insulin-resistant patients, this may allow for a greater amount of calories to be delivered over time (Krause & McKenzie, 2007).

All components of parenteral nutrition solutions must be mixed in a sterile manner prior to administration. Components should be added to a sterile bag using a closed system through gravity flow. In order to decrease the risk of bacterial contamination, optimally this process should be performed in a laminar flow hood. All injection ports should be cleaned with alcohol prior to puncture. Dextrose and amino acid solutions should be added to the infusion bag first, followed by lipids if they are being used. If lipids are added earlier, there is a risk

---

[1]Normosol-M®, Hospira, Inc., Lake Forest, IL, USA.
[2]Plasmalyte 148®, Baxter Healthcare Corp., Deerfield, IL, USA.

[3]Dextrose 50%, Baxter Healthcare Corp., Clintec Nutr. Div., Deerfield, IL, USA.
[4]Travasol® 8.5%, Baxter Healthcare Corp., Clintec Nutr. Div., Deerfield, IL, USA.
[5]Intralipid® 20%, Baxter Healthcare Corp., Clintec Nutr. Div., Deerfield, IL, USA.

of the lipids coming out of emulsion when the more acidic solutions are added. Once compounded, PN solutions should be refrigerated, and lipid-containing solutions must be used within 24 hours of compounding. During administration, the infusion bag containing the final PN solution should be covered with a brown plastic bag to protect it from light, which can degrade amino acids and vitamins within the solution. Typical daily costs for compounded PN solutions in the author's institution are $75–125 in foals and $300–450 in adult horses, depending upon the solution used and the final infusion rates.

Premixed standardized PN solutions formulated for human patients are also commercially available. These PN products are termed "multi-chamber bag" formulations because the dextrose and amino acid solutions are contained in separate compartments of a closed system, and they are mixed together immediately prior to administration by removing a barrier separating the two solutions. Lipid-containing premixed PN solutions are not available in the United States at this time, although they are available in Europe. Premixed PN products are shelf stable for 2 years, sterile, and accurately compounded. The shelf stable nature of these products makes it feasible to keep them in stock and readily available, thereby avoiding the need to wait for the preparation of compounded PN. Premixed PN solutions also reduce the risk of contamination as they are only exposed to the environment once when the bag is spiked for administration. A solution with the same composition as the lipid-free PN described above is readily available (4.25% amino acid, 25% dextrose)[6]. However, a range of other dextrose and amino acid concentrations (5–25% and 2.75–5%, respectively) are available, allowing the clinician some leeway in selecting a formulation. The simplicity and availability of these products makes them particularly appropriate for use in settings that lack full pharmacy support. The use of premixed PN in human hospitals has been associated with a reduction in the cost of PN therapy and in bloodstream infections, when compared to compounded PN (Turpin et al., 2011). The cost of premixed PN solutions in the author's institution is comparable to that of pharmacy-compounded solutions in the smaller volumes needed for foals, typically 2 L per day. Premixed PN is approximately 20% more expensive on a per liter basis when compared to large-volume compounded solutions for adult horses, which are usually made up in 4-liter bags.

Indications for parenteral nutrition

Enteral feeding always represents the primary means of nutrient delivery in horses and foals, as it is the most physiologic and efficient route, as well as the most cost-effective. Enteral feeding is contraindicated, however, in patients with anterior enteritis, postoperative ileus, gastrointestinal obstruction, or severe, persistent diarrhea due to malabsorption or maldigestion. Other contraindications to enteral feeding include situations where oral intake is not physically possible, as is the case with some oral and pharyngeal disorders, pharyngeal or esophageal obstructions, pyloric stricture or obstruction, botulism, tetanus, neurologic dysfunction, or the presence of space-occupying masses in the upper gastrointestinal tract.

Some animals may simply lack the desire or strength to eat, as is often the case with very weak neonatal foals. In many cases of neonatal sepsis there are also concerns that gastrointestinal function may be impaired secondary to severe systemic inflammation and possible splanchnic hypoperfusion. Recumbent animals of any age are often too weak to eat, and are at risk of gastrointestinal dysfunction and aspiration pneumonia if enteral feeding is used.

When the lower gastrointestinal tract is expected to function adequately, access may be gained by placement of a nasogastric tube or an esophagostomy tube. Unfortunately, these interventions may be associated with complications and could result in overload of a marginally functional lower gastrointestinal tract. A complete discussion of enteral feeding strategies can be found in Chapter 21.

The use of a simple decision tree can facilitate decision-making regarding implementation of nutritional support (Stratton-Phelps, 2008). First, is the patient consuming adequate energy and nutrients on a voluntary basis, defined as 70–80% of its resting daily energy requirement? If yes, then no intervention is required and the patient should continue to be closely monitored. If no, then the clinician must determine

---

[6]Clinimix® 4.25% Amino Acid in 25% Dextrose, Baxter Healthcare Corp., Clintec Nutr. Div., Deerfield, IL, USA.

if the gastrointestinal tract is functional. If the gastrointestinal tract is thought to be functional, then placement of a nasogastric tube should be considered. If the gastrointestinal tract is not thought to be functional, then PN should be considered.

Administration of parenteral nutrition

The solutions used for PN are hypertonic and can cause injury to the vascular endothelium, increasing the risk of thrombophlebitis. PN administration is associated with an increased risk of infectious complications in human patients, but one must keep in mind that patients requiring PN have been self-selected as high-risk patients for infectious side effects (Miller et al., 2011). In order to decrease the risk of catheter-associated complications, it is recommended that PN solutions be administered through polyurethane catheters, rather than catheters made of Teflon or other materials. In foals a 20-cm long polyurethane long-term guidewire style[7] catheter should be used, as the length of the catheter allows for the line to be considered central in most foals. In adult horses the jugular vein is large enough and has sufficient flow for it to tolerate infusions of hypertonic solutions. Indeed, the administration of dextrose solutions up to 25% concentration has been reported through the jugular vein in horses without the development of phlebitis (Spurlock & Ward, 1990).

The infused solutions should be as minimally hypertonic as possible. Tonicity can be lowered by delivering fluids with low tonicities through the same line as the PN. For example, if using a dedicated port in a multi-lumen catheter, sterile water can be concurrently administered with PN at a ratio of 1:3 water:PN (e.g., 150 mL/h of sterile water for a flow rate of 450 mL/h of PN) (Magdesian, 2010). While somewhat less effective at lowering the tonicity of the PN solution, one can also accomplish dilution by administering the PN solution via the same catheter through which the replacement or maintenance polyionic isotonic fluids are being delivered. Although this appears to contradict the ideal recommendations, this "piggybacking" of PN on the intravenous fluids is commonly performed in equine hospitals and appears to be well

tolerated (Carr & Holcombe, 2009; Hardy, 2003). While the final degree of dilution is not always well quantified with this approach, it usually provides at least a threefold dilution rate, which should be adequate in most cases.

The volume of fluid contained within PN formulations should be factored into the patient's overall fluid management plan, along with the volume of any concurrent fluids administered as diluents, particularly in patients where volume status is critical (e.g., foals with oliguria). Most PN formulas contain approximately 75% water, and if sterile water is used as a diluent as described above, it will represent an additional volume of 25% of the PN rate. Most patients will be able to easily eliminate this additional infused volume, but those with reduced renal function, cardiovascular disease, or increased endothelial permeability will be at risk for fluid retention. By factoring the volume of water from PN into the overall fluid therapy plan, the clinician can easily address this concern and decrease risks to the patient.

The use of multiple-lumen catheters can be beneficial when administering PN, as it will allow for one lumen to be dedicated to infusion of the PN solution, minimizing the risk of contamination. When using a dedicated lumen for PN administration in a multi-lumen catheter, it is imperative that the PN solution be diluted prior to reaching the vasculature, as there will be no dilutional effect from concurrent isotonic fluid administration. In adult horses, catheters may be of either the single-lumen stylet style[8], or single- or multiple-lumen long-term guidewire style[9]. Antiseptic-impregnated catheters are available[10], and these may aid in reducing the frequency of catheter site infections, but they are not yet widely used in equine medicine. In human medicine it is recommended that these specialized catheters only be used in centers with high rates of catheter site infections. Thorough skin antisepsis should be performed prior to placement of the intravenous catheter; human studies have demonstrated that chlorhexidine is superior to povidone-iodine for this purpose, and this appears to be the case in horses as well (Frasca et al., 2010; Geraghty et al., 2009).

---

[7]1410 or 1620, MILA International Inc., Erlanger, KY, USA.

[8]1411, MILA International Inc., Erlanger, KY, USA.
[9]1410 or 1620, MILA International Inc., Erlanger, KY, USA.
[10]API1410 or 1620, MILA International Inc., Erlanger, KY, USA.

The rate of PN administration in milliliters per day will always be calculated based upon the caloric density of the PN solution (kcal/mL: Table 25.1), the desired rate of caloric supplementation (kcal/kg/day: Table 25.2), and the body weight of the patient (kg). The calculation will be:

$$mL/day\,PN\,solution = (kcal/kg/day \times body\,weight\,in\,kg)/kcal/mL\,PN\,solution$$

$$(25.1)$$

For example, if a lipid-free PN with a caloric density of 1.02 kcal/mL is used, with a desired rate of caloric supplementation of 25 kcal/kg/day in a patient weighing 450 kg, the rate of administration will be 11,030 mL/day, or 460 mL/h. Using the lipid-containing PN formula 2, with a caloric density of 1.07 kcal/mL (Table 25.1), this would result in an infusion rate of 10,514 mL/day, or 438 mL/h.

Insulin resistance

Some degree of insulin resistance is frequently encountered in severely ill hospitalized human patients (Lazzeri et al., 2009). Insulin resistance evidenced as hyperglycemia is also commonly encountered during administration of nutritional support to severely ill horses and foals (Jose-Cunilleras et al., 2008; Krause & McKenzie, 2007; Lopes & White, 2002; Myers et al., 2009). Insulin resistance in critically ill patients is primarily due to the effects of severe systemic inflammation resulting from activation of the hypothalamic-pituitary-adrenal axis and the sympathetic system (Lazzeri et al., 2009; Toth et al., 2010).

Increased blood glucose concentrations occur secondary to increased production and decreased clearance. Glycogenolysis is increased under the influence of glucagon and epinephrine. Hepatic gluconeogenesis is increased despite the resulting increase in circulating blood glucose due to the activity of glucagon, epinephrine, growth hormone, and cortisol. At the same time the mechanisms for glucose uptake are downregulated, contributing to the development of hyperglycemia. Decreased glucose uptake in the adipose tissue, liver, and heart occurs due to both impaired insulin-dependent glucose uptake (through glucose-transporter 4) and impaired glycogen synthetase activity (Langouche & Van

den Berghe, 2006). While insulin-dependent glucose uptake is decreased, there is an increase of glucose uptake in tissues where uptake is passive. This passive process is not dependent on insulin. The central nervous system, hepatocytes, GI mucosa, endothelial cells, renal tubular cells, and immune cells all exhibit this passive, insulin-independent glucose uptake; therefore these tissues are not protected from the hyperglycemia associated with critical illness, and may be at risk of injury due to glucose toxicity (Langouche & Van den Berghe, 2006). The clinical significance of the adverse effects of hyperglycemia is supported by the evidence that hyperglycemia has been associated with worsened outcomes in critically ill horses and foals (Hassel et al., 2009; Hollis et al., 2007, 2008).

Interestingly, many septic foals are presented with hypoglycemia and decreased insulin concentrations (Barsnick & Toribio, 2011). While many of these foals will be intolerant of exogenous dextrose, true insulin resistance in this population is not well documented and requires further study (Barsnick & Toribio, 2011).

Insulin resistance appears to be increasing in frequency as a chronic condition in the general adult equine population, or at least it is being increasingly recognized. This phenomenon is most often associated with excessive body condition and decreased exercise, and has been termed equine metabolic syndrome (EMS) (Frank, 2011). Unfortunately the incidence of obesity is increasing in the adult horse population worldwide (Packer et al., 2011; Sillence et al., 2006; Wyse et al., 2008). Due to a pre-existing state of insulin resistance, these animals can be challenging to treat when they become sick and require nutritional support. In addition, these animals, along with ponies, donkeys, and miniature horses, appear predisposed to abnormal fat metabolism. In the presence of lipid metabolism derangements, there is excessive liberation of triglycerides in response to decreased nutrient availability; this leads progressively to hypertriglyceridemia, hyperlipidemia, and hyperlipemia (Dunkel & McKenzie, 2003). If not effectively controlled, these conditions can potentially progress to hepatic lipidosis and renal lipidosis, with resulting organ failure. Early nutritional support in the form of carbohydrates (i.e., dextrose) appears to be very beneficial in these cases, likely by increasing the endogenous production of insulin and thereby decreasing fat mobilization through inhibition of the activity of the enzyme hormone-sensitive lipase. Concurrent insulin therapy is required in more severe cases. This therapy is often effective in slowing or halting the progression of hyperlipemia and allowing for patient stabilization.

Parenteral nutrition in foals

Neonatal foals have very limited energy reserves. Therefore, if enteral intake is decreased for any reason, they require rapid institution of PN. This will prevent the development of protein/calorie malnutrition and substantial energy deficits (Buchanan, 2005). A reasonable initial goal for PN administration in the foal is 30–40 kcal/kg/day (Table 25.2). While this level of caloric support does not fully meet the theoretical energy requirements of the healthy neonate (up to 120 kcal/kg/day for the growing foal), it comes close to meeting the resting energy requirement in hospitalized foals (Ousey et al., 1996; Paradis, 2001). PN is used as a temporary support to prevent the foal from entering into a severely catabolic state; the goal is not to provide sufficient nutrition for growth (McKenzie & Geor, 2009).

When initiating PN administration to foals, the initial infusion rate should be 25% of the calculated final rate. The rate should gradually be increased every 1–4 hours following monitoring of blood glucose concentration, in order to confirm that hyperglycemia (blood glucose > 150 mg/dL) is not present. If the patient tolerates PN well and maintains blood glucose concentrations at or near normal levels, then consideration can be given to increasing the PN administration rate to 50–60 kcal/kg/day (Tillotson et al., 2002). However, many ill foals have difficulty tolerating this amount of parenteral supplementation as evidenced by the development of hyperglycemia and/or hypertriglyceridemia, and these foals will likely require insulin therapy when administered PN at higher rates. The clinician must decide if the additional complexity of treatment and monitoring associated with insulin therapy will be offset by a clinical benefit of a higher PN administration rate. Some references advocate PN administration rates of 100 kcal/kg/day or more (Spurlock & Ward, 1991), but there appears to be little benefit in using these higher rates of energy supplementation. The risk of complications such as hyperglycemia and hyperlipidemia is increased with higher PN rates.

An electronic infusion pump should always be used when administering PN solutions to foals. The rate of administration must be tightly controlled and adjustments to the infusion rate must be made easily and accurately. Excessive rates of administration can induce profound hyperglycemia, which has been shown in other species to be associated with severe complications and increased risk of death (Hays et al., 2006). Conversely, if a foal is receiving concurrent PN and insulin infusions, any interruption to the PN infusion can result in severe hypoglycemia. Interruption of an insulin infusion is likely to lead to marked hyperglycemia.

When PN is to be discontinued, the PN infusion rate should be decreased in 25% increments every 4–6 hours, while gradually introducing enteral feeding. Most foals can be removed from PN over a period of 24 hours, assuming that they tolerate the reintroduction of enteral nutrition. It is important that blood glucose monitoring be continued during the weaning process, in order to detect or prevent the development of severe hypoglycemia, particularly when foals have received insulin infusions. The insulin administration rate should be gradually titrated downward in parallel with the PN rate, but there can be a substantial lag between changes in the insulin infusion rate and the patient's response to this change. Some time should be allowed to account for this lag.

Table 25.2 Targeted goals for parenteral nutrition administration

Case type	Duration	Calories (kcal/kg/day)	Amino acid (g/kg/day)	Lipid (g/kg/day)
Foal	Short	30–40	0–1	0
Foal	Long	50–60	0.5–1.5	0.5–1.5
Adult	Short	20–25	0	0
Adult	Long	30–35	0.5–1	0.5–1
Adult – hypertriglyceridemia	Short	5–10	0.5–1	0

It is critical that foals being weaned from insulin infusions receive some form of enteral nutrition during this time period. It may be wise to wean them from PN and insulin over longer periods of time (24–36 hours) than would be required for a foal receiving PN alone, in order to prevent glucose derangements.

Monitoring the foal receiving parenteral nutrition

Frequent monitoring is particularly important during the initial phase of PN therapy. This should include a general physical examination, with close attention paid to neurologic status and respiratory function. Parenteral nutrition solutions contain carbohydrates, causing an increase in endogenous CO_2 production. Foals with decreased pulmonary function or decreased respiratory drive are at risk for hypercapnea, and this risk is increased when PN is administered. A blood gas sample should be analyzed in order to assess the P_aCO_2 and acid–base status in any foal with compromised respiratory function.

Rectal temperature should also be closely monitored, as fever is a common early manifestation of systemic infection. Blood glucose concentrations should be initially assessed on an hourly basis, until the patient has stabilized with the appropriate rate of PN infusion. This can be followed by blood glucose monitoring every 3–6 hours for the first day of therapy.

The frequency of blood glucose monitoring is dependent upon the stability of the patient. It may need to be more frequent in the very critically ill, up to once an hour, whereas it may not need to be more than every 12 hours in the stable patient.

Urine output should be monitored continuously where possible, in combination with intermittent monitoring of urine glucose concentration, due to the risk of hyperglycemia-induced diuresis and glucosuria. While the actual renal threshold for glucose is not well described in foals, glucosuria and diuresis will usually be observed when blood glucose levels exceed 180 mg/dL. Serum electrolytes should be monitored at least twice daily. Particular attention should be paid to serum potassium concentrations as they can fall rapidly, especially in foals receiving insulin therapy. Additional clinicopathologic monitoring should consist of daily complete blood counts and serum chemistry profiles

in critical cases, whereas these can be performed every 48 hours in more stable patients. Ideally, body weight should be assessed on a daily basis, in order to ensure that the foal is maintaining body weight while receiving PN. Foals receiving PN solutions containing lipids should be monitored for the development of hypertriglyceridemia (Krause & McKenzie, 2007; Myers et al., 2009).

If hypertriglyceridemia develops, it is often associated with PN formulations containing lipids. Hypertriglyceridemia can be addressed by changing to a PN formulation containing only dextrose and amino acids. If this is not clinically appropriate, or if the hypertriglyceridemia is severe, then the patient should be treated with exogenous insulin.

Parenteral nutrition in adult horses

The caloric needs of adult horses are lower than those for foals, as there is no nutritional requirement for growth. The estimated daily maintenance energy requirement (DEm) for adult horses is approximately 32–35 kcal/kg/day (Furr, 2002; Hansen et al., 1988), but this is an overestimation of the actual requirements of hospitalized horses, which are largely physically inactive. Daily resting energy requirements (DEr) are typically estimated at 70% of DEm, which yields a range of 23–25 kcal/kg/day. This range of values represents a reasonable target for PN caloric support in order to avoid overfeeding of calories (Table 25.2). This target is also consistent with the average rate of caloric support in both a retrospective report of PN in adult horses (24.5 kcal/kg/day; range 15–42 kcal/kg/day) (Lopes & White, 2002), and a prospective report investigating PN administration in postoperative colic cases (18 kcal/kg/day) (Durham et al., 2003, 2004). While it has been suggested to target DEm in horses that are tolerating PN administration, it is often not necessary to do so and a more conservative rate of supplementation may avoid harmful calorie overfeeding, although this requires study in horses. Exceptions include patients in very poor body condition, lactating mares, or patients likely to require prolonged PN therapy.

When considering how to set a target PN rate, it is helpful to consider that one of the primary goals is to prevent hypermetabolism. An excellent indicator of hypermetabolism in anorexic or feed-deprived adult equids is the development of hypertriglyceridemia and/or hyperlipemia secondary to excessive mobilization of fat stores (Dunkel & McKenzie, 2003; Durham et al., 2006; McKenzie, 2011). The provision of even small amounts of energy in the form of enteral or PN carbohydrate supplementation (5–10 kcal/kg/day) has been reported to be effective in resolving hypertriglyceridemia (serum triglyceride concentration >500 mg/dL) in clinically ill horses (Dunkel & McKenzie, 2003). Given that many equids with fat dysmetabolism are inherently insulin resistant, using lower dosage rates for parenteral caloric support will also aid in avoiding hyperglycemia. Insulin therapy may also be indicated in these patients to aid in resolution of fat dysmetabolism; insulin may allow for infusion of greater amounts of energy if required (Durham et al., 2006; McKenzie, 2011). Considering that hyperinsulinemia has been receiving attention in terms of a possible role in the development of laminitis, the dose rates of exogenous insulin infusions should be conservative and titrated to clinical effect.

Monitoring of adult horses receiving parenteral nutrition

In horses receiving PN, frequent assessment (2–4 times daily) of the catheter site should be performed in order to detect heat, swelling, discharge, or evidence of thrombosis. Daily physical examinations are also indicated. Horses on PN should be closely monitored for the development of hyperglycemia. When initiating PN therapy the blood glucose concentration should be monitored hourly for 2–3 hours, then every 6 hours until the target infusion rate has been achieved, and it becomes clear that PN is being tolerated. Once stable, blood glucose monitoring can be decreased to twice daily, but the frequency should be increased if there is any clinical deterioration in patient status. Serum electrolytes should be monitored twice daily, decreasing to once daily if the horse's condition is stable and has been receiving PN for more than 2–3 days. A serum chemistry profile should be monitored on a daily basis for the first 2 days, evaluating for evidence of electrolyte abnormalities, renal dysfunction or hepatic dysfunction; if stable, serum biochemistry evaluation can be performed every other day after that. If respiratory function is of concern, blood gases should be monitored at least daily.

Serum triglyceride concentrations should be monitored daily in horses at risk for hypertriglyceridemia and those receiving lipid-containing PN. In individuals suffering from chronic malnutrition or anorexia, there is a risk of "refeeding syndrome". Hypomagnesemia, hypophosphatemia, and hypokalemia develop when PN is initiated in these horses. This necessitates close monitoring and appropriate supplementation of electrolytes in these patients.

Insulin therapy

The critically ill patient often demonstrates some degree of insulin resistance for the reasons described above, making it difficult to achieve even a conservative rate of administration of PN. This phenomenon can only be addressed by reducing the rate of PN administration, reformulating the PN solution using lipids, and/or beginning insulin therapy. However, the administration of insulin in critically ill patients should not be undertaken lightly, as this therapy places additional demands on both the clinician and nursing staff in order to ensure that profound hypoglycemia does not occur. In addition, recent attention has been focused on insulin as a possible contributor to the development of laminitis, which many of these patients are predisposed to anyway (Parsons et al., 2007).

Intermittent dosing of subcutaneous insulin may offer some advantages in terms of simplicity of administration and moderation of effects; however, it does not allow for changes in dosage over the short term and can be challenging to regulate. Intermittent boluses of intravenous insulin can also be used, but this approach tends to produce dramatic swings in blood glucose concentrations and is also difficult to regulate. Intravenous bolus administration should probably be limited to initial therapy of cases with profound hyperglycemia and/or hyperlipemia. The use of continuous rate infusion (CRI) for the administration of insulin allows for a fairly rapid onset of action while also providing a simple and timely means of adjustment of the dosage. A summary of insulin routes, forms, and dosages is provided in Table 25.3.

The use of intermittent bolus intravenous or subcutaneous administration of insulin is associated with reduced cost of the insulin; it eliminates the need for a carrier solution for the dilution of insulin and the

Table 25.3 Insulin dosage protocols

Horse type	Route	Insulin formulation	Dosage	Frequency
Foal	SC	Regular	0.1–0.5 IU/kg	12 hours
			0.02–0.1 IU/kg	6–24 hours
Foal	IV	Regular	0.01–0.07 IU/kg/hr	Starting dose
	Continuous rate infusion		0.015–0.2 IU/kg/hr	Maintenance dose
Adult	SC	Protamine zinc	0.1–0.3 IU/kg	12 hours
Adult – hypertriglyceridemia	SC	Ultralente	0.4 IU/kg	24 hours
Adult – hypertriglyceridemia	IV	Regular	0.2 IU/kg	6 hours (as often as q 1 hour in hyperlipemia)
Adult	IV	Regular	0.07 IU/kg/h	Starting dose
	Continuous rate infusion			

associated intravenous administration sets and lines. Close monitoring of blood glucose concentrations is still required, however, and the risks of hypoglycemia and hyperglycemia are the same or greater as with continuous rate infusions. In the author's experience, it can be more challenging to achieve stable blood glucose concentrations when using intermittent bolus insulin therapy, particularly in foals. As mentioned above, intravenous bolus administration has limited application, but there is one report describing the use of insulin and PN in the treatment of hypertriglyceridemia in horses, ponies, and donkeys (Waitt & Cebra, 2009). Regular insulin at 0.2 IU/kg was given intravenously as often as hourly, but more typically every 6 hours, during initial treatment.

It is important to remember that hyperlipemic patients are inherently insulin-resistant, which explains why such high doses of insulin were required in the study mentioned above. The subcutaneous route of administration has broader applications as it allows for slow absorption that moderates the variations in blood glucose over time. Subcutaneous administration may be slightly more useful in adults than foals. Adult horses seem more resistant to hypoglycemia secondary to excessive insulin dosages, likely as a result of their greater energy reserves. One recommended dosage for subcutaneous insulin in foals is 0.1–0.5 IU of regular insulin every 12 hours for an average sized foal (Stratton-Phelps, 2008). A retrospective report of foal PN described subcutaneous insulin dosage rates of 0.02

to 0.1 IU/kg given every 6–24 hours (Myers et al., 2009). In adult horses subcutaneous insulin can be administered at 0.1–0.3 IU/kg of protamine zinc insulin every 12 hours (Durham, 2006; Stratton-Phelps, 2008). The use of ultralente insulin at 0.4 IU/kg subcutaneously every 24 hours has also been described (Waitt & Cebra, 2009). Glargine insulin would have the advantage of continuous release of insulin after subcutaneous administration, along with more stable glucose concentrations, but requires study in horses.

When using CRI of insulin, the maximal effect on blood glucose concentration is not typically seen until approximately 90 minutes after initiation of the infusion. It is thought that this may be due to the gradual saturation of cellular insulin receptors. The response to alterations in the rate of infusion occurs over a similar time frame. Altering the rate of infusion of PN solutions too rapidly after changing the rate of insulin infusion should be avoided. An initial insulin infusion rate of 0.07 IU/kg/h of regular insulin is generally well tolerated in the author's experience, and may represent a reasonable starting point in both foals and adults intolerant of PN (Han et al., 2011; McKenzie & Geor, 2009). This dosage was derived from a retrospective study of foals treated with PN, which reported initial insulin doses ranging from 0.014 to 0.2 IU/kg/h, with a mean of 0.065 IU/kg/h (Krause & McKenzie, 2007). Interestingly, the final insulin dose range remained very similar from 0.015 to 0.2 IU/kg/h, with a mean of 0.07 IU/kg/h.

Some authors advocate starting at lower dosages in foals, such as 0.01 IU/kg/h (Buechner-Maxwell, 2005). This conservative approach is very safe, with less risk of hypoglycemia than the higher dosage rate, but may require a longer period of time before the dose is titrated to a high enough level to control hyperglycemia. Even lower dosage rates of insulin have been reported, with a recent retrospective report describing insulin infusions at dosages of 0.0016 to 0.018 IU/kg/h (Myers et al., 2009).

When administering insulin as a CRI it is best to avoid simultaneous alterations in both the insulin and PN infusion rates. This practice can lead to a "roller-coaster ride" wherein the blood glucose concentration is rising and falling wildly due to the delay in the body's response to simultaneous changes in both PN and insulin. Using a protocol where changes in blood glucose concentration are primarily addressed by altering the insulin infusion rate can aid in minimizing dramatic alterations in blood glucose concentration (McKenzie & Geor, 2009). Blood glucose monitoring should be performed at least hourly for the first 2–3 hours after initiation of the insulin CRI. If hyperglycemia (blood glucose >150 mg/dL) is persistent beyond the first 2 hours of insulin therapy, then the insulin infusion rate may be increased by 50%, followed by hourly blood glucose monitoring for a further 2–3 hours. This procedure for increasing the insulin infusion rate may be repeated if hyperglycemia persists. Conversely, if hypoglycemia (blood glucose <60 mg/dL) is noted, then a bolus of 0.25–0.5 mL/kg of 50% dextrose solution should be administered intravenously over 3–5 minutes. The blood glucose level should then be reassessed every 30 minutes for at least 90 minutes in order to ensure that hypoglycemia does not recur. If hypoglycemia does recur, then a second bolus of dextrose is administered and the insulin infusion rate is decreased by 50%. Close monitoring will be required for a further 60–90 minutes in order to ensure that hypoglycemia does not recur, or hyperglycemia does not develop. Further changes to the insulin infusion rate are usually unnecessary once a steady state has been achieved, with the blood glucose concentration stable and the desired rate of PN administration having been reached. The frequency of blood glucose monitoring can also be decreased as the patient stabilizes, first to every 6 hours and then every 12 hours. The frequency of monitoring should not be less frequent than 12-hourly intervals in patients receiving insulin therapy.

Patient reassessment is indicated if the patient has become even more insulin resistant (requiring additional insulin administration in order to avoid hyperglycemia). Such a change may be an early indicator of an overall deterioration in the patient's condition accompanied by increasing systemic inflammation.

The protocol described above does not attempt to maintain strict control over blood glucose concentration, unlike the intensive insulin therapy (IIT) protocols that have been advocated for human patients over the last decade. In IIT, the goal is to maintain age-appropriate normoglycemia, because of the risks associated with hyper- and hypoglycemia (Gunst & Van den Berghe, 2010; Hollis et al., 2007, 2008; Vlasselaers et al., 2009). Early studies reporting beneficial effects of IIT were performed in human ICU patients receiving PN (van den Berghe et al., 2001). These studies compared the patients on IIT to patients where blood glucose was allowed to range up to the renal threshold (215 mg/dL). Later studies also reported the use of this intervention in hyperglycemic patients receiving PN and/or enteral nutrition. In some of these studies, the incidence of profound hypoglycemia was high. Profound hypoglycemia appeared to eliminate any beneficial effects of IIT overall, and in patients not receiving PN IIT actually appeared to increase the risk of death (Marik & Preiser, 2010). The concept of IIT has become controversial as a result.

More recent assessments have suggested that the goals for insulin therapy should be revised to maintain blood glucose concentrations as close to normal as possible, while avoiding periods of hypoglycemia or hyperglycemia (Gunst & Van den Berghe 2010). In equine patients, it is extremely unusual to use insulin therapy in patients that are not receiving PN, as true diabetes mellitus is rare in horses (Durham et al., 2009; Navas de Solis & Foreman, 2010; Ruoff et al., 1986).

Conclusions

While concerns regarding the complexity, expense, and potential for complications have discouraged the use of PN in both adult horses and foals, it may be time to reconsider. If more conservative rates of PN administration are utilized, it is possible to minimize the expense and lessen the risk of hyperglycemia, while improving the support of patients during periods of anorexia or food withdrawal. Combining conservative

PN administration with small-volume enteral support may decrease the likelihood of complications associated with both of these interventions, while providing superior nutritional support.

References

Barsnick RJ, Toribio RE. (2011) Endocrinology of the equine neonate energy metabolism in health and critical illness. *Vet Clin North Am Equine Pract* **27**:49–58.

Barton RG. (1994) Nutrition support in critical illness. *Nutr Clin Pract* **9**:127–39.

Bercier DL. (2003) How to use parenteral nutrition in practice. In: Proceedings of the 49th Annual Convention of the American Association of Equine Practitioners. AAEP, pp. 268–73.

Boitano M. (2006) Hypocaloric feeding of the critically ill. *Nutr Clin Pract* **21**:617–22.

Buchanan BR, Sommardahl CS, Rohrbach BW, et al. (2005) Effect of a 24-hour infusion of an isotonic electrolyte replacement fluid on the renal clearance of electrolytes in healthy neonatal foals. *J Am Vet Med Assoc* **227**:1123–9.

Buechner-Maxwell VA. (2005) Nutritional support for neonatal foals. *Vet Clin North Am Equine Pract* **21**:487–510, viii.

Carr EA, Holcombe SJ. (2009) Nutrition of critically ill horses. *Vet Clin North Am Equine Pract* **25**:93–108, vii.

Corley K. (2008) *Common treatments: Fluid therapy* In: Corley K, Stephen J (eds) The Equine Hospital Manual. Chichester, West Sussex: John Wiley & Sons, Ltd., pp. 365–92.

Cruz AM, Cote N, McDonell WN, et al. (2006) Postoperative effects of anesthesia and surgery on resting energy expenditure in horses as measured by indirect calorimetry. *Can J Vet Res* **70**:257–62.

Dan A, Jacques TC, O'Leary MJ. (2006) Enteral nutrition versus glucose-based or lipid-based parenteral nutrition and tight glycaemic control in critically ill patients. *Crit Care Resusc* **8**:283–8.

Dandona P, Mohanty P, Chaudhuri A, et al. (2005) Insulin infusion in acute illness. *J Clin Invest* **115**:2069–72.

Dunkel B, McKenzie HC 3rd. (2003) Severe hypertriglyceridaemia in clinically ill horses: diagnosis, treatment and outcome. *Equine Vet J* **35**:590–5.

Dunkel BM, Wilkins PA. (2004) Nutrition and the critically ill horse. *Vet Clin North Am Equine Pract* **20**:107–26.

Durham AE. (2006) Clinical application of parenteral nutrition in the treatment of five ponies and one donkey with hyperlipaemia. *Vet Rec* **158**:159–64.

Durham AE, Phillips TJ, Walmsley JP, et al. (2003) Study of the clinical effects of postoperative parenteral nutrition in 15 horses. *Vet Rec* **153**:493–8.

Durham AE, Phillips TJ, Walmsley JP, et al. (2004) Nutritional and clinicopathological effects of post operative parenteral nutrition following small intestinal resection and anastomosis in the mature horse. *Equine Vet J* **36**:390–6.

Durham AE, Hughes KJ, Cottle HJ, et al. (2009) Type 2 diabetes mellitus with pancreatic beta cell dysfunction in 3 horses confirmed with minimal model analysis. *Equine Vet J* **41**:924–9.

Eve R, Sair M. (2008) Nutritional support in the critically ill. *Anaesth Intens Care Med* **10**:127–30.

Finck C. (2000) Enteral versus parenteral nutrition in the critically ill. *Nutrition* **16**:393–4.

Frank N. (2011) Equine metabolic syndrome. *Vet Clin North Am Equine Pract* **27**:73–92.

Frasca D, Dahyot-Fizelier C, Mimoz O. (2010) Prevention of central venous catheter-related infection in the intensive care unit. *Crit Care* **14**:212.

Furr MO. (2002) Intravenous nutrition in horses: clinical applications. In: Proceedings of the 20th Annual ACVIM Forum. American College of Veterinary Internal Medicine, pp. 186–7.

Geraghty TE, Love S, Taylor DJ, et al. (2009) Assessing techniques for disinfecting sites for inserting intravenous catheters into the jugular veins of horses. *Vet Rec* **164**:51–5.

Gomaa N, Koeller G, Schusser G. (2009) Triglycerides, free fatty acids and total bilirubin in horses with left ventral colon impaction. *Pferdeheilkunde* **25**:137–40.

Greatorex JC. (1975) Intravenous nutrition in the treatment of tetanus in horses. *Vet Rec* **97**:498.

Gunst J, Van den Berghe G. (2010) Blood glucose control in the intensive care unit: benefits and risks. *Semin Dialysis* **23**:157–62.

Han JH, McKenzie HC, McCutcheon LJ, et al. (2011) Glucose and insulin dynamics associated with continuous rate infusion of dextrose solution or dextrose solution and insulin in healthy and endotoxin-exposed horses. *Am J Vet Res* **72**:522–9.

Hansen TO. (1986) Parenteral nutrition in foals. In: Proceedings of the 32nd Annual Convention of the American Association of Equine Practitioners. AAEP, pp. 153–6.

Hansen TO, White NA 2nd, Kemp DT. (1988) Total parenteral nutrition in four healthy adult horses. *Am J Vet Res* **49**:122–4.

Hardy J. (2003) Nutritional support and nursing care of the adult horse in intensive care. *Clin Tech Equine Pract* **2**:193–8.

Hassel DM, Hill AE, Rorabeck RA. (2009) Association between hyperglycemia and survival in 228 horses with acute gastrointestinal disease. *J Vet Intern Med* **23**:1261–5.

Hays SP, Smith EO, Sunehag AL. (2006) Hyperglycemia is a risk factor for early death and morbidity in extremely low birth-weight infants. *Pediatrics* **118**:1811–18.

Hoffer RE, Barber SM, Kallfelz FA, et al. (1977) Esophageal patch grafting as a treatment for esophageal stricture in a horse. *J Am Vet Med Assoc* **171**:350–4.

Hollis AR, Boston RC, Corley KT. (2007) Blood glucose in horses with acute abdominal disease. *J Vet Intern Med* **21**:1099–103.

Hollis AR, Furr MO, Magdesian KG, et al. (2008) Blood glucose concentrations in critically ill neonatal foals. *J Vet Intern Med* **22**:1223–7.

Jose-Cunilleras E, Hinchcliff K, Nout YS, et al. (2008) Glucose metabolism in five septic neonatal foals. *J Vet Emerg Crit Care* **18**:404–8.

Klein CJ, Stanek GS, Wiles CE 3rd. (1998) Overfeeding macronutrients to critically ill adults: metabolic complications. *J Am Diet Assoc* **98**:795–806.

Krause JB, McKenzie HC 3rd. (2007) Parenteral nutrition in foals: a retrospective study of 45 cases (2000–2004). *Equine Vet J* **39**:74–8.

Kuwahara T, Shimono K, Kaneda S, et al. (2010) Growth of microorganisms in total parenteral nutrition solutions containing lipid. *Int J Med Sci* **7**:101–9.

Langouche L, Van den Berghe G. (2006) Glucose metabolism and insulin therapy. *Crit Care Clin* **22**:119–29, vii.

Lazzeri C, Tarquini R, Giunta F, et al. (2009) Glucose dysmetabolism and prognosis in critical illness. *Int Emerg Med* **4**:147–56.

Lopes MA, White NA 2nd. (2002) Parenteral nutrition for horses with gastrointestinal disease: a retrospective study of 79 cases. *Equine Vet J* **34**:250–7.

Lunn JJ, Murray MJ. (1998) Nutritional support in critical illness. *Yale J Biol Med* **71**:449–456.

Magdesian KG. (2003) Nutrition for critical gastrointestinal illness: feeding horses with diarrhea or colic. *Vet Clin North Am Equine Pract* **19**:617–44.

Magdesian KG. (2010) Parenteral nutrition in the mature horse. *Equine Vet Educ* **22**:364–71.

Marik PE, Preiser JC. (2010) Toward understanding tight glycemic control in the ICU: a systematic review and metaanalysis. *Chest* **137**:544–51.

McKenzie HC 3rd. (2011) Equine hyperlipidemias. *Vet Clin North Am Equine Pract* **27**:59–72.

McKenzie HC 3rd, Geor RJ. (2009) Feeding management of sick neonatal foals. *Vet Clin North Am Equine Pract* **25**:109–19, vii.

Miller KR, Lawson CM, Smith VL, et al. (2011) Carbohydrate provision in the era of tight glucose control. *Curr Gastroenterol Rep* **13**:388–94.

Mok E, Hankard R. (2011) Glutamine supplementation in sick children: is it beneficial? *J Nutr Metab* **2011**:Art. ID 617597.

Myers CJ, Magdesian KG, Kass PH, et al. (2009) Parenteral nutrition in neonatal foals: clinical description, complications and outcome in 53 foals (1995–2005). *Vet J* **181**:137–44.

Navas de Solis C, Foreman JH. (2010) Transient diabetes mellitus in a neonatal Thoroughbred foal. *J Vet Emerg Crit Care* **20**:611–15.

Ousey J. (1994) Total parenteral nutrition in the young foal. *Equine Vet Educ* **6**:316–17.

Ousey JC, Holdstock NB, Rossdale PD, et al. (1996) How much energy do sick neonatal foals require compared with healthy foals? *Pferdeheilkunde* **12**:231–7.

Ousey JC, Prandi S, Zimmer J, et al. (1997) Effects of various feeding regimens on the energy balance of equine neonates. *Am J Vet Res* **58**:1243–51.

Packer MJ, German AJ, Hunter L, et al. (2011) Adipose tissue-derived adiponectin expression is significantly associated with increased post operative mortality in horses undergoing emergency abdominal surgery. *Equine Vet J* **43**(Suppl. 39):26–33.

Paradis MR. (2001) Caloric needs of the sick foal: determined by the use of indirect calorimetry. In: *Proceedings of the 3rd Dorothy Havemeyer Foundation Neonatal Septicemia Workshop.* Newmarket, Suffolk: R & W Publications (Newmarket) Ltd., pp. 1–5.

Parsons CS, Orsini JA, Krafty R, Capewell L, Boston R. (2007) Risk factors for development of acute laminitis in horses during hospitalization: 73 cases (1997–2004). *J Am Vet Med Assoc* **230**:885–9.

Pichard C, Thibault R, Heidegger C-P, et al. (2009) Enteral and parenteral nutrition for critically ill patients: A logical combination to optimize nutritional support. *Clin Nutr Suppl* **4**:3–7.

Ruoff WW, Baker DC, Morgan SJ, et al. (1986) Type II diabetes mellitus in a horse. *Equine Vet J* **18**:143–4.

Scurlock C, Mechanick JI. (2008) Early nutrition support in the intensive care unit: a US perspective. *Curr Opin Clin Nutr Metab Care* **11**:152–5.

Seron-Arbeloa C, Puzo-Foncillas J, Garces-Gimenez T, et al. (2011) A retrospective study about the influence of early nutritional support on mortality and nosocomial infection in the critical care setting. *Clin Nutr* **30**:346–50.

Sillence M, Noble G, McGowan C. (2006) Fast food and fat fillies: the ills of western civilisation. *Vet J* **172**:396–7.

Skipper A, Tupesis N. (2005) Is there a role for nonprotein calories in developing and evaluating the nutrient prescription? *Nutr Clin Pract* **20**:321–4.

Spurlock SL, Donaghue S. (1990) Weight gains in foals on parenteral nutrition. In: Proceedings of the 2nd International Society of Veterinary Perinatology Scientific Conference. International Society of Veterinary Perinatology, p. 61.

Spurlock SL, Ward DL. (1990) Providing parenteral nutritional support for equine patients. *Vet Med* **85**:883–90.

Spurlock SL, Ward MV. (1991) Parenteral nutrition in equine patients: Principles and theory. *Comp Cont Educ Pract Vet* **13**:461–9.

Stratton-Phelps M. (2008) Nutritional management of the hospitalised horse. In: Corley K, Stephen J (eds) *The Equine Hospital Manual.* Oxford: Blackwell Publishing, pp. 261–311.

Suann CJ. (1982) Oesophageal resection and anastomosis as a treatment for oesophageal stricture in the horse. *Equine Vet J* **14**:163–4.

Tillotson K, Traub-Dargatz JL, Morgan PK. (2002) Partial parenteral nutrition in equine neonatal clostridial enterocolitis. *Comp Cont Educ Pract Vet* **24**:964–9.

Toth F, Frank N, Geor RJ, et al. (2010) Effects of pretreatment with dexamethasone or levothyroxine sodium on endotoxin-induced alterations in glucose and insulin dynamics in horses. *Am J Vet Res* **71**:60–8.

Turpin RS, Canada T, Liu FX, et al. (2011) Nutrition therapy cost analysis in the US: pre-mixed multi-chamber bag vs compounded parenteral nutrition. *Appl Health Econ Health Policy* **9**:281–92.

van den Berghe G, Wouters P, Weekers F, et al. (2001) Intensive insulin therapy in critically ill patients. *N Engl J Med* **345**:1359–67.

Vanek VW, Matarese LE, Robinson M, et al. (2011) A.S.P.E.N. position paper: parenteral nutrition glutamine supplementation. *Nutr Clin Pract* **26**:479–94.

Vlasselaers D, Milants I, Desmet L, et al. (2009) Intensive insulin therapy for patients in paediatric intensive care: a prospective, randomised controlled study. *Lancet* **373**: 547–56.

Waitt LH, Cebra CK. (2009) Characterization of hypertriglyceridemia and response to treatment with insulin in horses, ponies, and donkeys: 44 cases (1995–2005). *J Am Vet Med Assoc* **234**:915–19.

Wernerman J. (2011) Glutamine supplementation. *Ann Intens Care* **1**:25.

Wyse CA, McNie KA, Tannahill VJ, et al. (2008) Prevalence of obesity in riding horses in Scotland. *Vet Rec* **162**:590–1.

CHAPTER 26

Advanced hemodynamic monitoring

Kevin Corley

Veterinary Advances Ltd, The Curragh, Co. Kildare, Ireland

Introduction

Most equine patients respond to fluid therapy in a fairly predictable manner. For these horses, basic hemodynamic monitoring is sufficient. This consists of monitoring the heart rate, jugular fill, pulse pressure, frequency of urination, and intermittent blood samples for lactate concentration. In animals with dynamic disease processes, such as critically ill foals, and in animals that are not responding to treatment as expected, hemodynamic monitoring is stepped up to an intermediate level. This includes measurement of arterial blood pressure, urine output and specific gravity, and venous oxygen saturation in addition to basic monitoring detailed above. With specific disease processes, such as nephropathy leading to oliguria or anuria and congestive heart failure, the addition of central venous pressure monitoring is essential.

Advanced hemodynamic monitoring consisting of cardiac output monitoring and/or perfusion monitoring is reserved for the most complicated patients and for research. The addition of cardiac output monitoring allows calculation of several parameters such as cardiac stroke volume, systemic vascular resistance, global oxygen delivery, and global oxygen uptake, which give a large volume of information about whole body hemodynamics. In contrast, perfusion monitoring allows estimation of the blood flow through specific organs, which can vary dramatically from whole body blood flow.

Cardiac output measurement

Definitions and normal values

Cardiac output measures the amount of blood pumped by the heart per minute. Cardiac output in resting, conscious, adult horses ranges from approximately 32 to 41 L/min (Clark et al., 1991; Hedenstierna et al., 1987; Hinchcliff et al., 1991; Muir, 1992; Muir et al., 1976; Skarda & Muir, 1996; Steffey et al., 1987). The normal cardiac output in foals increases from 7.1 L/min at 2 hours old to 15.5 L/min at 12 days of age (Thomas et al., 1987).

For serial monitoring of an individual horse, the cardiac output in liters per minute is the appropriate measurement. However, given the great size differentials between different breeds of horses, the raw cardiac output number can be difficult to interpret when comparing different horses. The cardiac index normalizes the cardiac output for the size of the animal. In humans and some small animals, cardiac output is divided by body surface area of the animal to calculate cardiac index. Body surface area is considered a better measure of metabolic mass than body weight (Holliday et al., 1967) and therefore a better measure to normalize cardiac output. However, there is no well-accepted formula for calculating body surface area in horses, and cardiac output is normally divided by body weight to calculate the cardiac index (Bonagura & Reef, 1998; Corley et al., 2003).

Equine Fluid Therapy, First Edition. Edited by C. Langdon Fielding and K. Gary Magdesian.
© 2015 John Wiley & Sons, Inc. Published 2015 by John Wiley & Sons, Inc.

Methods of measurement

Many different methods have been used in horses to measure cardiac output and these have been described in detail elsewhere (Corley et al., 2003). In the clinical patient, the ideal method of measuring cardiac output would be non-invasive, quick to set up, accurate, provide continuous real-time data, and require little or no expertise to operate. For veterinary patients, low capital cost and low cost per patient would also be ideal attributes. Unfortunately, no currently available method meets all of these criteria.

Ultrasound methods

Ultrasound methods, such as the "Bullet Method" (Giguere et al., 2005; McConachie et al., 2013), are perhaps the closest to meeting these criteria. They are non-invasive, have a small cost per patient, and provide close to real-time information. However, they require considerable expertise to achieve repeatable measurements, and the capital costs of ultrasound machines are not small.

The Bullet Method is based on estimation of stroke volume (SV) from ultrasonographic measurements of the short-axis view of the left ventricle at the papillary muscle level just below the mitral valve for measurement of the left ventricular area in diastole (LVASAd), the left ventricular length in diastole (LVLRd), and the equivalent measurements in systole (LVASAs and LVLRs). The equation for calculating stroke volume is:

$$SV = (5/6 \times LVASAd \times LVLRd) - (5/6 \times LVASAs \times LVLRs)$$

$$(26.1)$$

This is then multiplied by heart rate to give the cardiac output. This method is relatively accurate in the foal, where the method overestimated the cardiac output measured by lithium dilution by 4.2%, and less than 10% of measurements varied from the lithium dilution measurement by more than 30% of the measured cardiac output (Giguere et al., 2005).

In the adult horse, the required ultrasound views are more technically challenging. In adults, the Bullet Method overestimated cardiac output measured by lithium dilution by an average of 6.9 L/min (22.6%) and the limits of agreement were between an overestimation of 25 L/min and an underestimation of 11 L/min (McConachie et al., 2013). Given that the normal cardiac output of the adult horse is approximately 32–40 L/min (Corley et al., 2003), it is a matter of debate whether the Bullet Method is accurate enough for monitoring clinical cases in adult horses.

Other ultrasound techniques for measuring cardiac output have been used in adult horses. Different methods of calculation of cardiac output from transthoracic ultrasound and Doppler ultrasound have been compared to lithium dilution (McConachie et al., 2013). The methods have varying agreement with lithium dilution, but none is close enough to stand out as a suitable method for use in clinical cases. In contrast, transesophageal Doppler measurements of blood flow are very accurate (Young et al., 1995, 1996) but have the disadvantage that they require a specialized probe (these have been made by combining an endoscope and a Doppler probe made for human medicine) and considerable technical skill. Furthermore, the probe needs to be passed down the esophagus, preventing its use in most conscious, unsedated horses.

Indicator dilution methods

Indicator dilution methods have been used for many years in horses, mainly as a research tool. These methods rely on rapidly injecting an indicator on one side of the heart and measuring the concentration of the indicator against time on the other side of the heart. The cardiac output can be calculated from the indicator dilution curve. The more blood that is being pumped by the heart, the more the indicator will be diluted. Therefore a higher cardiac output results in a smaller curve (Corley et al., 2003).

Indicator dilution methods are very accurate if correctly performed. The main limitation concerns the indicator used. The ideal indicator would not be a normal component of blood; it would be dispersed rapidly and proportionally between the plasma and the cellular components of the blood, be non-toxic, and not accumulate. Furthermore, injecting the indicator would not change the cardiac output. If the indicator accumulates, it limits the number of sequential measurements that can be performed. Indicators that do not enter the cellular components of the blood can be used, if a hematocrit is taken with each measurement. The hematocrit allows the amount of blood pumped by the heart per minute (cardiac output) to be calculated from the amount of plasma pumped by the heart per minute (which is what is measured by an indicator that stays completely within the plasma). An indicator that partly enters the cellular component during the measurement window could not be used.

The indicator that comes closest to matching the properties of an ideal indicator is a change in temperature. Thermodilution is based on the rapid injection of ice cold saline into the right atrium. The change in temperature is then detected by a thermistor in the pulmonary artery (i.e., the other side of the right ventricle). Unfortunately there are several limitations to thermodilution that have restricted its use in clinical cases. The most important of these is that it requires a pulmonary artery catheter, which can cause marked morbidity in horses. Schlipf et al. (1994) reported right atrial, right ventricular, and pulmonary fibrinous endothelial lesions in nine adult horses in which multiple thermodilution cardiac output determinations were performed using a pulmonary artery catheter over a 5–6 h period. One horse also had a solitary thrombus in the pulmonary artery. Contact of the catheter with the ventricular wall can induce life-threatening ventricular arrhythmias particularly in anesthetized horses. A further limitation with thermodilution in the horse is the large cardiac output of the adult horse, particularly at exercise. In adult horses at rest or under anesthesia, it is necessary to use ice-cold saline to improve the signal-to-noise ratio (Corley et al., 2003). However, any warming of the saline before or during injection decreases the accuracy of the measurement. Even holding the syringe briefly in a hand can be enough to warm the saline. Higher volumes of injectate also improve the signal-to-noise ratio, but also increase the preload of the heart thereby altering the cardiac output. Automated injectors further improve the signal-to-noise ratio by ensuring a rapid, smooth injection of the cold saline (Corley et al., 2003). Usually three to four measurements are taken at end expiration, with the cardiac output being taken as the average of the two or three closest results. The need to take repeated measurements and average can also decrease accuracy when the cardiac output is not in a steady state. Thermodilution is not suitable for measurement of cardiac output during exercise in horses, as the signal-to-noise ratio at these very high cardiac outputs is not sufficient to obtain reliable readings.

An adaptation of this technique is transpulmonary thermodilution, where the change of temperature is detected in the femoral artery or a peripheral artery (Shih et al., 2009). This method avoids a pulmonary artery catheter, but decreases the signal-to-noise ratio and is therefore only likely to be suitable in foals and not adult horses. In one experiment in anesthetized neonatal foals, transpulmonary thermodilution using an arterial catheter in a metatarsal failed to produce a reading in 4 out of 18 attempts (Shih et al., 2009).

Lithium dilution is an indicator dilution method based on rapid injection of lithium chloride, and detection of the lithium–time concentration curve with the use of a lithium-specific sensor (Corley et al., 2002; Linton et al., 2000). The technique requires a catheter in a major vein such as the jugular vein, a peripheral arterial catheter, and measurement of hemoglobin and sodium. The advantages of this system over thermodilution are that a pulmonary artery catheter is not necessary, lower volumes of injectate can be used, only a single measurement is needed for each reading, and an adapted technique can be used to measure cardiac output during exercise (Durando et al., 2008). The disadvantages compared to thermodilution are that if very many measurements are made lithium accumulation can decrease the accuracy (Mason et al., 2002) and that measurements may not be accurate during infusion treatment with xylazine, ketamine, lidocaine, and rocuronium (Ambrisko et al., 2013). It is also not possible to use the lithium sensors on more than one animal, and this may also explain part of the inaccuracy noted in a recent study (Ambrisko et al., 2012). Other studies of lithium dilution in horses and foals have found it to be extremely accurate (Linton et al., 2000). The method has been used in several experimental studies in horses (de Vries et al., 2009; Hallowell & Corley, 2006; Hollis et al., 2006a, 2006b, 2008; Schauvliege et al., 2007) and in clinical patients. An adaptation of the technique can give accurate measurements of cardiac output during treadmill exercise. However, the number of measurements that can be taken during an exercise session is limited (Durando et al., 2008).

Pulse contour analysis

Pulse contour analysis calculates cardiac output from arterial pressure waveforms. The area under the arterial pressure tracing during systole represents blood flow in the catheterized vessel and therefore reflects the cardiac output (Corley et al., 2003). The advantage of these systems is that they provide real-time beat-to-beat analysis of cardiac output either following intermittent use of another measurement technique to calibrate the machine or uncalibrated using only an arterial catheter. The disadvantage of the systems is a question about their accuracy, especially in the face of changing hemodynamics (Ambrisko et al., 2012; Shih et al., 2009). At the time of this writing, three devices that require intermittent calibration and five devices that are used without calibration are marketed for human medicine (Ramsingh et al., 2013). Two devices have been tested in horses. These devices use proprietary algorithms based on power analysis of flow within the human radial artery (PulseCO, LiDCO, London, UK) or the area under the curve prior to the dicrotic notch and calculated aortic impedance (PiCCO, Pulsion Medical Systems, Munich, Germany) (Ambrisko et al., 2012; Shih et al., 2009).

In adult horses, pulse contour analysis (PulseCO) calibrated with lithium dilution was found to be fairly accurate over 30 minutes during stable hemodynamics under anesthesia (Hallowell & Corley, 2005), but not when vasoactive drugs were used in another study (Schauvliege et al., 2009). In anesthetized neonatal foals in which the hemodynamics were varied by changing inhaled concentrations of isoflurane and use of vasoactive drugs, PulseCO was relatively accurate but pulse contour analysis calibrated by transpulmonary thermodilution was not (Shih et al., 2009).

The Fick method

Cardiac output can be calculated by using the Fick principle, named after Adolph Fick (Fick, 1870). This method was used in the horse as early as 1894 (Zuntz & Hagemann, 1894). The Fick principle is based on the uptake of oxygen by blood as it flows through the lungs. The fundamental assumption is that all of the oxygen removed from inspired air is taken up by the blood as it passes through the lungs (Corley et al., 2003). The cardiac output is calculated from the arterial and mixed venous oxygen contents together with the rate of oxygen uptake in the lungs.

The disadvantages of the Fick method are the requirements for a pulmonary arterial catheter to measure mixed venous blood oxygen content (Edwards & Mayall, 1998; Wetmore et al., 1987) and either a closed airway system to measure oxygen uptake or an expensive open-circuit system (Corley et al., 2003; Fedak et al., 1981). It is also necessary to measure blood gases and oxygen percentage in air.

The Fick method is very accurate when meticulously performed under ideal conditions. However, the requirement for a pulmonary artery catheter, a closed airway system such as an endotracheal tube or a facemask, and the expense limit its utility in clinical patients,

with the exception of treadmill exercise tests where the facilities are available (Corley et al., 2003).

Bioimpedance

Bioimpedance uses the naturally occurring charges on molecules in the body to measure blood flow. Blood has a relatively high electrical conductivity compared to solid tissues and air. Arterial blood flow is pulsatile. The pulsatile flow in the great arteries results in changes in thoracic impedance, with the magnitude of change corresponding to the amount of blood flowing and therefore cardiac output (Corley et al., 2003; Kubicek et al., 1974). The accuracy of bioimpedance for measuring cardiac output in human critical care is only moderate (Ramsingh et al., 2013; Raval et al., 2008; Squara et al., 2007). Whereas the use of bioimpedance to measure cardiac output has not been published in horses, the technique has been used to estimate the values for total body water, intracellular fluid, and extracellular fluid in horses and foals (Fielding et al., 2004, 2007, 2011; Forro et al., 2000; Waller & Lindinger, 2006).

Which technique should be used in clinical patients?

Unfortunately there is no optimal technique for measurement of cardiac output in horses. In foals, lithium dilution and the Bullet ultrasound method appear to be the most practical methods that have shown reasonably good accuracy in validation studies. Pulse contour analysis calibrated by lithium dilution may also find a place in the clinic for neonatal foals. For adult horses, lithium dilution or perhaps transesophageal ultrasound methods represent the best available methods. There is much innovation in the area of noninvasive cardiac output measurement in human medicine (Faraoni & Barvais, 2013; Fischer et al., 2013). Although none of these techniques is immediately applicable to the horse, it might be possible to adapt these or future technologies so that cardiac output measurements are readily available in the equine hospital.

Derived parameters from cardiac output

Several hemodynamic variables can be calculated from cardiac output, heart rate, blood pressure, and blood gases. These include stroke volume, systemic vascular

Table 26.1 Calculations for hemodynamic variables.

Parameter	Calculation	Units	Normal values for 1-day-old foals
Cardiac index (CI)	$\dfrac{\text{Cardiac output (L/min)} \times 1000}{\text{Bodyweight (kg)}}$	mL/kg/min	197.3 ± 12.0
Stroke volume (SV)	$\dfrac{\text{Cardiac output (L/min)} \times 1000}{\text{Heart rate}}$	mL	107 ± 6.4
Stroke volume index (SVI)	$\dfrac{\text{Stroke volume}}{\text{Body weight (kg)}}$	mL/kg	2.35 ± 0.14
Systemic vascular resistance (SVR)	$\dfrac{(\text{MAP} - \text{CVP}) \times 80}{\text{Cardiac output}}$	dynes.s.cm^{-5}	708 ± 74
Arterial oxygen content (C_aO_2)	$1.34 \times [\text{Hb}] \times S_aO_2 + 0.0031\, P_aO_2$	mL/L	158 ± 13[a]
Venous oxygen content (C_vO_2)	$1.34 \times [\text{Hb}] \times S_vO_2 + 0.0031\, P_vO_2$	mL/L	130 ± 13[a]
Global oxygen delivery (DO$_2$)	$\dfrac{C_aO_2 \times \text{Cardiac index}}{1000}$	mL O$_2$/kg/min	31[b]
Global oxygen uptake (VO$_2$)	$\dfrac{(C_aO_2 - C_vO_2) \times \text{Cardiac index}}{1000}$	mL O$_2$/kg/min	5.6[b]
Oxygen extraction ratio (O$_2$ER)	$\dfrac{(C_aO_2 - C_vO_2) \times 100}{C_aO_2}$	%	18.0 ± 0.02[a]
Pulmonary vascular resistance (PVR)	$\dfrac{(\text{PAP} - \text{PAOP}) \times 80}{\text{Cardiac output}}$	dynes.s.cm^{-5}	194 ± 37

MAP, mean arterial pressure; CVP, central venous pressure; [Hb], hemoglobin concentration (g/L); S_aO_2, arterial hemoglobin saturation (%); P_aO_2, arterial oxygen tension (mmHg); S_vO_2, venous oxygen saturation (%); P_vO_2, venous oxygen tension (mmHg); PAP, mean pulmonary arterial pressure (mmHg); PAOP, pulmonary arterial occlusion pressure (mmHg).
Normals from Thomas et al. (1987), except as specified below:
[a] Data from five conscious, healthy 30–46-hour-old mixed breed foals in lateral recumbency.
[b] Calculated from other data presented. Intended as a guide only.

resistance, oxygen extraction ratio, global oxygen delivery, and global oxygen uptake (Table 26.1).

Stroke volume is an indirect indicator of myocardial contractile function and should be interpreted in light of the fluid status and central venous pressure of the animal. A low stroke volume, despite a high central venous pressure or in spite of an adequate fluid challenge, is consistent with cardiac failure. A greater than normal stroke volume suggests that hypovolemia is unlikely.

Systemic vascular resistance is an indicator of vasodilation or constriction. It is a useful parameter to determine the root cause of hypotension and the response to drugs. However, since this is a derived parameter, treatments should be titrated to mean arterial pressure, not systemic vascular resistance (Hollenberg et al., 1999).

Global oxygen delivery is a measure of the amount of oxygen delivered from the heart per minute and is an indicator of both cardiovascular and respiratory system function. It only describes the rate at which oxygen is entering the systemic circulation and not its distribution to the various tissues, which varies markedly between individual organs in both normal as well as disease states.

Global oxygen uptake is the amount of oxygen removed in the systemic circulation and indicates overall tissue oxygen utilization. It indicates whether organs are able to utilize the delivered oxygen. In normal animals, the oxygen uptake reflects metabolic oxygen requirements, and increasing oxygen delivery will not increase oxygen uptake when there is no increase in oxygen demand by the tissue. In diseased animals, treatments that increase oxygen uptake are, in general, likely to be beneficial. There are two situations in which increasing oxygen delivery will not increase a reduced oxygen uptake. The first is where there is significant shunting of blood past some organs. If some organs are adequately perfused, but local vascular constriction or dilation is preventing perfusion of other organs, increasing cardiac output may simply increase flow through the already perfused organs. The second situation is sepsis. Biochemical changes to the cells may reduce oxygen uptake in sepsis despite adequate oxygen delivery (Fink, 1997). As in the case of global oxygen delivery, individual organs may vary markedly from the global parameter in both normality and disease.

The oxygen extraction ratio describes the percent of oxygen delivered that is utilized by the tissues. Its main advantage over the global oxygen delivery and uptake parameters is that it does not require cardiac output measurement. The disadvantage is that it cannot distinguish between the contribution of these two factors to the ratio. A decreasing oxygen extraction ratio may result from decreased oxygen uptake without a change in oxygen delivery, or increased oxygen delivery without a change in oxygen uptake. Conversely a high oxygen extraction ratio may represent decreased relative oxygen delivery or increased relative oxygen uptake.

Tissue perfusion monitoring

Cardiac output and the derived hemodynamic parameters give very useful information about global hemodynamics. However, the distribution of blood flow to different tissues is not equal and global hemodynamics may mislead the veterinarian. A classic example of this is endogenous epinephrine release during the "fight or flight" reaction, where blood is distributed preferentially to the heart, brain, and muscles and away from the gastrointestinal tract and skin (Mohrman & Heller, 1997). This uneven distribution of blood flow and therefore oxygen delivery happens also in disease and with the use of vasoactive drugs. When there is uneven distribution of blood flow, both blood pressure and cardiac output can be normal and yet there may be serious cardiovascular compromise to individual organs (Heard, 2003).

In septic shock, microcirculatory dysfunction appears to be the key element in pathogenesis (van Griensven, 2013), likely as a result of thrombosis within the microvasculature (Semeraro et al., 2012). The microcirculation dysfunction can result in continued regional hypoxia despite apparently successful therapeutic correction of the systemic circulation (van Griensven, 2013). This has led to efforts to measure and monitor regional circulation and the microvasculature itself.

A particular concern in clinical equine practice is blood flow to the gastrointestinal tract. As stated above, epinephrine, released during physiologic stress, results in decreased blood flow in the splanchnic circulation. This can lead to local ischemia. The consequences of this can be marked, from gastric ulceration in neonatal foals (Elfenbein & Sanchez, 2012; Sanchez et al., 2008), to bacterial translocation with endotoxemia or septicemia in horses of all ages (Hurcombe et al., 2012; Vendrig & Fink-Gremmels, 2012). Because of similar concerns in human medicine, tools have been developed to measure blood flow in the gastrointestinal tract (Heard, 2003).

Measuring gastrointestinal perfusion

Gastric tonometry attempts to determine the perfusion status of the gastric mucosa using measurements of local P_{CO_2} (Heard, 2003). The principle is based on local CO_2 diffusing into a balloon that is in contact with the mucosa. The balloon contents can be saline or air (Heard, 2003) The CO_2 will equilibrate with the balloon contents over time, so that the balloon contents can then be aspirated and measured to give a measure of the gastric mucosal P_{CO_2} (Boda & Muranyi, 1959). The initial method for assessing gastric mucosal perfusion was to calculate the intramucosal pH (pHi) using arterial bicarbonate concentration from an arterial blood gas sample. Based on the assumption that the mucosal bicarbonate concentration is equivalent to the arterial bicarbonate concentration, pHi is calculated from the Henderson–Hasselbach equation (Heard, 2003):

$$pHi = log([HCO_3]art / 0.03(P_{CO_2}muc)) \qquad (26.2)$$

where $P_{CO_2}muc$ is the CO_2 partial pressure in the tonometer balloon and $[HCO_3]$ art is the arterial bicarbonate concentration.

The lower the pHi or the bigger the difference between arterial pH and pHi, the lower the mucosal perfusion. Unfortunately, the central assumption for the calculation of pHi, that arterial bicarbonate concentrations can be substituted for mucosal bicarbonate, is flawed (Morgan et al., 1999). The error is greatest when there is significant mucosal ischemia, during which the pHi is significantly overestimated from the arterial bicarbonate (i.e., the mucosal perfusion is calculated to be better than it is). For this reason, the directly measured mucosal P_{CO_2} (or the difference from arterial P_{CO_2}) is now used in preference to the calculated value for pHi (Schlichtig et al., 1996).

Tonometry has been found to be very useful in human patients. When compared to global parameters such as cardiac index, oxygen delivery, and oxygen uptake, tonometry was considerably superior at predicting outcome in 83 critically ill patients (Maynard et al., 1993). In patients admitted as an emergency for acute circulatory or respiratory failure, an increased difference between arterial and mucosal Pco_2 (ΔCO_2) was associated with increased mortality at admission (mortality 51% vs 5% in patients with normal ΔCO_2; $P < 0.0001$) (Jakob et al., 2008). Despite these very promising results, gastric tonometry has not been widely adopted in human medicine because placing instrumentation and performing measurements in clinical patients is cumbersome (Chung et al., 2012).

Gastric tonometry was used during a study of inopressors in anesthetized neonatal foals (Valverde et al., 2006). The authors found that they were able to measure mucosal Pco_2 and calculate ΔCO_2 in five of six foals that completed the experiment. In one foal, there was equipment failure during one of three experiments and the tonometry readings could not be obtained. They also found an increase in ΔCO_2 with hypotension and with infusion of vasopressin (Valverde et al., 2006), suggesting that it could be a useful measurement and that interpretation will be similar to that in humans.

Although gastric tonometry was used in this experimental study in foals (Valverde et al., 2006), there are several limitations to its use in clinical cases and in adult horses. In foals, the variation in the values obtained in normal animals is so large as to make the changes expected in clinical cases impossible to interpret. Furthermore the values obtained are altered by both feeding (which reduces ΔCO_2, possibly because of increased mucosal perfusion or perhaps an effect of the milk in the stomach on measurement) and treatment with omeprazole treatment (which increases ΔCO_2) (Sanchez et al., 2008).

Potential limitations in adult horses include the length of probe required and the heavy sedation usually required for passage of a gastroscope (and therefore presumably for a tonometer). The probes made for human use are not long enough for placement in adult horses. A further theoretical limitation is the large area of non-glandular mucosa in the adult horse, which could affect the results if the probe were in contact with this area rather than the glandular mucosa. However, in humans esophageal (rather than gastric) tonometry has been

used successfully (Sato et al., 1997), suggesting that it may not be important which area of the stomach the probe is in contact with.

Sublingual capnometry is an alternative to gastric tonometry that has been used in human medicine (Weil et al., 1999). The advantage is that the probe is simply placed under the tongue, rather than passed into the stomach. The sublingual mucosa is the most proximal and accessible part of the gastrointestinal tract, potentially allowing for rapid measurement.

The sublingual technique has been shown to be useful in human medicine. Increases in sublingual Pco_2 measurements were shown to reflect inadequate perfusion, and improvements in sublingual Pco_2 were seen prior to decreases in circulating lactate concentrations (Weil et al., 1999). It has been shown to be equivalent to lactate measurement in terms of prognostic ability in hypovolemic humans with hemorrhagic shock (Baron et al., 2007). In contrast, however, an experimental progressive reduction in central blood volume caused by lower body negative pressure was not detected by sublingual capnometry (Chung et al., 2012).

No published work could be found detailing the use of sublingual capnometry in horses. Its use in conscious animals may be limited by possible damage to the sensor from the teeth and, in adult horses, by the limited length of sensors made for the human market.

Other new technologies are now being applied in an attempt to define the microcirculation in human medicine. These include capillary microscopy, laser Doppler, intravital videomicroscopy, side stream dark field imaging, and orthogonal polarization spectral imaging (van Griensven, 2013). Of these, only laser Doppler has been used in horses to date (Adair et al., 1994; Serteyn et al., 1986). Laser Doppler measures regional perfusion, but does not give any information about heterogeneity of flow within the microvasculature. In a recent study in human patients with sepsis, the proportion of perfused small vessels was a strong predictor of outcome (De Backer et al., 2013).

The main use of laser Doppler in the horse has been to investigate muscle blood flow during anesthesia with an aim to reduce the incidence of post-anesthetic myopathy (Raisis et al., 2000; Serteyn et al., 1986, 1988). A further use of laser Doppler has aimed at defining blood flow in the hooves during models of laminitis (Adair et al., 2000; Ingle-Fehr & Baxter, 1998) or the effect of various drugs on laminar blood flow (Castro et al., 2010; Ingle-Fehr & Baxter, 1999). The primary problem with laser Doppler is that it is difficult to obtain consistent, repeatable readings (McGorum et al., 2002). This has prevented its routine use in equine clinical cases to date.

Near-infrared spectroscopy (NIRS)

Near-infrared spectroscopy is a light-based method of monitoring tissue oxygen status (Pellicer & Bravo Mdel, 2011). It works on the principle that biological tissue is relatively transparent to light in the near-infrared range (700–1000 nm). Changes in the oxidation-reduction level of cytochrome aa3, in the oxygenation state of hemoglobin, and in tissue blood volume can be assessed by differential absorbance of near-infrared light (Brazy et al., 1985). Cerebral blood flow can be calculated with NIRS if the patient responds to increased inspired oxygen concentration by increasing the oxygen content in the blood. This allows oxygen to be used as a tracer for blood flow, allowing for calculation of cerebral blood flow by a modification of the Fick method. The reproducibility of each measurement varies between 17% and 24% (Pellicer & Bravo Mdel, 2011). The major drawback to NIRS is that 80% of the total attenuation of near-infrared light in tissue is due to scattering rather than absorption (Pellicer & Bravo Mdel, 2011). This means that the noise-to-signal ratio can be large, reducing the ability to make quantitative measurements. This is exacerbated in humans with pigmented skin, as melanin absorbs near-infrared light in the same spectrum as hemoglobin (Pellicer & Bravo Mdel, 2011; Wassenaar & Van den Brand, 2005). These two factors, scatter and pigmented skin, may limit its usefulness in equine clinical cases; both haired and pigmented skin are likely to interfere with the signal in horses.

Despite these potential limitations, near-infrared spectroscopy has been used for measurement of hoof and skeletal blood flow and regional cerebral oxygenation in horses (Hinckley et al., 1995; McConnell et al., 2013; Pringle et al., 2000). In each experiment, the skin was clipped or shaved prior to application of the sensor and the sensor was covered with lightproof tape or cloth. The need for close clipping may limit the usefulness of NIRS to some situations where it is used in humans, such as monitoring during cardio-pulmonary-cerebro resuscitation (CPCR) (Meex et al., 2013).

Regional cerebral oxygenation has been measured using a probe placed over the dorsal sagittal sinus.

Although there were changes in the measured values for regional cerebral oxygenation during different manipulations (sedation, anesthesia, and drug infusions), the greatest variation in value was between individual horses (McConnell et al., 2013). Based on these results, it appears that NIRS is most useful for following trends in regional cerebral oxygen in individual horses rather than for obtaining exact values or for comparing horses. NIRS was found to detect the expected changes in blood flow both in muscles (Pringle et al., 2000) and hooves (Hinckley et al., 1995) of horses, where a tourniquet was applied to the limb. These latter three studies have shown the feasibility of using NIRS to measure blood flow, but the usefulness for prognostication or directing therapy in clinical cases remains to be elucidated.

Conclusions

Tissue perfusion monitoring is likely to be become an integral part of equine critical care in the future. However, in order for tissue monitoring to gain widespread use in equine clinical patients, it needs to be accurate, repeatable, low cost per measurement, easy to perform, and have low capital cost. At the present time, none of the existing methods meet these criteria.

Advanced hemodynamic monitoring has a place in complicated cases to guide fluid therapy and inotropic and pressor support. Current applications in equine clinical cases are limited by the available technologies.

References

Adair HS 3rd, Goble DO, Shires GM, Sanders WL. (1994) Evaluation of laser Doppler flowmetry for measuring coronary band and laminar microcirculatory blood flow in clinically normal horses. *Am J Vet Res* **55**:445–9.

Adair HS 3rd, Goble DO, Schmidhammer JL, Shires GM. (2000) Laminar microvascular flow, measured by means of laser Doppler flowmetry, during the prodromal stages of black walnut-induced laminitis in horses. *Am J Vet Res* **61**:862–8.

Ambrisko TD, Coppens P, Kabes R, Moens Y. (2012) Lithium dilution, pulse power analysis, and continuous thermodilution cardiac output measurements compared with bolus thermodilution in anaesthetized ponies. *Br J Anaesth* **109**:864–9.

Ambrisko TD, Kabes R, Moens Y. (2013) Influence of drugs on the response characteristics of the LiDCO sensor: an in vitro study. *Br J Anaesth* **110**:305–10.

Baron BJ, Dutton RP, Zehtabchi S, et al. (2007) Sublingual capnometry for rapid determination of the severity of hemorrhagic shock. *J Trauma* **62**:120–4.

Boda D, Muranyi L. (1959) Gastrotonometry; an aid to the control of ventilation during artificial respiration. *Lancet* **i**:181–2.

Bonagura JD, Reef VB. (1998) Cardiovascular diseases. In: Reed SM, Bayly WM (eds) *Equine Internal Medicine*, 1st edn. Philadelphia: W.B. Saunders, pp. 290–370.

Brazy JE, Lewis DV, Mitnick MH, Jobsis vander Vliet FF. (1985) Noninvasive monitoring of cerebral oxygenation in preterm infants: preliminary observations. *Pediatrics* **75**:217–25.

Castro JR, Adair HS 3rd, Radecki SV, Kiefer VR, Elliot SB, Longhofer SL. (2010) Effects of domperidone on digital laminar microvascular blood flow in clinically normal adult horses. *Am J Vet Res* **71**:281–7.

Chung KK, Ryan KL, Rickards CA, et al. (2012) Progressive reduction in central blood volume is not detected by sublingual capnography. *Shock* **37**:586–91.

Clark ES, Gantley B, Moore JN. (1991) Effects of slow infusion of a low dosage of endotoxin on systemic haemodynamics in conscious horses. *Equine Vet J* **23**:18–21.

Corley KTT, Donaldson LL, Furr MO. (2002) Comparison of lithium dilution and thermodilution cardiac output measurements in anaesthetised neonatal foals. *Equine Vet J* **34**:598–601.

Corley KT, Donaldson LL, Durando MM, Birks EK. (2003) Cardiac output technologies with special reference to the horse. *J Vet Intern Med* **17**:262–72.

De Backer D, Donadello K, Sakr Y, et al. (2013) Microcirculatory alterations in patients with severe sepsis: impact of time of assessment and relationship with outcome. *Crit Care Med* **41**:791–9.

de Vries A, Brearley JC, Taylor PM. (2009) Effects of dobutamine on cardiac index and arterial blood pressure in isoflurane-anaesthetized horses under clinical conditions. *J Vet Pharmacol Ther* **32**:353–8.

Durando MM, Corley KT, Boston RC, Birks EK. (2008) Cardiac output determination by use of lithium dilution during exercise in horses. *Am J Vet Res* **69**:1054–60.

Edwards JD, Mayall RM. (1998) Importance of the sampling site for measurement of mixed venous oxygen saturation in shock. *Crit Care Med* **26**:1356–60.

Elfenbein JR, Sanchez LC. (2012) Prevalence of gastric and duodenal ulceration in 691 nonsurviving foals (1995–2006). *Equine Vet J Suppl* **44**(Suppl. 41):76–9.

Faraoni D, Barvais L. (2013) Correlation between esCCO and transthoracic echocardiography in critically ill patients. *Br J Anaesth* **110**:139–40.

Fedak MA, Rome L, Seeherman HJ. (1981) One-step N2-dilution technique for calibrating open-circuit VO2 measuring systems. *J Appl Physiol* **51**:772–6.

Fick A. (1870) Ueber die Messung des Blutquantums in den Herzventrikeln. *Sitzber Physik Med Ges Würzburg* **2**:16.

Fielding CL, Magdesian KG, Elliott DA, Cowgill LD, Carlson GP. (2004) Use of multifrequency bioelectrical impedance analysis for estimation of total body water and extracellular and intracellular fluid volumes in horses. *Am J Vet Res* **65**:320–6.

Fielding CL, Magdesian KG, Carlson GP, Ruby RE, Rhodes DM. (2007) Estimation of acute fluid shifts using bioelectrical impedance analysis in horses. *J Vet Intern Med* **21**:176–83.

Fielding CL, Magdesian KG, Edman JE. (2011) Determination of body water compartments in neonatal foals by use of indicator dilution techniques and multifrequency bioelectrical impedance analysis. *Am J Vet Res* **72**:1390–6.

Fink M. (1997) Cytopathic hypoxia in sepsis. *Acta Anaesth Scand Suppl* **110**:87–95.

Fischer MO, Coucoravas J, Truong J, et al. (2013) Assessment of changes in cardiac index and fluid responsiveness: a comparison of Nexfin and transpulmonary thermodilution. *Acta Anaesthesiol Scand* **57**:704–12.

Forro M, Cieslar S, Ecker GL, Walzak A, Hahn J, Lindinger MI. (2000) Total body water and ECFV measured using bioelectrical impedance analysis and indicator dilution in horses. *J Appl Physiol* **89**:663–71.

Giguere S, Bucki E, Adin DB, Valverde A, Estrada AH, Young L. (2005) Cardiac output measurement by partial carbon dioxide rebreathing, 2-dimensional echocardiography, and lithium-dilution method in anesthetized neonatal foals. *J Vet Intern Med* **19**:737–43.

Hallowell GD, Corley KT. (2005) Use of lithium dilution and pulse contour analysis cardiac output determination in anaesthetized horses: a clinical evaluation. *Vet Anaesth Analg* **32**:201–11.

Hallowell GD, Corley KTT. (2006) Preoperative administration of hydroxyethyl starch or hypertonic saline to horses with colic. *J Vet Int Med* **20**:980–6.

Heard SO. (2003) Gastric tonometry: the hemodynamic monitor of choice (Pro). *Chest* **123**:469S–74S.

Hedenstierna G, Nyman G, Kvart C, Funkquist B. (1987) Ventilation-perfusion relationships in the standing horse: an inert gas elimination study. *Equine Vet J* **19**:514–19.

Hinchcliff KW, McKeever KH, Muir WW. (1991) Hemodynamic effects of atropine, dobutamine, nitroprusside, phenylephrine, and propranolol in conscious horses. *J Vet Int Med* **5**:80–6.

Hinckley KA, Fearn S, Howard BR, Henderson IW. (1995) Near infrared spectroscopy of pedal haemodynamics and oxygenation in normal and laminitic horses. *Equine Vet J* **27**:465–70.

Hollenberg SM, Ahrens TS, Astiz ME, et al. (1999) Practice parameters for hemodynamic support of sepsis in adult patients in sepsis. *Crit Care Med* **27**:639–60.

Holliday MA, Potter D, Jarrah A, Bearg S. (1967) The relation of metabolic rate to body weight and organ size. *Pediatr Res* **1**:185–95.

Hollis AR, Ousey JC, Palmer L, Stoneham SJ, Corley KT. (2006a) Effects of norepinephrine and a combined norepinephrine and dobutamine infusion on systemic hemodynamics and indices of renal function in normotensive neonatal thoroughbred foals. *J Vet Intern Med* **20**:1437–42.

Hollis AR, Ousey JC, Palmer L, Stoneham SJ, Corley KTT. (2006b) Effects of fenoldopam mesylate on systemic hemodynamics and indices of renal function in normotensive neonatal foals. *J Vet Int Med* **20**:595–600.

Hollis AR, Ousey JC, Palmer L, et al. (2008) Effects of norepinephrine and combined norepinephrine and fenoldopam infusion on systemic hemodynamics and indices of renal function in normotensive neonatal foals. *J Vet Intern Med* **22**:1210–15.

Hurcombe SD, Mudge MC, Daniels JB. (2012) Presumptive bacterial translocation in horses with strangulating small intestinal lesions requiring resection and anastomosis. *J Vet Emerg Crit Care (San Antonio)* **22**:653–60.

Ingle-Fehr JE, Baxter GM. (1998) Evaluation of digital and laminar blood flow in horses given a low dose of endotoxin. *Am J Vet Res* **59**:192–6.

Ingle-Fehr JE, Baxter GM. (1999) The effect of oral isoxsuprine and pentoxifylline on digital and laminar blood flow in healthy horses. *Vet Surg* **28**:154–60.

Jakob SM, Parviainen I, Ruokonen E, Kogan A, Takala J. (2008) Tonometry revisited: perfusion-related, metabolic, and respiratory components of gastric mucosal acidosis in acute cardiorespiratory failure. *Shock* **29**:543–8.

Kubicek WG, Kottke J, Ramos MU, et al. (1974) The Minnesota impedance cardiograph – theory and applications. *Biomed Eng* **9**:410–16.

Linton RA, Young LE, Marlin DJ, et al. (2000) Cardiac output measured by lithium dilution, thermodilution and transesophageal Doppler echocardiography in anesthetized horses. *Am J Vet Res* **61**:731–7.

Mason DJ, O'Grady M, Woods JP, McDonell WN. (2002) Effect of background serum lithium concentrations on the accuracy of lithium dilution cardiac output determination in dogs. *Am J Vet Res* **63**:1048–52.

Maynard N, Bihari D, Beale R, et al. (1993) Assessment of splanchnic oxygenation by gastric tonometry in patients with acute circulatory failure. *J Am Med Assoc* **270**:1203–10.

McConachie E, Barton MH, Rapoport G, Giguere S. (2013) Doppler and volumetric echocardiographic methods for cardiac output measurement in standing adult horses. *J Vet Intern Med* **27**:324–30.

McConnell EJ, Rioja E, Bester L, Sanz MG, Fosgate GT, Saulez MN. (2013) Use of near-infrared spectroscopy to identify trends in regional cerebral oxygen saturation in horses. *Equine Vet J* **45**:470–5.

McGorum BC, Milne AJ, Tremaine WH, Sturgeon BP, McLaren M, Khan F. (2002) Evaluation of a combined laser Doppler flowmetry and iontophoresis technique for the assessment of equine cutaneous microvascular function. *Equine Vet J* **34**:732–6.

Meex I, De Deyne C, Dens J, et al. (2013) Feasibility of absolute cerebral tissue oxygen saturation during cardiopulmonary resuscitation. *Crit Care* **17**:R36.

Mohrman DE, Heller LJ. (1997) Regulation of arterial pressure. In: *Cardiovascular Physiology*. New York: McGraw Hill, pp. 151–73.

Morgan TJ, Venkatesh B, Endre ZH. (1999) Accuracy of intramucosal pH calculated from arterial bicarbonate and the Henderson–Hasselbalch equation: assessment using simulated ischemia. *Crit Care Med* **27**:2495–9.

Muir WW. (1992) Cardiovascular effects of dopexamine HCl in conscious and halothane-anaesthetised horses. *Equine Vet J Suppl* **11**:24–9.

Muir WW, Skarda RT, Milne DW. (1976) Estimation of cardiac output in the horse by thermodilution techniques. *Am J Vet Res* **37**:697–700.

Pellicer A, Bravo Mdel C. (2011) Near-infrared spectroscopy: a methodology-focused review. *Semin Fetal Neonatal Med* **16**:42–9.

Pringle J, Roberts C, Art T, Lekeux P. (2000) Assessment of muscle oxygenation in the horse by near infrared spectroscopy. *Equine Vet J* **32**:59–64.

Raisis AL, Young LE, Taylor PM, Walsh KP, Lekeux P. (2000) Doppler ultrasonography and single-fiber laser Doppler flowmetry for measurement of hind limb blood flow in anesthetized horses. *Am J Vet Res* **61**:286–90.

Ramsingh D, Alexander B, Cannesson M. (2013) Clinical review: Does it matter which hemodynamic monitoring system is used? Crit. *Care* **17**:208.

Raval NY, Squara P, Cleman M, Yalamanchili K, Winklmaier M, Burkhoff D. (2008) Multicenter evaluation of noninvasive cardiac output measurement by bioreactance technique. *J Clin Monit Comput* **22**:113–19.

Sanchez LC, Giguere S, Javsicas LH, Bier J, Walrond CJ, Womble AY. (2008) Effect of age, feeding, and omeprazole administration on gastric tonometry in healthy neonatal foals. *J Vet Intern Med* **22**:406–10.

Sato Y, Weil MH, Tang W, et al. (1997) Esophageal PCO2 as a monitor of perfusion failure during hemorrhagic shock. *J Appl Physiol* **82**:558–62.

Schauvliege S, Van den Eede A, Duchateau L, Gasthuys F. (2007) Cardiovascular effects of enoximone in isoflurane anaesthetized ponies. *Vet Anaesth Analg* **34**:416–30.

Schauvliege S, Van den Eede A, Duchateau L, Pille F, Vlaminck L, Gasthuys F. (2009) Comparison between lithium dilution and pulse contour analysis techniques for cardiac output measurement in isoflurane anaesthetized ponies: influence of different inotropic drugs. *Vet Anaesth Analg* **36**:197–208.

Schlichtig R, Mehta N, Gayowski TJ. (1996) Tissue-arterial PCO2 difference is a better marker of ischemia than intramural pH (pHi) or arterial pH–pHi difference. *J Crit Care* **11**:51–6.

Schlipf JW, Dunlop CI, Getzy DM, Wagner AE, Wertz EM. (1994) Lesions associated with cardiac catheterization and thermodilution cardiac output determination in horses. In: *Proceedings of the 5th International Congress of Veterinary Anesthesia*, Guelph, Ontario, Canada. p. 71.

Semeraro N, Ammollo CT, Semeraro F, Colucci M. (2012) Sepsis, thrombosis and organ dysfunction. *Thromb Res* **129**:290–5.

Serteyn D, Mottart E, Michaux C, et al. (1986) Laser Doppler flowmetry: muscular microcirculation in anaesthetized horses. *Equine Vet J* **18**:391–5.

Serteyn D, Lavergne L, Coppens P, et al. (1988) Equine post anaesthetic myositis: muscular post ischaemic hyperaemia measured by laser Doppler flowmetry. *Vet Rec* **123**:126–8.

Shih AC, Giguere S, Sanchez LC, Valverde A, Jankunas HJ, Robertson SA. (2009) Determination of cardiac output in anesthetized neonatal foals by use of two pulse wave analysis methods. *Am J Vet Res* **70**:334–9.

Skarda RT, Muir WW. (1996) Analgesic, hemodynamic, and respiratory effects of caudal epidurally administered xylazine hydrochloride solution in mares. *Am J Vet Res* **57**:193–200.

Squara P, Denjean D, Estagnasie P, Brusset A, Dib JC, Dubois C. (2007) Noninvasive cardiac output monitoring (NICOM): a clinical validation. *Intensive Care Med* **33**:1191–4.

Steffey EP, Dunlop CI, Farver TB, Woliner MJ, Schultz LJ. (1987) Cardiovascular and respiratory measurements in awake and isoflurane-anesthetized horses. *Am J Vet Res* **48**:7–12.

Thomas WP, Madigan JE, Backus KQ, Powell WE. (1987) Systemic and pulmonary haemodynamics in normal neonatal foals. *J Reprod Fert Suppl* **35**:623–8.

Valverde A, Giguere S, Sanchez LC, Shih A, Ryan C. (2006) Effects of dobutamine, norepinephrine, and vasopressin on cardiovascular function in anesthetized neonatal foals with induced hypotension. *Am J Vet Res* **67**:1730–7.

van Griensven M. (2013) Has the cat got your tongue? Evaluation of circulation by microcirculation. *Crit Care Med* **41**:920–1.

Vendrig JC, Fink-Gremmels J. (2012) Intestinal barrier function in neonatal foals: options for improvement. *Vet J* **193**:32–7.

Waller A, Lindinger MI. (2006) Hydration of exercised standardbred racehorses assessed noninvasively using multi-frequency bioelectrical impedance analysis. *Equine Vet J Suppl Aug*(**36**):285–90.

Wassenaar EB, Van den Brand JG. (2005) Reliability of near-infrared spectroscopy in people with dark skin pigmentation. *J Clin Monit Comput* **19**:195–9.

Weil MH, Nakagawa Y, Tang W, et al. (1999) Sublingual capnometry: a new noninvasive measurement for diagnosis and quantitation of severity of circulatory shock. *Crit Care Med* **27**:1225–9.

Wetmore LA, Derksen FJ, Blaze CA, Eyster GE. (1987) Mixed venous oxygen tension as an estimate of cardiac output in anesthetized horses. *Am J Vet Res* **48**:971–6.

Young LE, Blissit KJ, Clutton RE, Molony V, Darke PGG. (1995) Feasibility of transoesophageal echocardiography for evaluation of left ventricular performance in anaesthetised horses. *Equine Vet J Suppl* **19**:63–70.

Young LE, Blissit KJ, Bartram DH, Clutton RE, Molony V, Jones RS. (1996) Measurement of cardiac output by transoesophageal Doppler echocardiography in anaesthetized horses: comparison with thermodilution. *Br J Anaesth* **77**:773–80.

Zuntz N, Hagemann O. (1894) Untersuchungen über den Stoffwechsel des Pferdes bei Ruhe und Arbeit. *Landw Jh* **27**:284–301.

CHAPTER 27

Peritoneal dialysis

Laurie Gallatin

Gallatin Veterinary Services LLC, Marysville, OH, USA

Introduction

Peritoneal dialysis (PD) has been described as a renal replacement therapy in human medicine since the 1920s and in veterinary medicine since the 1970s. In horses, it has traditionally been considered only as a therapy for acute renal failure. However, in humans and small animals, PD is used as a treatment modality for intoxications, a route of administration for medications, a means for nutritional support, and may have a future role in gene therapy (Chaudhary et al., 2010).

Peritoneal lavage procedures have been described and performed in horses since the late 1970s (Valdez & Wallace, 1979). Only more recently, however, has PD (both intermittent and continuous flow) been described in horses (Gallatin et al., 2005; Han & McKenzie, 2008; Reuss et al., 2006). Procedurally, peritoneal lavage and PD are very similar. Peritoneal lavage is typically defined as "to wash out" and is often used for the treatment of peritonitis. Dialysis is defined as "the separation of smaller molecules from larger molecules or of dissolved substances from colloidal particles in a solution by selective diffusion through a semipermeable membrane."

In 2005, the first case of continuous-flow peritoneal dialysis (CFPD) was described in an equine patient (Gallatin et al., 2005). Dialysis was used in the treatment of a 15-year-old Paso Fino gelding that developed acute renal failure following an episode of exertional rhabdomyolysis. Continuous-flow peritoneal dialysis was used after intermittent peritoneal dialysis (IPD) was deemed ineffective. Three additional cases of PD were reported over the next three years in the treatment of acute renal

failure in horses (Han & McKenzie, 2008; Reuss et al., 2006). All four of the reported cases of equine PD had successful outcomes and the patients were ultimately discharged from the hospital with normal renal values (Gallatin et al., 2005; Han & McKenzie, 2008; Reuss et al., 2006).

Physiology of peritoneal dialysis

The peritoneum makes an excellent natural dialyzer membrane using diffusive and convective transport as well as osmosis simultaneously (Chaudhary & Khanna, 2010; Devuyst, 2010). It has been suggested that transport across the peritoneal membrane involves three different-sized pores. Large (20–40 nm radius) and small (4–6 nm radius) pores are responsible for the transport of the larger solutes, whereas the ultrapores (aquaporins, radius <0.8 nm) allow for water movement only (Chaudhary & Khanna, 2010; Rippe, 1993). Dialysis itself occurs during the dwell time for the dialysate solution. For intermittent peritoneal dialysis, the dwell time is the period that the solution remains in the abdomen. A 30–60 min dwell time per exchange has been reported in horses undergoing IPD (Gallatin et al., 2005; Han & McKenzie, 2008). For CFPD, a certain amount of fluid remains in the abdomen, which is determined by the height of the egress collection bag.

There are many factors affecting the rate of peritoneal transport, most of which have not been investigated in horses. Dose, temperature, peritoneal blood flow, contact area, contact time, and inflammation are just a

Equine Fluid Therapy, First Edition. Edited by C. Langdon Fielding and K. Gary Magdesian.
© 2015 John Wiley & Sons, Inc. Published 2015 by John Wiley & Sons, Inc.

few of the variables. In humans, some of these factors can be manipulated to improve effectiveness. Fortunately in equine medicine there is a large contact surface area (approximately $6.3\,m^2$) compared to humans ($2\,m^2$) (Gallatin et al., 2005). Another variable easily addressed is the concentration gradient. It has been shown that simply increasing the dwell time alone is inefficient as the concentration gradient can quickly dissipate. However, maintaining a high concentration gradient by constantly replenishing the dialysate solution (i.e., CFPD) or performing multiple IPD exchanges per day can improve transfer. The goal is to achieve a 30–50% decline in blood urea nitrogen (BUN) daily. A more significant decline can lead to "disequilibrium syndrome" causing nausea and neurologic symptoms (M. Bercovitch, unpublished). This syndrome is more pronounced in hemodialysis (HD) due to its improved efficiency over PD.

There are limited reports of hemodialysis (HD) being successfully performed in horses (Vivrette et al., 1993). Hemodialysis is used in human and small animal medicine, although PD is available in these areas of medicine as well. Hemodialysis requires a patient to be immobilized with reliable vascular access, additional equipment such as a dialysate exchanger, and specially trained personnel with constant monitoring. Patients may need to be kept on heparin, or other medications as well. Although time consuming, PD in horses can be performed while the patient is restrained in the stocks or moving freely within the stall.

Indications for peritoneal dialysis in horses

The primary indication for PD in horses appears to be moderate to severe azotemia refractory to traditional medical management. In small animals, guidelines for institution of dialysis are based on one or more of the following (Lane & Carter, 2000):
- BUN >100 mg/dL;
- serum creatinine >10 mg/dL;
- life-threatening hyperkalemia;
- refractory fluid overload;
- persistent oliguria.

To date, no similar recommendations have been made in equine medicine. In the reported cases, patients had BUNs ranging from 32.5 to 136 mg/dL, and creatinine values ranging from 5.1 to 19.0 mg/dL.

Case selection of horses for peritoneal dialysis

Patient selection and timing of treatment is important for the success of PD in horses. Peritoneal dialysis has traditionally been viewed as a last resort treatment. Not every horse in acute renal failure (ARF) will need PD, but those who remain refractory to traditional treatments for more than 1–3 days (M. Bercovitch, unpublished; Reuss et al., 2006) should be considered candidates. Other non-renal related issues such as intoxication with a dialyzable substance, severe metabolic or electrolyte abnormality, fluid overload, uroabdomen, pancreatitis, and hyper/hypothermia may also be indications for PD in horses (Labato, 2000; Lane & Carter, 2000). Peritoneal dialysis of either type is contraindicated in patients with abdominal wall trauma or recent abdominal surgery.

Hypoproteinemia, severe peritoneal adhesions, and other types of abdominal disease may complicate the use of PD in horses and lead to unfavorable outcomes. Twenty-four hour monitoring is required for facilities where PD will be performed. As evident from the reported PD cases, treatment may last 6 days or longer. This can represent a significant expense for the client.

Technical aspects of peritoneal dialysis in horses

Catheters
There are several types of peritoneal dialysis catheters available. Most of these options have multiple fenestrations and configurations; however, a large-bore thoracic catheter can work as well. In all four of the described cases a 28–32-Fr indwelling thoracic catheter was used as at least one of the ports, but typically the egress port. Other catheters available for use are the de Pezzer mushroom tip catheter, Ash Advantage T-Fluted catheter, Cook Spiral catheter, and the Tenckhoff Straight or Coiled catheter. There are new catheters currently being designed and tested (S.R. Ash, personal communication).

Dialysate
The recommended typical dialysate fluid used in equine PD is 1.5% dextrose in warmed, sterile, balanced, lactate-based, polyionic fluid. Polyionic fluids would include

Normosol™-R, lactated Ringer's solution, Hartmann's solution, and 0.9% sodium chloride. A 0.9% sodium chloride solution should be chosen if hyperkalemia is present. In small animal medicine, the recommended dialysate dose is 30–40 mL/kg per exchange (Labato, 2000; Lane & Carter, 2000). Dextrose is used as an osmotic agent. Hypertonic dextrose-containing fluids (2.5% or 4.25% dextrose) are used in overhydrated or edematous patients (Labato, 2000; Lane & Carter, 2000). In human patients there is concern over the dextrose and its glucose degradation products leading to peritoneal membrane changes and ultimately failure of peritoneal dialysis (Chaudhary & Khanna, 2010). This is typically observed in cases where PD is utilized for more than 3–5 years. In equine patients, PD has been performed only for less than six consecutive days in the published case reports, and this phenomenon therefore did not appear to be a problem. Other osmotic agents such as amino acids and other large molecular sized polymers (icodextrin) are being investigated in humans. Although the non-dextrose osmotic agents provide relief from the glucotoxic side effects of the dextrose-containing dialysates, they have other complications such as increased inflammatory responses. A combination dialysate fluid containing dextrose and other osmotic agents could provide a more "biocompatible" dialysate solution in the future.

Procedure

Intermittent peritoneal dialysis requires only a ventral abdominal catheter placed to serve as both the ingress and egress port. The catheter is placed at the most pendulous point of the abdomen, just to the right of the midline (similar to the location for performing an abdominocentesis) (Figure 27.1). Catheter placement can be performed via ultrasound guidance or based only on the anatomic landmarks. The catheter is held in place by a pursestring suture followed by a Chinese fingertrap suture pattern. Bandaging over the catheter is optional. Ten to fifteen liters of warmed 1.5% dextrose polyionic fluid is instilled into the abdomen. In the few reports describing IPD in horses, the dwell time has typically been 30–60 minutes (Gallatin et al., 2005; Han & McKenzie, 2008; Kritchevsky et al., 1984). The transperitoneal concentration gradient can dissipate quickly, and in humans solute transfer at 6-hour dwell is minimal (Amerling et al., 2003). There is currently no information regarding adequate dwell times for IPD in

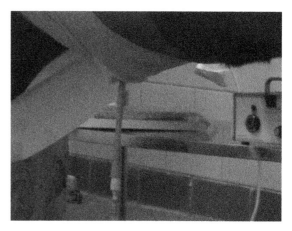

Figure 27.1 Location of the egress catheter.

horses. A twice-daily exchange with a 1-hour dwell time was clinically successful in one report in horses (Han & McKenzie, 2008). At the end of the dwell time, the used dialysate is allowed to drain via the ventral abdominal catheter. The catheter can either then be clamped or a one-way valve can be attached to allow for further passive drainage.

Continuous flow peritoneal dialysis maintains a large volume of intraperitoneal fluid that is continually being replenished, thus keeping fluid with a high transperitoneal concentration gradient in constant contact with the peritoneal membrane (Amerling et al., 2003). By placing the ingress and egress catheters far apart and maintaining a modest amount of intraperitoneal dialysate fluid, better mixing and contact time of the dialysate fluid can be achieved. In a human study, ingress and egress catheters placed side by side allowed for 50% port-to-port "streaming", but catheters placed in a "one up, one down" configuration (similar to reported CFPD cases) allowed only 11% streaming. Even when intrapelvic catheters were placed as far apart as possible, there was still 40% "streaming" (Amerling et al., 2003). For CFPD, placement of the egress catheter is the same as for IPD. The ingress catheter is placed in the left flank either blindly or by peritoneoscopic assistance (Figure 27.2). Care must be taken that the catheter is truly intraperitoneal and not in the retroperitoneal space. Using a sterile closed system, infuse the dialysate at 3 L/h and collect the used dialysate back into the sterile fluid bags. Placement of the "catch" bag will help regulate the amount of intraperitoneal fluid that will be maintained. Placement at

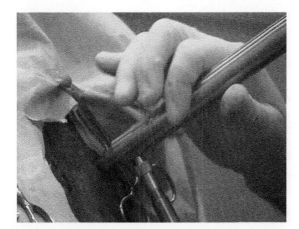

Figure 27.2 Placement of the ingress catheter.

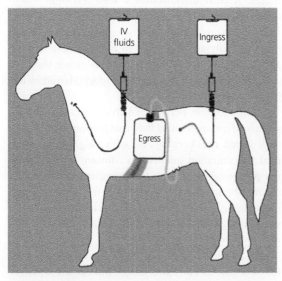

Figure 27.3 Placement of the "catch" bag slightly below the height of the withers.

the approximate height of the withers or slightly below may be appropriate (Figure 27.3).

Peritoneal dialysis, regardless of type, should be continued until there is no further improvement in BUN and creatinine. There is no recommended length of treatment; however, in the equine IPD and CFPD cases reported, dialysis lasted for 3–6 days (Gallatin et al., 2005; Han & McKenzie, 2008; Reuss et al., 2006). A creatinine clearance rate of 80 L/week was reported with IPD and would likely be greater with CFPD (Gallatin et al., 2005; Han & McKenzie, 2008; Reuss et al., 2006).

Patient monitoring

There are currently no universally accepted recommendations for monitoring horses undergoing PD. In some of the reported cases, patients underwent physical examinations two to four times per day in addition to body weight measurements and packed cell volume (PCV)/total protein (TP) monitoring at similar intervals. Serum BUN, creatinine, and electrolyte concentrations should also be monitored daily (or more frequently as indicated) in all patients. Effluent fluid BUN and creatinine levels should also be checked at least once daily to chart improvement. Repeated complete blood counts and cytology of effluent fluid can help monitor for early signs of peritonitis. Blood pressure and central venous pressure monitoring can be useful if available. Periodic urinalysis should also be considered.

Complications of peritoneal dialysis in horses

Complications are typically mild and can be easily addressed if recognized early. Peritonitis (septic or aseptic), localized cellulitis, and catheter failure were the most commonly reported complications in equine PD (Gallatin et al., 2005; Han & McKenzie, 2008; Reuss et al., 2006). Monitoring of the complete blood count and abdominal fluid cytology will aid in determining the appropriate clinical course of treatment. Gram stain and culture of the fluid may also be indicated. It has been reported that 22% of small animal patients undergoing PD develop peritonitis, likely from the handling of the bag spikes or tubing (Labato, 2000). All of the equine PD cases were either started on antibiotics prophylactically or after cytologic examination of the peritoneal fluid revealed inflammation (Gallatin et al., 2005; Han & McKenzie, 2008; Reuss et al., 2006).

Other considerations for horses undergoing peritoneal dialysis

The majority of the cases currently reported describe horses in acute renal failure. Appropriate therapy to correct acid–base and electrolyte dyscrasias as well as alterations in hydration should be instituted. Proper nutritional support, laminitis prevention/treatment, and other supportive care modalities should also be used. Nutritional requirements may also need to be addressed depending on the length of time that horses remain hospitalized and their concurrent caloric intake.

References

Amerling R, lGlezerman I, Savransky E, et al. (2003) Continuous flow peritoneal dialysis: principles and applications. *Semin Dialysis* **16**:335–40.

Chaudhary K, Khanna R. (2010) Biocompatible peritoneal dialysis solutions: do we have one? *Clin J Am Soc Nephrol* **5**:723–32.

Chaudhary K, Haddadin S, Nistala R, et al. (2010) Intraperitoneal drug therapy: an advantage. *Curr Clin Pharmacol* **5**:82–88.

Devuyst O. (2010) Water channels in peritoneal dialysis. *J Nephrol* **23**:S170–S174.

Gallatin LL, Couetil CL, Ash SR. (2005) Use of continuous-flow peritoneal dialysis for the treatment of acute renal failure in an adult horse. *J Am Vet Med Assoc* **226**:756–9.

Han JH, McKenzie III HC. (2008) Intermittent peritoneal dialysis for the treatment of acute renal failure in two horses. *Equine Vet Educ* **20**:256–64.

Kritchevsky JE, Stevens DL, Christopher J, et al. (1984) Peritoneal dialysis for presurgical management of ruptured bladder in a foal. *J Am Vet Med Assoc* **185**:81–2.

Labato MA. (2000) Peritoneal dialysis in emergency and critical care medicine. *Clin Tech Small Anim Pract* **15**:126–35.

Lane IF, Carter L. (2000) Peritoneal dialysis and hemodialysis. In: Wayne E, Wingfield MS (eds) *Veterinary Emergency Medicine Secrets*, 2nd edn. Philadelphia: Hanley & Belfus, pp. 350–4.

Reuss SM, Franklin RP, Peloso JG, et al. (2006) How to perform continuous flow peritoneal dialysis in an adult horse. *AAEP Proceedings* **52**:96–100.

Rippe B. (1993) A three-pore model of peritoneal transport. *Periton Dialysis Int* **13**:35–8.

Valdez H, Wallace MK. (1980) American Association of Equine Practitioners 26th annual proceedings. 239–242.

Vivrette S, Cowgill LD, Pascoe J, et al. (1993) Hemodialysis for treatment of oxytetracycline-induced acute renal failure in a neonatal foal. *J Am Vet Med Assoc* **203**:105–7.

Index

Note: Page references in *italics* refer to Figures; those in **bold** refer to Tables and Boxes

Equine Fluid Therapy, First Edition. Edited by C. Langdon Fielding and K. Gary Magdesian.
© 2015 John Wiley & Sons, Inc. Published 2015 by John Wiley & Sons, Inc.

Printed and bound by CPI Group (UK) Ltd, Croydon, CR0 4YY

16/04/2025

14658462-0001